Neurocultural Health and Wellbeing

Series Editors
Lorenzo Lorusso, Neurology Unit
A.S.S.T. Lecco-Merate
Merate, Italy

Bruno Colombo, DIMER, Neurologia
Ospedale San Raffaele
Milano, Italy

Alessandro Porro, Dip. di Scienze Cliniche e di Comunità
University of Milan
Milano, Italy

Nicholas Wade, Department of Psychology
University of Dundee
Dundee, UK

Aim of this devoted book Series in neurology is to highlight the relationship between neuroscience and culture. Nowadays, there is more evidence of how our brain is influenced by the various artistic and cultural disciplines, both in the form of entertainment as well as – and above all – through the emotions and gratification which lead to wellbeing. The emotional mechanisms, the different cultural manifestations provided, are due to the activation of a perceptual and cognitive range that constitute the basis of the social behaviors. All this makes us aware of the benefits the arts have on personal and collective health.

This concept was already known to philosophers in ancient times, who were convinced that inner balance was influenced by culture and in particular by music.

During the centuries, men understood that the *cultivation of the spirit*, or *humanitas*, had a certain role on behavior and from the beginning of modern experimental science, in the fifteenth, the spread of the notions of neuroanatomy allowed artists to get closer to the knowledge of the brain's mechanisms and reveal the emotional and empathic responses at the basis of creativity, and indeed of their own psychophysical wellbeing. A dialogue between the science of the mind and artistic disciplines was born. The results of this meeting made it possible to better define which mental processes are involved when we come into contact with the various humanistic disciplines, and how they can be applied, for instance, to the treatment of mental disorders and neuropsychiatric diseases.

The goal of this Series is both to prove the role of biological brain mechanisms and the influence of various artistic forms on clinical practice, especially in neuro-psychiatric disorders, as well as to trace different therapeutic and psycho-physical well-being applications based on scientific evidence from medical literature.

Volumes of the Series will be edited by experts under the supervision of an international editorial committee. Each book, focused on a specific discipline, will provide knowledge on relationship between the brain activity and different forms of language, communication, art. This close inter-relationship with specific focus on different forms of art will explain the effectiveness of this kind of approaches in neuro-psychiatric diseases.

This Series will allow to understand how the culture is one of the fundamental tools to improve general well-being, quality of life and motivation in neurological diseases.

This Series also find a correlation with SDG3 goal "ensuring healthy lives and promoting wellbeing for all at all ages" for the progress of the health and wellbeing considering that neurological diseases are on the rise worldwide including in the developing countries.

Gunter Kreutz • Günther Bernatzky
Editors

Music and Medicine

Complementing and Enhancing Prevention, Therapy, Rehabilitation and Education

Springer

Editors
Gunter Kreutz
Systematic Musicology
Carl von Ossietzky University Oldenburg
Oldenburg, Lower Saxony, Germany

Günther Bernatzky
Department of Biosciences and
Medical Biology
University of Salzburg
Salzburg, Austria

ISSN 2731-4464 ISSN 2731-4472 (electronic)
Neurocultural Health and Wellbeing
ISBN 978-3-662-72174-2 ISBN 978-3-662-72175-9 (eBook)
https://doi.org/10.1007/978-3-662-72175-9

This book is a translation of the original German edition "Musik und Medizin," 2nd edition, by Günther Bernatzky and Gunter Kreutz, published by Springer-Verlag GmbH, DE in 2024. The translation was done with the help of an artificial intelligence machine translation tool. A subsequent human revision was done primarily in terms of content, so that the book will read stylistically differently from a conventional translation. Springer Nature works continuously to further the development of tools for the production of books and on the related technologies to support the authors.

This Springer imprint is published by the registered company Springer-Verlag GmbH, DE, part of Springer Nature.
The registered company address is: Heidelberger Platz 3, 14197 Berlin, Germany

Contents

Part V Musical Education and Well-Being

Introduction

1

Gunter Kreutz and Günther Bernatzky

Music has accompanied and shaped human cultural evolution for thousands of years. It is part of our everyday affairs across the entire lifespan. Music eludes any attempt of definition, as it exists only in our minds, memories, and feelings, and in social experiences and interaction. It encompasses a wide range of behaviors such as singing, playing instruments, dancing, composing, improvising, and much more. All these behaviors interact with our well-being and our health. The chapters of this volume examine implications of this basic idea from a wide range of perspectives. It turns out that the medical significance of music extends far beyond specific psychotherapeutic treatment, as laid out in music therapy. Instead, the expertise of the authors provides deep insights into how music-related knowledge can be helpful for prevention, therapy and rehabilitation thus exhibiting its potentials for evidence-based clinical practice and health policy. Finally, they remind us about the importance of cultural capital as a health resource, in general, and the benefits that arise from the power of music, in particular.

The chapters in this volume offer one key message: musical education is a societal task to build individual and social cultural capital, and it functions at the same time as a health resource. Thus, enabling cultural participation by means of musical

G. Kreutz (✉)
Systematic Musicology, Carl von Ossietzky University Oldenburg, Oldenburg, Lower Saxony, Germany
e-mail: gunter.kreutz@uni-oldenburg.de

G. Bernatzky
Department of Biosciences and Medical Biology, University of Salzburg, Salzburg, Austria

G. Kreutz, G. Bernatzky (eds.), *Music and Medicine*, Neurocultural Health and Wellbeing, https://doi.org/10.1007/978-3-662-72175-9_1

practices offers the opportunity to promote individual well-being and improve the quality of life of many, if not all, people in a society in one way or another. That is, in our view, a rather positive message in an era in which numerous crises and uncertainty about the future course of life affairs dominate at many levels.

The authors of the chapters in this volume are high-ranking experts in the fields of music psychology, medicine, neurosciences, and related disciplines. The six sections discuss essential facets of the relationships between music and medicine. They point out that musical activities, learning, and development characterize a human basic need in many life situations. Albeit such activities mainly comprise lay or amateur music culture, those need to be valued equally with the artistic-aesthetic goals and demands of high culture music. To this end, all chapters share the idea that a contemporary medical care should tie in with the cultural identity of both care staff and patients, and take musical needs, experiences, and potentials for well-being and quality of life into their accounts.

Part I sheds light on the "Socio-cultural, genetic, and neuro-biological foundations." Their deep roots in the humanities, and the social and natural sciences tie in with the increasing importance of epidemiology and brain research for the understanding of health potentials of musical activities. The investigation of key questions with regard to how music can influence health-related processes at individual and societal levels seems only possible in interdisciplinary, bio-cultural, and medical, contexts.

Part II, "Music in clinical and pedagogical inclusion practice," introduces application-oriented research of musical practices in traditional music, medical, and therapeutic contexts. For example, a substantial body of research suggests that the quality of life of patients in emotionally aversive and pain-dominated situations could be improved by means of music-based interventions. There seem to be few restrictions, if any, to consider music in severe neurological diseases, such as Parkinson's disease, depression, stroke, and dementia. Further chapters address children with hearing impairments and inclusion needs. In addition to primarily pedagogical and therapeutic goals, artistic development plays an important role. The medical tasks in the care of professional singers are quite different. Yet all the diverging questions of the chapters are united by the close interlocking of medical problems and musical practice.

The third part, titled "Music Therapy in Transition," is dedicated to innovative and pioneering areas of application for medical-musical interventions in the coming years and decades. A key to the successful design of this change lies in the specification of both the forms of interventions and the target groups, as well as understanding specific disease patterns. It turns out that musical interventions as adjuvant forms of therapy in some areas are confronted with great challenges, yet they sometimes have unique potentials, especially when it comes to reaching people with brain damage.

Part IV, "Listening to Music, Amateur Music Making and Dancing," puts the emotionality of music at the center of different explorations. Listening to music in everyday life and under the special conditions of the Covid-19 pandemic, music as a trigger for strong reactions, and health aspects of common musical activities mark research areas with no less high methodological requirements, such as those found in epidemiological and brain research.

The chapters in Part V, “Musical Education and Well-being,” reflect musical activities primarily in educational contexts. Complementary and, in a sense, contrary to the selective and competitive paradigm focusing on talent and deliberate practice, which largely shapes the reality of music education, personal development and well-being are more in the foreground here. As a result, all forms of music-making, not least professional musicianship are shaped by the idea of promoting well-being.

The final part, “Health Strains through Music,” sheds light on the health risks and the abuse that are associated with exposure to music and maladaptive musical activities. Musical preferences and mental health are in a complex relationship with each other. The consumption of loud music, which can cause hearing damage both in the short and long term, is no less ambivalent. People need protection from the abuse of music as a means of humiliation and torture. Finally, we must learn our lessons from the pandemic, which has shown that more needs to be done to protect individual and social music engagement in times of health crises.

Part I

Socio-cultural, Genetic and Neurobiological Foundations

Music and Well-Being: A Dynamically Advancing Field of Research

2

Gunter Kreutz and Günther Bernatzky

Musical activities have increasingly become the subject of empirical studies in health science contexts in recent times. Listening to music as well as creative approaches such as singing, dancing, and learning and playing instruments solo or in groups have predominantly positive effects on psychological, physical, social, and mental levels, often regardless of clinical or nonclinical contexts. Nevertheless, music-induced changes are mostly unspecific and may occur in a similar form also in nonmusical activities. At the center of this contribution are some basic assumptions and the development of models that could be useful for the orientation and development of current and future investigations.

2.1 What Is Music?

Obviously, beyond pragmatic definitions of music as "sound art" or as a human cultural technique widespread in all ethnic groups, there is no sufficient delimitation of what the term "music" means (Gerigk 1957). An a priori basic understanding requires almost inevitably a neurobiological orientation in the health context, which goes beyond the traditional field of music therapy (Kreutz and Lotze 2007; Panksepp and Bernatzky 2002). In this article, music stands for a totality of musical activities. These include the *active* listening to music (as an overarching and independent

G. Kreutz (✉)
Systematic Musicology, Carl von Ossietzky University Oldenburg, Oldenburg, Lower Saxony, Germany
e-mail: gunter.kreutz@uni-oldenburg.de

G. Bernatzky
Department of Biosciences and Medical Biology, University of Salzburg, Salzburg, Austria

G. Kreutz, G. Bernatzky (eds.), *Music and Medicine*, Neurocultural Health and Wellbeing, https://doi.org/10.1007/978-3-662-72175-9_2

activity), playing of musical instruments, singing and dancing, as well as *creative* forms of musical expression, thinking, and acting in improvisation and composition. Instead of specific features that prescribe musical objects in terms of structural parameters, music here is understood as a product of intentions that intentionally or unintentionally arise from these activities or can make up a significant part of the activity (such as when dancing).

A number of authors have begun to outline such phenomena, which we attribute musical content to, with terms like "Community music" (Kraus et al. 2014; MacDonald 2013) or "Musicking" (Batt-Rawden and Tellnes 2011; Krueger 2014; O'Callaghan et al. 2012; Pavlicevic et al. 2014). This reflects a therapeutically and socio-pedagogically motivated holistic view, which avoids subordinating the aesthetic experience to a functional view. Although a rigorous experimental approach to the specific effects of musical activities is complicated in these approaches, they are especially significant because they represent spaces of experience between clinical and nonclinical areas. People who are discharged from psychiatric or other medical treatments find informal support in music-oriented communities such as singing groups when returning to everyday life. Systematic studies on this issue are, to our knowledge, still rare. Nevertheless, anecdotal evidence provides enough reason to consider cultural offerings as facilitating factors in healing processes (Theorell and Kreutz 2012).

In addition to the reevaluations of musical activities based on life-world reasons, specifically oriented therapeutic concepts emerge, such as the "Melodic Intonation Therapy" (MIT; Zumbansen et al. 2014), which is primarily aimed at defined treatment situations for stroke patients. Despite mixed findings and open questions regarding MIT (Stahl and Kotz 2014), it provides a good example of how music-related therapies regarding neurological damage and diseases have become part of clinical everyday life. They can now reach a wide range of syndromes very often as adjuvant, non-pharmacological therapy options (Benoit et al. 2014; Bernatzky and Hesse 2003; Bernatzky et al. 2004; Haro-Martínez et al. 2021).

An immediate consequence of this perspective is that no longer the historically transmitted and updated object of music is in the foreground, but rather *the human being*, whose musicality unfolds under equally significant genetic and cultural conditions (Oikkonen and Järvelä 2014; Savage et al. 2021; Tan et al. 2014). This brings individual characteristics such as demographic characteristics of a person, cultural backgrounds, educational and developmental status, and not least the health status and emotional well-being into the foreground. It is important to note that musical behaviors, experiences and effects are also culturally justified in the neurobiological focus, as they are based on individual biographical acculturation. The majority of authors assume that the effects of music are significantly influenced by individual preferences and cultural backgrounds (MacDonald 2013).

Thus, it is assumed that every human being has genetic and experience-based resources that enable him or her, at the latest from the day of birth, to develop a musical-cultural participation, to initiate this themselves, and to develop individual skills and abilities (Hambrick and Tucker-Drob 2014; Trevarthen 2008). Understanding these musical resources in their significance for the well-being, quality of life, and health of a person not only is a concern of the emerging research field (MacDonald et al. 2012) but also entails societal responsibilities to accommodate these resources by providing institutional and educational frameworks to bring those to life (Reyes 2019).

The connection between music and well-being has a far-reaching cultural-historical tradition that goes back thousands of years and is particularly tangible in the unbroken relevance of music therapy (see Spahn et al. in this volume). It is crucial, that music and well-being are put into a much broader context of effects, which is pragmatically aimed at asking to what extent musical activities are or can be causal for changes in this well-being. This results in the further consequence that these relationships of effects can be derived from empirically tangible and thus also from concrete action situations and contexts accessible to social science and experimental methods of psychological research.

2.2 From Human to Music

The demographic change as well as increasing or high-level stagnating life expectancy, combined with a steadily growing proportion of the population in higher age groups, stands for individual, peace, and social prosperity in Western industrial nations, regardless of the warning pandemic, Russia's war of aggression on Ukraine, and many other conflicts. However, this development is associated with an extremely high consumption of resources, which seems necessary to maintain the standard of living.

The high life expectancy is also reflected in high health costs. These continue to be influenced by lifestyle factors (e.g., lack of exercise, poor nutrition, alcohol and nicotine addiction, and legal and illegal drug use). The extent to which these burdens in total affect social life is also evident in the comparison between the available health resources both between the more or less industrialized countries and within the individual societies (Clift et al. 2010). It therefore seems necessary at this point to reevaluate individual cultural resources in the interest of health, well-being, and quality of life.

In recent years, for example, research interest has been growing in the effects of musical activities on individual well-being and the quality of life of people who are mainly involved in nonprofessional areas of singing, dancing, or playing music instrumentally. In this context, model ideas about diverse potentials for change of musical activities on cognitive, emotional, and social levels are beginning to develop. These potentials concern clinical as well as nonclinical populations and thus justify a comprehensive health science research area between prevention and care (MacDonald et al. 2012).

2.3 Why Music?

The special feature of music, especially for health science concerns, can be justified in various ways. This should not obscure a latent lack of dedicated research programs, although concerted, long-term research efforts do exist (e.g., Clift

2012). The heterogeneity of the research landscape reveals a wide spectrum, within which a number of basic motivations can be identified: Music, in its different forms, is part of the experiential treasure of almost all people. It demands and promotes cognitive, emotional, and social processes that are predominantly perceived and processed as gratifying. In addition, music has the potential to influence behaviors that do not necessarily have to turn out positive (Fischer and Greitemeyer 2006), but can usually encourage people to receive health-relevant messages at all and to distance themselves from negative behavior (Burkhardt and Brennan 2012).

2.4 Well-Being and Health

The term "well-being" is conspicuously at the center of a scientifically and politically highly significant definition of health, namely, according to the statutes of the widely known World Health Organization (WHO):

> "Health is a state of complete physical, mental and social well-being and not merely the absence of disease or infirmity"

This definition from the preamble to the WHO constitution followed an expert conference in New York and was signed by government representatives from 61 countries on July 22, 1946 (Official Records of the World Health Organization, no. 2, p. 100). It came into force on April 7, 1948. Later, the definition was expanded to include the term spiritual well-being.

What is striking about this definition is the positive view of health as comprehensive well-being due to individual and collective state of being. The salutogenic approach of Aaron Antonovsky (1997), which focuses on those influences of life that promote health and convalescence, as well as reduce the risks of diseases, is particularly close to the spirit of the WHO definition. It is not surprising that the so-called salutogenesis has particularly caught on in the theory formation on the health effects of musical activities (Clift and Hancox 2001).

2.5 Models

The development of a robust model conception has noticeably progressed in recent years. There seems to be a consensus that mechanisms which underly health-promoting effects, and the health-related impacts per se are to be considered as equal research areas. However, opinions vary widely as to the extent to which structural properties of the music itself are attributed or not attributed to specific causalities in these contexts.

Västfjäll et al. (2012), for example, characterize in their model the effects of listening to music as the result of a complex interplay between situational-contextual variables, which are inextricably intertwined with the everyday listening experience itself. However, it is essential that music-induced emotional processing be triggered. In short, the contents of musical experiences play a subordinate role for the subjective experience as well as the physical reactions. This model derives its plausibility primarily from its derivation from the "classical" emotion research on the one hand and its approach to the "modern" psychoendocrinology on the other hand (Panksepp and Bernatzky 2002). However, the focus on listening to music without considering other musical activities seems to be a disadvantage. In addition, musical contents, styles, genres, and production and reception aspects are far in the background.

Koelsch and Stegemann (2012) agree with most authors that both the evocation of (positive) emotions via specific networks in the midbrain and the modulation of existing emotional states are crucial when it comes to the health effects of music and especially of listening to music. In particular, music-induced modulations of the endocrine system are at the center of their discussion. The authors also strive to systematically capture contextual factors (so-called seven c's). (1) contact between individuals as a basic human need; (2) social cognition as specifically communal thinking; (3) co-pathy in the sense of an emotionally homogeneous group dynamic; (4) communication as an exchange of information on emotional, cognitive, and social levels; (5) rhythmic coordination of actions to an external beat; (6) cooperation between group members to build and strengthen trust; and finally (7) increase social cohesion to protect all members (Koelsch and Stegemann 2012, p. 439ff.). Without discussing the specifications, overlaps and empirical validations of the *seven c's* in more detail here, these play a prominent role especially with regard to musical health effects. In other words, even a seemingly private activity like listening to music unfolds effects on well-being and health through its implicitly communicative character (Kreutz et al. 2012; Quiroga Murcia et al. 2011).

Bernardi and colleagues (2006, 2009) assume that listening to music, and especially the rhythmicity of complex musical processes, triggers physiological adaptation processes of the cardiovascular system. In this context, musical tempo and tempo fluctuations play a similarly important role as patterns of changes in volumes. The authors assume that the modulation of bodily rhythms is driven by temporal structures of musical parameters. These modulations can occur synchronously, but also with a time delay. They found, for example, evidence that physiological indicators for relaxation and calming *after* the fading of a piece of music were more pronounced than during the listening itself. It seems, therefore, that a multitude of temporal levels, starting with the rhythms formed by the shortest note values of a piece of music, through rhythmic-metric units, patterns of tension and relaxation through modulations of tempo and dynamics, up to the highest level in the temporal sequence, which only captures a sequence of pieces of music with breaks in between, need to be considered in terms of psychophysiological effects.

The models just discussed are more or less limited to listening to music. This seems somewhat justified, as every musical activity contains an element of listening (including vibro-tactile stimulation through airborne sound via the eardrum as well as bone conduction through the skin and the musculoskeletal system). Nevertheless, extensions of these models are necessary to also consider possible repercussions of musical activities in singing, dancing, and playing instruments on the body and psyche of the musically active individuals. This also opens up to a much greater extent than in listening to music alone the social dimension of musical thinking, feeling, and acting, as the systematization by Koelsch (see above) puts it.

Figure 2.1 extends the spectrum of musical activities as well as that of health effects compared to Västfjäll et al. (2012). In addition, the potential mechanisms that initiate a relationship between musical stimulation and health effects encompass a range of processes at psychological, physical, and social levels that interact in complex ways.

Healing in the narrower sense of the complete restoration of all physical, psychological, and mental resources is certainly the legitimate goal of any kind of medical-therapeutic treatment. Nevertheless, the reduction or complete cessation of symptoms, the improvement of general well-being or the increase in quality of life through more or less extensive care measures and rehabilitation are also important. And finally, in a modern health system it is not only about treating existing diseases and injuries and providing the best possible care, but also about preventing or delaying their onset.

Empirical studies indicate rather positive psychophysiological effects across the three domains sketched on the right side of Fig. 2.1. This view is not only supported by similar orientations of classical music therapy (Bruhn 2000), but also, for example, by studies aimed more at the area of public health and prevention about the effects of choir singing among amateurs (Clift 2012).

Regardless of the simplicity and plausibility of models, which suggest psychophysiological and psychosocial effects of music activities, there is still considerable influence of contextual and situational factors. Also, the implied causality in the association pattern must be treated with some caution. After all, individual mental and physical resources are needed to engage in music in the first place. Figure 2.2 therefore shifts the focus more toward the self and self-awareness, which are attributed pivotal roles. This model is inspired by the salutogenic approach to health (Antonovsky 1997). The basis of his concept are so-called

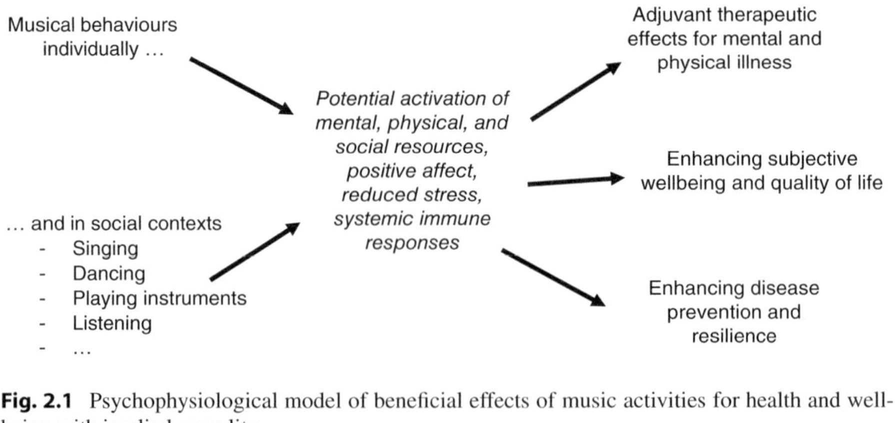

Fig. 2.1 Psychophysiological model of beneficial effects of music activities for health and well-being with implied causality

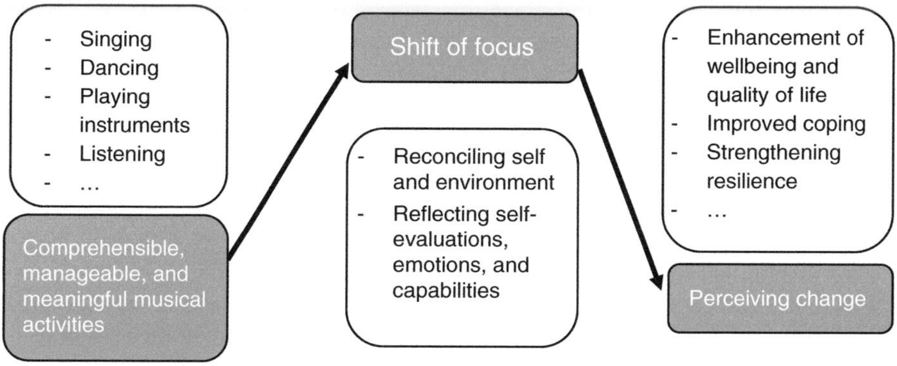

Fig. 2.2 Salutogenetical model of beneficial effects of music activities with implied shift of focus on self and perceived change

coherence feelings. These enable individuals to cope under adverse life circumstances. Actions must be subjectively understandable, manageable and meaningful in order to trigger coherence feelings. Health, quality of life and well-being are thus products of inner attitudes and dealing with experiences in a sometimes stressful environment. Implicitly, this model also suggests an avoidance of health-damaging behaviors.

The so-called diseases of affluence, prevalent in industrial societies, particularly those of the cardiovascular system, type II diabetes, and some forms of cancer (e.g., lung cancer), can be attributed to factors that individuals can influence themselves. These include lack of exercise, unbalanced diet, and the consumption of alcohol, tobacco, and drugs. Prevention programs are fundamentally designed to provide individuals with opportunities to reassess themselves and their perception of their environment. Musical activities can initiate such re-evaluations of self and environment, indirectly influencing attitudes and lifestyles. Such approaches are followed, for example, by prevention programs for children and adolescents from socially disadvantaged populations, who are supposed to be paved the way to more physical activity or better nutrition through cultural participation (Bungay and Vella-Burrows 2013).

Recently, Gustavson et al. (2021) have provided a comprehensive account of the potential benefits of music for mental health. Their review and framework place some emphasis on genetic factors and gene-environment interactions. Indeed, such approaches begin to move away from the genetics of musicality toward a genetics of healthy musicality, which puts mental sanity rather than achievement in the focus of the discussion.

The models presented are naturally idealized representations, which can facilitate the formulation and empirical testing of hypotheses. Finally, the relationships between musical activities on the one hand and health changes on the other, can be optimally investigated by hypothesis-supported, controlled procedures. However, there is considerable relevance of practical experience and knowledge, even before scientific knowledge of the mechanisms and mediating factors is established. This knowledge,, therefore, is an important source for both systematic inquiry and health policy. Vice versa, not all research-based claims on musical health effects are sustainable and generalizable to the extents being proclaimed (Clift et al. 2021).

2.6 Musical Needs, Preferences, and Resources

Every person undergoes a socialization characterized by musical elements under individual genetic as well as environmental conditions. Consequently, these musical activities are fundamentally holistic and human-centered. Targeted research questions that can reveal aspects and facets of complex relationships are always to be considered and formulated under these conditions. Both the preference or aversion to a music style or even a piece of music and the associated degree of familiarity are crucial for the emotional processing of music pieces.

Perhaps the most important conclusion to meet this dimension in research and application in health areas concerns the necessity of musical anamneses. Developing musical anamneses in the context of treatment and therapy concepts in a systematic way and incorporating them into music medical practice seems overdue against the background of a steadily growing number of clinical application areas. Based on already existing, extensive surveys in the general population (Müllensiefen et al. 2014), expectations of the musicality of hospitalized populations can be formulated and tested using suitable procedures. Musical preferences as well as abilities and skills, and finally, individual experiences with music can contain indications of resources such as self-efficacy and self-regulation, which could systematically be incorporated into treatment and rehabilitation concepts as soon as a research-based standardization of individual musical anamnesis is achieved (Bernatzky and Hesse 2003).

2.7 Health Opportunities and Risks

The problem of music-related health research is reflected in the opportunities and risks of differently musically active people. Simplifying, it can be stated that the risk-opportunity ratio for professional and nonprofessional musicians is almost reversed. It is evident that the musician's profession involves considerable strains, which can question the long-term practice of the profession itself. Amateur musicians, apart from the high volumes that are sometimes prevalent in leisure music listening and playing, are fundamentally much less exposed to psychological, mental, and physical (musculoskeletal system) strains. Therefore, in these (much larger) populations, far fewer disorders are to be expected that would be attributable to music practice. However, it should be noted that professional musicians are by no means excluded from any positive effects. Here, reduced occupational risks are also equated with health improvements.

2.8 Musical Activities and Health Status

The individual health status is, of course, a relevant dimension not only in terms of the professionalism of making music. However, amateur musicians, singers, dancers, and leisure music listeners are primarily of interest here. Obviously, music therapy as a form of psychotherapy is aimed at groups of patients with specific diagnoses and indications. However, this neither defines the reach of music therapeutic interventions, nor does it exclude quasi-therapeutic effects in nonclinical contexts. In other words, The applicability, form, and potential effects of musical activities are largely determined by a person's health status. But fundamentally, it is very difficult to determine under what circumstances the meaningfulness of musical interventions, even if therapeutic goals are not or only indirectly considered, must be regarded as exhausted.

Conclusion

The field of research of music in medicine is characterized by dynamically advancing knowledge bases that appear promising for the future. Nevertheless, scientific model formations and foundations through meta-analyses and systematic reviews are still rare. There is still the impression of a widely fragmented research landscape. The emergence of professional organizations and journals, congresses, and symposia on specific topics has apparently increased significantly in recent decades. The "*International Association for Music and Medicine (IAMM),*" for example, represents a coalition of scientists and practitioners that extends far beyond music therapeutic representatives and is collectively capable of sustainably improving the methodological quality and visibility of music medical research.

References

Antonovsky A (1997) Salutogenese. Dgvt Verlag, Tübingen

Batt-Rawden K, Tellnes G (2011) How music may promote healthy behaviour. Scand J Public Health 39(2):113–120. https://doi.org/10.1177/1403494810393555

Benoit C-E, Dalla Bella S, Farrugia N, Obrig H, Mainka S, Kotz SA (2014) Musically cued gait-training improves both perceptual and motor timing in Parkinson's disease. Front Hum Neurosci 8:494. https://doi.org/10.3389/fnhum.2014.00494

Bernardi L, Porta C, Sleight P (2006) Cardiovascular, cerebrovascular, and respiratory changes induced by different types of music in musicians and non-musicians: the importance of silence. Heart 92(4):445–452. https://doi.org/10.1136/hrt.2005.064600

Bernardi L, Porta C, Casucci G, Balsamo R, Bernardi NF, Fogari R, Sleight P (2009) Dynamic interactions between musical, cardiovascular, and cerebral rhythms in humans. Circulation 119(25):3171–3180. https://doi.org/10.1161/CIRCULATIONAHA.108.806174

Bernatzky G, Hesse H-P (2003) Musik in der Palliativmedizin. In: Schmerzbehandlung in der Palliativmedizin. Springer, Wien, pp 159–163

Bernatzky G, Bernatzky P, Hesse H-P, Staffen W, Ladurner G (2004) Stimulating music increases motor coordination in patients afflicted with Morbus Parkinson. Neurosci Lett 361(1–3):4–8. https://doi.org/10.1016/j.neulet.2003.12.022
Bruhn H (2000) Musiktherapie: Geschichte, Theorien, Methoden. Hogrefe, Göttingen
Bungay H, Vella-Burrows T (2013) The effects of participating in creative activities on the health and well-being of children and young people: a rapid review of the literature. Perspect Public Health 133(1):44–52. https://doi.org/10.1177/1757913912466946
Burkhardt J, Brennan C (2012) The effects of recreational dance interventions on the health and well-being of children and young people: a systematic review. Arts & Health 4(2):148–161. https://doi.org/10.1080/17533015.2012.665810
Clift S (2012) Singing, wellbeing and health. In: MacDonald RAR, Kreutz G, Mitchell LA (eds) Music, health, and wellbeing. Oxford University Press, Oxford, pp 113–124. https://doi.org/10.1093/acprof
Clift S, Hancox G (2001) The perceived benefits of singing: findings from preliminary surveys of a university college choral society. J R Soc Promot Heal 121(4):248–256. https://doi.org/10.1177/146642400112100409
Clift S, Camic P, Daykin N (2010) The arts and global health inequities. Arts & Health 2(1):3–7. https://doi.org/10.1080/17533010903421476
Clift S, Phillips K, Pritchard S (2021) The need for robust critique of research on social and health impacts of the arts. Cultural Trends 30(5):442–459. https://doi.org/10.1080/09548963.2021.1910492
Fischer P, Greitemeyer T (2006) Music and aggression: the impact of sexual-aggressive song lyrics on aggression-related thoughts, emotions, and behavior toward the same and the opposite sex. Personal Soc Psychol Bull. https://doi.org/10.1177/0146167206288670
Gerigk H (1957) Fachwörterbuch der Musik. Sikorski, Hamburg
Gustavson DE, Coleman PL, Iversen JR, Maes HH, Gordon RL, Lense MD (2021) Mental health and music engagement: review, framework, and guidelines for future studies. Transl Psychiatry 11(1):370. https://doi.org/10.1038/s41398-021-01483-8
Hambrick DZ, Tucker-Drob EM (2014) The genetics of music accomplishment: evidence for gene-environment correlation and interaction. Psychon Bull Rev. https://doi.org/10.3758/s13423-014-0671-9
Haro-Martínez A, Pérez-Araujo CM, Sanchez-Caro JM, Fuentes B, Díez-Tejedor E (2021) Melodic intonation therapy for post-stroke non-fluent aphasia: systematic review and meta-analysis. Front Neurol 12:700115. https://doi.org/10.3389/fneur.2021.700115
Koelsch S, Stegemann T (2012) The brain and positive biological effects in healthy and clinical populations. In: MacDonald RAR, Kreutz G, Mitchell LA (eds) Music, health, and wellbeing. Oxford University Press, Oxford, pp 436–456. https://doi.org/10.1093/acprof:oso/9780199586974.003.0029
Kraus N, Slater J, Thompson EC, Hornickel J, Strait DL, Nicol T, White-Schwoch T (2014) Music enrichment programs improve the neural encoding of speech in at-risk children. J Neurosci 34(36):11913–11918. https://doi.org/10.1523/JNEUROSCI.1881-14.2014
Kreutz G, Lotze M (2007) Neuroscience of music and emotion. In: Neurosciences in music pedagogy. Nova Science, New York, pp 143–167. https://doi.org/10.1002/biot.200690104
Kreutz G, Quiroga C, Bongard S (2012) Psychoneuroendocrine research on music and health: an overview. In: MacDonald RAR, Kreutz G, Mitchell L (eds) Music, health, and well-being. Oxford University Press, Oxford, pp 457–476. https://doi.org/10.1093/acprof:oso/9780199586974.003.0030
Krueger J (2014) Affordances and the musically extended mind. Front Psychol 4:1003. https://doi.org/10.3389/fpsyg.2013.01003
MacDonald RAR (2013) Music, health, and well-being: a review. Int J Qual Stud Health Well Being 8:20635
MacDonald RAR, Kreutz G, Mitchell L (eds) (2012) Music, health, and wellbeing. Music, health, and wellbeing. Oxford University Press, Oxford. https://doi.org/10.1093/acprof:oso/9780199586974.001.0001

Müllensiefen D, Gingras B, Musil J, Stewart L (2014) The musicality of non-musicians: an index for assessing musical sophistication in the general population. PLoS One 9(2):e89642. https://doi.org/10.1371/journal.pone.0089642

O'Callaghan C, Barry P, Thompson K (2012) Music's relevance for adolescents and young adults with cancer: a constructivist research approach. Support Care Cancer 20(4):687–697. https://doi.org/10.1007/s00520-011-1104-1

Oikkonen J, Järvelä I (2014) Genomics approaches to study musical aptitude. BioEssays 36(11):1102–1108. https://doi.org/10.1002/bies.201400081

Panksepp J, Bernatzky G (2002) Emotional sounds and the brain: the neuro-affective foundations of musical appreciation. Behav Process 60(2):133–155. https://doi.org/10.1016/s0376-6357(02)00080-3

Pavlicevic M, O'Neil N, Powell H, Jones O, Sampathianaki E (2014) Making music, making friends: long-term music therapy with young adults with severe learning disabilities. J Intellect Disabil 18(1):5–19. https://doi.org/10.1177/1744629513511354

Quiroga Murcia C, Kreutz G, Bongard S (2011) Endokrine und immunologische Wirkungen von Musik. In: Schubert C (ed) Psychoneuroimmunologie und Psychotherapie. Schattauer, Stuttgart, pp 248–262

Reyes E (2019) Music deserts: how social inequality affects accessibility to music resources important to actively participating in music. Ursidae 6(2):480–487

Savage PE, Loui P, Tarr B, Schachner A, Glowacki L, Mithen S, Fitch WT (2021) Music as a coevolved system for social bonding. Behav Brain Sci 44:e59. https://doi.org/10.1017/S0140525X20000333

Stahl B, Kotz SA (2014) Facing the music: three issues in current research on singing and aphasia. Front Psychol 5:1033. https://doi.org/10.3389/fpsyg.2014.01033

Tan YT, McPherson GE, Peretz I, Berkovic SF, Wilson SJ (2014) The genetic basis of music ability. Front Psychol 5. https://doi.org/10.3389/fpsyg.2014.00658

Theorell T, Kreutz G (2012) Epidemiological studies of the relationship between musical experiences and public health. In: MacDonald RAR, Kreutz G, Mitchell L (eds) Music, health, and wellbeing. Oxford University Press, Oxford, pp 424–435. https://doi.org/10.1093/acprof:oso/9780199586974.003.0028

Trevarthen C (2008) The musical art of infant conversation: narrating in the time of sympathetic experience, without rational interpretation, before words. Music Sci 12(Suppl 1):15–46. https://doi.org/10.1177/1029864908012001021

Västfjäll D, Juslin PN, Hartig T (2012) Music, subjective well-being, and health: the role of everyday emotions. In: MacDonald RAR, Kreutz G, Mitchell LA (eds) Music, health, and wellbeing. Oxford University Press, Oxford, pp 405–423

Zumbansen A, Peretz I, Hébert S (2014) The combination of rhythm and pitch can account for the beneficial effect of melodic intonation therapy on connected speech improvements in Broca's aphasia. Front Hum Neurosci 8:592. https://doi.org/10.3389/fnhum.2014.00592

Music and Medicine: An Overview

3

Claudia Spahn, Günther Bernatzky, and Gunter Kreutz

In recent years, music and medicine have come closer due to a significant increase in research activity and the stock of knowledge in many branches. Music therapy was long considered virtually the only link between the two subjects. This link is currently spreading out in a dynamic way, forming an innovative area of research characterized by a high degree of interdisciplinary and an evolved methodological quality; included here are both clinical and nonclinical contexts, as well as health promotion, quality of life and well-being over the span of a lifetime (e.g., MacDonald et al. 2013; Richter 2018).

3.1 Music in Medicine—Music Medicine

In the field of music in medicine, research is undertaken into the therapeutic effects of musical activities, such as listening to music, singing and dancing, or learning and playing musical instruments alone or in groups. The term "music medicine" was first coined in specialist German-language literature of the 1970s by the physicians Ralph Spintge and Roland Droh in the publications concerned (e.g., Spintge and Droh 1992). Today, the term is used synonymously with music and medicine. As part of expanding issues to include health promotion and prevention, the

C. Spahn (✉)
Freiburg Institute for Musicians' Medicine (FIM), University of Music Freiburg, Medical Faculty University Freiburg, University Clinic Freiburg, Freiburg, Germany
e-mail: claudia.spahn@uniklinik-freiburg.de

G. Bernatzky
Department of Biosciences and Medical Biology, University of Salzburg, Salzburg, Austria

G. Kreutz
Systematic Musicology, Carl von Ossietzky University Oldenburg, Oldenburg, Lower Saxony, Germany

G. Kreutz, G. Bernatzky (eds.), *Music and Medicine*, Neurocultural Health and Wellbeing, https://doi.org/10.1007/978-3-662-72175-9_3

short-term and long-term prophylactic effect of making and listening to music is also investigated and discussed in music medicine within the context of society and education. In so doing, overlaps occur with different areas of applied music psychology within the field of systematic musicology (MacDonald et al. 2013) and with the prevention and health promotion within music physiology and musicians' medicine (Spahn 2015).

Musical interventions have presumably been employed as remedies over centuries and in various human cultures. The use of music in healing is testified to both among primitive peoples and in the ancient high cultures up to Greek-Roman antiquity (Bernatzky and Hesse 2013). Greek mythology unites music, beauty and healing power through the genealogy of the gods: thus, Apollo was worshipped as the god of music and the art of healing. He conceived Orpheus, the greatest singer of antiquity, whom he taught to master the lyre, and Asclepius, the father of medicine, whom he instructed in medicine (Spahn and Richter 2007). According to Plato, making music and movement were considered basic elements in the ancient world of a healthy and balanced development, both physical and mental (cf. Plato's "Politeia," 1998). In the Christian world the traditional notions of the effect of music attracted little interest, for illness was considered divine punishment for sinful behavior. Fundamental change only came with the Age of the Enlightenment, in which efforts were made to attribute all natural phenomena to laws of nature in accordance with the principle of causality. While up to that point, music had been experienced as a medium of the word with a religious function, it also now became one of life's pleasures, along with the emancipation of the bourgeoisie (Bernatzky and Hesse 2013). The potential in musical performances to delight people, express affects and arouse a wide range of feelings was appreciated. Consequently, since the end of the seventeenth century, the therapeutic application of music in medicine has been the subject of intense discussion, too (ebd.). Athanasius Kircher, Jesuit priest and universal scholar, debates in his 1673 "Phonurgia nova" the healing effect of music:

> The nerves and musculi in the human body are moved by music like the strings of an instrument. (…) The spirits of life (…) which thus reside in the heart are touched by the movement of the external sound, (…) therefore a mind that is worn down by worries and as it were wilting, recovers once again and is refreshed. (Kirchner 1684, p. 133 and 138)

In the course of the eighteenth century, the therapeutic effect of music was increasingly employed in the area of mental disorders, out of which present-day music therapy developed.

Far-reaching research into music in medicine was carried out in the area of pain management (Kullich et al. 2003), so that nowadays a link can be reestablished again with this historical tradition, reaching far into the past, of therapeutically motivated listening to music. Bernatzky coined the term recently "Musikament" (which one could approximately translate as "musication") to refer to listening to music as a non-pharmacological form of medication. Specially produced music, as a kind of medication, can offer the chance for relaxation and diversion to groups of people who are at risk of stress or ill (Bernatzky 2013). The paradigm of "listening to music as medication" is also supported by research into the effect on depression and anxiety (DeMarco et al. 2012; Jarzok et al. 2013; MacDonald et al. 2013). The anxiolytic (i.e., anxiety-reducing) effect of music before and during diagnostic examinations and medical interventions could be demonstrated in scientific studies. The playing of music is today widespread in heart catheter examinations (Chang et al. 2011), MRI diagnostics (Walworth 2010), as well as in dental treatments (Thoma et al. 2014) and patients' waiting rooms (Hamel 2001) (summarized in Hesse and Bernatzky 2005). Furthermore, listening to music, along with being coached to actively practice musical rhythms, showed positive effects in the neurological rehabilitation of stroke patients (Särkämö and Soto 2012). On the basis of these and other relevant research results, Neurologic Music Therapy (NMT) has been able to take root in music medicine in recent years (Chap. 11). The basic neuro-scientific research into the cerebral processing of music-listening and music-making, as well as the influence of those two activities on the plasticity of the brain, is the basis for a growing number of application areas (Panksepp and Bernatzky 2002; MacDonald et al. 2013). In this context, research into the effect of music in terms of maintaining mental performance in old age and for the prevention of dementia plays an important role as well (Presch et al. 2011).

3.2 Music Therapy

Music therapy forms a distinct healing method in the area of clinical psychology and psychotherapy. Historically, it draws on the centuries-old experience of music being able to influence the human psyche in a positive way (Panksepp and Bernatzky 2002). As medicine evolved historically—depending on the degree of significance accorded to the psyche in how illness and health were understood—acceptance also shifted in terms of music being employed as a psychotherapeutic agent. Music therapy established itself after the Second World War as a distinct form of therapy for treating mental and psychosomatic illnesses.

Essentially, one should distinguish between receptive music therapy, in which the therapeutic effect is achieved through hearing music, and active music therapy, in which patients themselves produce musical sounds and rhythms. Today, music therapy in medicine is a fixed element in the inpatient treatment of psychosomatic and psychiatric illnesses. With regard to the underlying psychotherapeutic approach, different manifestations and independent procedures have developed within music therapy with varying degrees of closeness to different psychotherapy concepts, whether psychoanalytic psychotherapy, behavioral therapy/learning theory, or systemic, anthroposophical and humanistic approaches. Moreover, music therapy traditionally stretches into the area of personality development among children and adolescents, in the context of the so-called Orff Music Therapy, for example (Decker-Voigt 2001), and increasingly captures other social and medical fields of activity, too (Keller and Wolfram 2013; Bosse et al. 2013). This expansion into medical areas outside the domain of psychotherapy leads to an increasing convergence and overlap between music therapy and music medicine. This is conceptually logical, as music therapy, according to its name, is not limited to mental illnesses, but can essentially consist of making and listening to music as a form of therapy for a range of clinical conditions. One example of this is Neurologic Music Therapy (Thaut 2007; Chap. 11). Since 2009, the Music Therapy Law has existed in Austria. This law regulates in which fields music is applied as a form of therapy. Herein it is stipulated that music therapy provides proven assistance to people with psychoses, coma patients, patients with craniocerebral trauma, and children and adolescents suffering from cancer, among others. In Germany, music therapy is recommended in the guidelines for treatment of the Working Group of the Scientific Medical Specialized Companies (in German AWMF) as a form of therapy in the early rehabilitation of stroke patients and those suffering from dementia. In these guidelines, music therapy increasingly finds a fixed place in the field of psychosomatic and psychiatric illnesses, as well as in psycho-oncology.

3.3 Music in Hospitals

Developed substantially by Victor Flusser in Strasbourg, the concept of interactive music-making in hospitals and care homes represents a distinct concept as regards the presence of music in the medical field. Here, musicians specially trained for this make music with patients, family members and physicians in the hospital; the goal is to enliven the emotional setting (Grosse and Vogels 2007). The training to become a "musician intervenant" is offered in France at nine French universities with special training centers—the "Centres de Formation de Musiciens Intervenants" (CFMI). Another training center for professional musicians in clinical institutions that closely cooperates with France is run by the Royal Northern College of Music in Manchester, UK. In addition, mention should be made here of those vocal ensembles, growing in number for some years, that are affiliated with the international network "Singing Hospitals e.V." (Chap. 18).

3.4 Musicians' Medicine

In contrast with the therapeutic application of music, musicians' medicine, as a special field, includes the prevention, diagnostics and therapy of health problems that can arise through making music or have arisen, or which can have an impact on the music-making. Musicians' medicine is equally concerned with professional and amateur musicians, whether instrumentalists or singers. Musicians' medicine as a medical discipline that engages with the genesis and treatment of specific clinical conditions among musicians is proven by the first sources to have already existed in the fifteenth century. The physician Giovanni Michele Savonarola, who taught in Padua, dedicated himself in a 1486 tract to the possible causes of hernias among "trumpeters and flautists" in particular, who in his view represented a threatened occupational group (quoted from Breuer 1982, p. 4). In 1675, the Dutch anatomist Ysbrand van Diemerbroeck described disease patterns that could result from the high blowing pressure of the wind instruments of the period (Breuer 1982). An early major work in occupational medicine, in which a whole chapter is devoted to the "Diseases of Speakers, Singers and Other People of the Like"—the latter referring to instrumentalists—was published in 1700 written by Bernardino Ramazzini with the title "De morbis atrificum diatribe" (ibid.). In the course of the nineteenth century music medicine-related issues continued to grow in importance, as health complaints among musicians due to the increase in virtuosic playing and the intensified practice times. In this regard, reports from prominent musicians have come down to us, an example being Robert Schumann, who in 1831 developed impaired movement of the right hand after intense piano studies, or Alexander Scriabin, who in 1890 had to stop playing the piano with his right hand for many years on account of an overuse syndrome (Otte and Wink 2008). Singers, too, were exposed to greater strain—such as the Wagnerian tenor Ludwig Schnorr von Carolsfeld, for example, whose early and sudden death in 1865 was attributed by some contemporaries to the exertions of the title role of "Tristan." An early comprehensive publication on musicians' medicine was published in 1831 titled "Ärztlicher Ratgeber für Musiktreibende" (Medical Guide for Music Players) by Karl Sundelin. It was followed in 1925 by the book "Berufskrankheiten des Musikers" (Occupational Diseases of the Musician) by the physician Julius Flesch. In the 1920s, the Berlin neurologist, musicologist and music critic Kurt Singer attempted for the first time to integrate the subject of musicians' medicine into the university education of music students (Singer 1926). Since 1923, he had held a teaching position for this subject at the "Staatliche Akademische Hochschule für Musik" (State Academic University for Music) in Berlin. These beginnings at establishing, both substantively and institutionally, musicians' medicine as a discipline and a specialized medical area were again destroyed by the National Socialists on account of the Jewish origins of Kurt Singer. After the Second World War, musicians' medicine was continued in East Germany. An example of this is the "Bühnenambulatorium" (Stage Out-Patient Clinic) for treating artists in East Berlin.

In the USA in the 1980s, "Performing Arts Medicine" emerges, which sets itself the task of medical care for all performing artists—including dancers and actors alongside instrumentalists and singers. In Europe, societies for musicians' medicine have likewise been created to date, i.a., in Germany, England, the Netherlands, France and Austria. These regularly hold symposia and congresses on themes relating to musicians' medicine. In the last 10–15 years, the network of offerings for treating musicians medically has continued to take root internationally. In Germany, musicians' medicine treatment offers exist both at some university clinics and music universities, as well as among resident doctors.

It has proven possible in the care of musicians within musicians' medicine to develop specific treatments over the last 10 years. Examples including treating music performance anxiety (Spahn et al. 2011) and disorders among singers (Richter 2018), as well as new findings concerning clinical conditions such as focal dystonia among musicians (Altenmüller and Jabusch 2011). The current knowledge on diagnostics, prevention and treatment of musician-specific diseases is reflected in the textbook titled "Musikermedizin" (2011), edited by Spahn, Richter and Altenmüller.

In Germany, physicians working in the field of musicians' medicine do so on the basis of their respective specialist disciplines (e.g. phoniatrics, psychosomatic medicine, neurology, etc.). To ensure quality assurance in the further training of physicians and therapeutes working in the field of musicians' medicine, a certification course of advances studies in musicians' medicine for physicians and therapeutes was launched and offered for the first time in 2023 (Spahn et al. 2025).

3.5 Music Physiology

Expanding upon musicians' medicine, music physiology is concerned with the physiological and psychological foundations of *healthy* music-making. Its goal is thus equally to prevent health problems that may arise through practicing music.

Historical roots of music physiology in Germany reach back to the 1960s. In East Germany, the "Studio for Voice Research" was founded by Harry Schwickardi in 1959 at the Hochschule für Musik in Dresden (University for Music in Dresden), which established the link between vocal teaching and scientific research in the area of the singing voice. In West Germany, the physician and conductor Christoph Wagner (1931–2013) had engaged since the 1960s with the healthy physiological processes in music-making from both the medical and scientific perspective, thus forging the notion of music physiology. In 1974, Christoph Wagner was appointed to the first professorial chair for "music physiology" at the Hochschule für Musik und Theater Hannover (University for Music and Theater Hannover).

In 1994, together with Jochen Blum, he founded the "Deutsche Gesellschaft für Musikphysiologie und Musikermedizin" (DGfMM) or "German Society for Music Physiology and Musicians' Medicine" and combined, in terms of content, music physiology as an academic discipline with musicians' medicine as a specific discipline for treating patients. Accordingly, those members of the society are physicians and therapists as well as musicians. Today, the DGfMM is one of the internationally largest and most active societies in the field of music physiology and musicians' medicine.

Meanwhile, courses in music physiology are on offer at nearly all music universities in Germany and Austria. These are especially comprehensive at music universities with separate institutes in the field of music physiology and musicians' medicine, such as those in Freiburg, Dresden, Hannover, Munich, among others. At the Hochschule für Musik Freiburg, the subject can be studied as a separate minor subject—Minor Music Physiology—as part of the Bachelor of Music and since 2023 Music Physiology as a main subject in the Master of Music. Academic qualifications such as a Dr. phil. and PhD in Music Physiology and a Habilitation with a venia legendi in Music Physiology are also possible for musicians, e.g. at the Freiburg University of Music in the Freiburg Institute for Musicians' Medicine.

Today, in music physiology as a subject, physiological foundations of singing and making music—the basics of functional anatomy, the study of movement and motoric learning—concerning their application to singing and instrumental playing (Wasmer and Eickhoff 2011; Spahn et al. 2013, Spahn 2011) are taught. Besides theoretical knowledge, practical skills for improving performance (Steinmüller

2008; Spahn 2017; Spahn, 2015) are taught. Voice physiology forms a separate, highly specialized discipline within music physiology (Richter 2018).

In the spirit of the prevention, students are prepared for the health challenges presented by their occupation to come. The course material here is the prevention of hearing damage among musicians by means of hearing protection (Richter et al. 2007), as well as prevention of hearing impairments through leisure noise (Chap. 16). Communication and leadership skills in the orchestral profession as well as the teaching of healthy music making and singing in instrumental and vocal pedagogy are also covered (Chap. 21 and Chap. 26).

Music physiology includes musical-psychological content, too, which has to do with the musician's personality and the process of music making. The focus here is on how music performance anxiety is handled, as well as during examinations and auditions, for which students these days are taught the relevant measures to take (Spahn 2012).

Overall, it can be demonstrated that carrying out prevention-oriented teaching programs yields a positive effect on the student's performance during their studies (Spahn 2006, 2015, 2017; Zander 2006; Spahn et al. 2017).

In the context of transferring scientific research results on the fundamentals of music making, the specialized subject of music physiology also includes subjects relating to the health promotion through making music (Chap. 25) and advocates preserving music culture in society.

3.6 Related Areas of Expertise

As a branch of Systematic Musicology, music psychology creates a link in its applied research to questions of music education and the effect of music. Its research themes include the effects and meanings of musical taste, as well as examining the pedagogical and socio-cultural basics of musical activities and their implications. It is within this context that the critical debate takes place as to whether the means available for the provision of our musical life reaches all members of society to a sufficient degree—regardless of whether any special musical talent is present or not, or whether any individual limitations exist, be they emotional, physical or mental (Chap. 9). A series of scientific examinations have shown that music in general, and active music making in particular, have health-promoting effects (Bygren et al. 1996; Kreutz et al. 2004; Biegl 2006). Choral singing in particular could be shown to have positive psychosocial effects (Clift and Hancox 2001; Chap. 18 and Chap. 19). The scientific research activities in the field of music psychology are represented by the Deutsche Gesellschaft für Musikpsychologie (DGM) or German Society for Music Psychology, among others. In existence since 1983, the DGM is the largest national society in this sector and is closely associated with the European Society for Music Perception and Cognition (ESCOM).

3.7 Conclusion

The differentiated consideration of the thematically diverse areas located between music and medicine illustrates the variety and vibrancy of this field of research. Viewed from a range of perspectives, the importance of music in its historically established role for the well-being of mankind is thus enhanced.

References

Altenmüller E, Jabusch H-C (2011) Neurologie. In: Spahn C, Richter B, Altenmüller E (eds) Musikermedizin. Diagnostik, Therapie und Prävention von musikerspezifischen Erkrankungen. Schattauer, Stuttgart, pp 187–223

Bernatzky G (2013) Das "Musikament". Arzt & Praxis 994:112–114

Bernatzky G, Hesse HP (2013) Musik in der Palliativmedizin. In: Bernatzky G, Likar R, Sittl R (eds) Schmerzbehandlung in der Palliativmedizin, 3rd edn. Springer, Vienna/New York, pp 175–179

Biegl T (2006) Singen macht glücklich. Tagungsreader der Jahrestagung der Deutschen Gesellschaft für Musikpsychologie

Bosse J, Stegemann T, Schmidt HU, Timmermann T (2013) Dem Aufmerksamkeitsdefizit mit Aufmerksamkeit begegnen—was die Musiktherapie Kindern und Jugendlichen mit einer ADHS-Diagnose bieten kann. Musikther Umsch 34(1):7–22

Breuer R (1982) Berufskrankheiten von Instrumentalmusikern aus medizinhistorischer Sicht (vom 15. Jahrhundert bis 1930). Dissertation. Johannes-Gutenberg-Universität, Mainz

Bygren LO, Konlaan BB, Johansson SE (1996) Attendance at cultural events, reading books or periodicals, and making music or singing in a choir as determinants for survival: Swedish interview survey of living conditions. Br Med J 313(7072):1577–1580

Chang HK, Peng TC, Wang JH, Lai HL (2011) Psychophysiological responses to sedative music in patients awaiting cardiac catheterization examination: a randomized controlled trial. J Cardiovasc Nurs 26(5):E11–E18

Clift S, Hancox G (2001) The perceived benefits of singing: findings from the preliminary surveys of a university college choral society. J R Soc Promot Heal 121(4):248–256

Decker-Voigt H-H (2001) Schulen der Musiktherapie. Ernst Reinhardt Verlag, Munich

DeMarco J, Alexander JL, Nehrenz G, Gallagher L (2012) The benefit of music for the reduction of stress and anxiety in patients undergoing elective cosmetic surgery. Music Med 4(1):44–48

Flesch J (1925) Berufskrankheiten des Musikers. Niels Kampmann, Celle

Grosse T, Vogels R (eds) (2007) Interaktives Musizieren. Beiträge zu einem deutschen Modellprojekt an Krankenhäusern und Pflegeeinrichtungen. Blumhardt, Hannover

Hamel WJ (2001) The effects of music intervention on anxiety in the patient waiting for cardiac catheterization. Intensive Crit Care Nurs 17(5):279–285

Hesse H-P, Bernatzky G (2005) Musik im Alter. In: Likar R, Bernatzky G, Pipam W, Janig H, Sadjak A (eds) Lebensqualität im Alter. Therapie und Prophylaxe von Altersleiden. Springer, Vienna/New York, pp 161–166

Jarzok MN, Koenig J, Schuster AK, Thayer JF, Fischer JE (2013) Nighttime heart rate variability, overnight urinary norepinephrine, and glycemic status in apparently healthy human adults. Int J Cardiol 168(3):3025–3026

Keller R, Wolfram I (2013) Instrumente in der Gruppenmusiktherapie mit traumatisierten Flüchtlingen. Musikther Umsch 34(4):383–386

Kircher A (1684) Phonurgia nova. Neue Hall- und Thonkunst. Friedrich Schultes Noerdlingen (Reprint 1983, Th. Schäfer, Hannover)

Kreutz G, Bongard S, Rohrmann S, Hodapp V, Grebe D (2004) Effects of choir singing or listening on secretory immunoglobulin A, cortisol, and emotional state. J Behav Med 27:623–635

Kullich W, Bernatzky G, Hesse H-P, Wendtner F, Likar R, Klein G (2003) Musiktherapie—Wirkung auf Schmerz, Schlaf und Lebensqualität bei Low Back Pain. Wien Med Wochenschr 153:217–221

MacDonald R, Kreutz G, Mitchell L (2013) Music, health, and wellbeing, 2nd edn. Oxford University Press, Oxford
Otte A, Wink K (2008) Kerners Krankheiten großer Musiker. Schattauer, Stuttgart
Panksepp J, Bernatzky G (2002) Emotional sounds and the brain: the neuro-affective foundations of musical appreciation. Behav Proc 60:133–155
Platon (1998) Der Staat. Deutscher Taschenbuch Verlag, Munich
Presch M, Hartl L, Tucek G, Minnich B, Kullich W, Bernatzky G (2011) Einflüsse von aktiver und rezeptiver Musiktherapie auf Kognition, Verhalten, Schlaf und allgemeine Befindlichkeit von Demenzpatienten—eine Pilotstudie. Schweiz Z Ganzheitsmed 28:218–223
Richter B (2018) Die Stimme, 3rd edn. Henschel, Leipzig
Richter B, Zander MF, Spahn C (2007) Gehörschutz im Orchester. In: Spahn C (ed) Freiburger Beiträge zur Musikermedizin, vol 4, Bochum/Freiburg
Särkämö T, Soto D (2012) Music listening after stroke: beneficial effects and potential neural mechanisms. Ann N Y Acad Sci 1252:266–281
Singer K (1926) Die Berufskrankheiten der Musiker. Max-Hesses, Berlin
Spahn C (2006) Gesundheit für Musiker—Entwicklung des Freiburger Präventionsmodells. In: Spahn C (ed) Freiburger Beiträge zur Musikermedizin, vol 1, Bochum/Freiburg
Spahn C (2011) Prävention und Gesundheitsförderung. In: Spahn C, Richter B, Altenmüller E (eds) MusikerMedizin. Diagnostik, Therapie und Prävention von musikerspezifischen Erkrankungen. Schattauer, Stuttgart, pp 50–79
Spahn C (2012) Lampenfieber. Handbuch für den erfolgreichen Auftritt. Henschel, Leipzig
Spahn C (2015) Musikergesundheit in der Praxis. Grundlagen. Prävention. Übungen. Henschel, Leipzig
Spahn C (2017) Körperorientierte Ansätze für Musiker. Huber, Bern
Spahn C, Leiner J, Richter B (2025) Freiburger Zertifizierungslehrgang Musikermedizin (CAS) in Hinsken A, Bodo-Hartmann A-M, Ehinger J. (Hg) Qualität in der wissenschaftlichen und künstlerischen Weiterbildung, Evalag wbv, pp. 225–232
Spahn C, Richter B (2007) Gesundheitliche Aspekte des Singens und Musizierens. In: Gauger JD, Wilske H (eds) Bildungsoffensive Musikunterricht. Rombach, Freiburg, pp 133–141
Spahn C, Richter B, Altenmüller E (2011) Musikermedizin. Diagnostik, Therapie und Prävention von musikerspezifischen Erkrankungen. Schattauer, Stuttgart
Spahn C, Richter B, Pöppe J, Echternach M (2013) Das Blasinstrumentenspiel: Physiologische Vorgänge und Einblicke ins Körperinnere/Physiological insights for players of wind instruments. DVD-ROM Helbling, Esslingen
Spahn C, Voltmer E, Mornell A, Nusseck M (2017) Health status and preventive health behavior of music students during university education: merging prior results with new insights from a German multicenter stud. Musicae Scientiae 21:213–229
Spintge R, Droh R (1992) Musik-Medizin. Physiologische Grundlagen und praktische Anwendungen. G, Fischer, Stuttgart
Steinmüller W (2008) Körperbewusstheit für Musiker. Die Feldenkrais-Methode im Freiburger Präventionsmodell. In: Spahn C (ed) Freiburger Beiträge zur Musikermedizin, vol 3, Bochum/Freiburg
Sundelin K (1831) Ärztlicher Ratgeber für Musiktreibende. Grobenschütz & Seiler, Berlin
Thaut M (2007) Rhythm, music, and the brain. Scientific foundations and clinical applications. Routledge, New York
Thoma MV, Zemp M, Kreienbühl L, Hofer D, Schmidlin PR, Attin T, Ehlert U, Nater UM (2014) Effects of music listening on pretreatment anxiety and stress levels in a dental hygiene recall population. Int J Behav Med 22(4):498–505
Walworth DD (2010) Effect of live music therapy for patients undergoing magnetic resonance imaging. J Music Ther Winter 47(4):335–350
Wasmer C, Eickhoff F (2011) Vergleichende Untersuchungen zur Spielbewegung bei Geigern. In: Spahn C (ed) Freiburger Beiträge zur Musikermedizin, vol 7, Bochum/Freiburg
Zander MF (2006) Musiker zwischen Gesundheit und Krankheit—Evaluation des Freiburger Präventionsmodells. In: Spahn C (ed) Freiburger Beiträge zur Musikermedizin, vol 2, Bochum/Freiburg

4 Epidemiological Studies on Music and Health

Töres Theorell

4.1 What Are Epidemiological Studies?

By "epidemiological studies" I am referring to studies of the distribution of conditions in different groups of the general population. Typically, an epidemiological study aims at the establishment of exposures associated with illness, for instance, cigarette smoking in relation to cardiovascular disease (Berkman et al. 2014; Rothmann 2012). Here, I will limit this broad definition of epidemiology to studies using statistical methods and standardized assessments of musical activities and experiences in relation to possible relationships between music and various aspects of health. A typical epidemiological study includes thousands of participants, so the studies reviewed in this text will only include studies of large number of participants.

Of course, health can be defined in many ways. A broad range of different aspects of health will be discussed, from self-reports by means of standardized scales assessing well-being and loneliness to more objective assessments of illness development, including morbidity and mortality. An epidemiological study may be confined to a limited part of the general population. There are epidemiological studies that are limited to one specific age group, women only, health care workers, and car mechanics, for instance. Accordingly, in epidemiological music research, there are studies of children, of health care workers, of the elderly and of patients with various illnesses. A requirement for epidemiological studies is that the studied group's representativeness should be described and discussed. How was the target group

T. Theorell (✉)
Department of International Health, Karolinska Institutet, Solna, Sweden

Stress Research Institute, Stockholm University, Stockholm, Sweden

Royal College of Music, Stockholm, Sweden
e-mail: Tores.theorell@su.se

G. Kreutz, G. Bernatzky (eds.), *Music and Medicine*, Neurocultural Health and Wellbeing, https://doi.org/10.1007/978-3-662-72175-9_4

defined? How were participants invited, and what were the reasons for possible refusal to take part?

One example of large-scale studies of the relationship between music experiences and health is the mostly network-based convenience studies of the health of choral singers—studies that mostly do not fulfil criteria for epidemiological studies. Studies based on convenience sampling often provide insufficient in-depth information on individual differences. This means that they do not provide a representative basis for conclusions about associations between music experiences and health in the general population. In addition, by comparing singers and non-singers, it is still difficult to draw even tentative conclusions about causal effects of such musical activities on health measures. Men and women who participate regularly in choir singing comprise a highly selected group. Many choristers may have stopped singing due to health problems, such as lung and heart diseases affecting breathing capacity; or they may have encountered problems with the vocal cords, back pain, or psychiatric conditions that make participation difficult. Therefore, a selection bias might explain good health in a group of choir singers rather than the choral singing itself. Accordingly, conclusions about a possible causal relationship may require a prospective design—that subjects in the population are followed over time and assessments are made on several occasions and that some in the population are exposed to cultural experiences while others are not. In addition, since health is the outcome variable one needs to know how the health was at start. Is the health improved, unchanged or deteriorated at the end of the follow-up? Similarly, it is necessary to have information about socioeconomic factors and relevant health-related behavioral variables such as smoking, alcohol consumption, and physical activity. Finally, information about previous music experiences both on an individual and a group level is needed. Despite limitations, descriptions of health variables in national choir singer groups may be of great interest, but the limitations have to described and discussed.

It should also be pointed out that even large epidemiological studies with a good design cannot provide definite proof regarding causality. One needs a combination of many types of studies ranging from qualitative to epidemiological and experimental for final conclusions regarding causality.

4.2 The Importance of Gene–Environment Interactions

The possible influence of arts experiences constitutes a complex interplay between environmental and genetic factors (see Fig. 4.1). Music experiences to the left are perceived by our personal music program (in the center), which translates it into reactions (to the right) in the form of movement, emotions, and bodily (hormonal and cardiovascular, for instance) reactions (Theorell et al. 2014). The personal program is constantly changing due to influences of genes (above) and environment. As indicated in the diagram, the arrows are bidirectional. Accordingly, an adverse or positive reaction to a musical experience may result in a change in the personal music program. In addition, the activity in the genes may also change. A gene responsible for stress reactions, for instance, can be "sensitized" or "desensitized"

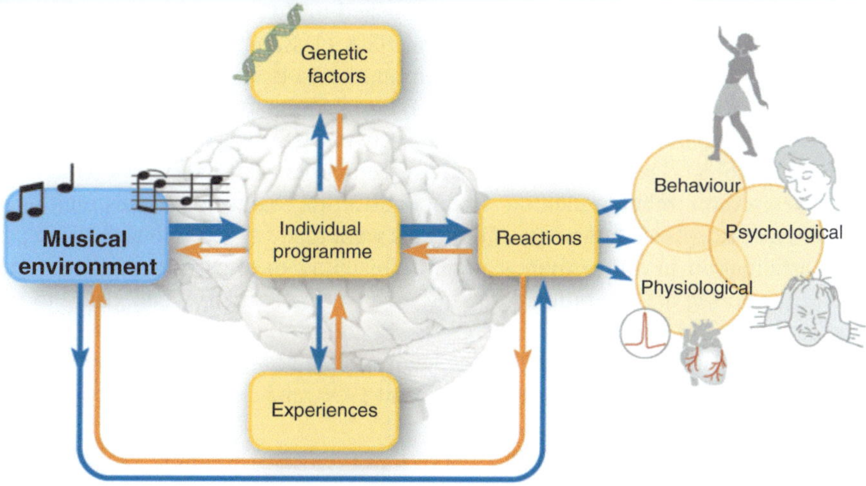

Fig. 4.1 Flowchart describing the complex relationships between exposure to music, individual program, and reactions. (Adapted from Theorell 2014)

by the environment. This is being increasingly discussed in modern epigenetics (Nair et al. 2021; Podlipniak 2021). Therefore, genes are not so stable as is often assumed. This emphasizes the importance of interaction between genes and environment.

As already mentioned, establishing causality from epidemiological data is challenging. There may be *confounders* which are factors that might generate spurious relationships. For instance, if musicians of a specific genre are prone to excessive alcohol consumption and associated health risks, it is clear that not the music genre, but the alcohol must be seen as the cause of poorer health in that group. Therefore, linking musical activities with both positive and negative health outcomes needs rather careful methodological considerations and caution with respect to interpreting correlational data.

Finally, if relationships are established in an epidemiological scientifically credible study between a specified kind of cultural activity and some aspect of health—even after adjustment for confounders—there may be genetic factors still influence any observed association. If a joint genetic factor explains the relationship we talk about *pleiotropy*, a concept that is discussed in another chapter of this book.

4.3 General Perspectives on Arts Experiences, Music, and Health

That participation in cultural activities may be good for health has been assumed for a long time. In the literature, it is often referred to the use in ancient cultures of arts activities, such as listening to and making music as health promoting. Strict epidemiological studies, however, have not existed for such a long time. One of the first epidemiological population studies was published in Sweden (Bygren et al. 1996). The study was performed during the early 1980s (1982–1983) when participation rates in population studies were higher (around 80%) than they are today and particularly so in the Scandinavian countries. The 12,982 participants were randomly selected individuals in the general population (Swedish Survey of Living Conditions) in the aged 16–84. Data collection was based upon personal interviews which may have been a more reliable method for data collection than self-administered questionnaires or telephone interviews. Questions were made about both active and passive participation in arts activities, such as listening to music/playing or singing regularly, visiting art exhibitions/drawing, or painting regularly, and going to theater/regular participation in a theater group. In addition, participants were asked in detail about health problems as well as health-related habits such as smoking and drinking. Participants were then followed until 1996, and deaths were recorded during the follow-up period.

The results in the Bygren study showed that subjects who rarely visited the cinema, concerts, museums, or art exhibitions compared with participants who visited such events most often had a significant excess mortality, with a relative risk of 1.57. This means that there was a 57% increase in risk of dying among those with no reported cultural activities compared to the others. These results were adjusted for age, gender, long-term disease, income, educational level, smoking, and physical exercise. The findings were met with considerable skepticism at the time, because the underlying biological mechanisms were unknown. This has changed during later years. In particular, there is accumulating evidence that cultural activities can stimulate brain development and regeneration in the body, as described later in this chapter.

One of the observations in the Bygren study that drew attention in subsequent discussions was that there was no observable survival effect related specifically to music making. In the discussion on this theme, it has been pointed out that the professional musicians constituting part of the music-making group may be at a disadvantage with regard to longevity and health due to drug and alcohol problems. Later a prospective study (Bellis et al. 2007) was performed on extraordinarily successful pop musicians ($n = 1064$, All Time Top 1000 albums) in the USA and in the United Kingdom. The survival of this cohort was compared to that of the general population, and it was shown that this group of musicians had an elevated mortality (relative risk 1.7) during the period three to 25 years after they achieved their fame. This is of course not immediately applicable to the general population, but it illustrates that extreme fame in music making could lead to health risks. It also illustrates that a cultural activity like music making could have dramatically different effects on health in different parts of the population (see also Kenny and Asher (2017) for a related study).

The Bygren et al. study of the Swedish population has been followed by similar studies in other countries. A large similar study was performed in Norway. There were 33,467 participants in a study of all inhabitants aged 20 years and above in part of the county area Nord Tröndelag (Løkken et al. 2018). This study was based upon a mailed questionnaire and there was a 50% participation rate. Participants were followed up with regard to mortality until the end of 2015. The participants made a self-rating of their general health using a standardized scale. After adjustments for education, marital status and long-lasting illness there were significant gender-specific findings. The hazard ratio of mortality among men who did not participate in music, singing and theater was significantly higher (HR = 1.40) than in men who participated in such activities. The hazard ratio decreased to 1.26 and became only borderline significant when the adjustments included participation in other leisure activities as well, the tentative conclusion being that participation in leisure activities in general may be the crucial variable.

For women there was no association between such cultural activities and subsequent mortality. On the other hand, among women there was a significant tendency to report poorer subjective health among nonparticipants in music, singing, and theater than among participants. This association became strongly attenuated and nonsignificant after adjustment for other creative activities, illustrating that the crucial variable may be creative activities in general.

A Finnish prospective study (Väänänen et al. 2009) comprised 7922 industrial employees. They completed in 1986 a questionnaire about engagement in cultural activities (arts and culture, activities in associations, societal action, reading literature, and studying). They were followed up for mortality rates until 2004. High engagement in cultural activities was independently associated with a reduced all-cause mortality after controlling for sociodemographic factors including age and sex, socioeconomic status, work stress and social characteristics as well as diabetes and hypertension. The hazard ratio was 0.71. High engagement was also associated with a reduced risk of cardiovascular mortality after adjustment for sociodemographic factors and stress.

Accordingly, in the Nordic countries during the early 1980s, several prospective studies were performed which examined the possible association between cultural participation and health in general, including mortality. The results showed that, statistically, high participation in cultural activities is associated with good health during follow-up. The findings could not be "explained away" by chronic disease, socioeconomic factors, or life style. However, first of all the largest study (the Norwegian) showed that there may be a gender difference with a stronger effect on mortality for men and a stronger effect on self-rated health for women. Second, it was difficult to establish more specific results indicating whether any form of cultural activity or other leisure activities is more important than other forms. Nor did these studies clarify whether active participation was more important than passive consumption of arts (making music versus listening, writing poetry versus reading, painting vs. viewing art, etc.,).

4.4 Population-Based Studies

Taking a step back, we might ask what strata of the general population are active participants in creative arts activities. A recent epidemiological study (Bone et al. 2021) based upon the General Social Survey (GSS), which is a survey of the general population in the USA (n = 8684 for arts events, 4372 for arts activities, 4268 for creative groups, and 2061 non-attendees), showed that more education, higher education in parents, and being female were factors consistently associated with higher participation in all types of arts activities. The authors noted that there was a difference between *attendance* at arts events and *active participation* in arts activities or creative groups. The difference between socioeconomic groups was evident for attendance but not for active participation.

Already in Bygren's first study and in all the subsequent Nordic population studies, the researchers were fully aware of the potential importance of socioeconomic gradients. Small financial resources are associated with poor health, and access to cultural activity is limited by being poor. These factors together could create spurious associations between participation in cultural activity and health, thus confounding them. Accordingly, the hazard ratios were adjusted for education or income (or both). In Bygren's study, it was observed that adjustment for income reduced the magnitude of the association between cultural participation and subsequent mortality. It was not nullified, however, so although participation in cultural activities is reduced by lack of financial resources, a statistical effect of cultural participation on health seems to remain. Similar observations were made in the other Nordic studies.

Although the socioeconomic differences in cultural participation have been observed in all countries where such studies have been performed, they are not completely stable. In a Swedish study (Theorell 2012), it was possible to study changing trends during the period 1976 to 2006 in a large survey of living conditions (ULF) in the Swedish general adult population. The study was performed with face-to-face interviews and a high participation rate between 70 and 80%. It was shown that attendance at theater performances and concerts was three times more likely among high- level white-collar workers in 1976 than among workers without secondary education. In 2006, this ratio had decreased to 1.5, indicating that it was then only 50% more common among high-level white collars than among blue collars with short education to attend theater performances. This is a dramatic change. Similar trends albeit not so strong were found for library visits and study groups. Visits in art museums were more common in the higher social strata throughout the whole study period, with no changes in trends. Accordingly, social patterns may change due to societal change but there are differences in such trends between different types of arts activities. It is of interest that the Swedish society had shown a strong development towards an increasing degree of social equality before and during the initial part of these 30 years.

In the Danish population study (Ekholm and Bonde 2018), more specific questions were examined regarding the possible relationships between musical activities and health. This was a cross-sectional study which had a participation rate of 57%—relatively high according to international standards at the time. Participants were 14,265 randomly selected Danes in ages from 16 and older. The authors separately analyzed musicians in four groups (active professionals, passive professionals, active amateur and passive amateurs). Many health outcomes were studied ranging from subjective health to diagnostic groups such as hypertension, asthma, and tinnitus. Among the objective diagnoses, tinnitus was the only one that deviated significantly in musicians in comparison to others—tinnitus was more common in musicians, particularly among professionals. Alcohol use was significantly more common among professional musicians but in contrast significantly *less* common among amateur musicians than in the general population. Cannabis use was reported more often among musicians, particularly among active professional ones, than in the general population. Interestingly, the professional active musicians described their subjective health as significantly better than other participants did, *despite also reporting more sleeping problems and more pain in neck and back than others.* These findings are particularly interesting because the distinction was made between groups who earn their living by making music and groups who make music for fun. Some of the results explain why music making in general may not be related to health in any simple way.

The authors of the Danish report also studied musicking (Ekholm et al. 2016)—a concept including all kinds of music making in everyday life, thus, for instance, singing in the shower, in the kitchen, and while soothing babies but also organized rehearsals in choirs and instrument groups. An important criterion was that musicking should have been performed during at least 1 h per day. Using subjective health as an outcome, the results indicated that both men and women who practiced musicking were more likely than others to report good self-rated health than other participants. There was, however, a gender difference: Only women were less likely than other women to report poor physical and mental health. In men, there was no such finding.

The Danish population study will continue and prospective results will thus be available in the future.

4.5 Twin Studies

When these epidemiological studies were published and the societal discussion regarding the role of experiences of arts was vitalized, a parallel development in physiology and brain research had been going on (see Theorell 2014). This is described in other parts of this book. It seemed more and more reasonable to assume that indeed frequent and continued participation in cultural activities could influence bodily functions of significance to health in a broad sense. But what about different arts? Is music more important than poetry? What about visual arts compared to dance? In the Norwegian study referred to above (Løkken et al. 2018) there was a hint that all creative activities may be important. It was assumed that one of the underlying themes in all of this would be how emotions are handled. In epidemiological studies based upon the Swedish Twin Registry the concept alexithymia was used (Theorell et al. 2019). Alexithymia means inability to handle emotions, and this has been shown to be associated with certain illnesses, mainly hypertension and alcohol abuse. Since experiences of art influence emotions, is logical to explore whether they have a beneficial effect on ability to handle emotions and accordingly reduce the prevalence of alexithymia. Alexithymia is assessed in population studies by means of a short questionnaire with questions about ability to differentiate emotions, ability to put words on them, and finally ability to communicate emotions to others. A high score indicates a poor ability to handle emotions and this correlates with poor ability to identify emotions visualized in faces that are shown on a screen.

At first, the association between amount of music practice in a life-long perspective on one hand and degree of alexithymia was studied. The Twin Registry was first used as a population study. This means that in all participating twin pairs one sibling is randomly excluded. After this procedure, in this study the 2000 men and 3700 women who had ever played or sung and reported number of hours practicing during different age periods were analyzed separately. There was a relatively low participation rate in the order of 30%. This means that it would be difficult to estimate population prevalence of different variables but since there was sufficient contrast within the study sample the analyses of associations were judged to be reliable. The total number of lifetime music practices was calculated from self-estimates in different age periods, and the subjects were divided into tertiles of music practice hours. All the analyses were adjusted for age. Indeed, there was a highly significant association between the amount of music practice and alexithymia in the expected direction, the more music practice, the lower the alexithymia score (Theorell et al. 2019). In addition, information was used regarding ensemble or no ensemble playing during the practice of music, and the presence of an ensemble during practice strengthened the association. Both in men and women, those in the low tertile of music practice and without ensemble playing had a higher (half a standard deviation) alexithymia score than those in the highest tertile with the addition of ensemble playing. A high educational level was correlated with a low alexithymia score whereas general intelligence was not correlated with alexithymia.

It was possible to analyze a possible genetic component of the association between number of music practice hours and alexithymia, using the full twin sample. This showed that the association between number of music practice hours and alexithymia was pleiotropic—which means that it could be explained by the genetic component in alexithymia overlapping with the genetic component in likelihood of practicing music. Such a finding does not mean that alexithymia could not be influenced by external factors. As with development of musical expertise, it is likely that there is an interaction between genetic and environmental variables. In the case of alexithymia, this will be discussed later.

It was also possible to use the population part in the twin study to examine different kinds of active creative arts experiences (writing, music, theater, dance, visual arts) in relation to alexithymia (Lennartsson et al. 2017). The explanatory variable in that study was "creative achievement," a scale with seven steps. The lowest step corresponds to no experience at all and step seven to professional activity resulting in mass media reviews. After adjustment for age, it was found both for men and women, that participants who reported no creative arts experience compared to those who defined themselves as experienced amateurs or professionals had higher scores (on average two points higher) for the different kinds of arts that showed significant differences. For dance, there was no significant difference and for theater there was significant difference only for women. Correspondingly, for visual arts there was significant difference only for men. When achievement scores from the different kinds of arts were added to one another for each individual, it became possible to examine the relationship between multiple arts practice experiences and alexithymia. Participants (both men and women, analyzed separately) in the lowest multiple creative achievement tertile had significantly higher alexithymia scores (5 points) than those in the highest tertile. Since professionals constitute a small part of the sample these comparisons mainly reflect differences between non-active and multi-active amateurs. The genetic components were not examined. Our previous study had shown a strong genetic component in the association between amount of music practice and ability to handle emotions and it could be assumed that genetics may be of importance not only for music but also for the other creative arts. However, the main conclusion from this study is that other creative activities, not only music, are associated with ability to handle emotions. Writing and music were those creative activities that showed the strongest negative associations with alexithymia scores. In addition, for theater and visual arts there seemed to be sex differences. For dance there were no significant differences between the achievement for the total alexithymia scores, but a more detailed analysis (Bojner Horwitz et al. 2015) showed that professional dancers had a better ability to communicate emotions than subjects without artistic dance experience.

The importance of alexithymia as a possible central variable in associations between arts experiences and health lies in the fact that arts may help the individual to interpret emotions. Subjects who are unable to differentiate, to translate emotions into words and to communicate emotions are handicapped in many stressful situations in life, particularly in a social context. Training ability to handle emotions by means of creative activities might thus have potential in improving the relationship between such activities and health in general.

The direct question—whether there is any relationship between alexithymia and depressive scores—was also explored in the twin study of alexithymia. Both in men and women (Theorell et al. 2014), there was a significant positive correlation in the order of 0.3 (same for men and women) between alexithymia and depressive symptoms—good ability to handle emotions thus correlated with a *higher* propensity to report depressive feelings. This finding is hard to interpret, first of all since it is based upon cross-sectional observations which do not allow conclusions regarding causality and second because a well-developed ability to handle emotions in a person increases the likelihood that this individual has a better ability to identify depressive feelings than others. It should finally be pointed out that depressive feelings should not be equated with illness.

In another study based upon the same music twin cohort (Wesseldijk et al. 2023), episodes of psychiatric disease were identified for each individual during their life from hospital registries (depression, anxiety, schizophrenia, bipolar disease, stress-related exhaustion). Music engagement and practice were not associated with risk of having registry-based diagnosis of depression, anxiety, and psychosis. In an analysis of "polygenic scores" for mental health problems, it was shown that a high polygenic score for bipolar disorder was associated with engagement, practice, and achievement in music, however.

Wesseldijk et al. (2019b) also examined psychological symptom reporting by means of co-twin analyses. They showed that the *increased* symptom reporting among participants who had been making music could be explained away by interacting genetic variables. This is again an example of genetic pleitropy, which means that music practice does not "cause" increased reporting of mental symptoms although it is associated with them. This is in line with my previous reasoning about music practice being associated with emotional competence which is itself related to a better-than-average ability to recognize mental symptoms. The authors concluded that mental health problems observed in musically active subjects are partly explained by preexisting genetic risk for depression and bipolar disorder.

These Swedish twin studies provided information of the relative importance of genes and environment in the development of musical expertise (Wesseldijk et al. 2019a). It was confirmed that musical enrichment in childhood is associated with musical achievement in adulthood but that genes are important, especially for the development of excellency. Thus, excellency arises in interplay between genetic factors and enrichment of music practice.

4.6 Flow

The music twin study identified an important potential intermediary variable, namely flow. The concept flow has been described as effort-less attention. When an individual experiences flow, he/she is doing something requiring effort (because it may be a difficult task and may have required considerable training), but it runs smoothly and gives rise to a joyful feeling. Physiologically it has been shown to be associated with sympathetic arousal (high heart rate), slow deep breathing and electrophysiological activity in laughing muscles (de Manzano et al. 2010). Flow experiences are important for musicians and other stage artists. In the twin project, a flow scale was developed. Correlations were computed between proneness to flow experiences on one hand and depressive and exhausted feelings on the other hand. The results (Mosing et al. 2018) showed that there were significant negative correlations between flow proneness and depressive feelings as well as between flow proneness and feelings of exhaustion. In other words, the more flow proneness the less depressive and exhaustive feelings. Interestingly, these associations were not fully explained by pleiotropy. There was a significant contribution both from genetic factors and from non-shared (factors not related to shared childhood) environmental conditions—approximately half-half. Since musical experiences may contribute to flow experiences this may reveal a truly environmental pathway from music practice to reduced prevalence of exhaustion and depression. This has to be tested in prospective studies, however. What may be particularly attractive in a model using flow experiences as a central intermediary variable is that this appeals to the artists themselves. When musicians describe what they consider important it seems that flow experiences in themselves and in their audiences play a decisive role.

Although the twin epidemiology research has shown that there is a strong genetic component in the association between amount of music practice and degree of alexithymia, there has been other research which indicates that extensive music practice may stimulate the growth of specific emotion-related areas in the brain. de Manzano and Ullén (2018) identified monozygotic twin pairs that were piano-discordant. This means that one of the siblings in such pairs had been playing the piano extensively from childhood to adult life, whereas the other one had not. There were nine such pairs that could be examined with magnetic resonance imaging of the brain. The importance of this study lies in the fact that the music-discordant monozygotic twin siblings have an identical genetic makeup, but they differ in music experience. If there are differences in the brain, these differences cannot be explained as genetic. The observations showed that the piano-playing twin had a statistically significantly higher volume of structures of relevance for motor functions of the right hand, for functions that coordinate finger movements, and for structures that connect hearing with emotional functions. Of particular importance was the observation that the anterior part of the corpus callosum was enlarged in the playing twins. The corpus callosum connects the right and left hemispheres of the brain, and is very important for emotional competence. Sperry (Nobel Prize winner 1981) observed that a missing corpus callosum results in an extreme lack of ability to handle emotions. The observation of the brains in music-discordant monozygotic twin pairs and the previous observation that there is an association between lack of music practice and alexithymia may be put together. Perhaps the association between music practice and emotional skill arises in an interplay between genetic liability and environmental music stimulation.

An additional perspective was used in the music twin study in Sweden (Theorell et al. 2015). The question was whether it was possible to identify predictors of continued playing or singing lasting until adult years. Only those who reported that they had ever played an instrument or had trained singing in addition to the regular school curriculum during school years participated. 3820 subjects (after random exclusion of one twin when both twins participated) had responded to questions regarding cultural childhood stimulation. Half of them continued during adult years. In multivariate analysis the following significant positive predictors were identified: Male gender (boys were less likely to start music practice during school years but more likely to continue if they did!), early start, exposure to music (music makers in the environment), and other kinds of culture (attendance at concerts and other cultural events) during childhood/adolescence and own choice of instrument (or singing). A separately analyzed factor that had a very strong predictive value was number of hours of music practice during the age period 12–17. There were also negative predictors, such as more than 100 music recordings at home during childhood. Special music schools increased the likelihood of continued playing.

Some of the predictors of continued playing are family factors and it is impossible to know whether they are genetic or environmental in nature. It is quite clear that some of them could be influenced by parents as role models and by parental decisions, such as early start and own choice of instrument as well as number of hours of practice. The main perspective in this study was not development of musical expertise but rather maintenance of a habit that is assumed to be health promoting. Development of musical expertise is discussed in other parts of this book.

In another study based upon the Swedish twin cohort, a phenotypic analysis (with random exclusion of co-twins) was performed of the relationship between objectively measured musicality and the likelihood of working in a creative occupation (Theorell et al. 2019). Separate analyses were made for men and women. "Creative occupation" was identified by means of an occupational matrix. Accordingly, it was not based upon the participant's own assessment of creativity of their job. After adjustment for a measure of general intelligence, age, and education, it was shown that men with a high score for pitch (ability to differentiate between high and low notes) were more likely to work in creative (nonmusician) occupations than other men. Similar correlations were found for women, but they were more confounded by general intelligence. Instead, a low score on alexithymia was a predictor of working in creative occupations in women. Regardless of causality, it is evident that musical aptitude among children could be a predictor of creative work in adult years.

In my presentation so far, twin studies have occupied an important position. It could be argued that the population of twins differs from people in general although this argument is mostly refuted in discussions about the relevance of twin research. In addition, estimates of heritability from twin studies should be seen as proxy measures. Discussions regarding possible over- and underestimation of genetic contribution in twin studies have been going on for many years (see for instance Hawkes 1997). Both over- and underestimation of the importance of genetic factors could occur in such studies. One other problem is that the participation rates in the detailed twin studies that I have described here are relatively low, around 30%. This means that studies of relationships between music experiences and health are likely to be meaningful as long as there are sufficient contrasts both in music experiences and in health, but that prevalence estimates may be unreliable. Accordingly, prevalences were not described.

4.7 Segments of the General Population

4.7.1 Working Population

It is popular in daily newspapers to speculate about the possibility of using art experiences in efforts to create a good working environment. The underlying hypothesis is that cultural experiences can stimulate creativity and cohesiveness which may in turn be health promoting (Theorell et al. 2013). A study based upon a cohort of working men and women in Sweden (SLOSH) followed every second year longitudinally and with successive addition of participants was used for a crude test of this hypothesis (Theorell and Nyberg 2019). When the study was designed, there was awareness of the possibility that relationships between creative cultural experiences organized through work and health might be bidirectional. On one hand, such experiences could benefit health, but on the other hand, participants with poor health might also withdraw from such activities in the work place. A statistical path modelling technique was used which allows for bidirectional application. The health variable was represented by a standardized score for depressive symptoms. The question about cultural participation was: Are cultural activities (movie, theater, concert, or art exhibition) arranged for the employees by your job organization? 0 = never, 1 = once per year, 2 = once per month, 3 = once per week or more). Figure 4.2 illustrates the results, based upon 9313 female and 7193 male 2-year follow-up periods. The path coefficients are relative linear regression coefficients between scores before and after follow-up which means that they correspond to standard deviation changes.

First, it is seen that both cultural activity and depression scores are relatively stable for both men and women—with beta coefficients indicating pre-post stability between 0.4 and 0.6. Second, there is a significantly negative association between cultural activity before start and change in depression score after 2 years with beta coefficients in the order of −0.02 for both men and women, indicating a protective role of "culture at work" against development of increased depressive feelings among employees. But there is also a significantly negative association of similar magnitude between depression score at start and change in cultural activity 2 years later. Thus, according to these results subjects with a high depression score are likely to avoid participation in cultural activities organized by the work organization. Both depression-preventive effects of culture at work and reduction of cultural activity *due to* depression may thus occur at the same time. The associations are small, but it should be born in mind that they are potentially important when translated to the general population of working men and women. Interestingly, they are slightly stronger for men than for women. A weakness in this study is that the explanatory variable, cultural activity through work, is a general one and it is impossible to disentangle specific contributions of different kinds of art. A previous similar study showed that ratings of leadership and psychosocial work environment variables co-varies with frequency of cultural activities organized by the work site (Theorell et al. 2013), although significant association remained after adjustments. Accordingly, these studies suggest that cultural activities in work-sites may have a role in preventing mental ill health among employees and that depressed employees may need extra intensive invitation to cultural activity at work—when they may need such activity the most.

4.7.2 Amateur Musicians and Singers

Although inferences to the general population regarding the importance of musical activities cannot be drawn from studies based upon separate music groups who are defined by uncontrollable selection effects, it is still interesting to study relationships between various aspects of the musical activity and health within such subgroups. One of the first studies of choir singers was performed in Great Britain by Clift et al. (2010). There were 600 choral singers who were asked by means of standardized questionnaires about physical, psychological, social, and environmental well-being. A 12-item questionnaire about well-being and choral singing. Qualitative data were also collected. Among the findings there were several sex

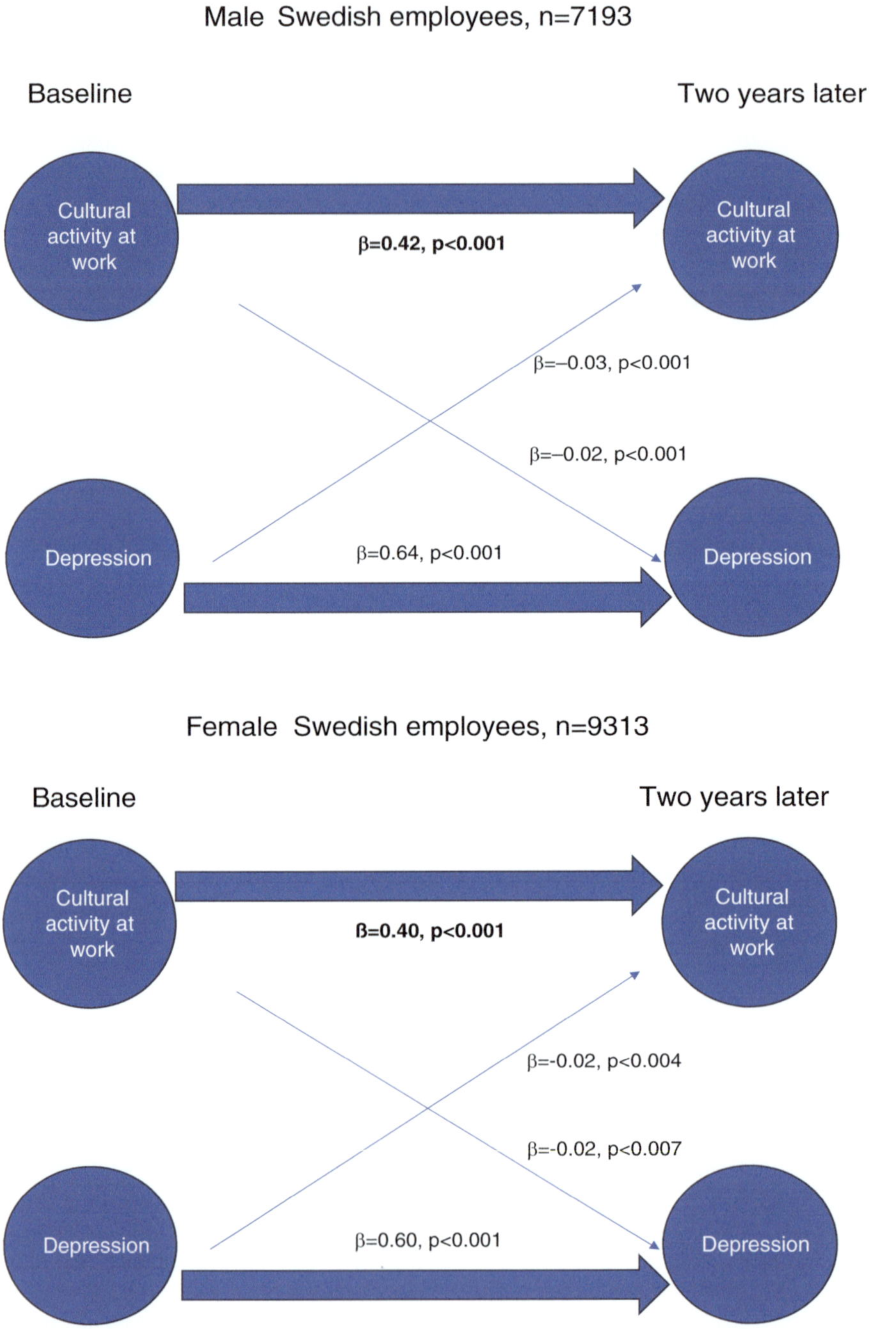

Fig. 4.2 (**a**, **b**) Weighted regression (*β*) for culture at work and depression, baseline and 2 years later. (**a**) Swedish male employees (n = 7.193); (**b**) Swedish female employees (n = 9.313). (Data from SLOSH-study Theorell and Nyberg 2019)

differences. Women seemed to endorse the well-being effects of singing more strongly than men. The social dimension in choir singing was prominent in the results of this study.

Questionnaire studies of choral singers have also been performed in other countries. A large study of 1000 choristers in Australia, England and Germany was published by Clift et al. (2009). The study was based upon one single question that was carefully formulated: What effects, if any, does singing in a choir have on your physical health? There was a wide spectrum of answers ranging from "no effects on physical health" to relaxation and stress relief, physical activity and energy, effects on breathing and lung function and finally on posture and body control.

These studies will be described more in detail in another chapter of this book. A recent questionnaire study of 5000 choir singers in Sweden and Norway was focusing on health related losses due to the lockdown of all choral activity in these countries as it appeared to the singer during the first half-year of the Covid-19 pandemic. Possible health related consequences were divided into effects broadly related to the artistic experiences (flow and aesthetic experiences), physical aspects (physical exercise as well as breathing and voice training), and finally social factors (social bonding as well as something to look forward to in the life routine). The question was: *Now, when you are not allowed to participate in choir singing, what is it that you miss the most? Rate your answer from 1(missing the least) to 5 (missing the most).*

It is impossible to know how representative the participants may have been for choir singers in general in this study. But the distribution of different genres among these participants is similar to the distribution of different genres of choir singers in Sweden and Norway. Some interesting observations were made. In general, the social component seemed to be the most crucial aspect for most singers. However, with increasing number of years as a choir singer and among professional choir singers there was an increasing emphasis on aesthetics, flow, and physical aspects whereas among starters with few years of experience the social aspect was particularly important. The social component seemed to be particularly important among gospel singers. As in the British study, women seemed to experience the loss of all the health aspects of choir singing as more important than did men.

The potential importance of using choir singing in communities for improved public health work has been described by Stige (2018) who introduced the concept musicking for public health. It is possible to utilize the social bonding in music activities for strengthening motivation for public health in a community.

4.7.3 Older Adults

There is considerable attention to the potential of experiences of art to improve the health of elderly. Two different studies have recently been published that are based upon the English Longitudinal Study of Ageing (ELSA). One of these studies (Tymoszuk et al. 2020a) was focused on the effect of art experiences on feelings of loneliness. At start in this study of randomly selected British men and women there has been a participation rate between 60 and 70%. Both cross-sectional and 10-year follow-up analyses were performed. In the cross-sectional analyses there was a statistically significant association between several kinds of art experiences (visits to cinema, museums/galleries/exhibitions, theater/concerts) and loneliness. In a cross-sectional analysis it is always difficult to know what is cause and what is effect, but the 10-year follow-up analysis also showed a significant finding, namely that after all adjustments (for instance, for socioeconomic factors) regular visits to museums had a significant protective effect whereas visits to theater/concerts did not. One interpretation of this could be that visits at museums may be more interactive with other people than the others. Frequency of visits was important: Those who responded that they made visits "every few months" had stronger effects than the others. The most reliable finding, the prospective result with adjustments, indicated an odds ratio of 0.68 for those who visited museums every few months of feeling lonely compared to the others. This corresponds to 30% reduction of loneliness. Since loneliness has been shown to be related to increased mortality and morbidity in high age this is a potentially interesting finding in the field of arts and health.

In the other study based upon the ELSA cohort the same starting point and the same participants were included as well as the same 10-year follow-up (Tymoszuk et al. 2020b). This study is of even more interest from a music and health perspective because of the findings. Information from the 2-year interval waves were used for calculation of intensity and frequency of participation throughout the follow-up period. The most intensive participation, "sustained," was equal to frequent reported visits "every few months" in at least four waves. The prospective findings were very clear for "visits to theater or concerts" after adjustments for socioeconomic factors with regard to positive affect, eudaimonic well-being (happiness) and self-realization. Such findings were not found with regard to cinema or museum visits. The observation is not clean-cut only in favor of music, however, since theater visits were included in the same group.

4.7.4 Ethnic Minorities

An interesting hypothesis based upon studies of ethnic subgroups in populations is that small minority groups with a strong historically founded social capital may have health advantages from this. The most extensive epidemiological studies are the ones published on the Swedish-speaking minority in East Bothnia. Studies have shown that this group has a better survival and better health in general than their Finnish- speaking neighbors. The studies also show that this difference cannot be statistically explained by differences in genetic makeup or in prevalence of widely accepted risk factors such as smoking, overweight or alcohol consumption patterns (Hyyppä and Mäki 2001). The authors have drawn the conclusion that the most likely explanation is the strong social capital in the Swedish-speaking group. The capital is linked to cultural activities. Among those, choir singing is prominent. It is hypothesized that not only the singers themselves but also listeners to the choirs during Swedish-speaking gatherings appreciate the choirs and feel strengthened in their cohesiveness with the whole group.

4.7.5 Young People and Self-Esteem

An aspect of life that is central to health in a general way is self-esteem which is often founded in childhood circumstances. The potential importance of arts activities in childhood for development of a good self-esteem was examined by Mak and Fancourt (2019) in a study of 6209 children participating in the United Kingdom Millenium Cohort study. Children´s arts engagement was specified into (1) listening to or playing music, (2) drawing, painting, or making things, and finally (3) reading for enjoyment. The association between such activities and self-esteem (Rosenberg self-esteem scale) at age 11 was examined. It was shown that all three kinds of engagement were associated, after adjustments for socioeconomic factors, with development of good self-esteem.

This study was cross-sectional and it would be interesting to see whether the results hold in a prospective analysis.

4.8 Conclusions

This review shows that a growing number of epidemiologists are interested in the associations between cultural activities and their relationship to health. I have emphasized that health is a multifaceted concept and that health outcomes associated with cultural activities could range from basic behavioral patterns such as ability/inability to handle emotions to intermediary variables related to health such as flow experiences that could be regarded as central in a healthy life. Of course, also morbidity, mortality and brain development should be and have been used as outcomes.

Many of the published studies do support the general idea that cultural activities may be beneficial for health, but research so far has reminded researchers that conventional health definitions (such as depressive states) are not easy to use in this kind of research. For instance, ability to recognize depressive feelings may indicate a healthy attitude to life. To recognize that genetic variables may influence both experience and practice of music is important. There seems to be gene-environment interaction. In general, the music-health associations that are found in large epidemiological studies are modest but still of considerable importance in a population perspective. In the first Swedish study, 24% of the participants had cultural experiences very infrequently. The excess risk of dying during the 10-year follow-up was 57% (Relative risk 1.57 after adjustments for health habits, age, sex, health, and socioeconomic factors). On the basis of these numbers it is possible to calculate the "attributable fraction" for death during the follow-up associated with nonparticipation (defined in this way) according to a formula (with prevalence of risk factor = p and relative risk of death = RR), attributable fraction = p*(RR-1)/[p*(RR−1) + 1].

This calculation tells us that theoretically 12% of deaths could be prevented by means of participation in cultural activities during the follow-up. There are many sources of error in such a calculation, and it should therefore be regarded as a rough approximation. However, it does provide an idea of the potential. It does not separate different kinds of mortality or different kinds of cultural activity. Nor does it take into account individual differences in vulnerability. Music does not seem to play a unique role. Research on other creative activities such as visual arts, theater and writing shows that these could also play an important role in population health work.

References

Bellis MA, Hennell T, Lushey C, Hughes K, Tocque K, Ashton JR (2007) Elvis to Eminem: quantifying the price of fame through early mortality of European and North American rock and pop stars. J Epidemiol Community Health 61(10):896–901. https://doi.org/10.1136/jech.2007.059915

Berkman LF, Kawachi I, Maria Glymour M (eds) (2014) Social Epidemiology. Oxford University Press, Oxford

Bojner Horwitz E, Lennartsson A-K, Theorell T, Ullén F (2015) Engagement in dance is associated with emotional competence in interplay with others. Front Psychol 6. https://doi.org/10.3389/fpsyg.2015.01096

Bone JK, Bu F, Fluharty ME, Paul E, Sonke JK, Fancourt D (2021) Who engages in the arts in the United States? A comparison of several types of engagement using data from the general social survey. BMC Public Health 21(1):1349. https://doi.org/10.1186/s12889-021-11263-0

Bygren LO, Konlaan BB, Johansson SE (1996) Attendance at cultural events, reading books or periodicals, and making music or singing in a choir as determinants for survival: Swedish interview survey of living conditions. BMJ 313(7072):1577–1580. https://doi.org/10.1136/bmj.313.7072.1577

Clift S, Hancox G, Morrison I, Hess B, Kreutz G, Stewart D, De S (2009) What do singers say about the effects of choral singing on physical health? Findings from a survey of choristers in Australia, England and Germany. In: 7th triennial conference of European Society for the Cognitive Sciences of music (ESCOM), pp 52–59

Clift S, Hancox G, Morrison I, Hess B, Kreutz G, Stewart D (2010) Choral singing and psychological wellbeing: quantitative and qualitative findings from English choirs in a cross-national survey. J Appl Arts Health 1(1):19–34. https://doi.org/10.1386/jaah.1.1.19/1

de Manzano Ö, Ullén F (2018) Same genes, different brains: neuroanatomical differences between monozygotic twins discordant for musical training. Cereb Cortex 28(1):387–394. https://doi.org/10.1093/cercor/bhx299

de Manzano Ö, Theorell T, Harmat L, Ullén F (2010) The psychophysiology of flow during piano playing. Emotion 10(3):301–311. https://doi.org/10.1037/a0018432

Ekholm O, Bonde LO (2018) Music and health in everyday life in Denmark: associations between the use of music and health-related outcomes in adult Danes. In: Music and public health. Springer, Cham, pp 15–31. https://doi.org/10.1007/978-3-319-76240-1_2

Ekholm O, Juel K, Bonde LO (2016) Associations between daily musicking and health: results from a nationwide survey in Denmark. Scand J Public Health 44(7):726–732. https://doi.org/10.1177/1403494816664252

Hawkes CH (1997) Twin studies in medicine—what do they tell us? QJM 90(5):311–321. https://doi.org/10.1093/qjmed/90.5.311

Hyyppä MT, Mäki J (2001) Why do Swedish-speaking Finns have longer active life? An area for social capital research. Health Promot Int 16(1):55–64. https://doi.org/10.1093/heapro/16.1.55

Kenny DT, Asher A (2017) Gender differences in mortality and morbidity patterns in popular musicians across the lifespan. Med Probl Perform Art 32(1):13–19. https://doi.org/10.21091/mppa.2017.1004

Lennartsson A-K, Horwitz EB, Theorell T, Ullén F (2017) Creative artistic achievement is related to lower levels of alexithymia. Creat Res J 29(1):29–36. https://doi.org/10.1080/10400419.2017.1263507

Løkken BI, Rangul V, Merom D, Ekholm O, Krokstad S, Sund ER (2018) Are playing instruments, singing or participating in theatre good for population health? Associations with self-rated health and all-cause mortality in the HUNT3 study (2006–2008), Norway. In: Bonde LO, Theorell T (eds) Music and public health. Springer, London, pp 33–54. https://doi.org/10.1007/978-3-319-76240-1_3

Mak HW, Fancourt D (2019) Arts engagement and self-esteem in children: results from a propensity score matching analysis. Ann N Y Acad Sci 1–10. https://doi.org/10.1111/nyas.14056

Mosing MA, Butkovic A, Ullén F (2018) Can flow experiences be protective of work-related depressive symptoms and burnout? A genetically informative approach. J Affect Disord 226:6–11. https://doi.org/10.1016/j.jad.2017.09.017

Nair PS, Raijas P, Ahvenainen M, Philips AK, Ukkola-Vuoti L, Järvelä I (2021) Music-listening regulates human microRNA expression. Epigenetics 16(5):554–566. https://doi.org/10.1080/15592294.2020.1809853

Podlipniak P (2021) The role of canalization and plasticity in the evolution of musical creativity. Front Neurosci 15. https://doi.org/10.3389/fnins.2021.607887

Rothmann KJ (2012) Epidemiology: an introduction. Oxford University Press, Oxford

Stige B (2018) Partnerships for health musicking: a case for connecting music therapy and public health practice. In: Bonde LO, Theorell T (eds) Music and public health. A Nordic perspective. Springer, Berlin, pp 115–128

Theorell T (2012) Kulturella aktiviteter, sociala förhållanden och folkhälsa [Cultural activities, social conditions and public health]. In: Rostila M, Toivanen S (eds) Den orättvisa hälsan [The unfair health]. Liber, Stockholm, pp 221–239

Theorell T (2014) Psychological health effects of musical experiences. Springer, Dordrecht. https://doi.org/10.1007/978-94-017-8920-2

Theorell T, Nyberg A (2019) Cultural activity at work: reciprocal associations with depressive symptoms in employees. Int Arch Occup Environ Health 92(8):1131–1137. https://doi.org/10.1007/s00420-019-01452-1

Theorell T, Osika W, Leineweber C, Magnusson Hanson LL, Bojner Horwitz E, Westerlund H (2013) Is cultural activity at work related to mental health in employees? Int Arch Occup Environ Health 86(3):281–288. https://doi.org/10.1007/s00420-012-0762-8

Theorell T, Lennartsson A-K, Mosing MA, Ullén F (2014) Musical activity and emotional competence—a twin study. Front Psychol 5. https://doi.org/10.3389/fpsyg.2014.00774

Theorell T, Lennartsson AK, Madison G, Mosing MA, Ullén F (2015) Predictors of continued playing or singing—from childhood and adolescence to adult years. Acta Paediatr Int J Paediatr. https://doi.org/10.1111/apa.12870

Theorell T, Madison G, Ullén F (2019) Associations between musical aptitude, alexithymia, and working in a creative occupation. Psychol Aesthet Creat Arts 13(1):49–57. https://doi.org/10.1037/aca0000158

Tymoszuk U, Perkins R, Fancourt D, Williamon A (2020a) Cross-sectional and longitudinal associations between receptive arts engagement and loneliness among older adults. Soc Psychiatry Psychiatr Epidemiol 55(7):891–900. https://doi.org/10.1007/s00127-019-01764-0

Tymoszuk U, Perkins R, Spiro N, Williamon A, Fancourt D (2020b) Longitudinal associations between short-term, repeated, and sustained arts engagement and well-being outcomes in older adults. J Gerontol B Psychol Sci Soc Sci 75(7):1609–1619. https://doi.org/10.1093/geronb/gbz085

Väänänen A, Murray M, Koskinen A, Vahtera J, Kouvonen A, Kivimäki M (2009) Engagement in cultural activities and cause-specific mortality: prospective cohort study. Prev Med 49(2–3):142–147. https://doi.org/10.1016/j.ypmed.2009.06.026

Wesseldijk LW, Mosing MA, Ullén F (2019a) Gene-environment interaction in expertise: the importance of childhood environment for musical achievement. Dev Psychol 55(7):1473–1479. https://doi.org/10.1037/dev0000726

Wesseldijk LW, Ullén F, Mosing MA (2019b) The effects of playing music on mental health outcomes. Sci Rep 9(1):12606. https://doi.org/10.1038/s41598-019-49099-9

Wesseldijk LW, Lu Y, Karlsson R, Ullén F, Mosing MA (2023) A comprehensive investigation into the genetic relationship between music engagement and mental health. Transl Psychiatry 13(1):15. https://doi.org/10.1038/s41398-023-02308-6

Music and Brain Plasticity

5

Lutz Jäncke

5.1 Why Musicians

The brains of musicians are special. The neural networks controlling music behavior and cognition have adapted to the specific demands of the unique and usually intensive practicing required to develop musical expertise. This adaptation leads to an increase in the processing efficiency of the neural networks involved in music-making and music-processing. These adaptations manifest themselves in distinctive anatomical and neurophysiological features.

5.2 Why Musicians?

One of the most interesting findings in the past 30 years from cognitive neuroscience is that the human brain is tremendously plastic. This phenomenon, called brain plasticity, neuroplasticity, or simply plasticity, has only come into focus with the use of modern methods to study the human brain noninvasively.

5.2.1 Functional Neuroplasticity

Functional neuroplasticity refers to changes in neurophysiological activity in neuronal cell assemblies due to experience and learning. These changes can occur locally as altered activity patterns in specific neuronal networks, and are often the result of an optimization process. Consequently, only those neurons that are used to control

L. Jäncke (✉)
Department of Psychology, Division Neuropsychology, University Zurich,
Zürich, Switzerland
e-mail: ljaencke@icloud.com

G. Kreutz, G. Bernatzky (eds.), *Music and Medicine*, Neurocultural Health and Wellbeing, https://doi.org/10.1007/978-3-662-72175-9_5

the trained function become active (principle of optimization). Furthermore, it is possible that the functional coupling to other neuron groups changes as a result of learning (principle of network modulation). This may result in certain cell assemblies working together efficiently due to training, or cell assemblies connecting to form a new cell assembly as a result of training or specific experience (principle of network construction and modulation).

5.2.2 Structural Neuroplasticity

Structural neuroplasticity refers to structural changes in the brain as a result of experience. These can be changes in gray and white matter, which may present as gray matter volume changes, increases, or decreases in cortical thickness, and cortex surface area. Changes in the anatomical connectivity pattern as a function of experience and learning have also been reported. The cellular basis of structural plasticity is still unclear. However, the following mechanisms have been discussed: Neuron enlargements (surface enlargement), an increase in dendritization and glial processes (enlargement of the neuropil), synaptogenesis, and an increase in capillarization.

Neuroplasticity has been discussed in several review articles in the past (Jäncke 2009a, b; Jerison 2000; May 2011; Pascual-Leone et al. 2005, Zatorre et al. 2012, Münte et al. 2002). Inevitably, neuroplasticity must also be considered in the context of genetic bases or frameworks. Influences from the "environment" and "genetics" always interact with each other. The general conditions for the brain's development and its ability to be influenced by experience are determined via genetic influences. Some brain areas (e.g., the primary motor and sensory areas) are likely to be less plastic than others, and the opportunity for plasticity is significantly greater in early childhood than in adulthood. Fundamentally, however, it has been shown that despite all genetic determinations, the adult brain is also remarkably plastic. Brain plasticity is probably also the basis for the enormous learning capacity of humans (Jäncke 2024).

How does one study neuroplasticity? Primarily, cross-sectional and longitudinal approaches are used. In the cross-sectional approach, individuals who are experts in a particular field are studied at a specific point of time. These experts are compared with nonexperts in terms of neurophysiological and neuroanatomical characteristics. The differences between these two groups are then attributed to expertise. This approach is relatively economical and quite plausible. Specifically, it is plausible because expertise research indicates that experts sometimes have to expend considerable effort to acquire the respective expertise. Ericsson, for example, has shown that excellent professional musicians have practiced for more than 10,000 h by the age of 20 (Ericsson et al. 1993; Ericsson 2004). In comparison, amateur musicians of the same age had expended a more modest 1500 training hours. When professional musicians invest a high amount of training effort, the involved neural networks should adapt and change accordingly. Musicians—and professional musicians in particular—are often studied as experimental groups because they start their music training very early and sometimes practice intensively until they are old. This high intensity of training makes them ideal subjects for the study of expertise-dependent neuroplasticity (Jäncke 2009a, b; Münte et al. 2002; Schlaug 2015).

In longitudinal approaches, subjects (experts and laypersons) are repeatedly studied over short or extended periods, with various interventions occurring during the study. By choosing appropriate control groups and control conditions, researchers can examine whether these interventions lead to anatomical and neurophysiological changes. This approach is quite costly because of the repeated measurement and the need to introduce appropriate control groups. Despite the expense, this approach is particularly useful for identifying causal influences of learning and experience. Cross-sectional studies in which biographical characteristics or learning characteristics are included in the analyses occupy a somewhat special position. Typical examples of these characteristics are the age of onset of music training or the frequency of music training. If such parameters are included in cross-sectional studies, causal relationships are more likely to be assumed (e.g., Amunts et al. 1997; Bengtsson et al. 2005).

In this chapter, I will mainly refer to findings from longitudinal studies and mention cross-sectional studies only briefly. Results from cross-sectional studies have been extensively discussed in various reviews. I will present some functional systems in more detail, specifically the auditory and sensorimotor, before discussing the basic principles of plasticity. In summary, cross-sectional studies comparing musicians with nonmusicians have uncovered the following basic findings (Herholz and Zatorre 2012; Jäncke 2008a, b, 2009a, b; Herholz and Zatorre 2012; Kraus and Chandrasekaran 2010; Münte et al. 2002; Schlaug 2015):

- In string players, the overall sensory representation (in Area 3) of the five fingers of the left, nondominant hand is larger than in nonmusicians. The strength of the neural response in the sensory cortex to tactile stimulation of the little finger of the left hand is particularly strong in string players. The strength of the neural response correlates with the age of onset of music training. The earlier the string players started to practice, the stronger the little finger's neural responses (Elbert et al. 1995). In this study, Magnetencephalography (MEG) was used as a neurophysiological measurement method. The strength of the neuronal response measured by MEG is generally taken as an indicator of the number of neurons responding synchronously.
- Neuroanatomically, several distinctive features stand out in musicians compared to nonmusicians. Anatomical landmarks in the hand motor area (particularly the depth of the central sulcus) are substantial and less asymmetrical. The horizontal length of the sulcus centralis correlates with the age of onset of music training (Amunts et al. 1997). The anterior part of the corpus callosum is particularly large in musicians who had begun music training before age 7 (Schlaug et al. 1995a). Many brain areas involved in the control of music-making demonstrate greater gray matter density. These include the primary motor cortex, Heschl's gyrus, parts of the cerebellum and premotor cortex, and the inferior temporal lobe (Gaser and Schlaug 2003; Schneider et al. 2002, 2005, 2006; Specht et al. 2002). The white matter system is different in musicians indicating a more effi-

cient information transfer within the brain. Particularly transcallosal connections between the auditory cortex of both hemisphere, tracts connecting the auditory cortex with one hemisphere to frontal and temporal areas are more efficient. The integrity of these anatomical connections correlate with the age of commencement of musical training (Leipold et al. 2021).

- Furthermore, musicians at rest show a more pronounced functional inter- and intrahemispheric connectivity than nonmusicians (Leipold et al. 2021), indicating that anatomical and functional connectivity is better overall in musicians. These connections are partly similar to those identified in anatomical studies. Hemodynamic fluctuations (indication neural activity) in the auditory cortex (Heschl's Gyrus and Planum temporale) correlate positively with the performance in musical perception and labeling tests.
- Aging amateur musicians exhibit significantly less neuroanatomical aging than nonmusicians and professional musicians. When biological age is estimated using neuroanatomical characteristics, amateur musicians' estimated biological age is considerably younger than their chronological age. Professional musicians seem to age somewhat faster concerning neuroanatomical characteristic values, which is speculatively associated with increased stress and pressure to perform (Rogenmoser et al. 2018).
- Absolute listeners demonstrate an excessive left>right volume asymmetry of the secondary auditory cortex (planum temporale) (Keenan et al. 2001; Luders et al. 2004; Schlaug et al. 1995b). Furthermore, the primary auditory cortex (Heschl's gyrus) in the right hemisphere is enlarged in absolute listeners and the volume of the right-sided Heschl's gyrus correlates with the quality of absolute hearing (Wengenroth et al. 2014; Leipold et al. 2021). The volume asymmetries in the auditory cortex are related to specific processing strategies for musical stimuli (Schneider et al. 2006). The network architecture in the perisylvian brain areas is fundamentally different in musicians and especially in absolute listeners compared to control subjects (Jäncke et al. 2012, Leipold et al. 2021). In addition, individual association fibers are also specifically distinct even in professional pianist differing in applied practice hours (Bengtsson et al. 2005). In particular, these include the arcuate fasciculus (Loui et al. 2011, 2012; Oechslin et al. 2009b), as well as the corticospinal tract (Imfeld et al. 2009). The anatomical connections from the planum temporale and auditory cortex to the frontal cortex are more pronounced in absolute listeners compared to non-absolute listeners (Brauchli et al. 2019; Burkhard et al. 2020; Wengenroth et al. 2014).
- The neural responses (measured with MEG and EEG) in the auditory cortex to tones are generally stronger in musicians than in nonmusicians. The strength of the neural response in the auditory cortex depends on the age of onset of music training. The earlier the musicians started music training, the stronger the neural responses in the auditory cortex (Baumann et al. 2008; Pantev et al. 1998, 2001). These neural responses are very specific in professional musicians. String players respond more strongly to violin tones than to trumpet tones, while trumpet players respond more strongly to trumpet tones (Pantev et al. 2001). This specialization of the auditory system can also be seen in conductors, who have signifi-

cantly improved auditory spatial perception, accompanied by characteristic auditory evoked potentials (Münte et al. 2001). In general, musicians process auditory information more efficiently (Kraus and Chandrasekaran 2010; Pantev and Herholz 2011).

- When musicians or music-trained individuals passively listen to music, they often show stronger functional connectivities than nonmusicians as evaluated by EEG activity measured on the cranial surface (Bhattacharya and Petsche 2001). However, in regard to intracortical sources, musicians reveal weaker functional connectivities, indicating more efficient processing of music stimuli (Brauchli et al. 2020).
- In early childhood, the auditory cortex adjusts to specific experiences with musical sounds. Children who intensively practice playing the violin at the age of 8–9 years react with stronger neuronal responses of the auditory cortex to violin tones than to sine tones after a certain training period. Quasi incidentally, they also seem to develop absolute hearing ability (Meyer et al. 2011).
- The way the auditory cortex processes phonemes is also altered in musicians. Even at the initial and early processing stages of the auditory processing chain, phonemes' presentation leads to different neurophysiological processing patterns than in nonmusicians (Kühnis et al. 2013a, b, 2014; Ott et al. 2011). Music expertise also affects visual processing of letters (Proverbio et al. 2013).
- Processing of syntax, prosody, and semantics is associated with altered neural activations in the inferior frontal gyrus, auditory cortex, superior temporal sulcus, and posterior part of the medial temporal gyrus in musicians (Koelsch et al. 2004; Oechslin et al. 2009a). Simultaneously, evoked potentials elicited by word and syntax stimuli are markedly different in individuals with music experience (Magne et al. 2006; Marie et al. 2011). In this context, a more efficient functional connectivity of ventral and dorsal information processing has been shown (Dittinger et al. 2018).
- When musicians perform motor activities, especially those that are similar to music-making activities, the motor system is often significantly less activated than in nonmusicians. In particular, premotor areas are significantly less involved in motor control in musicians (Jäncke et al. 2000; Meister et al. 2005). Even within the group of musicians, experience-related specializations have been identified. For example, brain activations typical for opera singers have been found in the basal ganglia, insula, and thalamus, but also in premotor brain areas (Kleber et al. 2010). Imagining singing or playing a musical instrument is also associated with brain activations typical for musicians (Kleber et al. 2007; Lotze et al. 2003). Overall, it can be concluded that musicians or those experienced in music can more efficiently combine and integrate sensory and spatial information to accomplish the complex spatiotemporal movement patterns involved in music-making (Ladda et al. 2020).
- Some studies have also found distinctive neurophysiological activation patterns in professional dancers when viewing and imagining dance movements. Some authors identified altered functional connectivities (Poikonen et al. 2018) or striking evoked potentials during these activities (Orlandi and Proverbio 2019).

Others observed mainly parietal alpha-band activity increases in the EEG of dancers compared to nondancers (Fink et al. 2009). Some anatomical peculiarities were found in ballet dancers compared to nondancers, which were related to the age of onset of ballet training. In particular, the premotor cortex, basal ganglia, and corpus callosum were specific (Hänggi et al. 2010).
- The functional coupling between the auditory cortex and the frontal premotor cortex is stronger in musicians than in nonmusicians (Bangert et al. 2006b; Baumann et al. 2007; Jäncke et al. 2012).

5.3 The Auditory System

Meanwhile, a wealth of papers have been published applying a longitudinal approach to study the influence of musical training on various functional systems. Since the amount is too large, it is impossible to summarize them in the context of this book chapter. In addition, these studies widely differ in terms of study length (from several minutes to decades), used methodology (MRI, fMRI, EEG, MEG, tMS, tDCS, and NIRS), applied tasks and measurement setting (resting states and task related measures), and examined different subject groups (children, adults). Thus, it is difficult to summarize them here. The reader is advised to have a look at a recent review trying to summarize most of these papers (Olszewska et al. 2021).

The auditory system is essential for musicians because music-making is about producing and understanding acoustic signals. In this respect, it is evident that the musician's auditory system works efficiently and precisely. According to current knowledge, these special skills are developed based on neuroanatomical and neurophysiological predispositions in interaction with musicians' specific experiences. Animal studies using electrophysiological single-cell recordings of neurons in the auditory system (mostly in monkeys, cats, and rodents) have demonstrated that the auditory system is strongly influenced by experience or learning. A commonly reported experience-dependent change in animal studies is the enlargement or reduction of "tonotopic maps" in the auditory cortex associated with tone discrimination tasks. These changes are task-specific and most robust when the trained auditory task is behaviorally relevant (Fritz et al. 2005; Ohl and Scheich 2005). Experience-induced activation changes in the auditory cortex are strongly influenced by existing reinforcers and reward mechanisms (Bakin and Weinberger 1996; Bao et al. 2001; Blake et al. 2006). Thus, it is clear that dopamine released in the reward system (nucleus accumbens, orbitofrontal cortex, and ventromedial prefrontal cortex) is important for reorganization in the auditory system. Further animal studies have shown that plastic changes are rapid and efficient during specific critical periods (de Villers-Sidani et al. 2007, 2008).

The human auditory system is probably much more plastic than the auditory systems of all animal species studied. The reason for the more remarkable plasticity is perhaps the special ability of humans to learn different languages that has developed in the course of evolution. In principle, humans can learn all the world's languages, which means that they can learn 6000 languages and 20,000 dialects.

Humans acquire understanding of the different speech sounds and the prosody to a large extent via the principle of "statistical learning"(Saffran et al. 1996, 1999). In statistical learning, the frequency of presentation and the presence of the material to be learned plays an essential role. The more frequently an event is processed in the auditory system's neural network, the better it is anchored there. It is irrelevant whether this event is processed consciously. Unconsciously processed information establishes itself in this way very efficiently and, above all, very early in development (Kuhl 2004). Via this learning principle, the foundations for understanding the mother tongue are already laid down in the young child at the age of 6–9 months. Understanding of and preference for musical stimuli are also likely laid down very early in the auditory system. Children recognize deviations from conventional musical rules, even if they have no particular musical aptitude (Koelsch et al. 2000). Furthermore, they seem to particularly like music that they have heard frequently (Soley and Hannon 2010). In this respect, unconscious statistical learning is essential for the auditory system and, above all, is effective at a very early age.

In this context, it is remarkable that these mostly implicit learning processes occur in the entire auditory system, i.e., not only the auditory core system, but also the primary and secondary auditory cortex. The extended auditory system includes the auditory pathway in the brainstem and frontal and parietal brain areas. In this respect, it is not surprising if these extended system parts are also affected by statistical learning (Koelsch et al. 2000; Tillmann et al. 2006; Wong et al. 2009).

Pantev et al. (1999) demonstrated that the human auditory system could adapt to changing acoustic stimulation conditions in as little as 3 h. They presented music to subjects through headphones, filtering out a specific frequency range from the music during the presentation. After this 3-h stimulation, they presented tones in the filtered-out frequency range and found that subjects' neural responses (as measured with evoked potentials) to these tones were greatly reduced.

In other work, subjects were instructed to actively discriminate tones or speech stimuli. In summary, these studies showed that discrimination performance improved significantly with this training and that neural responses to the trained auditory stimuli changed. In general, neural responses to the trained stimuli were stronger after training (Alain et al. 2007; Bosnyak et al. 2004; Gaab et al. 2003; Jäncke et al. 2001; Menning et al. 2000; Schulte et al. 2002). This stronger response is generally associated with optimized neural processing. It is likely that after training, more of those neurons that are useful for auditory processing stimuli are involved in processing, while neurons that do not contribute to processing are eliminated from the neural network. This could lead to more neurons firing synchronously and in phase.

The work presented above has shown that experiential influences at the cortical level are possible. However, recent work demonstrates that experience-related changes also occur within the auditory pathway in the brainstem. For instance, a French research group (Carcagno and Plack 2011a, b) demonstrated that in the course of intensive pitch discrimination training, the "frequency-following response" changed significantly. Brainstem mechanisms drive this neural response.

It is thus well-established that auditory training affects activity in the auditory system.

Whether formal music training elicits similar auditory system effects has been investigated, using longitudinal studies. However, these studies are relatively rare. One reason for the dearth of such studies is that longitudinal studies are lengthy and not easy to handle. However, the few studies that use this methodological approach provide evidence for the auditory system's plasticity in the context of music stimulation. Fujioka et al. (2006) studied 4- to 6-year-old children for 1 year of music training in a Suzuki music school. In these schools, children practice frequently and intensively, focusing on the implicit learning of music-making. The authors demonstrated that children from Suzuki music schools showed altered amplitudes and latencies of auditory evoked potentials to tones and sounds after 1 year of music training compared to control children who did not receive formal and hands-on music instruction. Shahin and colleagues (Shahin et al. 2008) further demonstrated that gamma-band energy increased after tone presentation due to music instruction. The gamma band (30–120 Hz) is considered a frequency band of the EEG and MEG signal that occurs particularly when feature binding and/or conscious awareness occurs.

Four other longitudinal neurophysiological studies have been published in recent years reporting studies with children who engaged in formal music training over an extended period. The most comprehensive study was conducted by the Finnish research group led by Mari Tervaniemi (Putkinen et al. 2014a, b, 2019). All three studies examined changes in the mismatch negativity (MMN) to sounds throughout 5 years using a relatively large sample of children. They found that the MMN and the P300 amplitude developed more with age in children who participated in formal music instruction. These changes were taken as evidence that music instruction optimizes the neurophysiological processing of acoustic stimuli. These findings are particularly interesting because the MMN is a component of the evoked potential that is independent of attention and other top-down cognitive processes. A similar but equally important finding has been reported by Chobert and colleagues (2014). In this 2-year longitudinal study, the authors presented syllables and vowels as auditory stimuli. Only the group with music training was found to have larger MMN amplitudes, especially in response to the hard-to-discriminate acoustic stimuli. An extensive longitudinal study by Habibi and Damasio, which is still ongoing, also demonstrates neurophysiological activity changes associated with formal music training (Habibi et al. 2016).

These findings correspond with a previously mentioned paper (Meyer et al. 2011) in which EEG mismatch negativity (MMN) was registered to sine tones and violin tones. The MMN is an evoked potential that signals pre-attentive auditory processing. This MMN is more pronounced in Suzuki-taught children when they hear the sounds of the instrument they use (in this particular case, violin tones). No difference in MMN is exhibited when these children are presented with sine tones, which have not been particularly practiced, compared to the control group. It is also interesting to note that the frequency of practice in the Suzuki music school correlates with performance on tests of absolute pitch. The more frequently the children had practiced in the Suzuki school, the better their absolute hearing test performance.

Overall, these longitudinal studies provide evidence for the auditory system's plasticity and confirm the particular features of the auditory system of individuals with music expertise that have been repeatedly reported in cross-sectional studies. The expertise acquired longitudinally leads not only to neurophysiological but also to macroanatomical changes. This was demonstrated by a Boston research group led by Gottfried Schlaug in a longitudinal anatomical study of 8- to 9-year-old children (Hyde et al. 2009). Two groups of children were studied: one group underwent normal music training with 1 h of music lessons per week (piano lessons) and usual training at home. The other group consisted of children from the same social class who did not receive piano training. Before and after the one-year piano training, the authors measured the children's brain anatomy and found that specific brain areas showed marked changes in gray matter density in the children who underwent the piano training. These were brain areas typically involved in the control of music-making. Children with piano lessons also showed marked increases in gray matter density in the right auditory cortex.

The research group led by Assal Habibi and Antonio Damasio is currently working on a longitudinal project. They are studying a group of children aged 5–8 years over a 5-year period and collecting a range of neuroanatomical, neurophysiological, and psychometric data. Their study uses an experimental design with three groups, one group receiving regular music training and another group receiving regular sports training. A third group is a passive control group. The researchers evaluated whether any differences in the measured variables existed at the start of the study, so as to better relate possible changes to the music training. Although the longitudinal project has not yet been completed, interim results already exist. After 2 years, children with music training show changes in cortical thickness in brain areas involved in processing auditory information (e.g., the posterior superior temporal gyrus with the planum temporale). Furthermore, particular characteristics of the corpus callosum's integrity (increased fractional anisotropy: FA) were also revealed, indicating that the corpus callosum is more efficiently primed for interhemispheric exchange (Habibi et al. 2018). A subsequent paper, published by the same group working only with the music training group and one control group reports the results obtained over a period of 4 years (Habibi et al. 2020). The authors identified that the cortical thickness of the secondary auditory cortex (the posterior part of the superior temporal gyrus) changes differently in children receiving musical training im placating a specific influence of music practice on the maturation of the auditory cortex.

A recently published paper from an Austrian research group presented data from a 12-years lasting longitudinal study including more than 100 subjects (Schneider et al. 2023). In this study, the authors obtained structural and functional data of the auditory system from kids being in primary school until they reached adolescence. They identified that those subjects with musical training experience demonstrated larger volumes of the Heschl's gyrus and planum temporale than found in nonmusicians even in the beginning of the study implying a trait-like structural difference maybe favoring this group for music learning. During the course of the 10–12 years, the auditory cortex value increases in musicians as well as in nonmusicians, while the slope of volume increase did not differ between both groups. However, the authors identified strong differences between both groups in terms of auditory performances. These differences even increase favoring the musicians during the course of the study.

Overall, this work demonstrates that the auditory system is significantly affected by music-specific training in children. However, it is possible that a genetically driven influence might affect the auditory system, both anatomically and neurophysiologically favoring specific subjects for music performance.

If auditory information is coupled with motor commands during practice, such as when learning to play the piano, the training succeeds comparatively better than auditory practice only, when actions are not coupled to the motor system (Lappe et al. 2008). A fundamental principle of learning emerges here. Information is best stored when it is coupled with other information, preferably multimodally. In addition to audio-motor coupling, there is robust audio-visual coupling, which also can be further extended by training and which can be demonstrated by means of the mismatch negativity responses (Paraskevopoulos et al. 2012a, b, c). Bangert and Altenmüller (2003) examined audio-motor coupling in learning to play the piano and found that this coupling also establishes itself neurophysiologically after only a few training sessions, as determined on the basis of EEG coherence patterns (Bangert and Altenmüller 2003).

Finally, musicians recognize auditory irregularities in tone sequences quite quickly, even when they are not familiar with the sequences (Herholz et al. 2009). Musicians also can learn rules of tone sequences faster than nonmusicians (Herholz et al. 2011).

5.4 The Sensorimotor System

Neurophysiological and neuroanatomical changes in the motor system due to practice have been demonstrated in many studies using a wide variety of methods in animals and humans. In humans, it has been shown that different parts of the motor system adapt depending on the intensity of practice and the task practiced. Longitudinal studies show an increase in excitation in the primary motor cortex (M1) during the first days of motor training, decreasing with continued training. New neurons or groups of neurons likely become involved in motor control as training progresses, with optimization then occurring. Only those groups of neurons that are optimally suited for control are retained. This activation pattern in the primary motor cortex during motor training is well documented in nonmusicians (Koeneke et al. 2006; Pascual-Leone et al. 1995). Initial studies in individuals learning to play the piano have yielded a similar finding (D'Ausilio et al. 2006). The long-term neuroanatomical consequences of piano playing were also demonstrated in the aforementioned study by Hyde and colleagues, who demonstrated an increase in gray matter density in the motor cortex and premotor cortex only in children who received piano lessons.

Perhaps more interesting are the findings concerning long-term exercise for the sensorimotor system, because the motor system virtually never acts without being connected to the sensory system. Therefore, some scientists speak of a sensorimotor system to express that motor and sensory systems are closely intertwined. Practicing an instrument is a specific form of sensorimotor training. When learning to play the piano, sensory signals (visual or auditory) must be coupled with motor commands. Thus, the musician must have an auditory goal (implicit or explicit) to achieve with his motor skills. If the musician plays at sight, the musician must be able to translate the visual cues into motor commands.

Tight audio-motor couplings have been described multiple times in musicians. For example, Baumann and colleagues showed that the auditory cortex is active in pianists even when they are playing the piano without hearing themselves play (Baumann et al. 2007). Using new mathematical methods, it is possible to calculate whether neural activity in the auditory cortex influences activity in the premotor cortex. To this end, Jäncke et al. (2012) estimated intracerebral activity in the auditory cortex and premotor cortex in pianists during piano playing and calculated whether activity in the premotor cortex can be predicted from activity in the auditory cortex. Indeed, it was shown that activity in the premotor cortex could be predicted based on the time course of neurophysiological activity in the auditory cortex.

These tight audio-motor couplings do not necessarily require decades of training (Bangert et al. 2006a). They can be "built-up" even in music laymen within 20 min of exercise and stabilize after about 5 weeks of further training. In another study, pianists demonstrated increased motor cortex excitability after piano practice when they heard the piece of music they had practiced. When they were presented with a flute piece that they could not play, there was no change in motor cortex excitability (D'Ausilio et al. 2006).

These audio-motor couplings are probably "just" a special case of multimodal cross-modal couplings common in the human brain. Much, if not all, sensory, motor, and cognitive information can be coupled or, in the language of systems theory, correlated. Depending upon which simultaneously activated networks strengthen their connections or couplings, these couplings are probably established via a Hebb mechanism. Here, the coupling strength depends on the frequency of simultaneous activations. Making music requires several multimodal couplings, including audio-motor couplings as well as tactile-motor and tactile-auditory couplings. However, couplings between auditory and cognitive information (audio-cognitive) also are common in musicians, such as when musical pieces evoke particular memories.

Few extensive and well-controlled longitudinal studies with children who received music instruction have been published. One, already briefly discussed, is the Boston research group's work above (Hyde et al. 2009). In this work, children showed increases in gray matter density in the motor cortex and cerebellum after 1 year of music training. The authors attributed these anatomical changes to the music-making practiced in music classes. However, only a passive control group was used in this study. That is, this group did not practice in addition to regular school lessons over the year. A study by Hudziak et al. (2014), published 5 years later, used a quasi-experimental longitudinal design and analyzed data from a relatively large sample of 232 children and adolescents aged 6–18. These participants were intensively studied neuroanatomically and psychometrically on three occasions over 2 years. Statistical analyses revealed that the children with music instruction had faster maturation of cortical thickness in those brain areas involved in the control of motor planning and coordination (M1, PMC, SMA, and parietal lobes).

5.5 Transfer

In cognitive psychology, learning transfer occurs when training or learning in one functional area influences an individual's performance in another untrained functional area. Positive transfer occurs when these influences are favorable and benefit the performance of the untrained function. Conversely, negative transfer occurs when training in the practiced function unfavorably influences the performance of the untrained function. The similarity of the trained and untrained functions determines whether there is near transfer or far transfer.

In general, the more similar the functions, the closer the transfer of learning between them. Transfer effects of music education or training have been reported primarily for near transfer. We have described typical examples involving auditory and sensorimotor systems in previous chapters. Whether music training affords far transfer effects on higher-level cognitive functions (e.g., general intelligence, memory, attention, executive functions, emotions, social behavior, etc.) is currently the subject of intensive research and controversy. A recent meta-analysis concluded that music education would not elicit beneficial far transfer effects (Sala and Gobet 2020). The authors argued that most research conducted to date did not use randomized control group experiments, in which subjects were randomly assigned to experimental and control groups and then studied longitudinally.

Glenn Schellenberg (2004), however, did employ such a study design in his now-famous paper. He randomly assigned 144 children from the same socioeconomic class to one of four experimental groups, three of which were offered different supplementary lessons (piano lessons, singing lessons, acting lessons, or no additional intervention) for 1 year in addition to their regular schooling. With this study, Schellenberg demonstrated that children receiving supplementary music lessons showed a slight increase in IQ after 1 year. It is possible that Schellenberg succeeded in this random assignment, but in principle, it is hard to imagine that both children and adults would accept a random assignment to a particular intervention that does not suit them—especially when the intervention occurs over such a long period. One might imagine eagerly wishing to learn to play an instrument but being prevented from taking music lessons for a year due to an artificial experimental design. One would probably follow the forcibly imposed intervention without motivation. In this respect, we must assume that such experiments are nearly impossible to conduct in real school and education settings and are associated with high subject dropout rates (see also Tervaniemi et al. 2018 for a review). Other experimental designs and statistical evaluation techniques are therefore necessary for such intervention studies.

Despite these experimental challenges, several longitudinal studies have been published in recent years investigating the impact of formal music training on various psychological aspects (Ilari 2020). Although perfect experimental designs cannot be realized in these studies for the reasons mentioned above, more and more findings support the notion that music education and training can exert beneficial effects on higher-level psychological functions.

In particular, it is likely that transfer effects from music training to language skills are observed due to musicians'special expertise in auditory functions. Since they are particularly well trained to perceive, distinguish, and remember tones, tone sequences, and melodies, their auditory systems are especially "trained" and prepared in this regard (Fig. 5.1). In this respect, those with music training also find it easy to learn and discriminate speech stimuli and to sort them into new contexts (Jäncke 2012a). Musicians also learn new language stimuli somewhat faster than others (Kühnis et al. 2013a, b; Elmer et al. 2014; Dittinger et al. 2016, 2018, 2019),

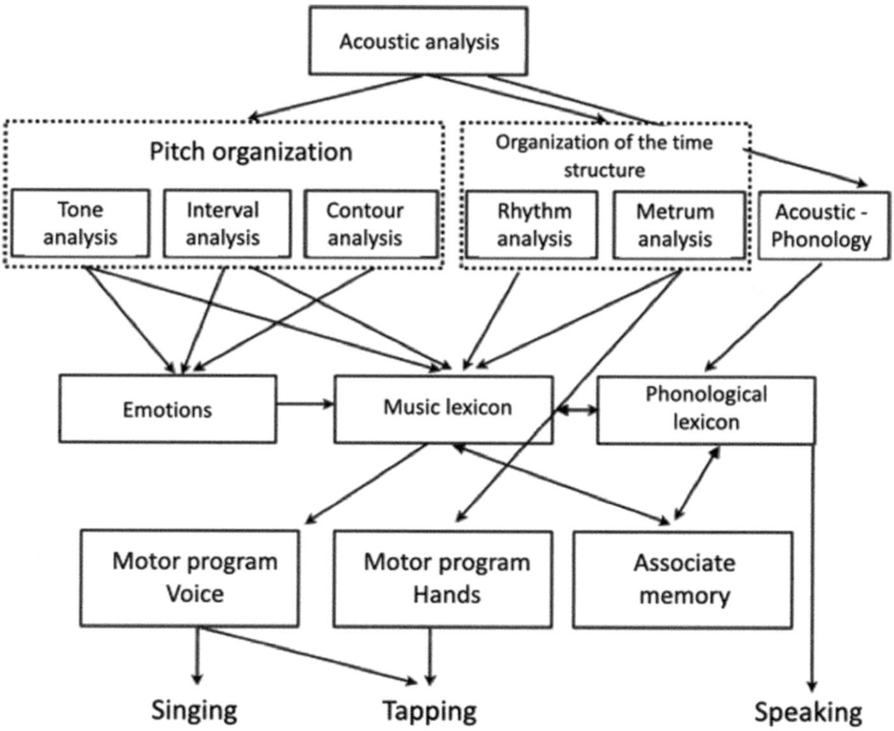

Fig. 5.1 Schematic representation of the auditory analysis processes associated with both music and speech processing (after Jäncke 2008a, b). As seen here, acoustic analysis is also linked to higher-level functions (such as emotions, music lexicon, phonological lexicon, motor programs, and associative memory). These relationships are not fixed from birth but are acquired and stabilized during learning

which may also be why musicians seem to have less trouble acquiring foreign languages (Slevc and Miyake 2006). Favorable effects on reading and speech perception have also been brought to light (Moreno and Besson 2006; Moreno et al. 2009; Carpentier et al. 2016).

In addition to overlaps between speech and music perception for elementary auditory perceptual processes, remarkable similarities also exist between speech and music syntax. Both systems are controlled by overlapping brain structures and functional modules (Koelsch et al. 2000). Music can also convey meaning (semantics) and address semantic networks, albeit not as precisely as language. Thus, it can "pre-activate" information retrieval in the addressed network, so that this information can be preferentially accessed (Koelsch et al. 2004). An interesting and relatively new concept is the consideration that typical English and French music use certain peculiarities of the respective languages (Patel and Iversen 2007). This can be recognized by the sequential order of music intervals and the sequence of important stress-bearing elements of the respective languages. Typically, French-sounding music is characterized by less variability of successive intervals and smaller semitone steps. The French language is also characterized by lower vowel duration variability. Whether such correlations can be found for languages other than French and English remains an avenue for further research. Finally, it should be noted that connections between music and reading skills have recently been addressed. In particular, phonological awareness is associated with music skills (tone, sound, rhythm, and melody perception) (Dege and Schwarzer 2011).

Music training also appears to have a beneficial effect on executive functions, as evidenced by the results of several cross-sectional and longitudinal studies. In the cross-sectional studies, musicians (or musically trained individuals) were compared to nonmusicians. In the research published to date, musicians often performed better on executive function tests than control subjects (Moreno et al. 2014; Moussard et al. 2016). Also, some longitudinal studies found that music training exerts a beneficial effect on executive functions, particularly on inhibition of irrelevant actions (Moreno et al. 2011; Janus et al. 2016; Hennessy et al. 2019). Of particular note is Hennessy and colleagues' 3-year longitudinal study, in which children with music training exhibited better performance on the Flanker task, which required them to inhibit inappropriate actions. Similarly, they demonstrated superior ability in terms of delayed gratification relative to children in the control group. Hemodynamic responses during the performance of these tasks, as measured by MRI, revealed stronger bilateral responses in brain areas involved in controlling executive functions in the children with music training (Hennessy et al. 2019). It is hypothesized that music training reorganizes neural networks to more efficiently control these executive functions.

Finally, it is important to mention that music-trained individuals perform better in various memory (Jäncke 2008a, b, 2018). These better memory performances are probably also related to the somewhat more efficiently operating executive functions, which support encoding and retrieval. However, specific abilities in auditory and visual perception may also have a beneficial effect on memory performance (for a more detailed discussion see Jäncke 2018).

Due to the close proximity of language and music functions, attempts are currently being made to use music or music-specific interventions for the therapy of Broca's aphasia (Schlaug et al. 2010) and autism (Wan and Schlaug 2010; Wan et al. 2011). Whereas choral speaking and singing in stutterers results in only temporary success, Melodic Intonation Therapy has yielded interesting and promising findings in those with Broca's aphasia. For dyslexia patients, elementary music skills training offers an interesting alternative or supplemental therapy to improve basic skills regarding phonological awareness.

One important psychological variables has not been mentioned so far, which is entirely neglected particularly in neuroscience research and that is "self-efficacy." Kreutz and his colleagues (2023) describe this personality trait as the belief in one's perceived capabilities for learning and performing actions at designated levels. This is a fundamental psychological attitude fostering motivation and learning, and is thus the basis for academic success. Music and also sports and book promote this important attitude, while modern variants of computer gaming not.

Nevertheless, as Glenn Schellenberg correctly stated, we have to be careful and reluctant not to overemphasize the above-mentioned findings (Schellenberg 2015). Most of these studies are correlative in nature and do not control essential variables, which might also have substantial influences on transfer effects. However, it is difficult if not even impossible to design and conduct the perfect longitudinal experiment with a kind of music intervention. For this, it would be necessary to allocate a set of subjects randomly to different groups, while one group would be the music intervention group. In real life, the subjects will somehow react to the group allocation. Some will like them others not, which in turn will evoke specific psychological reactions associated with underlying changes in neurophysiological underpinnings. Thus, we have to live with the applied approaches and do our best to interpret the findings conservatively and to the best of our scientific knowledge.

5.6 Theoretical Foundations of Neuronal Plasticity

Currently, the neuroanatomical and neurophysiological features of the musicians' brains presented in the preceding sections are understood to be the consequence of gene-environmental interactions (see also Schellenberg 2015; Swaminathan and Schellenberg 2018). Although the detailed biological and cellular processes driving experiential changes in brain structures involved in music-making are not yet fully understood, the fundamental mechanisms can be described using ideas from systems theory.

All information is stored in neural networks (neural assemblies), comprised of a few neurons or many. It is conceivable that various smaller neural networks are interconnected to form larger ones (Jäncke 2024). The networks consist of neurons that are connected via synaptic contacts. For the storage of information, the number of synaptic contacts is of particular importance. The more synaptic connections in a neural network, the more information can be stored in that network.

Suppose a network consists of four input neurons and four output neurons. If each input neuron were connected to one output neuron, this would result in 16 connections (4 × 4 = 16, see Fig. 5.2). If there were eight input neurons and eight output neurons, one would analogously arrive at 64 connections. With each linear increase in the number of neurons in the network, the number of possible synaptic contacts increases exponentially. Fig. 5.3 shows a hypothetical network with 16 × 16 neurons. Using the same connection logic as for the previous network results in 256 synaptic contacts. Large neural networks with many neurons and many synaptic connections therefore allow the storage of a lot of information.

How the respective network and the synaptic contacts within the network are established depends on the learning history. The Hebb mechanism, originally proposed by Canadian neuropsychologist Donald Hebb in 1949 and now recognized as a fundamental neurophysiological learning principle, is important in learning and establishing synaptic connections. According to this learning principle, connections between two neurons strengthen when both neurons are simultaneously active (Fig. 5.4). The more often this occurs, the stronger the connections between these neurons will be. Depending on which neurons are involved and how frequently they are simultaneously engaged, certain connection patterns are established within the network. Each piece of stored information is associated with a specific pattern of connection strengths or synaptic connection strengths. These connection patterns form the anatomical basis for neurophysiological activity within the network. Neuronal plasticity consequently plays out at these synaptic connections.

For example, when a pianist practices his motor skills to play complicated scores, he needs many specific, well-defined motor programs. In this respect, large neural networks in the motor system are advantageous, because they allow more efficient storage of these programs than would small neural networks. In this respect, practicing and training stimulates the motor system to create more synaptic connections.

Musical exercise stimulates different neurophysiological mechanisms in the following ways: (1) The surface areas of the neurons involved may be increased so that

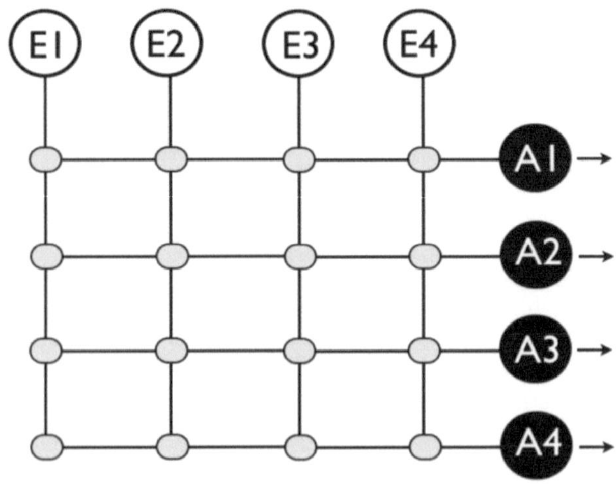

Fig. 5.2 Example of a neural network with four input neurons (E1 ... E4) and four output neurons (A1 ... A4). The small gray circles represent the connections (synaptic contacts) between the neurons. In this network, each neuron is assumed to be connected to all other neurons. Therefore, in a 4 × 4 network, there are 16 synaptic contacts

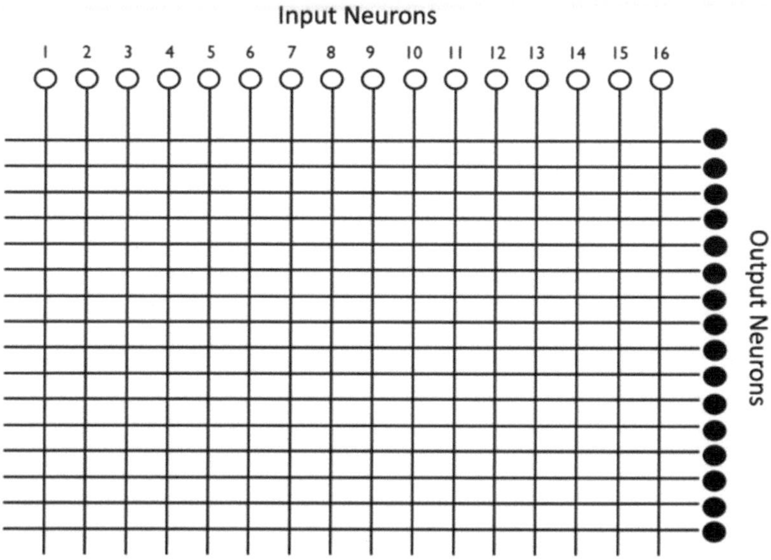

Fig. 5.3 The schematic representation of a 16 × 16 network follows the same logic as the 4 × 4 network. With 16 × 16 neurons, there are 256 synaptic contacts

Fig. 5.4 Schematic representation of Hebb's learning model

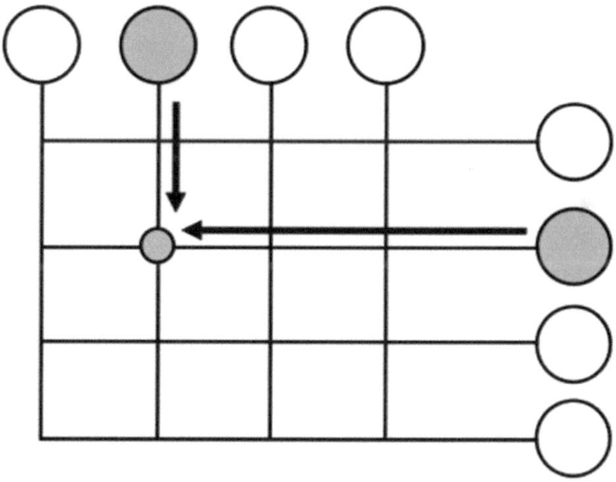

a larger area is available for synaptic contacts. (2) In this context, more receptors can also be established on the larger surface area, providing more unfolding opportunities for transmitters to cross into the synaptic cleft. (3) More synaptic contacts may also be established, as more receptors and vesicles have a greater opportunity to travel into the synaptic cleft; both pre- and postsynaptic neurons contribute to the increased synaptic area. (4) The formation, storage, and transport of neurotransmitters may also be enhanced; these changes may lead to volume increases in the brain areas involved. (5) Finally, the anatomical connections between brain areas can also be modulated. This can be accomplished by altering myelination or by forming new contacts at other neurons or networks so that overall, the network becomes more extensive and thus more differentiated.

In addition to the network architecture-associated anatomical changes, neurophysiological activation changes may also occur. These are manifested by:

- Stronger focal activities (e.g., larger N1 amplitudes of the evoked potential to tones)
- Reduced activities in secondary areas during simpler tasks
- More distributed activities within larger networks, usually in more complex expertise tasks

Stronger focal activations in the primary auditory and motor cortices during relatively simple auditory and motor tasks are typical for neurophysiological activity optimization. Here, fewer neurons are involved in neurophysiological control, although they "fire" more synchronously. Consequently, only very specific neurons (namely the important ones) would fire simultaneously during the required control processes. Due to intensive learning in musically trained individuals, strong synaptic contacts with little interference are established, so that only a few neurons need to be activated to retrieve the desired information. In an untrained person, on the other hand, the synaptic connections would be less strongly formed. As a consequence, information retrieval would not always lead to the same result, and more interference could exert its influence. Overall, this would lead to variable synchronicity in joint neuronal firing. Ultimately, the focal neurophysiological activations, which can be measured by evoked potentials, would be weaker.

For relatively simple tasks, secondary brain areas are less active in skilled musicians. This may be related to the fact that sufficient algorithms are stored in the primary areas for the expertise-related tasks. Therefore, musicians need not use secondary brain areas for relatively simple expertise-related activities. However, for control of more complex activities, secondary brain areas and/or other networks not previously used for the expertise-related activity must be made available. For this purpose, the network is enlarged through integration with other networks. For example, in musicians, temporo-parietal regions are involved in tone perception because these brain areas are essential for tone memory (Gaab et al. 2003).

Such networks are then used to establish multiple couplings between the different modalities (auditory, visual, motor, and tactile). One can also explain the typical cross-modal couplings that are so extraordinarily important for musicians. The basis for this is Kalveram's system-theoretical model, which is reproduced here in modified form (Kalveram 1998, 2000). The sensorimotor system can access the motor commands used to operate a musical instrument via an "inversion" (also called a "feedforward mechanism"). This inversion succeeds via a correlation memory in which sensorimotor couplings are stored. Each sensory event is associated with a specific motor command (see Fig. 5.5). These correlations are built and modulated by experience (i.e., by learning), and their strength depends on the quality of the mapping between them. In this example, the audio-motor couplings are particularly

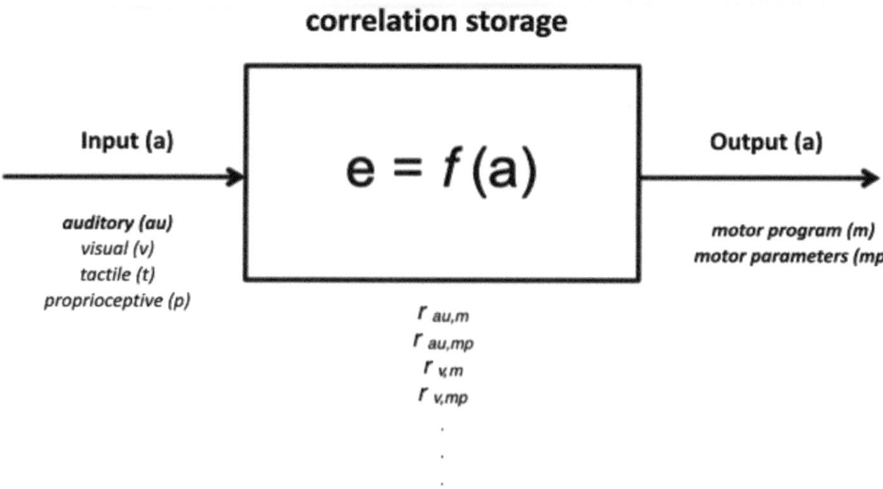

Fig. 5.5 Schematic representation of a correlation memory

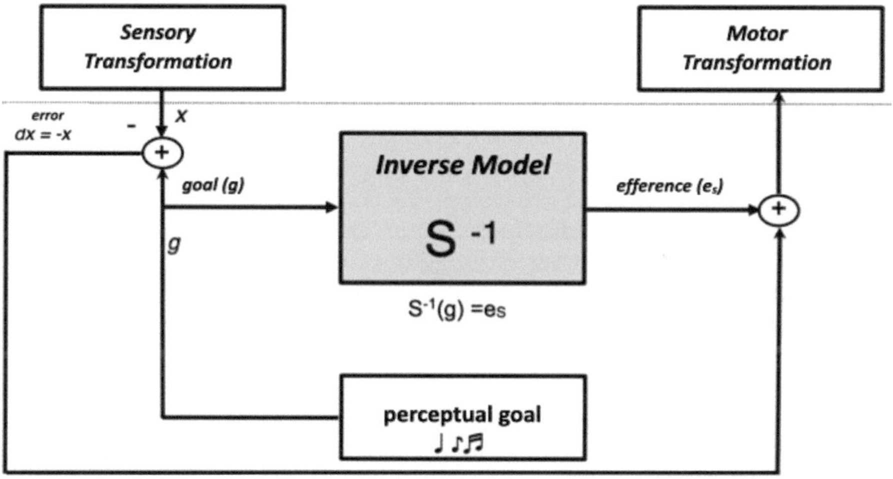

Fig. 5.6 Schematic representation of a sensorimotor model (Kalveram 1998, 2000)

emphasized, but in principle, one can imagine that many cross-modal couplings (e.g., visuomotor, tactile-motor, and audio-motor couplings) are stored in such a correlation memory (Fig. 5.6).

Of course, the audio-motor couplings are of particular interest for music-making. Let us assume that a pianist wants to play a piano piece or just strike a certain note. His brain can retrieve the auditory target ("g" in Fig. 5.6) from auditory memory and route it to correlation memory. The correlation memory then provides the inverse model for the efferents, which help relay the motor commands associated with the auditory target. These commands, in turn, can be used to determine the perceptual target (motor transformation) from which the appropriate motor program is retrieved and executed. Which motor program is retrieved and whether the same one is always retrieved for a given auditory target depends on the correlation strength. The higher the correlation, the better and more unambiguous the motor program's recall for producing a particular sensory event. The correlation strength depends on the frequency and quality of learning and the interference-free coupling between input and output (Kalveram 1998).

5.7 Medical Applications

Making music is a multimodal activity associated with numerous plastic changes in the brain. Therefore, it is unsurprising that attempts are made to apply the plasticity-initiating effects of music-making to everyday clinical practice. In the past 15 years, the field of research on neuroscience-oriented music therapy has developed tremendously. This new research direction was triggered by the work of the Finnish research group led by Teppo Särkämö. In their first paper (Särkämö et al. 2008), the authors studied stroke patients treated in a neurological rehabilitation clinic. Patients were randomly assigned to one of three groups. One group of patients listened to self-selected music for 1 h a day. A second group listened to self-selected audiobooks for 1 h a day. The third group received no further stimulation. All patients completed the same neurological and neuropsychological treatment over several months. After 3 and 6 months, only those patients who had listened to self-selected music for 1 h a day improved in verbal memory and focused attention. The underlying causes of the performance-enhancing effects of listening to music are not yet fully understood. However, it is suspected that listening to music triggers positive emotions, thus activating the ncl. accumbens and stimulating dopamine release, which may have increased the learning effect on memory and attention. If positive emotions and probable dopamine release were primarily responsible for the favorable learning effects, then other measures leading to mood elevation with concomitant dopamine release should also have learning-enhancing effects. However, this has not yet been investigated, and whether music-specific effects contribute to this phenomenon must be corroborated in future studies.

It is also interesting to note that even passive music listening leads to stronger activation in the perisylvian brain area around the auditory cortex in stroke patients in the long term (Särkämö et al. 2010). Passive stimulation appears to reactivate tissue in the perisylvian cortex that seems to be less active after stroke.

Music therapy interventions may also optimize motor training in stroke patients. Schneider and colleagues (2007) offered simple percussion training to a group of stroke patients with mildly paralyzed limbs and monitored motor performance improvement using standard motor tests. Compared with stroke patients who had undergone conventional motor training, there were significant advantages for the percussion training group.

Due to lack of space, a detailed review of current music therapy research cannot be provided here. However, in recent review articles by the Finnish research group, music therapy's effects have been excellently described and discussed (Särkämö 2018; Moumdjian et al. 2017; Sihvonen et al. 2017, 2020; Siponkoski et al. 2020). These papers describe the controlled studies that suggest potentially rehabilitative effects of music-based interventions, such as listening to music, singing, or playing an instrument, which are likely to be observed in various neurological conditions. Although the number of studies and the amount of available evidence are currently greatest for stroke and dementia, there is also evidence that music-based interventions exert effects that support cognition, motor function, or emotional well-being in people with Parkinson's disease, epilepsy, multiple sclerosis, depression, aphasia, tinnitus, traumatic brain injury, and disorders of consciousness, thereby favorably affecting motor function, speech, mood, or cognition in these patient groups. The neurobiological mechanisms underlying the effects of music interventions have not yet been clearly elucidated. However, what is certain is that neural networks involved in the control of reward, arousal, affect regulation, learning, and memory are primarily involved. Although further controlled studies are needed to demonstrate the efficacy of music in neurological recovery, music-based interventions are already emerging as promising rehabilitation strategies.

5.8 Music and Healthy Aging

As outlined above, playing music significantly modulates the anatomical and neurophysiological foundations of the brain and thus also the cognitive functions controlled by the brain. This places musical activities (and, to some extent, listening to music) among other activities that have been found to induce similar anatomical and neurophysiological changes (summarized in Jäncke 2008a, b, 2009a, b; May 2011; Zatorre et al. 2012). Ultimately, it can be assumed that all sensorimotor and/or multimodal activities that are learned and practiced over a long period trigger microstructural and macrostructural changes as well as neurophysiological adaptation processes in the brain.

Such anatomical and neurophysiological changes can then develop into anatomical and neurophysiological reserves that buffer age-related atrophy. In this respect, not only education and occupation (as frequently described, e.g., Hall et al. 2009; Hotz et al. 2021) but also lifestyle and leisure activities such as playing music and dancing contribute to this reserve. A series of longitudinal and postmortem studies have linked these activities (including playing music and dancing) to a reduction in age-related cognitive decline (Verghese et al. 2003) and dementia (Verghese et al. 2003; Scarmeas et al. 2001) or to a delayed (Hall et al. 2009) or diminished manifestation of symptoms in dementia patients (Scarmeas et al. 2001; Katzman 1993).

The frontal lobe is considered particularly relevant regarding the potentially age-decelerating function of playing music, as it is one of the brain regions most affected by early degeneration (Jäncke 2013). The frontal cortex plays a crucial role in core functions necessary for musical performance, including planning, preparation, and the controlled execution of fine motor actions, which are regulated by the primary and secondary motor areas as well as the premotor cortex. Audio-motor interactions and all executive functions (including attention and concentration) are controlled by the dorsal and ventral prefrontal cortex. Additionally, the primary and secondary auditory cortices, which are frequently stimulated by the processing of tones and melodies, should not be overlooked. The specific and long-term engagement of these regions during musical activity appears to stimulate neurovascular and metabolic activity, thereby enhancing synaptic plasticity and glial activity. Essentially, these processes can be summarized under the metaphor "use it or lose it." The long-term and intensive use of these brain regions appears to have protective effects against aging and dementia.

A particularly interesting recent study reexamined the neuroanatomical effects of playing music in the context of aging (Rogenmoser et al. 2018). The researchers employed an innovative method to parametrize the anatomical aging of the brain. Using MRI scans and specialized statistical analyses, they were able to estimate the biological age of individuals. This estimated biological age could then be compared to their chronological (i.e., actual) age. In amateur musicians, the biological age of the brain was significantly lower than their chronological age. In other words, amateur musicians had brains that were younger than their actual age, indicating less brain aging compared to nonmusicians.

In contrast to amateur musicians, this "rejuvenation" effect was not as pronounced in professional musicians. This may suggest that an intense focus on a single, albeit enriching, activity is not as beneficial as engaging in multiple activities, as is often the case with amateur musicians. Furthermore, professional-level musical engagement might also lead to stress-related disorders and a less enriching environment compared to amateur musicians, which could slightly diminish the otherwise positive effects of playing music.

Overall, the findings suggest that playing music has a stronger age-decelerating effect when it is pursued as a leisure activity rather than as a primary profession. It is possible that the multisensory, motor, and socio-affective experiences of making music, in addition to other main activities pursued by amateur musicians, contribute to these benefits. Clearly, the positive effects of playing music do not increase indefinitely with more intensive practice. Brain plasticity can also have unfavorable consequences. Nevertheless, it must be emphasized that playing music represents an interesting and rewarding strategy for successful and healthy aging.

5.8.1 Conclusion

In this overview article, the effects of making and listening to music on human brain plasticity and the related psychological functions have been addressed. Making music and listening to it can trigger various changes or better adaptations in the human brain. These changes manifest in larger brain volume, greater gray matter density, or better anatomical connectivity in the brain areas involved in the control of music-making and auditory appreciation. Anatomical changes and altered neurophysiological activation patterns can be detected in musicians when listening to and generating music. Likely, these neuroanatomical and neurophysiological experience-related changes are also associated with widespread changes in various cognitive domains. These findings open up new perspectives for research into medical applications of brain plasticity in the context of various neurological and psychiatric diseases.

References

Alain C, Snyder JS, He Y, Reinke KS (2007) Changes in auditory cortex parallel rapid perceptual learning. Cereb Cortex 17(5):1074–1084
Amunts K, Schlaug G, Jancke L, Steinmetz H, Schleicher A, Dabringhaus A et al (1997) Motor cortex and hand motor skills: structural compliance in the human brain. Hum Brain Mapp 5(3):206–215
Bakin JS, Weinberger NM (1996) Induction of a physiological memory in the cerebral cortex by stimulation of the nucleus basalis. Proc Natl Acad Sci USA 93(20):11219–11224
Bangert M, Altenmüller EO (2003) Mapping perception to action in piano practice: a longitudinal DC-EEG study. BMC Neurosci 4:26
Bangert M, Jurgens U, Hausler U, Altenmuller E (2006a) Classical conditioned responses to absent tones. BMC Neurosci 7:60
Bangert M, Peschel T, Schlaug G, Rotte M, Drescher D, Hinrichs H et al (2006b) Shared networks for auditory and motor processing in professional pianists: evidence from fMRI conjunction. NeuroImage 30(3):917–926
Bao S, Chan VT, Merzenich MM (2001) Cortical remodelling induced by activity of ventral tegmental dopamine neurons. Nature 412(6842):79–83
Baumann S, Koeneke S, Schmidt CF, Meyer M, Lutz K, Jancke L (2007) A network for audio-motor coordination in skilled pianists and non-musicians. Brain Res 1161:65–78
Baumann S, Meyer M, Jäncke L (2008) Enhancement of auditory-evoked potentials in musicians reflects an influence of expertise but not selective attention. J Cogn Neurosci 20(12):2238–2249
Bengtsson SL, Nagy Z, Skare S, Forsman L, Forssberg H, Ullén F (2005) Extensive piano practicing has regionally specific effects on white matter development. Nat Neurosci 8(9):1148–1150
Bhattacharya J, Petsche H (2001) Enhanced phase synchrony in the electroencephalograph gamma band for musicians while listening to music. Phys Rev E Stat Nonlinear Soft Matter Phys 64:012902
Blake DT, Heiser MA, Caywood M, Merzenich MM (2006) Experience-dependent adult cortical plasticity requires cognitive association between sensation and reward. Neuron 52(2):371–381
Bosnyak DJ, Eaton RA, Roberts LE (2004) Distributed auditory cortical representations are modified when non- musicians are trained at pitch discrimination with 40 Hz amplitude modulated tones. Cereb Cortex 14(10):1088–1099
Brauchli C, Leipold S, Jäncke L (2019) Univariate and multivariate analyses of functional networks in absolute pitch. NeuroImage 189:241–247
Brauchli C, Leipold S, Jäncke L (2020) Diminished large-scale functional brain networks in absolute pitch during the perception of naturalistic music and audiobooks. NeuroImage 216:116513
Burkhard A, Hänggi J, Elmer S, Jäncke L (2020) The importance of the fibre tracts connecting the planum temporale in absolute pitch possessors. NeuroImage 211:116590
Carcagno S, Plack CJ (2011a) Pitch discrimination learning: specificity for pitch and harmonic resolvability, and electrophysiological correlates. J Assoc Res Otolaryngol 12(4):503–517
Carcagno S, Plack CJ (2011b) Subcortical plasticity following perceptual learning in a pitch discrimination task. J Assoc Res Otolaryngol 12(1):89–100
Carpentier SM, Moreno S, McIntosh AR (2016) Short-term music training enhances complex, distributed neural communication during music and linguistic tasks. J Cogn Neurosci 28:1603–1612

Chobert J, François C, Velay J-L, Besson M (2014) Twelve months of active musical training in 8- to 10-year-old children enhances the preattentive processing of syllabic duration and voice onset time. Cereb Cortex 24:956–967
D'Ausilio A, Altenmuller E, Olivetti Belardinelli M, Lotze M (2006) Cross-modal plasticity of the motor cortex while listening to a rehearsed musical piece. Eur J Neurosci 24(3):955–958
de Villers-Sidani E, Chang EF, Bao S, Merzenich MM (2007) Critical period window for spectral tuning defined in the primary auditory cortex (A1) in the rat. J Neurosci 27(1):180–189
de Villers-Sidani E, Simpson KL, Lu YF, Lin RC, Merzenich MM (2008) Manipulating critical period closure across different sectors of the primary auditory cortex. Nat Neurosci 11(8):957–965
Dege F, Schwarzer G (2011) The effect of a music program on phonological awareness in preschoolers. Front Psychol 2:124
Dittinger E, Barbaroux M, D'Imperio M, Jäncke L, Elmer S, Besson M (2016) Professional music training and novel word learning: from faster semantic encoding to longer-lasting word representations. J Cogn Neurosci 28:1584–1602
Dittinger E, Valizadeh SA, Jäncke L, Besson M, Elmer S (2018) Increased functional connectivity in the ventral and dorsal streams during retrieval of novel words in professional musicians. Hum Brain Mapp 39:722–734
Dittinger E, Scherer J, Jäncke L, Besson M, Elmer S (2019) Testing the influence of musical expertise on novel word learning across the lifespan using a cross-sectional approach in children, young adults and older adults. Brain Lang 198:104678
Elbert T, Pantev C, Wienbruch C, Rockstroh B, Taub E (1995) Increased cortical representation of the fingers of the left hand in string players. Science 270(5234):305–307
Elmer S, Klein C, Kühnis J, Liem F, Meyer M, Jäncke L (2014) Music and language expertise influence the categorization of speech and musical sounds: behavioral and electrophysiological measurements. J Cogn Neurosci 26:2356–2369
Ericsson KA (2004) Deliberate practice and the acquisition and maintenance of expert performance in medicine and related domains. Acad Med 79(Suppl 10):S70–S81
Ericsson KA, Krampe RT, Clemens T (1993) The role of deliberate practise in the acquisition of expert performance. Psychol Rev 100(3):363–406
Fink A, Graif B, Neubauer AC (2009) Brain correlates underlying creative thinking: EEG alpha activity in professional vs. novice dancers. NeuroImage 46:854–862
Fritz J, Elhilali M, Shamma S (2005) Active listening: task-dependent plasticity of spectrotemporal receptive fields in primary auditory cortex. Hear Res 206(1–2):159–176
Fujioka T, Ross B, Kakigi R, Pantev C, Trainor LJ (2006) One year of musical training affects development of auditory cortical-evoked fields in young children. Brain 129(Pt 10):2593–2608
Gaab N, Gaser C, Zaehle T, Jancke L, Schlaug G (2003) Functional anatomy of pitch memory—an fMRI study with sparse temporal sampling. NeuroImage 19(4):1417–1426
Gaser C, Schlaug G (2003) Brain structures differ between musicians and non-musicians. J Neurosci 23(27):9240–9245
Habibi A, Cahn BR, Damasio A, Damasio H (2016) Neural correlates of accelerated auditory processing in children engaged in music training. Dev Cogn Neurosci 21:1–14
Habibi A, Damasio A, Ilari B, Veiga R, Joshi AA, Leahy RM, Haldar JP, Varadarajan D, Bhushan C, Damasio H (2018) Childhood music training induces change in micro and macroscopic brain structure: results from a longitudinal study. Cereb Cortex 28:4336–4347
Habibi A, Ilari B, Heine K, Damasio H (2020) Changes in auditory cortical thickness following music training in children: converging longitudinal and cross-sectional results. Brain Struct Funct 225(8):2463–2474
Hall CB, Lipton RB, Sliwinski M, Katz MJ, Derby CA, Verghese J (2009) Cognitive activities delay onset of memory decline in persons who develop dementia. Neurology 73(5):356–361
Hänggi J, Koeneke S, Bezzola L, Jäncke L (2010) Structural neuroplasticity in the sensorimotor network of professional female ballet dancers. Hum Brain Mapp 31:1196–1206
Hebb DO (1949) The organization of behavior. Wiley, New York

Hennessy SL, Sachs ME, Ilari B, Habibi A (2019) Effects of music training on inhibitory control and associated neural networks in school-aged children: a longitudinal study. Front Neurosci 13:1080

Herholz SC, Zatorre RJ (2012) Musical training as a framework for brain plasticity: behavior, function, and structure. Neuron 76(3):486–502

Herholz SC, Lappe C, Pantev C (2009) Looking for a pattern: an MEG study on the abstract mismatch negativity in musicians and nonmusicians. BMC Neurosci 10:42

Herholz SC, Boh B, Pantev C (2011) Musical training modulates encoding of higher-order regularities in the auditory cortex. Eur J Neurosci 34(3):524–529

Hotz I, Deschwanden PF, Mérillat S, Liem F, Kollias S, Jäncke L (2021) Associations of subclinical cerebral small vessel disease and processing speed in non-demented subjects: a 7-year study. NeuroImage Clin 32:102884

Hudziak JJ, Albaugh MD, Ducharme S, Karama S, Spottswood M, Crehan E, Evans AC, Botteron KN, Brain Development Cooperative Group (2014) Cortical thickness maturation and duration of music training: health-promoting activities shape brain development. J Am Acad Child Adolesc Psychiatry 53(11):1153–1161, 1161.e1–e2

Hyde KL, Lerch J, Norton A, Forgeard M, Winner E, Evans AC et al (2009) Musical training shapes structural brain development. J Neurosci 29(10):3019–3025

Ilari B (2020) Longitudinal research on music education and child development: contributions and challenges. Music Sci 3:2059204320937224

Imfeld A, Oechslin MS, Meyer M, Loenneker T, Jancke L (2009) White matter plasticity in the corticospinal tract of musicians: a diffusion tensor imaging study. NeuroImage 46(3):600–607

Jäncke L (2008a) Macht Musik schlau? Neue Erkenntnisse aus den kognitiven Neurowissenschaften und der Kognitiven Psychologie. Huber, Bern

Jäncke L (2008b) Music, memory and emotion. J Biol 7:21

Jäncke L (2009a) The plastic human brain. Restor Neurol Neurosci 27(5):521–538

Jäncke L (2009b) Music drives brain plasticity. F1000 Biol Rep 1:78

Jäncke L (2012a) The relationship between music and language. Front Psychol 3:123

Jäncke L (2013) Music making and the aging brain. Z Neuropsychol 24(2):113–121

Jäncke L (2018) Music and memory. In: Thaut M, Hodges DA (eds) The Oxford handbook of music and the brain. Oxford University Press, pp 1–32

Jäncke L (2024) Plastizität. In: Jäncke L, (ed) Lehrbuch Kognitive Neurowissenschaften. Hogrefe Verlag, pp 527–552

Jäncke L, Loose R, Lutz K, Specht K, Shah NJ (2000) Cortical activations during paced finger-tapping applying visual and auditory pacing stimuli. Brain Res Cogn Brain Res 10(1–2):51–66

Jäncke L, Gaab N, Wustenberg T, Scheich H, Heinze HJ (2001) Short-term functional plasticity in the human auditory cortex: an fMRI study. Brain Res Cogn Brain Res 12(3):479–485

Jäncke L, Langer N, Hanggi J (2012) Diminished whole-brain but enhanced Peri-sylvian connectivity in absolute pitch musicians. J Cogn Neurosci 24(6):1447–1461

Janus M, Lee Y, Moreno S, Bialystok E (2016) Effects of short-term music and second-language training on executive control. J Exp Child Psychol 144:84–97

Jerison HJ (2000) Evolution of intellgence. In: Sternberg G (ed) Handbook of human intelligence. Cambridge University Press, Cambridge, pp 216–244

Kalveram KT (1998) Wie das Individuum mit seiner Umwelt interagiert: Psychologische, biologische und kybernetische Betrachtungen über die Funktion von Verhalten. Pabst Science, Lengerich

Kalveram KT (2000) Sensorimotor sequential learning by a neural network based on redefined Hebbian Learning. In: Artificial Neural Networks in Medicine and Biology: Proceedings of the ANNIMAB-1 Conference, Göteborg, Sweden, 13–16 May 2000. Springer, London

Katzman R (1993) Education and the prevalence of dementia and Alzheimer's disease. Neurology 43(1):13–20. https://doi.org/10.1212/wnl.43.1_part_1.13

Keenan JP, Thangaraj V, Halpern AR, Schlaug G (2001) Absolute pitch and planum temporale. NeuroImage 14:1402–1408

Kleber B, Birbaumer N, Veit R, Trevorrow T, Lotze M (2007) Overt and imagined singing of an Italian aria. NeuroImage 36:889–900

Kleber B, Veit R, Birbaumer N, Gruzelier J, Lotze M (2010) The brain of opera singers: experience-dependent changes in functional activation. Cereb Cortex 20:1144–1152

Koelsch S, Gunter T, Friederici AD, Schroger E (2000) Brain indices of music processing: «nonmusicians« are musical. J Cogn Neurosci 12(3):520–541

Koelsch S, Kasper E, Sammler D, Schulze K, Gunter T, Friederici AD (2004) Music, language and meaning: brain signatures of semantic processing. Nat Neurosci 7(3):302–307

Koeneke S, Lutz K, Herwig U, Ziemann U, Jancke L (2006) Extensive training of elementary finger tapping movements changes the pattern of motor cortex excitability. Exp Brain Res 174(2):199–209

Kraus N, Chandrasekaran B (2010) Music training for the development of auditory skills. Nat Rev Neurosci 11(8):599–605

Kreutz G, Feldhaus M, Saarikallio S (2023) Leisure activities are associated with self-efficacy in childhood and adolescence. Leis Sci 0(0):1–18

Kuhl PK (2004) Early language acquisition: cracking the speech code. Nat Rev Neurosci 5(11):831–843

Kühnis J, Elmer S, Meyer M, Jancke L (2013a) Musicianship boosts perceptual learning of pseudoword-chimeras: an electrophysiological approach. Brain Topogr 26(1):110–125

Kühnis J, Elmer S, Meyer M, Jäncke L (2013b) The encoding of vowels and temporal speech cues in the auditory cortex of professional musicians: an EEG study. Neuropsychologia 51:1608–1618

Kühnis J, Elmer S, Jäncke L (2014) Auditory evoked responses in musicians during passive vowel listening are modulated by functional connectivity between bilateral auditory-related brain regions. J Cogn Neurosci 26:2750–2761

Ladda AM, Wallwork SB, Lotze M (2020) Multimodal sensory-spatial integration and retrieval of trained motor patterns for body coordination in musicians and dancers. Front Psychol 11:576120

Lappe C, Herholz SC, Trainor LJ, Pantev C (2008) Cortical plasticity induced by short-term unimodal and multimodal musical training. J Neurosci 28(39):9632–9639

Leipold S, Klein C, Jäncke L (2021) Musical expertise shapes functional and structural brain networks independent of absolute pitch ability. J Neurosci 41(11):2496–2511

Lotze M, Scheler G, Tan H-RM, Braun C, Birbaumer N (2003) The musician's brain: functional imaging of amateurs and professionals during performance and imagery. NeuroImage 20:1817–1829

Loui P, Li HC, Hohmann A, Schlaug G (2011) Enhanced cortical connectivity in absolute pitch musicians: a model for local hyperconnectivity. J Cogn Neurosci 23(4):1015–1026

Loui P, Zamm A, Schlaug G (2012) Enhanced functional networks in absolute pitch. Neuroimage 63(2):632–640

Luders E, Gaser C, Jancke L, Schlaug G (2004) A voxel-based approach to gray matter asymmetries. NeuroImage 22:656–664

Magne C, Schön D, Besson M (2006) Musician children detect pitch violations in both music and language better than nonmusician children: behavioral and electrophysiological approaches. J Cogn Neurosci 18:199–211

Marie C, Magne C, Besson M (2011) Musicians and the metric structure of words. J Cogn Neurosci 23:294–305

May A (2011) Experience-dependent structural plasticity in the adult human brain. Trends Cogn Sci 15(10):475–482

Meister I, Krings T, Foltys H, Boroojerdi B, Müller M, Töpper R et al (2005) Effects of long-term practice and task complexity in musicians and nonmusicians performing simple and complex motor tasks: implications for cortical motor organization. Hum Brain Mapp 25(3):345–352

Menning H, Roberts LE, Pantev C (2000) Plastic changes in the auditory cortex induced by intensive frequency discrimination training. Neuroreport 11(4):817–822

Meyer M, Elmer S, Ringli M, Oechslin MS, Baumann S, Jancke L (2011) Long-term exposure to music enhances the sensitivity of the auditory system in children. Eur J Neurosci 34(5):755–765
Moreno S, Besson M (2006) Musical training and language-related brain electrical activity in children. Psychophysiology 43:287–291
Moreno S, Marques C, Santos A, Santos M, Castro SL, Besson M (2009) Musical training influences linguistic abilities in 8-year-old children: more evidence for brain plasticity. Cereb Cortex 19:712–723
Moreno S, Bialystok E, Barac R, Schellenberg EG, Cepeda NJ, Chau T (2011) Short-term music training enhances verbal intelligence and executive function. Psychol Sci 22:1425–1433
Moreno S, Wodniecka Z, Tays W, Alain C, Bialystok E (2014) Inhibitory control in bilinguals and musicians: event related potential (ERP) evidence for experience-specific effects. PLoS One 9:e94169
Moumdjian L, Sarkamo T, Leone C, Leman M, Feys P (2017) Effectiveness of music-based interventions on motricity or cognitive functioning in neurological populations: a systematic review. Eur J Phys Rehabil Med 53:466–482
Moussard A, Bermudez P, Alain C, Tays W, Moreno S (2016) Life-long music practice and executive control in older adults: An event-related potential study. Brain Res 1642:146–153
Münte TF, Kohlmetz C, Nager W, Altenmüller E (2001) Neuroperception. Superior auditory spatial tuning in conductors. Nature 409:580
Münte TF, Altenmüller E, Jäncke L (2002) The musician's brain as a model of neuroplasticity. Nat Rev Neurosci 3(6):473–478
Oechslin MS, Meyer M, Jäncke L (2009a) Absolute pitch—functional evidence of speech-relevant auditory acuity. Cereb Cortex 20(2):447–455
Oechslin MS, Imfeld A, Loenneker T, Meyer M, Jancke L (2009b) The plasticity of the superior longitudinal fasciculus as a function of musical expertise: a diffusion tensor imaging study. Front Hum Neurosci 3:76
Ohl FW, Scheich H (2005) Learning-induced plasticity in animal and human auditory cortex. Curr Opin Neurobiol 15(4):470–447
Olszewska AM, Gaca M, Herman AM, Jednoróg K, Marchewka A (2021) How musical training shapes the adult brain: predispositions and neuroplasticity. Front Neurosci 15:630829
Orlandi A, Proverbio AM (2019) Bilateral engagement of the occipito-temporal cortex in response to dance kinematics in experts. Sci Rep 9:1000
Ott CG, Langer N, Oechslin M, Meyer M, Jancke L (2011) Processing of voiced and unvoiced acoustic stimuli in musicians. Front Psychol 2:195
Pantev C, Herholz SC (2011) Plasticity of the human auditory cortex related to musical training. Neurosci Biobehav Rev 35:2140–2154
Pantev C, Oostenveld R, Engelien A, Ross B, Roberts LE, Hoke M (1998) Increased auditory cortical representation in musicians. Nature 392(6678):811–814
Pantev C, Wollbrink A, Roberts LE, Engelien A, Lutkenhoner B (1999) Short-term plasticity of the human auditory cortex. Brain Res 842(1):192–199
Pantev C, Roberts LE, Schulz M, Engelien A, Ross B (2001) Timbre-specific enhancement of auditory cortical representations in musicians. Neuroreport 12(1):169–174
Paraskevopoulos E, Kuchenbuch A, Herholz SC, Pantev C (2012a) Evidence for training-induced plasticity in multisensory brain structures: an MEG study. PLoS One 7(5):e36534
Paraskevopoulos E, Kuchenbuch A, Herholz SC, Pantev C (2012b) Musical expertise induces audiovisual integration of abstract congruency rules. J Neurosci 32(50):18196–18203
Paraskevopoulos E, Kuchenbuch A, Herholz SC, Pantev C (2012c) Statistical learning effects in musicians and non-musicians: an MEG study. Neuropsychologia 50(2):341–349
Pascual-Leone A, Nguyet D, Cohen LG, Brasil-Neto JP, Cammarota A, Hallett M (1995) Modulation of muscle responses evoked by transcranial magnetic stimulation during the acquisition of new fine motor skills. J Neurophysiol 74(3):1037–1045
Pascual-Leone A, Amedi A, Fregni F, Merabet LB (2005) The plastic human brain cortex. Annu Rev Neurosci 28:377–401

Patel AD, Iversen JR (2007) The linguistic benefits of musical abilities. Trends Cogn Sci 11(9):369–372
Poikonen H, Toiviainen P, Tervaniemi M (2018) Dance on cortex: enhanced theta synchrony in experts when watching a dance piece. Eur J Neurosci 47:433–445
Proverbio AM, Manfredi M, Zani A, Adorni R (2013) Musical expertise afects neural bases of letter recognition. Neuropsychologia 51(3):538–549
Putkinen V, Tervaniemi M, Saarikivi K, de Vent N, Huotilainen M (2014a) Investigating the effects of musical training on functional brain development with a novel melodic MMN paradigm. Neurobiol Learn Mem 110:8–15
Putkinen V, Tervaniemi M, Saarikivi K, Ojala P, Huotilainen M (2014b) Enhanced development of auditory change detection in musically trained school-aged children: a longitudinal event-related potential study. Dev Sci 17:282–297
Putkinen V, Tervaniemi M, Huotilainen M (2019) Musical playschool activities are linked to faster auditory development during preschool-age: a longitudinal ERP study. Sci Rep 9:11310
Rogenmoser L, Kernbach J, Schlaug G, Gaser C (2018) Keeping brains young with making music. Brain Struct Funct 223:297–305
Saffran JR, Aslin RN, Newport EL (1996) Statistical learning by 8-month-old infants. Science 274(5294):1926–1928
Saffran JR, Johnson EK, Aslin RN, Newport EL (1999) Statistical learning of tone sequences by human infants and adults. Cognition 70(1):27–52
Sala G, Gobet F (2020) Cognitive and academic benefits of music training with children: a multi-level meta-analysis. Mem Cogn 48:1429–1441
Särkämö T (2018) Cognitive, emotional, and neural benefits of musical leisure activities in aging and neurological rehabilitation: a critical review. Ann Phys Rehabil Med 61:414–418
Särkämö T, Tervaniemi M, Laitinen S, Forsblom A, Soinila S, Mikkonen M et al (2008) Music listening enhances cognitive recovery and mood after middle cerebral artery stroke. Brain 131(Pt 3):866–876
Särkämö T, Pihko E, Laitinen S, Forsblom A, Soinila S, Mikkonen M et al (2010) Music and speech listening enhance the recovery of early sensory processing after stroke. J Cogn Neurosci 22(12):2716–2727
Scarmeas N, Levy G, Tang MX, Manly J, Stern Y (2001) Influence of leisure activity on the incidence of Alzheimer's disease. Neurology 57(12):2236–2242
Schellenberg EG (2004) Music lessons enhance IQ. Psychol Sci 15(8):511–514
Schellenberg EG (2015) Music training and speech perception: a gene–environment interaction. Ann N Y Acad Sci 1337:170–177
Schlaug G (2015) Musicians and music making as a model for the study of brain plasticity. Prog Brain Res 217:37–55
Schlaug G, Jancke L, Huang Y, Staiger JF, Steinmetz H (1995a) Increased corpus callosum size in musicians. Neuropsychologia 33(8):1047–1055
Schlaug G, Jancke L, Huang Y, Steinmetz H (1995b) In vivo evidence of structural brain asymmetry in musicians. Science 267(5198):699–701
Schlaug G, Norton A, Marchina S, Zipse L, Wan CY (2010) From singing to speaking: facilitating recovery from nonfluent aphasia. Future Neurol 5(5):657–665
Schneider P, Scherg M, Dosch HG, Specht HJ, Gutschalk A, Rupp A (2002) Morphology of Heschl's gyrus reflects enhanced activation in the auditory cortex of musicians. Nat Neurosci 5(7):688–694
Schneider P, Sluming V, Roberts N, Scherg M, Goebel R, Specht HJ et al (2005) Structural and functional asymmetry of lateral Heschl's gyrus reflects pitch perception preference. Nat Neurosci 8(9):1241–1247
Schneider P, Andermann M, Engelmann D, Schneider R, Rupp A (2006) Music in the head. Individual differences in sound perception and the cerebral symphony orchestra. Dtsch Med Wochenschr 131(51–52):2895–2897
Schneider S, Schonle PW, Altenmuller E, Munte TF (2007) Using musical instruments to improve motor skill recovery following a stroke. J Neurol 254(10):1339–1346

Schneider P, Engelmann D, Groß C, Bernhofs V, Hofmann E, Christiner M, Benner J, Bücher S, Ludwig A, Serrallach BL, Zeidler BM, Turker S, Parncutt R, Seither-Preisler A (2023) Neuroanatomical disposition, natural development, and training-induced plasticity of the human auditory system from childhood to adulthood: a 12-year study in musicians and nonmusicians. J Neurosci Off J Soc Neurosci 43(37):6430–6446

Schulte M, Knief A, Seither-Preisler A, Pantev C (2002) Different modes of pitch perception and learning-induced neuronal plasticity of the human auditory cortex. Neural Plast 9(3):161–175

Shahin AJ, Roberts LE, Chau W, Trainor LJ, Miller LM (2008) Music training leads to the development of timbre-specific gamma band activity. NeuroImage 41(1):113–122

Sihvonen AJ, Särkämö T, Leo V, Tervaniemi M, Altenmüller E, Soinila S (2017) Music-based interventions in neurological rehabilitation. Lancet Neurol 16:648–660

Sihvonen AJ, Leo V, Ripollés P, Lehtovaara T, Ylönen A, Rajanaro P, Laitinen S, Forsblom A, Saunavaara J, Autti T, Laine M, Rodríguez-Fornells A, Tervaniemi M, Soinila S, Särkämö T (2020) Vocal music enhances memory and language recovery after stroke: pooled results from two RCTs. Ann Clin Transl Neurol 7:2272–2287

Siponkoski S-T, Martínez-Molina N, Kuusela L, Laitinen S, Holma M, Ahlfors M, Jordan-Kilkki P, Ala-Kauhaluoma K, Melkas S, Pekkola J, Rodriguez-Fornells A, Laine M, Ylinen A, Rantanen P, Koskinen S, Lipsanen J, Särkämö T (2020) Music therapy enhances executive functions and prefrontal structural neuroplasticity after traumatic brain injury: evidence from a randomized controlled trial. J Neurotrauma 37:618–634

Slevc LR, Miyake A (2006) Individual differences in second-language proficiency: does musical ability matter? Psychol Sci 17(8):675–681

Soley G, Hannon EE (2010) Infants prefer the musical meter of their own culture: a cross-cultural comparison. Dev Psychol 46(1):286–292

Specht HJ, Gutschalk A, Rupp A (2002) Morphology of Heschl's gyrus reflects enhanced activation in the auditory cortex of musicians. Nat Neurosci 5(7):688–694

Swaminathan S, Schellenberg EG (2018) Musical competence is predicted by music training, cognitive abilities, and personality. Sci Rep 8:9223

Tervaniemi M, Tao S, Huotilainen M (2018) Promises of Music in Education? Frontiers in Education 3:74

Tillmann B, Koelsch S, Escoffier N, Bigand E, Lalitte P, Friederici AD et al (2006) Cognitive priming in sung and instrumental music: activation of inferior frontal cortex. NeuroImage 31(4):1771–1782

Verghese J, Lipton RB, Katz MJ, Hall CB, Derby CA, Kuslansky G, Ambrose AF, Sliwinski M, Buschke H (2003) Leisure activities and the risk of dementia in the elderly. N Engl J Med 348(25):2508–2516

Wan CY, Schlaug G (2010) Neural pathways for language in autism: the potential for music-based treatments. Future Neurol 5(6):797–805

Wan CY, Bazen L, Baars R, Libenson A, Zipse L, Zuk J et al (2011) Auditory-motor mapping training as an intervention to facilitate speech output in non-verbal children with autism: a proof of concept study. PLoS One 6(9):e25505

Wengenroth M, Blatow M, Heinecke A, Reinhardt J, Stippich C, Hofmann E, Schneider P (2014) Increased volume and function of right auditory cortex as a marker for absolute pitch. Cereb Cortex 24:1127–1137

Wong PC, Roy AK, Margulis EH (2009) Bimusicalism: the implicit dual enculturation of cognitive and affective systems. Music Percept 27(2):81–88

Zatorre RJ, Fields RD, Johansen-Berg H (2012) Plasticity in gray and white: neuroimaging changes in brain structure during learning. Nat Neurosci 15:528–536

Part II

Music in Clinical and Diversity Sensitive Practice

Music Medicine Against Pain, Anxiety, and Stress

6

Ralph Spintge

So-called medicofunctional music (music with intended therapeutic effects in medical settings) is used on a global scale for improving the psychophysic state of patients in emotionally aversive situations and situations marked by pain. While earlier studies emphasized therapeutic effects, it has been shown meanwhile that improvements can also be identified concerning cost containment, including parameters such as medication needed for analgesia and premedication to anesthesia, duration of in-patient treatment period after surgery, duration of NICU treatment for premature newborns, as well as efficacy and productivity of working staff. There are standards and definitions established for using medicofunctional music (recently also called music-based interventions to describe the fast growing number of applications of such concepts). Conducting research in the field, the standards established in medical science are adapted considering specific needs, such as use of mixed-methods research concepts combining quantitative and qualitative parameters as well. A growing number of physicians, hospitals another medical institutions enclose medicofunctional music and/or music-based interventions such as so-called anxioalgolytic (anxiety, pain, and stress relieving) music in their daily practice of patient care.

6.1 Introduction

Pain medicine deals with two different entities of pain, one is acute pain and the other one is chronic pain, with transitions. While in acute pain, the psychophysic status of a patient is marked by a trias of pain, distress, and anxiety for a limited period of time, chronic pain today is described as a chronic bio-psycho-social malady of its own. Furthermore, there are emotionally aversive situations in many

R. Spintge (✉)
Institute for Music Therapy, University for Music and Drama, Hamburg, Germany

G. Kreutz, G. Bernatzky (eds.), *Music and Medicine*, Neurocultural Health and Wellbeing, https://doi.org/10.1007/978-3-662-72175-9_6

medical settings where patient goes through invasive procedures, which themselves may create procedural pain and other unpleasant feelings. At the same time patients perceive such situations as basically dangerous, they are in a state of "emotional emergency" (Badner et al. 1990; Kain et al. 1997; Mondanaro and Sara 2013; Nijkamp 2004; Nolan 1992; Salimpoor et al. 2009; Spintge 1983; Spintge and Droh 1987; Wang et al. 2002). There exists a vicious circle of pain and stress in both entities, keeping patients in a state of general anxiety, enforced by fear of pain and sometimes fears of death. That combines with impaired conscious perception, decreased self-estimation, anger, helplessness, and disappointment (Tolksdorf 1997). Psychophysiological sequela of such feelings comprise disturbed central nervous (so-called neurovegetative) control of cardiovascular and cardio-respiratory systems, leading to increased energy turnover and oxygen demand, inadequate endocrinological control of metabolism with increased plasma-levels of catecholamines, steroids, and endogenous opioids (endorphins). This is combined with reduced pain tolerance, general hyperesthesia, and ephaptic spreading of pain (spreading of sensation to other nerve fiber qualities, for instance sympathetic nervous system fibers), which can be accompanied by vegetative dysfunction, such as nausea and vomiting, as well as by motor dysfunction such as tremor (Gellhorn 1964; Keller 1995; Spintge and Droh 1992). The entirety of such reactions leads to inadequate defense reactions, to aggressive behavior and reduced patient compliance—combined with increased demand of sedatives, anesthetics, and analgetics, especially preoperatively, up to prolonged postoperative rehabilitation (Buyukkocak et al. 2006; Caumo and Ferreira 2003; Grossi et al. 1999; Munafo 1998; Norman and Fink 1997; Schön et al. 2007; Stirling 2006; Thompson and Kam 2005; Tolksdorf 1997).

Studies in medical psychology show two main cognitive and emotional factors responsible for that »emotional emergency situation« mentioned above. On one hand it is a deficit in memorized information, at the other hand it is a lack in emotional support (Spintge 1983; Tolksdorf 1997; Trevena et al. 2006). Pharmacological interventions using analgetics and sedatives frequently offer only a limited effect in coping with stress responses or relieving fears and anxiety (Arts et al. 1994; Badner et al. 1990; Buyukkocak et al. 2006; Caumo and Ferreira 2003). At the same time there is the problem of undesired side effects of such drugs, as well as of causing reduced capacity of patients to collaborate (Jamison 1996; Sullivan et al. 2009).

6.2 Evaluations

Considering the clinical situation described above in 1977, we started to design specific musical interventions, first for perioperative use for psychophysiological preparation and support for patients in anesthesia and surgery. We called this kind of music-based intervention "medicofunctional music," or more specific, "anxioalgolytic" music AAM (1983). AAM comprised pieces of music specifically designed and selected to alleviate pain, distress, and anxiety. In situations where patients suffer from acute stress and pain, for instance, in anesthesia and surgery, in dental treatment, as well as in obstetrics under labor, it became clear that patients themselves should choose their music out of a wide repertoire offered via earphones. (Bernatzky et al. 2011; Spintge and Droh 1992). Such music is applied while aversive stimuli affect patients during treatment or perioperatively. In chronic pain, patients' musical interventions are used to prepare for treatment sessions, or to complement treatment sessions, as well as to conduct musically enhanced, self-administered postprocedural sessions, even at the workplace or in private environment (Spintge 1998a, 1998b, 1999, 2000). Our AAM concept has been continuously further developed and evaluated for both areas, including pre- and post-procedural questionnaires looking into subjective responses of patients amounting to data from 160.000 patients (surgery, obstetrics, dentistry, adult intensive care, Newborn Intensive Care Units, and pain medicine). At the same time, the use of AAM was evaluated in various clinical settings using standard study protocols from traditional medical scientific research, mainly conducted as dissertations in medicine or music therapy (Spintge and Droh 1992; Shin 2020). Study protocols include a selection of physiological and psychological monitoring parameters, such as open questionnaires, the Thematic Apperception Test (see also Westen 1991), behavioral observation and facial expression (facial action coding system; Ekman et al. 1983), stress hormone levels in blood plasma, EEG, positron emission tomography (PET), neurovegetative and cardiovascular parameters (cardiovascular rhythmicity, heart rate variability), drug consumption, duration of in-patient stay, and other economic parameters (Spintge and Droh 1992; Chlan 2018). Nowadays (but consider Rodt 1903) application of medicofunctional music as AAM is frequently used in surgery, anesthesia, dentistry, pain medicine and palliative care, intensive care, obstetrics, pediatrics, geriatrics, ophthalmology, as well as neurology, just to name some examples with scientific evidence and routine application (Arnon et al. 2006; Arts et al. 1994; Bradt 2010; Fowler-Kerry and Lander 1987; Leins 2006; Liu et al. 2007; Maranto 1991; Nelson et al. 2017; Nijkamp 2004; Pratt and Spintge 1996; Spintge 1983; Spintge and Droh 1987; Wulff et al. 2017). Those clinical randomized and controlled studies could demonstrate a wealth of desired effects in clinical settings listed with their recent references in Table 6.1. Such effects include:

- Decrease in heart rate and medium arterial blood pressure
- Harmonizing heart rhythm and elevation of heart rate variability (HRV)
- Decrease in respiratory minute-volume and oxygen demand
- Decrease of blood plasma levels of various stress hormones and neurotransmitters such as adrenalin, noradrenalin, ACTH, cortisol, β-endorphin, combined with reduction of basal metabolic rate and energy consumption, up to sleep induction

In addition, the following psychophysiological effects can be observed.

Table 6.1 Clinical settings and disciplines

Anesthesiology, induction room	Oyama et al. (1987), Bradt (2010)
Anesthesiology, recovery room	Fredriksson et al. (2009)
Anesthesiology, out-patient pediatric surgery	Kain et al. (1997), Wang et al. (2002)
Cardiac surgery	Bradt et al. (2013), Nilsson et al. (2009), Schwartz (2009)
Cardiology	Micci (1984), Thorgaard et al. (2004)
Dentistry	Bradt and Teague (2018), Wazzan et al. (2022)
Gastroenterology, abdominal surgery	Ovayolu et al. (2006)
Gynecological surgery	Binns-Turner et al. (2011), Ikonomidou et al. (2004)
Intensive care, adults	Conrad et al. (2007), Gilad and Arnon (2010), Nelson et al. (2008)
Intensive care, children	Arts et al. (1994), Coleman et al. (1997), Collins and Kuck (1991), Gilad and Arnon (2010), Golianu et al. (2007), Loewy et al. (2005), Lubetzky et al. (2010), Standley (2012), Standley and Moore (1995), Stewart (2009), Tramo et al. (2011)
Cesarean section	Laopaiboon et al. (2009)
Eye surgery, in-patient	Allen et al. (2001), Fernell (2002), Reilly (1999)
Orthopedic surgery	McCaffrey (2009))
Pain medicine	Chai et al. (2017), Campbell et al. (2019), Kullich et al. (2003), Lee (2016), Moss et al. (2023), Pando-Naude et al. (2019), Shim et al. (2017), Siedlecki (2009), Silvestrini et al. (2011), Usui et al. (2020), Shin (2020)
Palliative care, hospice	Canga et al. (2012), Clements-Cortes (2011), Dun (2011), Krout (2001), Stanczyk (2011), Warth et al. (2020)
General surgery, adults	DeMarco et al. (2012), Good et al. (1999), Leardi et al. (2007), Nilsson et al. (2005)
Pediatric surgery	Bradt (2010)

6.3 Psychophysiological Effects of AAM

- Reduction of vegetative nausea and vomiting occurs.
- Stimulation of neuro-immunological receptors for catecholamines, dopamine, and interleukin-6 can be observed leading to rise in antibody levels like IgA in saliva as well as to an increase in T cell-counts and of so-called killer cell activity.
- Pain threshold as well as general pain tolerance are increased. Even a reduction of inflammatory pain can be observed.
- Post-procedural cognitive disorientation and confusion in elder patients can be diminished while general compliance is enhanced.
- Motor behavior can be influenced in reducing restlessness, decreasing muscle tonus and spasms. At the same time, anxiety-driven restlessness is resolved.

Consequently, these psychophysiological effects produce economic advantages, such as decreased drug demand in premedication for anesthesia using

Benzodiazepines (50–100%) as well as postoperative requirement for analgesics (opioids). In our own studies we could demonstrate a reduction of in-patient treatment duration, amounting for instance to a medium of 3 days of incubator treatment in premature newborns, also a medium of 1 day in elderly patients undergoing cataract surgery. Another additional effect is improvement of staff work flow and a harmonization of work routine leading to lesser tension and stress in between staff members as well as in between staff and patients, both enhancing performance outcome and effectiveness at work (Table 6.1). In their review, Bernatzky et al. (2011) could also emphasize such psychophysiological background and desired effects.

6.4 Evidence

Many of our first clinical RCT (randomized controlled trials)—studies have been replicated by other research groups meanwhile. So today there is a wealth of RCTs in various clinical settings and numerous medical disciplines spreading knowledge and music-based intervention concepts on a global scale (Bernatzky and Kreutz 2024; Bernatzky et al. 2007, 2012; Spintge 2007). Through further studies, implementation of music-based interventions into standard regimes is steadily enlarged. That way standard treatment regimens during invasive or other emotionally aversive procedures were compared to medicofunctional music alone or in combination with other intervening variables such as environmental sounds, especially nature sounds. Clinical settings explored include a vast number of medically relevant applications and fields, as listed in Table 6.1.

In all these cases music is used either as a complementary medium in addition to pharmacological treatment to reduce pain, to relax, or to anesthetize patients, or in comparison or competing with drug treatment (Howlin and Rooney 2020). It must be mentioned here, that it is still an open question whether music has a direct positive effect during general anesthesia (Groß et al. 2003; Koelsch et al. 2006; Nilsson et al. 2003; Nilsson et al. 2005). Our knowledge about the operation and spectrum of applications of medicofunctional music becomes more and more complex, especially since brain imaging technologies are used to understand the processes involved. Only one aspect may be mentioned here, which is the question, which musical parameter may be most effective. Some studies, as well as our own research data and clinical experiences, point toward musical rhythm (Avanzini et al. 2005; Bernardi et al. 2009; Koepchen et al. 1992; Parncutt 2012; Rider 1985) and possibly timbre (Cook 2007). In 1939, Erich von Holst first observed a phenomenon he called "relative Koordination," later named entrainment, meaning that outer rhythms interact with inner rhythms of the body (Holst 1939). This happens, for example, with respect to heart rate variability (HRV) and cardio-respiratory rhythmicity (Koepchen et al. 1992; Kranz et al. 2011). However, further neurophysiological research is still necessary to finally identify the missing link between musical structure and biological function (Brown and Jordania 2011; Gomez and Danuser 2007; Koelsch and Friederici 2003; Koepchen et al. 1992; Saarikallio 2012; Spintge 1999). At present, research in that context especially looks into the significance of circadian rhythms and HRV (Jarczok et al. 2013; Koenig et al. 2014; Moser 2005; Moser et al. 1994; Park et al. 2014).

6.5 The Music: Quality, Selection, and Design

Quality standards for design and application of medicofunctional music have been consented after long lasting interdisciplinary discussions, publicized, and implemented (Maranto 1991; Robb and Carpenter 2009; Spintge and Droh 1992; Spintge and Loewy 2011). Table 6.2 comprises standards for receptive applications. It is of highest importance to describe in detail applied musical stimuli in order to secure reliability, validity, and reproducibility of concepts, methods, and research results as precondition for acknowledgement of therapeutic music-based interventions. That had often been impossible in the past before introduction of World Wide Web due to technical reasons. At present Good Scientific Publishing Practice demands in case of self-produced or individually produced pieces of musical stimuli to add an audio file to any manuscript submitted (see for instance Journal Music and Medicine, guidelines for submissions, http://mmd.iammonline.com).

6.6 Clinical Situations with Acute Pain and Anxiety

Beginning in late 1970s until 2020 in our hospital Sportklinik Hellersen, we routinely used AAM preoperatively as well as for patients with chronic pain. Analysis of more than 160.000 pre- and post-procedural patient questionnaires evaluated application of music-based intervention AAM from patient's viewpoint and staff as well. Results showed that it is most important in an acute emotionally aversive situation, that patient chooses his music. In our population a selection of ten different

Table 6.2 Quality standards for medicofunctional music for receptive application

Multidisciplinary team! Nothing without a Music Therapist!
Defined contents (title/source, notation, compository criteria, arrangement, interpretation, instruments, analog/digital, etc.)
Defined dosage (duration, loudness, vibrational impact)
Clear indication (specific to complaint/ailment, situation, target group)
Known effect profile in emotionally standardized situations (anxiolytic, stress reduction, pain decreasing, sleep induction, calming, relaxing, exciting, activating psyche and/or body, contemplative, enhancing focusing, increasing vigilance, enhancing motor/mental performance)
Known risk profile and undesired side effects with reference to setting and subjects, cave! Acoustic environmental pollution
Contraindications (general, specific, active psychic disorder, neurosis, borderline neurosis, suicidality, epileptic seizures, fluid drug addiction)
Technical items specific to situation (loudspeaker/headphones, stereo/mono, two-dimensional/three-dimensional, analog/digital, wired/wireless, foreground/background, receptive/active, subliminal, verbal suggestions)

music genres matches 95% of patient's preferences over that 40 years period. While frequency of choice for different genres varies over time, genre selection itself has stabilized. So patient controlled music ranges from Country Rock, Heavy Metal, Hip-Hop, Techno, House, over Swing to Baroque Music and music from romantic period (Spintge 2000). Today updates of music lists per genre every 3–4 months are necessary to meet rapidly changing trends of musical taste. Especially young patients up to 25 years become more and more sensitive and critical toward musical stimuli in medical settings. Unfortunately, technical aspects and copyright issues interfere with patients' preferences according to specific composer, conductor or music group. A Music Therapist in operating theaters communicating with each individual patient (and staff) has successfully been tested at several places on an anecdotal basis, rather it is unaffordable.

6.7 Clinical Situations with Chronic Pain and Anxiety

Patients with chronic pain, as chronically ill persons, suffer from feeling captured in a cage and thus avoid every additional, especially external restrictive structure. Therefore, music in a chronic situation is quite different from the musical selections mentioned above. Pain patients need musical stimuli opening new horizons, stimulating hope and enticing dreams, as well as facilitating catharsis of elevated stress levels. Pain patients avoid music with strong rhythmic structure. Our offer for pain patients embraces music from New Age, Enya, Nature Sound Scapes, Asian music for pre- and post-procedural waiting situations, as well as specifically designed music programs for specific treatment situations, or for individual self-treatment programs. The design of such musical stimuli addresses each specific treatment goal. Examples comprise stress relaxation via music-enhanced so-called emotional detonization exercise (Emotionales Abspanntraining), or behavioral control during unpleasant or painful treatment procedures aiming at supporting compliance, as well as control of biorhythm-directed activity levels during a 24-h day, and last but not least sleep induction (details in Spintge 1998a, b, 1999).

Among our own pain patients, three main target areas for music-based interventions have been identified and are routinely addressed in daily treatment regimes: myofascial pain, distress, and sleep disorders. To secure desired treatment outcomes in chronic patients, it is essential to transfer such programs as a means for self-support into daily life. Programs consist not only of musical stimuli, but offer a combination of music enhanced exercise programs, dream journey, Guided Imagery, and Nature Sound Scapes, such as for instance a night walk through Australian rain forest, isometric muscle exercises with verbal and musical guidance, and so forth. Patient is obliged by prescription to select their daily program with a mixture of music alone, music-enhanced exercise programs and other components as mentioned before. These personalized programs referring to daytime, weekday or season users gain support in controlling their pain at home and also at work. Finally, patients should be able to better control their ndividual pain perception over the course of the day and at night in various life situations aiming at improving quality of life in general. A word about music: design, composition, notation, instrumentation, technical and artistic performance, all these paramters must offer professional quality. Synthesizer should be avoided. In our own team, we collaborated with a multidisciplinary production team of experts from Music Therapy, medicine, composition (German and Chinese), studio technique and production. The latter with special experience in designing music and soundtracks for movies. Musicians performing were members of professional symphony orchestras such as Berliner Symphoniker, experienced sound technicians were responsible for excellent quality of music productions. Remarkebly, programs designed 20 years ago are still used successfully today, due to the "personal character" of support offered to patients. Details of designing such music programs are complex, as those programs themselves are, because composition parameters are ranging from musical description of circadian rhythms to central nervous connectome activity to compository means expressing certain emotions in a dynamic way. A selection of our developed medicofunctional programs is already described in more detail elsewhere (Spintge 1998a, 1998b, 1999). Bernatzky's research team at University of Salzburg is fostering developments in this area through designing further such therapeutic music programs (Bernatzky et al. 2011). In recent years, applied research has also focused on new areas and new clinical concepts. As examples, besides many other areas fibromyalgia shall be mentioned as a special so-called crux medicorum in pain medicine (Pando-Naude et al. 2019; Usui et al. 2020), also resilience in pain patients in general (Shim et al. 2017) and with special emphasis in palliative care (Warth et al. 2020), as well as with steadily growing significance the field of dementia care(Spintge 2019) and Parkinson's disease (Skogar and Lokk 2016). Each of them presenting their own pain problems hard to treat. New approaches of personalized multimodal pain treatment already embrace individual anti-pain-music programs, composed and recorded in direct active collaboration of each patient with their Music Therapist, and used as a means for self-support in daily life (Shin 2020).

Here, two points must be made clear. First of all, although considering the wealth and evidence of apparently valuable effects of such receptive medicofunctional programs, not at last our clinical experience from 40 years points out, that it is much more effective both for patient and staff to include Music Therapists offering active musical interventions on a regular basis. Trained Music Therapists as members of a multidisciplinary team can introduce their expertise in diagnostic evaluation as well as in treatment regimes in a vast number of medical settings. A most important field is pain medicine and palliative care. However, author is convinced, that it is impossible to create receptive music interventions and programs promising healing for every one, such as for instance a program for "music against headache for all." Groups of patients can be treated with identical therapeutic benefit solely in emotionally matching experienced situations as well as under condition of comparable social and psychological background using standardized music-based interventions. Permanent adaptation to changing environmental influences reaching from society to medical care is essential as demonstrated in case of recent pandemic, ravaging new wars in many regions of the world, and other ground shaking events on our globe.

6.8 Conclusion

Today music-based interventions such as medicofunctional music (AAM) are used on a global scale to improve the psychophysic state of patients in emotionally aversive and pain-driven situations (Cepeda et al. 2006; Dileo and Bradt 2005; Hilliard 2005; Maranto 1991; Moss and Fitzpatrick 2023; Pelletier 2004; Pratt and Spintge 1996; Standley 1986, 2002; Thompson and Kam 2005). While earlier studies focused on therapeutic effects, more recent studies also address economic outcome parameter (Chlan et al. 2018; DeLoach Walworth 2005; Kamioka et al. 2014; Romo and Gifford 2007; Schwartz et al. 1999; Rollins et al. 2009). It can be demonstrated that cost containment can be achieved, for instance, in drug demand, duration of in-patient treatment period in hospitals, effectiveness in staff deployment, as well as in general treatment time (Coleman et al. 1997; DeLoach Walworth 2005; Nilsson et al. 2005; Schwartz et al. 1999; Spintge and Droh 1981). As for any other medical treatment, also for the application of medicofunctional music/music-based interventions against anxiety and pain there do exist standards and definitions clearly described. Research is conducted today following guidelines of medical science appropriately, such mixed-method research concepts and RCTs. As a precondition for evidence-based music-based interventions and other music medicine concepts fact-based and consented guidelines are facilitating discussions about such intervention across professional borders (Loewy 2019; Maranto 1991; Robb and Carpenter 2009; Spintge and Droh 1992), leading to broad acceptance within traditional medical and scientific communities (MacDonald 2013; Spintge 2000). These achievements are the basis for a growing number of physicians and hospitals making use of medicofunctional music, such as AAM in their daily practice as well as in acute and chronic pain (Bernatzky et al. 2007; Campbell et al. 2019; MacDonald et al. 2012; Mathur et al. 2008; Moss and Fitzpatrick 2023; Pölkki et al. 2001; Sonntag et al. 2023; Warth et al. 2020; Wulff et al. 2017).

References

Allen K, Golden LH, Izzo JL, Ching MI, Forrest A, Niles CR et al (2001) Normalization of hypertensive responses during ambulatory surgical stress by perioperative music. Psychosom Med 63(3):487–492. https://doi.org/10.1097/00006842-200105000-00019

Arnon S, Shapsa A, Forman L, Regev R, Bauer S, Litmanovitz I, Dolfin T (2006) Live music is beneficial to preterm infants in the neonatal intensive care unit environment. Birth (Berkeley, Calif) 33(2):131–136. https://doi.org/10.1111/j.0730-7659.2006.00090.x

Arts SE, Abu-Saad HH, Champion GD, Crawford MR, Fisher RJ, Juniper KH, Ziegler JB (1994) Age-related response to lidocaine-prilocaine (EMLA) emulsion and effect of music distraction on the pain of intravenous cannulation. Pediatrics 93(5):797–801. Retrieved from http://www.ncbi.nlm.nih.gov/pubmed/8165081

Avanzini G, Lopez L, Koelsch S, Majno M (eds) (2005) The neurosciences and music II: from perception to performance, vol 1060. Wiley-Blackwell, New York

Badner NH, Nielson WR, Munk S, Kwiatkowska C, Gelb AW (1990) Preoperative anxiety: detection and contributing factors. Can J Anaesth/Journal Canadien d'anesthesie 37(4 Pt 1):444–447. https://doi.org/10.1007/BF03005624

Bernardi L, Porta C, Casucci G, Balsamo R, Bernardi NF, Fogari R, Sleight P (2009) Dynamic interactions between musical, cardiovascular, and cerebral rhythms in humans. Circulation 119(25):3171–3180. https://doi.org/10.1161/circulationaha.108.806174
Bernatzky G, Kreutz G (2024) Musik und Medizin, 2nd edn. Springer, Wien/Heidelberg
Bernatzky G, Likar R, Wendtner F, Wenzel G, Ausserwinkel M, Sittl R (2007) Nichtmedikamentöse Schmerztherapie. Springer, Wien
Bernatzky G, Presch M, Anderson M, Panksepp J (2011) Emotional foundations of music as a non-pharmacological pain management tool in modern medicine. Neurosci Biobehav Rev 35(9):1989–1999. https://doi.org/10.1016/j.neubiorev.2011.06.005
Bernatzky G, Strickner S, Presch M, Wendtner F, Kullich W (2012) In: MacDonald RAR, Kreutz G, Mitchell L (eds) Music as non-pharmacological pain management in clinics. Oxford University Press, London
Binns-Turner PG, Wilson LL, Pryor ER, Boyd GL, Prickett CA (2011) Perioperative music and its effects on anxiety, hemodynamics, and pain in women undergoing mastectomy. AANA J 79(Suppl 4):S21–S27. Retrieved from http://www.ncbi.nlm.nih.gov/pubmed/22403963
Bradt J (2010) The effects of music entrainment on postoperative pain perception in pediatric patients. Music Med 2(3):150–157. https://doi.org/10.1177/1943862110369913
Bradt J, Teague A (2018) Music interventions for dental anxiety. Oral Dis 24(3):300–306. https://doi.org/10.1111/odi.12615
Bradt J, Dileo C, Potvin N (2013) Music for stress and anxiety reduction in coronary heart disease patients. Cochrane Database Syst Rev 2013(12):CD006577. https://doi.org/10.1002/14651858.CD006577.pub3
Brown S, Jordania J (2011) Universals in the world's music. Psychol Music 41(2):229–248
Buyukkocak U, Caglayan O, Daphan C, Aydinuraz K, Saygun O, Agalar F (2006) Similar effects of general and spinal anaesthesia on perioperative stress response in patients undergoing haemorrhoidectomy. Mediat Inflamm 2006(1):97257. https://doi.org/10.1155/MI/2006/97257
Campbell E, Hynynen J, Burger B, Ala-Ruona E (2019) Exploring the use of Vibroacoustic treatment for managing chronic pain and comorbid mood disorders: a mixed methods study. Nord J Music Ther 28(5):1–24. https://doi.org/10.1080/08098131.2019.1604565
Canga B, Hahm CL, Lucido D, Grossbard ML, Loewy JV (2012) Environmental music therapy: a pilot study on the effects of music therapy in a chemotherapy infusion suite. Music Med 4(4):221–230. https://doi.org/10.1177/1943862112462037
Caumo W, Ferreira MBC (2003) Perioperative anxiety: psychobiology and effects in postoperative recovery. Pain Clin 15(2):87–101. https://doi.org/10.1163/156856903321579217
Cepeda MS, Carr DB, Lau J, Alvarez H (2006) Music for pain relief. Cochrane Database Syst Rev 2:CD004843. https://doi.org/10.1002/14651858.CD004843.pub2
Chai PR, Carreiro S, Ranney ML, Karanam K, Ahtisaari M, Edwards R, Boyer EW (2017) Music as an adjunct to opioid-based analgesia. J Med Toxicol 13(3):249–254. https://doi.org/10.1007/s13181-017-0621-9
Chlan LL, Heiderscheit A, Skaar DJ, Neidecker MV (2018) Economic evaluation of a patient-directed music intervention for ICU patients receiving mechanical ventilatory support. Crit Care Med 46(9):1430–1435. https://doi.org/10.1097/CCM.0000000000003199
Clements-Cortes A (2011) Portraits of music therapy in facilitating relationship completion at the end of life. Music Med 3(1):31–39. https://doi.org/10.1177/1943862110388181
Coleman JM, Pratt RR, Stoddard RA, Gerstmann DR, Abel H-H (1997) The effects of the male and female singing and speaking voices on selected physiological and behavioral measures of premature infants in the intensive care unit. Int J Arts Med 5(2):4–11
Collins SK, Kuck K (1991) Music therapy in the neonatal intensive care unit. Neonatal Netw 9(6):23–26. 2000074
Conrad C, Niess H, Jauch K-W, Bruns CJ, Hartl W, Welker L (2007) Overture for growth hormone: requiem for interleukin-6? Crit Care Med 35(12):2709–2713. https://doi.org/10.1097/01.ccm.0000291648.99043.b9
Cook ND (2007) The sound symbolism of major and minor harmonies. Music Percept 24(3):315–319. https://doi.org/10.1525/mp.2007.24.3.315

DeLoach Walworth D (2005) Procedural-support music therapy in the healthcare setting: a cost–effectiveness analysis. J Pediatr Nurs 20(4):276–284. https://doi.org/10.1016/j.pedn.2005.02.016
DeMarco J, Alexander JL, Nehrenz G, Gallagher L (2012) The benefit of music for the reduction of stress and anxiety in patients undergoing elective cosmetic surgery. Music Med 4(1):44–48. https://doi.org/10.1177/1943862111424416
Dileo C, Bradt J (2005) Medical music therapy: a meta-analysis & agenda for future research. Jeffrey Books, Cherry Hill
Dun B (2011) All in good time: a music therapist's reflection of providing a music therapy program in a pediatric cancer center over 20 years. Music Med 3(1):15–19. https://doi.org/10.1177/1943862110391470
Ekman P, Levenson R, Friesen W (1983) Autonomic nervous system activity distinguishes among emotions. Science 221(4616):1208–1210. https://doi.org/10.1126/science.6612338
Fernell J (2002) Listening to music during ambulatory ophthalmic surgery reduced blood pressure, heart rate, and perceived stress. Evid Based Nurs 5(1):16. https://doi.org/10.1136/ebn.5.1.16
Fowler-Kerry S, Lander JR (1987) Management of injection pain in children. Pain 30(2):169–175. https://doi.org/10.1016/0304-3959(87)91072-4
Fredriksson A-C, Hellström L, Nilsson U (2009) Patients' perception of music versus ordinary sound in a postanaesthesia care unit: a randomised crossover trial. Intensive Crit Care Nurs 25(4):208–213. https://doi.org/10.1016/j.iccn.2009.04.002
Gellhorn E (1964) Motion and emotion: the role of proprioception in the physiology and pathologyof the emotions. Psychol Rev 71(6):457–472
Gilad E, Arnon S (2010) The role of live music and singing as a stress-reducing modality in the neonatal intensive care unit environment. Music Med 2(1):18–22. https://doi.org/10.1177/1943862109357070
Golianu B, Krane E, Seybold J, Almgren C, Anand KJS (2007) Non-pharmacological techniques for pain management in neonates. Semin Perinatol 31(5):318–322. https://doi.org/10.1053/j.semperi.2007.07.007
Gomez P, Danuser B (2007) Relationships between musical structure and psychophysiological measures of emotion. Emotion 7(2):377–387. https://doi.org/10.1037/1528-3542.7.2.377
Good M, Stanton-Hicks M, Grass JA, Cranston Anderson G, Choi C, Schoolmeesters LJ, Salman A (1999) Relief of postoperative pain with jaw relaxation, music and their combination. Pain 81(1–2):163–172. https://doi.org/10.1016/s0304-3959(99)00002-0
Groß MAF, Nager W, Schalk F, Piepenbrock SA, Münte TF, Münte S (2003) Unbewusste Wahrnehmung bei Patienten im Operationssaal unter Allgemeinanästhesie: Eine Studie mit Ereigniskorrelierten Potentialen. In: Wissenschaftliche Arbeitstage der DGAI, p 755
Grossi EA, Zakow PK, Ribakove G, Kallenbach K, Ursomanno P, Gradek CE et al (1999) Comparison of post-operative pain, stress response, and quality of life in port access vs. standard sternotomy coronary bypass patients. Eur J Cardio Thorac Surg 16 Suppl 2:S39–S42. Retrieved from http://www.ncbi.nlm.nih.gov/pubmed/10613554
Hilliard RE (2005) Music therapy in hospice and palliative care: a review of the empirical data. Evid Based Complement Alternat Med 2(2):173–178. https://doi.org/10.1093/ecam/neh076
Holst EV (1939) Die relative Koordination als Phänomen und als Methode zentralnervöser Funktionsanalyse (relative coordination as phenomenon and as method for analysis of functioning of central nervous system). Ergeb Physiol Biol Chem Exp Pharmakol 42:228–306. https://doi.org/10.1007/BF02322567
Howlin C, Rooney B (2020) The cognitive mechanisms in music listening interventions for pain: a scoping review. J Music Ther 57(2):127–167. https://doi.org/10.1093/jmt/thaa003
Ikonomidou E, Rehnström A, Naesh O (2004) Effect of music on vital signs and postoperative pain. AORN J 80(2):269–274., 277–278. https://doi.org/10.1016/s0001-2092(06)60564-4
Jamison RN (1996) Psychological factors in chronic pain: assessment and treatment issues. J Back Musculoskelet Rehabil 7(2):79–95. https://doi.org/10.3233/BMR-1996-7202

Jarczok MN, Koenig J, Schuster AK, Thayer JF, Fischer JE (2013) Nighttime heart rate variability, overnight urinary norepinephrine, and glycemic status in apparently healthy human adults. Int J Cardiol 168(3):3025–3026. https://doi.org/10.1016/j.ijcard.2013.04.147

Kain ZN, Mayes LC, Cicchetti DV, Bagnall AL, Finley JD, Hofstadter MB (1997) The Yale preoperative anxiety scale: how does it compare with a "gold standard"? Anesth Analg 85(4) Retrieved from https://journals.lww.com/anesthesia-analgesia/Fulltext/1997/10000/The_Yale_Preoperative_Anxiety_Scale__How_Does_It.12.aspx

Kamioka H, Tsutani K, Yamada M, Park H, Okuizumi H, Tsuruoka K et al (2014) Effectiveness of music therapy: a summary of systematic reviews based on randomized controlled trials of music interventions. Patient Prefer Adherence 8:727–754. https://doi.org/10.2147/PPA.561340

Keller VE (1995) Management of nausea and vomiting in children. J Pediatr Nurs 10(5):280–286. https://doi.org/10.1016/S0882-5963(05)80045-4

Koelsch S, Friederici U (2003) Toward the neural basis of processing structure in music. Comparative results of different neurophysiological methods. Ann N Y Acad Sci 999:15–28

Koelsch S, Heinke W, Sammler D, Olthoff D (2006) Auditory processing during deep propofol sedation and recovery from unconsciousness. Clin Neurophysiol 117(8):1746–1759. https://doi.org/10.1016/j.clinph.2006.05.009

Koenig J, Jarczok MN, Ellis RJ, Hillecke TK, Thayer JF (2014) Heart rate variability and experimentally induced pain in healthy adults: a systematic review. Eur J Pain (London, England) 18(3):301–314. https://doi.org/10.1002/j.1532-2149.2013.00379.x

Koepchen H, Droh R, Spintge R, AbeL H, Kluessendorf D, Koralewski E (1992) Physiological rhythmicity and music in medicine. In: Spintge R, Droh R (eds) MusicMedicine, vol 1. MMB, St. Louis, pp 39–70

Kranz G, Kreutz G, Ericson M, Theorell T (2011) Bodily movements influence heart rate variability (HRV) responses to isolated melodic intervals. Music Med 3(2):108–113. https://doi.org/10.1177/1943862110387612

Krout RE (2001) The effects of single-session music therapy interventions on the observed and self-reported levels of pain control, physical comfort, and relaxation of hospice patients. Am J Hosp Palliat Care 18(6):383–390. https://doi.org/10.1177/104990910101800607

Kullich W, Bernatzky G, Hesse H-P, Wendtner F, Likar R, Klein G (2003) Musiktherapie—Wirkung auf Schmerz, Schlaf und Lebensqualitat bei Low back pain. Wien Med Wochenschr 153(9–10):217–221. https://doi.org/10.1046/j.1563-258X.2003.02081.x

Laopaiboon M, Lumbiganon P, Martis R, Vatanasapt P, Somjaivong B (2009) Music during caesarean section under regional anaesthesia for improving maternal and infant outcomes. Cochrane Database Syst Rev. https://doi.org/10.1002/14651858.CD006914.pub2

Leardi S, Pietroletti R, Angeloni G, Necozione S, Ranalletta G, Del Gusto B (2007) Randomized clinical trial examining the effect of music therapy in stress response to day surgery. Br J Surg 94(8):943–947. https://doi.org/10.1002/bjs.5914

Lee JH (2016) The effects of music on pain: a meta-analysis. J Music Ther 53(4):430–477. https://doi.org/10.1093/jmt/thw012

Leins AK (2006) Heidelberger Musiktherapiemanual: Migräne bei Kindern. uni-edition, Bochum

Liu RW, Mehta P, Fortuna S, Armstrong DG, Cooperman DR, Thompson GH, Gilmore A (2007) A randomized prospective study of music therapy for reducing anxiety during cast room procedures. J Pediatr Orthop 27(7):831–833. https://doi.org/10.1097/BPO.0b013e3181558a4e

Loewy J (2019) Efficacy of pain management: integration versus distraction. Music Med 11(1). https://doi.org/10.47513/mmd.v11i1.662

Loewy J, Hallan C, Friedman E, Martinez C (2005) Sleep/sedation in children undergoing EEG testing: a comparison of chloral hydrate and music therapy. J Perianesth Nurs 20(5):323–331. https://doi.org/10.1016/j.jopan.2005.08.001

Lubetzky R, Mimouni FB, Dollberg S, Reifen R, Ashbel G, Mandel D (2010) Effect of music by Mozart on energy expenditure in growing preterm infants. Pediatrics 125(1):e24–e28. https://doi.org/10.1542/peds.2009-0990

MacDonald RAR (2013) Music, health, and well-being: a review. Int J Qual Stud Health Well Being 8(1):20635. https://doi.org/10.3402/qhw.v8i0.20635

MacDonald RAR, Kreutz G, Mitchell L (2012) Music, health, and wellbeing. In: MacDonald R, Kreutz G, Mitchell L (eds) Music, health, and wellbeing. Oxford University Press, Oxford. https://doi.org/10.1093/acprof:oso/9780199586974.001.0001

Maranto CD (1991) Applications of music in medicine. National Association for Music Therapy, Silver Spring

Mathur A, Duda L, Kamat DM (2008) Knowledge and use of music therapy among pediatric practitioners in Michigan. Clin Pediatr 47(2):155–159. https://doi.org/10.1177/0009922807306777

McCaffrey RG (2009) The effect of music on the cognition of older adults undergoing hip and knee surgery. Music Med 1(1):22–28. https://doi.org/10.1177/1943862109335215

Micci NO (1984) The use of music therapy with pediatric patients undergoing cardiac catheterization. Arts Psychother 11(4):261–266. https://doi.org/10.1016/0197-4556(84)90023-6

Mondanaro J, Sara G (2013) Music and medicine: integrative models in the treatment of pain. Satchnote Press, New York. ISBN: 978-0-615-72042-8

Moser M (2005) Innovative Parameter zur Messung von Beanspruchung und Erholung in der Arbeitsmedizin. Österreichisches Forum Arbeitsmedizin:12–17

Moser M, Lehofer M, Sedminek A, Lux M, Zapotoczky HG, Kenner T, Noordergraaf A (1994) Heart rate variability as a prognostic tool in cardiology. A contribution to the problem from a theoretical point of view. Circulation 90(2):1078–1082. https://doi.org/10.1161/01.CIR.90.2.1078

Moss H, Fitzpatrick K (2023) "What do you need? And how can I help?" The role of music and music therapy in chronic pain. Music Med 15(2). https://doi.org/10.47513/mmd.v15i2.939

Moss H, Fitzpatrick K, O'Shea P (2023) An agenda for excellence: the role of music therapy for people living with chronic pain. Music Med 15(2). https://doi.org/10.47513/mmd.v15i2.925

Munafo MR (1998) Perioperative anxiety and postoperative pain. Psychol Health Med 3(4):429–433. https://doi.org/10.1080/13548509808400616

Nelson A, Hartl W, Jauch K-W, Fricchione GL, Benson H, Warshaw AL, Conrad C (2008) The impact of music on hypermetabolism in critical illness—a review. Cuur Opin Nutr Metab Care 11(6):790–794. https://doi.org/10.1097/MCO.0b013e328314dd01

Nelson K, Adamek M, Kleiber C (2017) Relaxation training and postoperative music therapy for adolescents undergoing spinal fusion surgery. Pain Manage Nurs 18(1):16–23. https://doi.org/10.1016/j.pmn.2016.10.005

Nijkamp MD (2004) Determinants of surgery related anxiety in cataract patients. Br J Ophthalmol 88(10):1310–1314. https://doi.org/10.1136/bjo.2003.037788

Nilsson U, Rawal N, Unosson M (2003) A comparison of intra-operative or postoperative exposure to music—a controlled trial of the effects on postoperative pain. Anaesthesia 58(7):699–703. https://doi.org/10.1046/j.1365-2044.2003.03189_4.x

Nilsson U, Unosson M, Rawal N (2005) Stress reduction and analgesia in patients exposed to calming music postoperatively: a randomized controlled trial. Eur J Anaesthesiol 22(2):96–102. https://doi.org/10.1017/s0265021505000189

Nilsson U, Lindell L, Eriksson A, Kellerth T (2009) The effect of music intervention in relation to gender during coronary angiographic procedures: a randomized clinical trial. Eur J Cardiovasc Nurs 8(3):200–206. https://doi.org/10.1016/j.ejcnurse.2009.01.001

Nolan P (1992) Music therapy with bone marrow transplant patients: reaching beyond the symptoms. In: Spintge R, Droh R (eds) MusicMedicine, vol 1. MMB, St. Louis, pp 209–212

Norman JG, Fink GW (1997) The effects of epidural anesthesia on the neuroendocrine response to major surgical stress: a randomized prospective trial. Am Surg 63(1):75–80. Retrieved from http://www.ncbi.nlm.nih.gov/pubmed/8985076

Ovayolu N, Ucan O, Pehlivan S, Pehlivan Y, Buyukhatipoglu H, Savas M-C, Gulsen M-T (2006) Listening to Turkish classical music decreases patients' anxiety, pain, dissatisfaction and the dose of sedative and analgesic drugs during colonoscopy: a prospective randomized controlled trial. World J Gastroenterol 12(46):7532–7536. https://doi.org/10.3748/wjg.v12.i46.7532

Oyama T, Sato Y, Kudo T, Spintge R, Droh R (1987) Effect of anxiolytic music on endocrine function in surgical patients. In: Music in medicine. Springer, Heidelberg, pp 169–174

Pando-Naude V, Barrios FA, Alcauter S, Pasaye EH, Vase L, Brattico E et al (2019) Functional connectivity of music-induced analgesia in fibromyalgia. Sci Rep 9(1):15486. https://doi.org/10.1038/s41598-019-51990-4

Park M, Gutyrchik E, Bao Y, Zaytseva Y, Carl P, Welker L et al (2014) Differences between musicians and non-musicians in neuro-affective processing of sadness and fear expressed in music. Neurosci Lett 566:120–124. https://doi.org/10.1016/j.neulet.2014.02.041

Parncutt R (2012) In: Hallam S, Cross I, Thaut M (eds) Prenatal development and the phylogeny and ontogeny of music, vol 1. Oxford University Press, Oxford. https://doi.org/10.1093/oxfordhb/9780199298457.013.0020

Pelletier CL (2004) The effect of music on decreasing arousal due to stress: a meta-analysis. J Music Ther 41(3):192–214. https://doi.org/10.1093/jmt/41.3.192

Pölkki T, Vehviläinen-Julkunen K, Pietilä A-M (2001) Nonpharmacological methods in relieving children's postoperative pain: a survey on hospital nurses in Finland. J Adv Nurs 34(4):483–492. https://doi.org/10.1046/j.1365-2648.2001.01777.x

Pratt RR, Spintge R (1996) MusicMedicine, vol 2. MMB, St. Louis

Reilly M (1999) Music, a cognitive behavioral intervention for anxiety and acute pain control in elderly cataract patients. Dissertation The University of Texas School of Biomedical Sciences, San Antonio

Rider MS (1985) Entrainment mechanisms are involved in pain reduction, muscle relaxation, and music-mediated imagery. J Music Ther 22(4):183–192. https://doi.org/10.1093/jmt/22.4.183

Robb SL, Carpenter JS (2009) A review of music-based intervention reporting in Pediatrics. J Health Psychol 14(4):490–501. https://doi.org/10.1177/1359105309103568

Rodt EV (1903) Musik und NARKOSE. Stämpfli & Cie, Basel; retrieved from University of California ; digitized, Jun 29, 2016

Rollins J, Sonke J, Cohen R, Boles A (2009) State of the field report: arts in healthcare 2009. NAAPPD State of the Field Committee, Washington, DC. https://www.artsandhealthalliance.org

Romo R, Gifford L (2007) A cost-benefit analysis of music therapy in a home hospice. Nurs Econ 25(6):353–358. Retrieved from http://www.ncbi.nlm.nih.gov/pubmed/18240837

Saarikallio S (2012) Development and validation of the brief music in mood regulation scale (B-MMR). Music Percept 30(1):30–105. https://doi.org/10.1525/mp.2012.30.1.97

Salimpoor VN, Benovoy M, Longo G, Cooperstock JR, Zatorre RJ (2009) The rewarding aspects of music listening are related to degree of emotional arousal. PLoS One 4(10):e7487. https://doi.org/10.1371/journal.pone.0007487

Schön J, Gerlach K, Hüppe M (2007) Einfluss negativer Stressverarbeitung auf postoperatives Schmerzerleben und -verhalten. Schmerz 21(2):146–153. https://doi.org/10.1007/s00482-006-0513-4

Schwartz F (2009) A pilot study of patients in postoperative cardiac surgery. Music Med 1(1):70–74. https://doi.org/10.1177/1943862109338189

Schwartz F, Ritchie R, Sacks L, Phillips C (1999) Music, stress reduction and medical cost savings in the neonatal care unit. In: Pratt RR, Grocke DE (eds) MusicMedicine, vol 3. University of Melbourne Press, Melbourne, pp 120–130

Shim M, Johnson RB, Gasson S, Goodill S, Jermyn R, Bradt J (2017) A model of dance/movement therapy for resilience-building in people living with chronic pain. Eur J Integr Med 9:27–40. https://doi.org/10.1016/j.eujim.2017.01.011

Shin HD (2020) Wenn Schmerzen sich in Musik verwandeln. Eine empirische Untersuchung zu einem neuen Konzept musiktherapeutischer Behandlung bei chronisch Schmerzkranken. Dissertation, Hochschule für Musik und Theater Hamburg, Hamburg

Siedlecki SL (2009) Racial variation in response to music in a sample of African-American and Caucasian chronic pain patients. Pain Manag Nurs 10(1):14–21. https://doi.org/10.1016/j.pmn.2008.08.003

Silvestrini N, Piguet V, Cedraschi C, Zentner MR (2011) Music and auditory distraction reduce pain: emotional or attentional effects? Music Med 3(4):264–270. https://doi.org/10.1177/1943862111414433

Skogar O, Lokk J (2016) Pain management in patients with Parkinson's disease: challenges and solutions. J Multidiscip Healthc 9:469–479. https://doi.org/10.2147/JMDH.S105857

Sonntag J, Preissler P, Treß J, Weymann E (2023) Establishing healing soundscapes through musical soundscape interventions in hospitals. Music Med 15(4):227–233. https://doi.org/10.47513/mmd.v15i4.928

Spintge R (1983) Psychophysiologische operations-fitness mit und ohne anxiolyti-sche Musik. In: Droh R, Spintge R (eds) Angst, Schmerz, Musik in der Anaesthesie. Editiones Roche, Grenzach, pp 77–88

Spintge R (1998a) Selbsthilfe bei Verspannungsschmerz. A handbook and audio program. Universal Music—Polymedia, Hamburg

Spintge R (1998b) Selbsthilfe zur Stressbewältigung. A handbook and audio program. Universal Music—Polymedia, Hamburg

Spintge R (1999) Selbsthilfe bei Schlafförderung. A handbook and audio program. Universal Music—Polymedia, Hamburg

Spintge R (2000) Musik in Anaesthesie und Schmerztherapie. AINS—Anästhesiologie · Intensivmedizin · Notfallmedizin · Schmerztherapie 35(04):243–261. https://doi.org/10.1055/s-2000-10852-5

Spintge R (2007) *Musik im Gesundheitswesen*. Schriftenreihe zur Gesundheitsanalyse. Gmünder Ersatzkasse, Schwäbisch Gmünd

Spintge R (2019) Musik und Demenz—Perspektiven einer wachsenden Beziehung. DMW—Deutsche Medizinische Wochenschrift 144(25):1810–1815. https://doi.org/10.1055/a-0988-3132

Spintge R, Droh R (1981) Die präoperative Angst. Intensivmedizinische Praxis/Intensivmedizinische Praxis 4:29–33

Spintge R, Droh R (1987) Musik in der Medizin/Music in medicine. Springer, Heidelberg

Spintge R, Droh R (1992) MusicMedicine, vol 1. MMB, St. Louis

Spintge R, Loewy JV (2011) At a crossroads: big questions—little knowledge in achievements, with issues of translation. Music Med 3(4):209–212. https://doi.org/10.1177/1943862111418121

Stanczyk MM (2011) Music therapy in supportive cancer care. Rep Pract Oncol Radiother 16(5):170–172. https://doi.org/10.1016/j.rpor.2011.04.005

Standley JM (1986) Music research in medical/dental treatment: meta-analysis and clinical applications. J Music Ther 23(2):56–122. https://doi.org/10.1093/jmt/23.2.56

Standley JM (2002) A meta-analysis of the efficacy of music therapy for premature infants. J Pediatr Nurs 17(2):107–113. https://doi.org/10.1053/jpdn.2002.124128

Standley JM (2012) Music therapy research in the NICU: an updated meta-analysis. Neonatal Netw 31(5):311–316. https://doi.org/10.1891/0730-0832.31.5.311

Standley JM, Moore RS (1995) Therapeutic effects of music and mother's voice on premature infants. Pediatr Nurs 21(6):509–512, 574. Retrieved from http://www.ncbi.nlm.nih.gov/pubmed/8700604

Stewart K (2009) PATTERNS—a model for evaluating trauma in NICU music therapy: part 1—theory and design. Music Med 1(1):29–40. https://doi.org/10.1177/1943862109338370

Stirling L (2006) Reduction and management of perioperative anxiety. Br J Nurs 15(7):359–361. https://doi.org/10.12968/bjon.2006.15.7.20896

Sullivan M, Tanzer M, Stanish W, Fallaha M, Keefe FJ, Simmonds M, Dunbar M (2009) Psychological determinants of problematic outcomes following total knee arthroplasty. Pain 143(1–2):123–129. https://doi.org/10.1016/j.pain.2009.02.011

Thompson JF, Kam PCA (2005) Music in the operating theatre. Br J Surg 82(12):1586–1587. https://doi.org/10.1002/bjs.1800821203

Thorgaard B, Henriksen BB, Pedersbæk G, Thomsen I (2004) Specially selected music in the cardiac laboratory—an important tool for improvement of the wellbeing of patients. Eur J Cardiovasc Nurs 3(1):21–26. https://doi.org/10.1016/j.ejcnurse.2003.10.001

Tolksdorf W (1997) Preoperative stress. Research approach and methods of treatment. Anasthesiologie, Intensivmedizin, Notfallmedizin, Schmerztherapie: AINS 32(Suppl 3):S318–S324. https://doi.org/10.1055/s-2007-995183

Tramo MJ, Lense M, Van Ness C, Kagan J, Settle MD, Cronin JH (2011) Effects of music on physiological and behavioral indices of acute pain and stress in premature infants: clinical trial and literature review. Music Med 3(2):72–83. https://doi.org/10.1177/1943862111400613

Trevena LJ, Davey HM, Barratt A, Butow P, Caldwell P (2006) A systematic review on communicating with patients about evidence. J Eval Clin Pract 12(1):13–23. https://doi.org/10.1111/j.1365-2753.2005.00596.x

Usui C, Kirino E, Tanaka S, Inami R, Nishioka K, Hatta K et al (2020) Music intervention reduces persistent fibromyalgia pain and alters functional connectivity between the insula and default mode network. Pain Med 21(8):1546–1552. https://doi.org/10.1093/pm/pnaa071

Wang S-M, Kulkarni L, Dolev J, Kain ZN (2002) Music and preoperative anxiety: a randomized, controlled study. Anesth Analg 94(6):1489–1494. https://doi.org/10.1213/00000539-200206000-00021

Warth M, Zöller J, Köhler F, Aguilar-Raab C, Kessler J, Ditzen B (2020) Psychosocial interventions for pain management in advanced cancer patients: a systematic review and meta-analysis. Curr Oncol Rep 22(1):3. https://doi.org/10.1007/s11912-020-0870-7

Wazzan M, Estaitia M, Habrawi S, Mansour D, Jalal Z, Ahmed H et al (2022) The effect of music therapy in reducing dental anxiety and lowering physiological stressors. Acta Bio Med: Atenei Parmensis 92(6):e2021393. https://doi.org/10.23750/abm.v92i6.11668

Westen D (1991) Clinical assessment of object relations using the TAT. J Pers Assess 56(1):56–74. https://doi.org/10.1207/s15327752jpa5601_6

Wulff V, Hepp P, Fehm T, Schaal N (2017) Music in obstetrics: an intervention option to reduce tension, pain and stress. Geburtshilfe Und Frauenheilkunde 77(09):967–975. https://doi.org/10.1055/s-0043-118414

Listening to Music in Depression and Dementia: From Brain Research to Clinical Application

7

Katarzyna Grebosz-Haring, Günther Bernatzky, Franz Wendtner, and Gunter Kreutz

There are numerous studies on the cerebral correlates of listening to music, with implications for music therapy and medical interventions. Depression and dementia are two such areas that, for different reasons, have become the focus of music interventions in health contexts. The chapter highlights how brain research has begun to inform this literature. However, there remain large research gaps between neurobiological foundations and clinical applications of music listening in clinical target groups.

K. Grebosz-Haring (✉)
Interuniversity Organisation Arts & Knowledges, Department of Art History, Musicology and Dance Studies, Mozarteum University Salzburg, University of Salzburg, Salzburg, Austria
e-mail: katarzyna.grebosz-haring@plus.ac.at

G. Bernatzky
Department of Biosciences and Medical Biology, University of Salzburg, Salzburg, Austria

F. Wendtner
Universitätsklinik für Psychiatrie, Psychotherapie und Psychosomatik, Universitätsklinik für Innere Medizin III, mit Hämatologie, internistischer Onkologie, Hämostaseologie, Infektiologie, Rheumatologie und Onkologisches Zentrum, University Hospital Salzburg (SALK), Salzburg, Austria
e-mail: f.wendtner@salk.at

G. Kreutz
Systematic Musicology, Carl von Ossietzky University Oldenburg, Oldenburg, Lower Saxony, Germany

G. Kreutz, G. Bernatzky (eds.), *Music and Medicine*, Neurocultural Health and Wellbeing, https://doi.org/10.1007/978-3-662-72175-9_7

7.1 Cerebral Correlates of Listening to Music

Empirical studies indicate that listening to music evokes positive emotions (Kallinen and Ravaja 2006; Salimpoor et al. 2009), can elevate mood (Völker 2021), and is experienced by individuals as both stimulating and relaxing (Bernardi et al. 2006; Greenberg et al. 2015; Panksepp and Bernatzky 2002). Moreover, listening to music can alleviate stress and anxiety (see Chap. 6 in this volume) and is associated with reduced cortisol levels (Dell'Anna et al. 2021; Fukui and Yamashita 2003; Kreutz et al. 2012). Such observations also form the basis for treatment approaches in adjunctive therapy for a variety of psychosomatic complaints and disorders (Bernatzky and Hesse 2013; Bernatzky et al. 2012). However, the transferability of these research results on the potential to activate or regulate emotions to possible rehabilitation therapies and relapse prophylaxes in patients with neurological disorders remains unclear.

The approaches of neurocognition provide key insights and neuronal foundations regarding musical processing and musical experiences, which are often associated with emotional or affective responses (e.g., Koelsch 2014). Imaging techniques (Positron Emission Tomography—PET, Functional Magnetic Resonance Imaging—fMRI) and electrophysiological methods (Electroencephalography—EEG, Magnetoencephalography—MEG) are particularly suitable for exploring brain physiological correlates of music perception and music cognition. These methods are increasingly used in music psychological and therapeutic research (Fachner and Stegemann 2013).

Existing functional imaging studies on music and emotion show that listening to music activates those limbic and paralimbic brain regions known to be heavily involved in the processing of reward and emotions, including the amygdala (Blood and Zatorre 2001; Koelsch 2014), the nucleus accumbens (NAc; Mavridis 2015), the hippocampus (Blood et al. 1999), the anterior cingulate and insula (Blood and Zatorre 2001; Menon and Levitin 2005), and the orbitofrontal and medial prefrontal cortex (OMPFC; Blood et al. 1999; Blood and Zatorre 2001; for an overview, see Koelsch 2014).

In a groundbreaking study by Blood et al. (1999), the authors used music excerpts that featured varying degrees of dissonance. These differences allowed the researchers to assign activations to different structures of the midbrain. By contrast, Blood and Zatorre (2001) used highly pleasurable music and exploited the fact that music perceived as intensely enjoyable by some participants did not elicit the same feelings in others. This demonstrated that differences in emotional processing are linked to specific brain structures. Peripheral physiological measurements (heart rate, muscle activity, and respiration rate) also corresponded with the emotional effects. Many follow-up studies reveal a differentiated picture of emotional music processing, including the activation of dopaminergic systems (Salimpoor et al. 2009; van den Bosch et al. 2013). The findings of music-evoked activation changes in the core structures of emotion processing in the brain provide an important basis for understanding cerebral music processing itself and for developing potential clinical applications (Koelsch and Stegemann 2012; Sihvonen et al. 2017).

7.2 Adjuvant Therapies for People Living with Depression

Depression is the most common mental illness (Kessler et al. 2003; Moussavi et al. 2007)[1] and one of the leading causes of the global disease burden (Vos et al. 2015). It impacts almost every aspect of life for those affected and is associated with severe consequences (see also Chap. 14 in this volume).

Depressive disorders are subject to multifactorial causes, with biological, psychological, and social factors clearly playing an important role (Kasper et al. 2012; Palazidou 2012). Research approaches from molecular biology, imaging, and neuroendocrinology have revealed that depressive disorders are apparently linked to and interact with many different organ and functional systems (Chechko et al. 2016; Herbert and Lucassen 2016; Riccelli et al. 2016).

The treatment of depression depends on its classification and primarily relies on psychopharmacological and psychotherapeutic strategies. Often, a combination of both therapies is recommended (Cipriani et al. 2018; Gartlehner et al. 2017). Particular challenges in the treatment of depressed patients arise from the high probability of relapse and the tendency toward chronicity, as 20–40% of patients do not or insufficiently respond to psychopharmacological therapy (Mathew and Charney 2009; Moret 2005; Pigott et al. 2010; Rief et al. 2009; Willner et al. 2013).

The search for supportive therapy measures that work in combination with various medications to relieve psychopathological symptoms in patients with depression is therefore essential. Given the complexity of depressive disorders, multimodal therapeutic approaches are indicated (Boeker 2009). Antidepressant pharmacotherapy is often supplemented or replaced by so-called complementary methods, such as sports and exercise therapies, physiotherapy, acupuncture, aromatherapy, herbal therapy, homeopathy, light therapy, yoga, mindfulness-based therapies, balneotherapy, and even art, music, and dance therapies (Chen et al. 2021; Haller et al. 2019; Lehofer and Stuppäck 2005).

7.3 Music Interventions in Depression

Music interventions are widely accepted in the treatment of depressive disorders. They have sparked significant research interest (see Chap. 14 for a comprehensive overview). Music-based activities address both individuals with primary psychiatric treatment needs and numerous groups of patients with other primary conditions (Aalbers et al. 2017; Dhippayom et al. 2022; Gold et al. 2009; Maratos et al. 2008).

Initial findings suggest that music therapy has more favorable effects on the depressive symptoms of patients than standard treatment alone (Dolle and Schulte-Körne 2014; Geipel et al. 2018; Gold et al. 2009; Heise et al. 2013; Maratos et al. 2008). It should be noted, however, that although active creative music therapy concepts show great potential (Albornoz 2011; Erkkilä et al. 2011; Fachner et al. 2013; Gold et al. 2009), that potential is rarely realized at the standards of clinical practice.

[1] http://www.who.int/mediacentre/factsheets/fs369/en/ (Accessed on 7.3.2023).

Review articles with meta-analyses examined the effectiveness of music-based treatments in older adults (Dhippayom et al. 2022; Zhao et al. 2016) and groups with heterogeneous conditions (Tang et al. 2020). They show the significance but also the challenges and problems of music-based interventions. In reviewing 15 randomized controlled studies of older adults (67–86 years), Dhippayom et al. (2022) found that short-term, low-dose interventions of less than 60 min per week could only alleviate depressive symptoms if the music therapy were combined with standard treatment. Music-based interventions with only a receptive format and short duration showed no measurable effect. These findings confirm observations by Zhao et al. (2016) and suggest that the interventions are to a certain extent effective for older people with depression but also observed a lack of methodologically high-quality studies.

Tang et al. (2020) included different patient groups in their research review and meta-analysis to delineate the effects of music therapeutic and music medical interventions. The latter include guided and free imagining to music, music-induced relaxation, and discussion groups about music. Key findings of the analysis were (a) the effectiveness of both forms of intervention, (b) an increased effectiveness over shorter, rather than longer, periods of time, and (c) a generally high methodological quality. The only aspect that was often neglected in studies was the use of blinding, i.e., the separation of information about group affiliation and measurement results during the conduct of the studies.

The findings discussed so far build on high methodological standards (Aalbers et al. 2017; Maratos et al. 2008). For example, Aalbers et al. (2017) recommend music therapy interventions (active and receptive forms) as an additional measure to standard treatment based on a Cochrane review. However, they recognize the need for further research, especially with regard to conditions such as duration, scope, and form of music therapy. According to these authors, there is a lack of detailed description and information about the music therapy practitioners with diverse music therapeutic backgrounds and training. Finally, they question to what extent music therapy can sustainably contribute to reduce depressive symptoms, such that individuals can keep their professions, partake in other activities, and maintain their social relationships. The number and scope of studies appear to be far too small to answer all of these questions.

So-called music medicine interventions, often in the form of listening to patient-selected music, are frequently because of a lack of trained music therapists. Such music interventions can be implemented by medical staff that has received additional training to facilitate access to music, or by organizing musical events. It is important, however, that opportunities for listening to music are accompanied by some guidance to support the convalescence and self-determination of individuals in the target groups as they manage their daily lives in the clinic.

7.4 Biomarkers

Recent neurobiological studies provide evidence of the effectiveness of musical interventions in helping to treat depression (see also Chap. 14, this volume). These studies investigate how people with mental illnesses process music and to what extent the music-induced activations on various levels can positively influence disease patterns (Koelsch 2009).

Field et al. (1998) examined female adolescents ($N = 14$) as they either listened to pop music or relaxed in silence for about 20 min. No statistically significant difference was found between the groups and in the pre- and post-surveys regarding their reported moods. However, the authors found a significant reduction in cortisol levels in members of the music group, associated with a reduced activation of the right frontal lobe during and after listening to music (measured by electroencephalogram, EEG). In a similar study, Tornek et al. (2003) examined the short-term effects of listening to music (20-min sessions of rock music and classical music) on 48 young mothers with depressive symptoms. Significant positive effects were found in the rock music group in anxiety reduction (measured with State Anxiety Inventory, STAI; Spielberger et al. 1983) and depressive mood (measured with Profile of Mood States, POMS; Mcnair et al. 1971). These results are consistent with the reduction of cortisol and the significant change in resting EEG.

Fachner et al. (2013) found a neuronal reorganization in frontotemporal areas in an EEG during active improvised music therapy, which was used as an additional treatment method to the usual standard treatment for depressive patients. After 3 months of music therapy interventions, a significant increase in alpha and theta amplitudes was observed in the left frontal lobe, which coordinates positive emotions and approach behavior. The activation of cortical processes in the left frontal lobe, which can be traced in an EEG, is discussed in the EEG literature as an indication of depression and anxiety in individuals. The changes in resting EEG correlated with clinically relevant reductions in depression (measured with MADRS; Rush Jr et al. 2009) and anxiety states (measured with HADS-A; Aro et al. 2004).

Some studies using imaging techniques for emotion induction by musical auditory stimuli suggest altered processes and mechanisms in subjects with depressive illness compared to healthy control subjects. Osuch et al. (2009) used functional MRI (fMRI) to investigate the neurophysiological reward sensation in preferred instrumental music compared to neutral music in healthy control subjects ($N = 15$) and depressive patients ($N = 16$). The authors found activations of the midbrain, particularly in the nucleus accumbens and ventral striatum, as well as in areas of the left medial orbitofrontal cortex in the healthy, but not in the depressive patients. The authors suspect a form of anhedonia in people with depressive disorders. It remains unclear to what extent this is a generalized or music-related disturbance of the reward sensation. Aust et al. (2013) found in another fMRI study that participants with a remitted depression showed less activation in the anterior cingulate cortex (ACC; regions responsible for changes in connectivity and activity in patients with depression) in response to both positive/pleasant and negative/unpleasant musical emotional stimuli (Aust et al. 2013). In addition, the authors point out that stress, coping style, and anxiety modulate these effects. Lepping et al. (2016) provided further evidence of divergent cerebral activation patterns in emotional musical and nonmusical stimuli in the ACC between subjects with depressive disorders and healthy control subjects. Particularly in the assessment of negative stimuli, the depressive patients showed a stronger reaction.

These results suggest that people with depression may process emotional auditory stimuli differently, based both on the type of stimulation and on the emotional content of this stimulation. This increases the possibility that music can be useful in retraining ACC function, which may lead to more effective and targeted treatments.

Recent studies propose a learning model for diagnosing and investigating "Major Depression"in the brain using receptive music and varying emotional content of this stimulation and fMRI data (Gui et al. 2019).

7.5 Music Interventions in Dementia

Dementia refers to various degenerative and chronically progressive diseases of the brain, which lead to memory problems and other behavioral disorders. Moreover, there is a high comorbidity with depressive symptoms (Livingston et al. 2014). Taking into account individual music preferences, listening to music can act as a carrier of emotions for people with dementia and evoke autobiographical memories associated with emotional reactions (El Haj et al. 2012; Sihvonen et al. 2017). In this context, Sihvonen and colleagues identified 17 randomized controlled studies with dementia patients in their review. In most of the studies, interventionists selected vocal or instrumental music that was presumably familiar to the patients, such as personal favorite songs, general popular music or well-known children's songs. Listening to music combined with cognitive training or physical movement led in some studies to the improvement of general cognitive performance compared to standard treatment. In addition, positive results were observed in terms of attention and executive functions, orientation, and verbal and episodic memory. In some studies, listening to music improved mood or reduced agitation, anxiety, and depression. The authors speculate that the cognitive-emotional gains could be explained by music-induced dopamine responses and the reward system in the brain. Another mechanism for the improvement of neuropsychiatric symptoms could be the music-induced activation of the parasympathetic nervous system. However, the causal link between music-induced mood improvement and neurological changes remains unclear (Sihvonen et al. 2017). Furthermore, the authors point out that familiar music activates the medial prefrontal cortex in healthy people and that the medial prefrontal cortex degenerates more slowly in people with Alzheimer's disease. This offers a possible explanation for why patients with Alzheimer's are able to recognize familiar songs even in the late stages of the disease, thereby retrieving personally meaningful episodic memories (see also El Haj et al. 2012; Eschrich et al. 2008; Janata 2009; Moreno-Morales et al. 2020; Pereira et al. 2011). Positive feelings can improve the memory of music pieces at least in the short term (Eschrich et al. 2008), as confirmed by a review with meta-analysis by Moreno-Morales et al. (2020).

However, it remains unknown how positive feelings toward music affect long-term memory, and which other factors promote the formation of relevant music autobiographical memories.

7.6 Brain Research on Music Listening and Dementia

The neurophysiological mechanisms behind musical interventions in dementia are increasingly the subject of imaging studies. King et al. (2019) used functional magnetic resonance imaging (fMRI) to investigate the cerebral correlates of preferred music in 17 Alzheimer's dementia patients based on excerpts that were also played backward. The authors found activations in the supplementary motor area when listening to preferred music excerpts, a region associated with memory for familiar music that is hardly affected in the early stages of Alzheimer's disease. They also found an increase in functional connectivity in both cortical and cerebellar networks associated with sensory and attention-related functions after the presentation of preferred music excerpts.

A study protocol by Flo et al. (2022) considers cerebral correlates of an active musical intervention (singing) compared to physical activity in a cohort of people with dementia and depressive moods as part of a 12-month, randomized-controlled clinical trial. In addition, cognition and activities of daily life are a primary focus. Such studies are suitable for determining the effectiveness of different interventions and providing indications of their clinical relevance.

7.7 Conclusions

Listening to music appears, according to existing findings, to be a sufficiently targeted and adjuvant effective intervention to supplement treatment and rehabilitation procedures. A prerequisite for this is the creation of suitable framework conditions. The development of a standard for musical anamnesis seems urgent in order to better define potential target groups.

It remains unclear how depressive and demented patients process musical stimuli based on the individual severity of the disease. Therefore, it would be important to capture the effect of the musical stimuli with regard to time-structuring features such as tempo and rhythm, as well as tonality, melody, and harmony, taking into account the different degrees of severity of the disease, and to analyze those in relation to synchronization and regulation processes. Further, there is a need to differentiate activation-promoting and relaxation-promoting elements in music interventions. Finally, the timing and duration of musical listening, for example, over the circadian cycle, could be important factors that systematically influence their effectiveness.

Taken together, the available studies so far confirm that listening to music may support the treatment of people living with depression, or dementia. The results refer to the average changes in psychological assessments and additional studies using biomarkers. In particular, there is little insight into short- or long-term neuronal changes due to music-receptive interventions. Psychobiological foundations of musical perception in mentally ill people are also largely uninvestigated. The challenge is to capture and evaluate behavioral and biological changes in the relevant real-life contexts.

References

Aalbers S, Fusar-Poli L, Freeman RE, Spreen M, Ket JC, Vink AC, Maratos A, Crawford M, Chen XJ, Gold C (2017) Music therapy for depression. Cochrane Database Syst Rev 11(11):CD004517. https://doi.org/10.1002/14651858.CD004517.pub3

Albornoz Y (2011) The effects of group improvisational music therapy on depression in adolescents and adults with substance abuse: a randomized controlled trial. Nord J Music Ther 20(3):208–224. https://doi.org/10.1080/08098131.2010.522717

Aro P, Ronkainen J, Storskrubb T, Bolling-Sternevald E, Svärdsudd K, Talley NJ et al (2004) Validation of the translation and cross-cultural adaptation into Finnish of the abdominal symptom questionnaire, the hospital anxiety and depression scale and the complaint score questionnaire. Scand J Gastroenterol 39(12):1201–1208. https://doi.org/10.1080/00365520410008132

Aust S, Filip K, Koelsch S, Grimm S, Bajbouj M (2013) Music in depression: neural correlates of emotional experience in remitted depression. World J Psychiatry 3(2):8–17. https://doi.org/10.5498/wjp.v3.i2.8

Bernardi L, Porta C, Sleight P (2006) Cardiovascular, cerebrovascular, and respiratory changes induced by different types of music in musicians and non-musicians: the importance of silence. Heart 92(4):445–452. https://doi.org/10.1136/hrt.2005.064600

Bernatzky G, Hesse H-P (2013) Musik in der Palliativmedizin. In: Schmerzbehandlung in der Palliativmedizin, 3rd edn. Springer, Wien, pp 175–179

Bernatzky G, Strickner S, Presch M, Wendtner F, Kullich W (2012) Music as non-pharmacological pain management in clinics*. In: MacDonald RAR, Kreutz G, Mitchell L (eds) Music, health, and wellbeing. Oxford University Press, New York, pp 258–275. https://doi.org/10.1093/acprof:oso/9780199586974.003.0019

Blood AJ, Zatorre RJ (2001) Intensely pleasurable responses to music correlate with activity in brain regions implicated in reward and emotion. Proc Natl Acad Sci USA 98(20):11818–11823. https://doi.org/10.1073/pnas.191355898

Blood AJ, Zatorre RJ, Bermudez P, Evans AC (1999) Emotional responses to pleasant and unpleasant music correlate with activity in paralimbic brain regions. Nat Neurosci 2(4):382–387. https://doi.org/10.1038/7299

Boeker H (2009) Selbst und Körper in der Depression: Herausforderungen an die Therapie. Zürich Open Science Repository and Archive, Zürich

Chechko N, Kellermann T, Augustin M, Zvyagintsev M, Schneider F, Habel U (2016) Disorder-specific characteristics of borderline personality disorder with co-occurring depression and its comparison with major depression: an fMRI study with emotional interference task. NeuroImage Clin 12:517–525. https://doi.org/10.1016/j.nicl.2016.08.015

Chen Y-J, Li X-X, Pan B, Wang B, Jing G-Z, Liu Q-Q et al (2021) Non-pharmacological interventions for older adults with depressive symptoms: a network meta-analysis of 35 randomized controlled trials. Aging Ment Health 25(5):773–786. https://doi.org/10.1080/13607863.2019.1704219

Cipriani A, Furukawa TA, Salanti G, Chaimani A, Atkinson LZ, Ogawa Y et al (2018) Comparative efficacy and acceptability of 21 antidepressant drugs for the acute treatment of adults with major depressive disorder: a systematic review and network meta-analysis. Lancet 391(10128):1357–1366. https://doi.org/10.1016/S0140-6736(17)32802-7

Dell'Anna A, Leman M, Berti A (2021) Musical interaction reveals music as embodied language. Front Neurosci 15. https://doi.org/10.3389/fnins.2021.667838

Dhippayom T, Saensook T, Promkhatja N, Teaktong T, Chaiyakunapruk N, Devine B (2022) Comparative effects of music interventions on depression in older adults: a systematic review and network meta-analysis. EClinicalMedicine 50:101509. https://doi.org/10.1016/j.eclinm.2022.101509

Dolle K, Schulte-Körne G (2014) Komplementäre Ansätze zur Behandlung von depressiven Störungen bei Kindern und Jugendlichen. Praxis Der Kinderpsychologie Und Kinderpsychiatrie 63(3):237–263. https://doi.org/10.13109/prkk.2014.63.3.237

El Haj M, Fasotti L, Allain P (2012) The involuntary nature of music-evoked autobiographical memories in Alzheimer's disease. Conscious Cogn 21(1):238–246. https://doi.org/10.1016/j.concog.2011.12.005

Erkkilä J, Punkanen M, Fachner J, Ala-Ruona E, Pöntiö I, Tervaniemi M et al (2011) Individual music therapy for depression: randomised controlled trial. Br J Psychiatry 199(2):132–139. https://doi.org/10.1192/bjp.bp.110.085431

Eschrich S, Münte TF, Altenmüller EO (2008) Unforgettable film music: the role of emotion in episodic long-term memory for music. BMC Neurosci 9:48. https://doi.org/10.1186/1471-2202-9-48

Fachner J, Stegemann T (2013) Electroencephalography and music therapy: on the same wavelength? Music Med 5(4):217–222. https://doi.org/10.1177/1943862113495062

Fachner J, Gold C, Erkkilä J (2013) Music therapy modulates fronto-temporal activity in rest-EEG in depressed clients. Brain Topogr 26(2):338–354. https://doi.org/10.1007/s10548-012-0254-x

Field T, Martinez A, Nawrocki T, Pickens J, Fox NA, Schanberg S (1998) Music shifts frontal EEG in depressed adolescents. Adolescence 33(129):109–116. Retrieved from http://www.ncbi.nlm.nih.gov/pubmed/9583665

Flo BK, Matziorinis AM, Skouras S, Sudmann TT, Gold C, Koelsch S (2022) Study protocol for the Alzheimer and music therapy study: an RCT to compare the efficacy of music therapy and physical activity on brain plasticity, depressive symptoms, and cognitive decline, in a population with and at risk for Alzheimer's disease. PLoS One 17(6):e0270682. https://doi.org/10.1371/journal.pone.0270682. PMID: 35771851; PMCID: PMC9246122

Fukui H, Yamashita M (2003) The effects of music and visual stress on testosterone and cortisol in men and women. Neuro Endocrinol Lett 24(3–4):173–180. Retrieved from http://www.ncbi.nlm.nih.gov/pubmed/14523353

Gartlehner G, Wagner G, Matyas N, Titscher V, Greimel J, Lux L et al (2017) Pharmacological and non-pharmacological treatments for major depressive disorder: review of systematic reviews. BMJ Open 7(6):e014912. https://doi.org/10.1136/bmjopen-2016-014912

Geipel J, Koenig J, Hillecke TK, Resch F, Kaess M (2018) Music-based interventions to reduce internalizing symptoms in children and adolescents: a meta-analysis. J Affect Disord 225:647–656. https://doi.org/10.1016/j.jad.2017.08.035

Gold C, Solli HP, Krüger V, Lie SA (2009) Dose-response relationship in music therapy for people with serious mental disorders: systematic review and meta-analysis. Clin Psychol Rev 29(3):193–207. https://doi.org/10.1016/j.cpr.2009.01.001

Greenberg DM, Baron-Cohen S, Stillwell DJ, Kosinski M, Rentfrow PJ (2015) Musical preferences are linked to cognitive styles. PLoS One 10(7):e0131151. https://doi.org/10.1371/journal.pone.0131151

Gui R, Chen T, Nie H (2019) The impact of emotional music on active ROI in patients with depression based on deep learning: a task-state fMRI study. Comput Intell Neurosci 2019:1–14. https://doi.org/10.1155/2019/5850830

Haller H, Anheyer D, Cramer H, Dobos G (2019) Complementary therapies for clinical depression: an overview of systematic reviews. BMJ Open 9(8):e028527. https://doi.org/10.1136/bmjopen-2018-028527

Heise S, Steinberg H, Himmerich H (2013) Die Diskussion um die Anwendung und die Wirksamkeit von Musik bei depressiven Störungen in Geschichte und Gegenwart. Fortschr Neurol Psychiatr 81(08):426–436. https://doi.org/10.1055/s-0033-1335341

Herbert J, Lucassen PJ (2016) Depression as a risk factor for Alzheimer's disease: genes, steroids, cytokines and neurogenesis—what do we need to know? Front Neuroendocrinol 41:153–171. https://doi.org/10.1016/j.yfrne.2015.12.001

Janata P (2009) The neural architecture of music-evoked autobiographical memories. Cereb Cortex 19(11):2579–2594. https://doi.org/10.1093/cercor/bhp008

Kallinen K, Ravaja N (2006) Emotion perceived and emotion felt: same and different. Music Sci 10(2):191–213. https://doi.org/10.1177/102986490601000203

Kasper S, Lehofer M, Doering S, Geretsegger C, Frey R, Haring C, Hausmann A, Hofmann P, Jelem H, Kalousek M, Kapfhammer HP, Klier C, Oberlerchner H, Rados C, Rothenhäusler HB, Sachs GM, Praschak-Rieder N, Psota G, Rainer M, Windhager E, Winkler D, Wrobel M (2012) Depression—Medikamentöse Therapie. CliniCum neuropsy Sonderausgabe

Kessler RC, Berglund P, Demler O et al (2003) The epidemiology of major depressive disorder: results from the national comorbidity survey replication (NCS-R). JAMA 289:3095–3105. https://doi.org/10.1001/jama.289.23.3095

King JB, Jones KG, Goldberg E, Rollins M, MacNamee K, Moffit C, Naidu SR, Ferguson MA, Garcia-Leavitt E, Amaro J, Breitenbach KR, Watson JM, Gurgel RK, Anderson JS, Foster NL (2019) Increased functional connectivity after listening to favored music in adults with alzheimer dementia. J Prev Alzheimers Dis 6(1):56–62. https://doi.org/10.14283/jpad.2018.19. PMID: 30569087; PMCID: PMC12280822

Koelsch S (2009) A neuroscientific perspective on music therapy. Ann N Y Acad Sci 1169:374–384. https://doi.org/10.1111/j.1749-6632.2009.04592.x

Koelsch S (2014) Brain correlates of music-evoked emotions. Nat Rev Neurosci 15(3):170–180. https://doi.org/10.1038/nrn3666

Koelsch S, Stegemann T (2012) The brain and positive biological effects in healthy and clinical populations. In: MacDonald RAR, Kreutz G, Mitchell LA (eds) Music, health, and wellbeing. Oxford University Press, Oxford, pp 436–456. https://doi.org/10.1093/acprof:oso/9780199586974.003.0029

Kreutz G, Quiroga C, Bongard S (2012) Psychoneuroendocrine research on music and health: an overview. In: MacDonald RAR, Kreutz G, Mitchell L (eds) Music, health, and wellbeing. Oxford University Press, Oxford, pp 457–476. https://doi.org/10.1093/acprof:oso/9780199586974.003.0030

Lehofer M, Stuppäck C (eds) (2005) Depressionstherapien. Thieme Verlag, Stuttgart

Lepping RJ, Atchley RA, Chrysikou E, Martin LE, Clair AA, Ingram RE et al (2016) Neural processing of emotional musical and nonmusical stimuli in depression. PLoS One 11(6):e0156859. https://doi.org/10.1371/journal.pone.0156859

Livingston G, Kelly L, Lewis-Holmes E, Baio G, Morris S, Patel N, Omar RZ, Katona C, Cooper C (2014) A systematic review of the clinical effectiveness and cost-effectiveness of sensory, psychological and behavioural interventions for managing agitation in older adults with dementia. Health Technol Assessment (Winchester, England) 18(39):1–vi. https://doi.org/10.3310/hta18390

Maratos A, Gold C, Wang X, Crawford M (2008) Music therapy for depression. Cochrane Database Syst Rev. https://doi.org/10.1002/14651858.CD004517.pub2

Mathew SJ, Charney DS (2009) Publication bias and the efficacy of antidepressants. Am J Psychiatry 166(2):140–145. https://doi.org/10.1176/appi.ajp.2008.08071102

Mavridis IN (2015) Music and the nucleus accumbens. Surg Radiol Anat 37(2):121–125. https://doi.org/10.1007/s00276-014-1360-0

Mcnair, D.M., Lorr, M., & Droppleman, L.F. (1971). Manual for the profile of mood states

Menon V, Levitin DJ (2005) The rewards of music listening: response and physiological connectivity of the mesolimbic system. NeuroImage 28(1):175–184. https://doi.org/10.1016/j.neuroimage.2005.05.053

Moreno-Morales C, Calero R, Moreno-Morales P, Pintado C (2020) Music therapy in the treatment of dementia: a systematic review and meta-analysis. Front Med 7:160. https://doi.org/10.3389/fmed.2020.00160

Moret C (2005) Combination/augmentation strategies for improving the treatment of depression. Neuropsychiatr Dis Treat 1(4):301–309. 18568111

Moussavi S, Chatterji S, Verdes E, Tandon A, Patel V, Ustun B (2007) Depression, chronic diseases, and decrements in health: results from the world health surveys. Lancet 370(9590):851–858. https://doi.org/10.1016/S0140-6736(07)61415-9

Osuch EA, Bluhm RL, Williamson PC, Théberge J, Densmore M, Neufeld RWJ (2009) Brain activation to favorite music in healthy controls and depressed patients. Neuroreport 20(13):1204–1208. https://doi.org/10.1097/WNR.0b013e32832f4da3
Palazidou E (2012) The neurobiology of depression. Br Med Bull 101(1):127–145. https://doi.org/10.1093/bmb/lds004
Panksepp J, Bernatzky G (2002) Emotional sounds and the brain: the neuro-affective foundations of musical appreciation. Behav Process 60(2):133–155. https://doi.org/10.1016/s0376-6357(02)00080-3
Pereira CS, Teixeira J, Figueiredo P, Xavier J, Castro SL, Brattico E (2011) Music and emotions in the brain: familiarity matters. PLoS One 6(11):e27241. https://doi.org/10.1371/journal.pone.0027241
Pigott HE, Leventhal AM, Alter GS, Boren JJ (2010) Efficacy and effectiveness of antidepressants: current status of research. Psychother Psychosom 79(5):267–279. https://doi.org/10.1159/000318293
Riccelli R, Passamonti L, Cerasa A, Nigro S, Cavalli SM, Chiriaco C et al (2016) Individual differences in depression are associated with abnormal function of the limbic system in multiple sclerosis patients. Mult Scler J 22(8):1094–1105. https://doi.org/10.1177/1352458515606987
Rief W, Nestoriuc Y, Weiss S, Welzel E, Barsky AJ, Hofmann SG (2009) Meta-analysis of the placebo response in antidepressant trials. J Affect Disord 118(1–3):1–8. https://doi.org/10.1016/j.jad.2009.01.029
Rush AJ Jr, First MB, Blacker D (2009) Handbook of psychiatric measures. American Psychiatric Publication
Salimpoor VN, Benovoy M, Longo G, Cooperstock JR, Zatorre RJ (2009) The rewarding aspects of music listening are related to degree of emotional arousal. PLoS One 4(10):e7487. https://doi.org/10.1371/journal.pone.0007487
Sihvonen AJ, Särkämö T, Leo V, Tervaniemi M, Altenmüller E, Soinila S (2017) Music-based interventions in neurological rehabilitation. Lancet Neurol 16(8):648–660. https://doi.org/10.1016/S1474-4422(17)30168-0
Spielberger CD, Gorsuch RL, Lushene R, Vagg PR, Jacobs GA (1983) Manual for the state-trait anxiety inventory. Consulting Psychologists Press, Palo Alto
Tang Q, Huang Z, Zhou H, Ye P (2020) Effects of music therapy on depression: A meta-analysis of randomized controlled trials. PLoS One 15(11):e0240862. https://doi.org/10.1371/journal.pone.0240862
Tornek A, Field T, Hernandez-Reif M, Diego M, Jones N (2003) Music effects on EEG in intrusive and withdrawn mothers with depressive symptoms. Psychiatry 66:234–243
van den Bosch I, Salimpoor VN, Zatorre RJ (2013) Familiarity mediates the relationship between emotional arousal and pleasure during music listening. Front Hum Neurosci 7. https://doi.org/10.3389/fnhum.2013.00534
Völker J (2021) Personalising music for more effective mood induction: exploring activation, underlying mechanisms, emotional intelligence, and motives in mood regulation. Music Sci 25(4):380–398. https://doi.org/10.1177/1029864919876315
Vos T, Barber RM, Bell B, Bertozzi-Villa A, Biryukov S, Bolliger I et al (2015) Global, regional, and national incidence, prevalence, and years lived with disability for 301 acute and chronic diseases and injuries in 188 countries, 1990–2013: a systematic analysis for the global burden of disease study 2013. Lancet 386(9995):743–800. https://doi.org/10.1016/S0140-6736(15)60692-4
Willner P, Scheel-Krüger J, Belzung C (2013) The neurobiology of depression and antidepressant action. Neurosci Biobehav Rev 37(10):2331–2371. https://doi.org/10.1016/j.neubiorev.2012.12.007
Zhao K, Bai ZG, Bo A, Chi I (2016) A systematic review and meta-analysis of music therapy for the older adults with depression. Int J Geriatr Psychiatry 31(11):1188–1198. https://doi.org/10.1002/gps.4494

Musical Potential of Children with Hearing Loss

8

Eva Mittmann

The following contribution is based on 10 years of professional experience and teaching research at a school for children with hearing losses. Within the framework of scientific findings and practical teaching experience, the central question is investigated under which conditions can hearing-impaired children best develop their basic musical potential in the context of positive teaching experiences with practical instrumental playing and singing. Of research interest was how musical learning processes can impact hearing abilities, cognitive performance, speech effect recognition, and voice development in these children. The following test procedures were used for this purpose: Musicality (Jungbluth), Intelligence (K-ABC), Speech-Affect Test (Mittmann), as well as extensive audio and video recordings of vocal improvisation and instrumental playing during the test period.

8.1 Introduction

> Currently there are only two reasons why I wear my eavesdroppers (CI):
>
> 1. communication with those who cannot sign
> 2. musiiiiiiiiiiiiiiiic ... (man, I missed this)! (Christine T., former student of the Johannes-Vatter-School)

Making music together with hard of hearing children requires a variety of musical differentiation skills. The ability to differentiate between pitches of a melody and to grasp the temporal interrelationships between the tonal events is necessary. The acquisition of these basic musical skills is therefore associated with increasing differentiation of the dimensions of pitch and time. Empirical research with normal

E. Mittmann (✉)
Institute for Music Education, Johann Wolfgang Goethe University, Frankfurt am Main, Germany

G. Kreutz, G. Bernatzky (eds.), *Music and Medicine*, Neurocultural Health and Wellbeing, https://doi.org/10.1007/978-3-662-72175-9_8

hearing children of primary school age supports this assumption and suggests that fundamental musical abilities are positively influenced by musical practice in qualified music lessons at school (Klemm 1987; Bastian 2000; Bähr 2001).

The results presented here relate to the presentation of the development of musical listening skills, cognitive performance, and voice development over a 3-year period in which a curriculum including instrumental instruction and singing was evaluated. Thirty-one children aged 8–12 years with different hearing care (HA = 13, CI = 18) from two support centers for the hard of hearing (MG = 21, CG = 10) participated in the study. The results demonstrate an overall positive development of musical hearing abilities through musical support. In addition, the linkage of instrumental playing and singing proves to be a favorable influencing factor for expanding the modulation abilities of the voices. Especially children with CI benefit significantly in their voice development (MG/CI: $p = 0.4$; $d = 1.2$).

Studies involving music-making with hard of hearing children have been known from the Anglo-American language area since the 1980s. They demonstrate that these children can, in principle, learn musical instruments and develop their general musicality (Prause 2001). When playing instruments, it should be noted that instruments with a clear pitch definition (e.g., keyboard and guitar) are used (Brockmeier 2005).

> Regardless of the type of hearing device used, most students with hearing losses learn best through active participation in music making. Learning music through performing, reading and writing music is essential for the student with hearing loss. (Adamek and Darrow 2005, p. 249)

Hard of hearing children undoubtedly have musical potential, which deserves special consideration due to the rapid progress in hearing technology made possible by digital hearing aids and cochlear implants (Kießling et al. 2008). This enables these children to perceive music and speech in a much more differentiated way, with enormous potential for enhancing their development through music education (Darrow 2013; Torppa and Huotilainen 2019).

8.2 Music Perception with Hearing Aids

Since the beginning of the twenty-first century, the possibilities of music enjoyment for people with hearing impairments have become increasingly interesting. The reason for this is the achievements in the field of hearing technology, which have created the conditions for hearing-impaired children to pick up acoustic signals primarily through the sense of hearing. This has been made possible by technical hearing aids such as digital hearing aids (HA) or the cochlear implant (CI) (Chasin and Russo 2004; Wessel et al. 2007). Among the innovations in the hearing technology of digital hearing aids, special functions that support “useful sound” in contrast to “background noise” and directional hearing, as well as approaches to compensate for high-frequency losses, should be highlighted. Digital hearing aids are capable of reproducing high tones octave by octave in lower frequency ranges, allowing melody contours to be perceived that were previously located in so-called dead zones.

Binaural and bimodal stimulation offer further improvements in hearing technology regarding the auditory perception of musical parameters. This ensures both-sided stimulation of the residual hearing; thus, the auditory impressions of both ears can complement each other (Ching et al. 2004; Limberger et al. 2005). With bimodal fitting, a hearing aid is worn in addition to the implanted ear, which can effectively complement the auditory impression of music, especially in the low frequency ranges that the CI is unable to reach (EAS = combination of electrical and acoustic stimulation). It has been determined that the pitch discrimination under bimodal fitting, meaning cochlear implant plus hearing aid, is significantly better than with the CI alone (Pflug 2011). Further studies document that the ability to discriminate pitch correlates positively with the duration of musical training on the instrument (Chen et al. 2010). In addition, research suggests that musical intervention can improve melody recognition (Galvin et al. 2007, 2009). Musical experience before and after implantation is also considered a strong positive influence on pitch discrimination and accurate melody recognition (ibid.). From this, it can be concluded that music education can contribute significantly to the improvement of functional hearing. This is especially true since improved hearing technology can now train pitch discrimination even more precisely than before (Sammler and Elmer 2020).

Looking at the possibilities of music reception of hearing-impaired children at special schools, it has to be considered especially that the learning groups to be taught are basically very inhomogeneous in their composition. On the one hand, because they are primarily divided according to age groups and not according to their different degrees of hearing loss, and on the other hand because of their different levels of previous support. Generally, we distinguish five very different degrees of hearing impairment (see p. 157 Kießling et al. 2008; Adamek and Darrow 2005, p. 238), whose effects on the ability to communicate are of immense diversity. Therefore, at the Johannes-Vatter-Schule in Friedberg, Germany, students with a hearing loss of up to 75 dB and appropriate technical hearing aids were taught in spoken language according to the so-called hearing-directed approach, those with a hearing loss of more than 80 dB were taught in sign language).

8.3 Promoting Potential Listening Skills in Music and Speech

To reach children with divergent hearing impairments through suitable musical support programs in the best possible way, positive emotional preconditions must be met before any other educational intervention. Here it is necessary to sensitively prepare small-step processes of musical learning, since a selection and filtering of incoming stimuli is always carried out after an initially emotional appraisal. From this results, the premise: “Music should first and foremost be fun!” In this context, research studies on the theoretical foundation of successful teaching emphasize the high value of the teacher's personality (Hattie et al. 2013). If learning is to succeed, school must become a "resonating space"; a space in which students feel that the material and the teacher are appealing (Rosa 2014). It is the spark of enthusiasm that needs to be ignited, since "learning always occurs when positive experiences are made" (Spitzer 2002). For this reason, it is necessary to consider "resonance axes" in the communication between teacher and student. Such resonance axes include self-efficacy expectations, intrinsic interests, recognition and mutual appreciation (Rosa ibid.).

8.3.1 Training of the Auditory Memory Through Multisensory Experiences

A resource-oriented approach aims in particular at the component of sensorimotor learning, which enables children to perceive music in their entire bodies—beyond unisensory critical hearing experiences in such a way that they do not experience themselves as deficient. They therefore need aesthetic fields of experience in the sense of multisensory learning opportunities—"the staging of aesthetic experiential spaces" (Rolle 2010), in order to provide auditory impressions with meanings and to network them holistically. It is about meaningful and sensual connections of different physical experiences, so that sensorimotor integration can succeed. This is not to be evaluated as compensation for hearing impairment, but in the sense of assigning, memorizing and structuring holistically experienced sensory experiences. Through this form of "appropriation" of originally deficient aural sound experiences, abstract musical parameters can acquire meaning on the basis of repetitions. Pictorial-emotional assignments can lead to the development of a secure auditory memory or vocabulary through assignments: Listening patterns are successively developed and reliable mental representations are built up. "Experiencing music not only as sound, but as a physical process," i.e., initiating contact with music on the level of physical sensations, is regarded as decisive and appreciative for all children (Gruhn 2003). This is especially true for children with hearing loss. An offer of multi-sensory sensorial experiences of different modes of perception that complement each other is therefore the basis for optimally stimulating the auditory memory.

Accordingly, practical teaching interventions are required that shape aesthetic spaces of experience so that multisensory learning processes in the sense of intermedial cross-connections can complement and condense beyond the interactional structure of hearing, moving and generating sounds (cf. Stadler-Elmer 2000; Jank 2005). Experiences in such aesthetic contexts prepare the differentiation abilities of musical parameters (loud-quiet, fast-slow, high-low, short-long), which can be added to the body schema through dance and movement games and finally be intensively trained and improved through the use of instrumental playing and singing.

The training of the auditory memory is thus a **multisensory stabilizing memory performance**.

8.3.2 Auditory Attention as an Indicator for Improved Speech Recognition

The training of these very skills is of particular relevance because the hearing system recognizes three primary elements that are crucial for the degree and quality of both music and speech recognition: Frequency (pitch), intensity (volume), and time (duration). These similarities in the acoustic and structural characteristics of music and speech reflect common evolutionary roots. Musical auditory training can thus lead to improved extraction of the sound characteristics of speech and thus also enable improved speech recognition. For example, the musical means of expression during a melody finds its equivalent in the speech prosody of a spoken question or answer sentence. Furthermore, it should be noted that negative effects of hearing impairment go far beyond the problem of language development deficits, since acoustic access to intelligible speech is considered essential for general brain development (see Gertner and Schraer-Joiner 2016). Music can therefore be considered a fundamental stimulus for general hearing training. In this sense, current research results indicate that musical training for hearing-impaired people has a positive influence on auditory-cortical representations, the temporal processing of the offered stimuli as well as the general recognition of acoustic information. Overall, this can lead to a significant improvement in auditory attention and thus also to significantly improved speech recognition, e.g., the pattern of strong and weak syllables can be better recognized, which facilitates speech perception in background noise (Torppa and Huotilainen 2019).

The conception of the music curriculum at the Johannes-Vatter-Schule at that time, in contrast to conventional rhythmic instruction, primarily pursued learning goals immanent to music and was based on teaching materials from the elementary level of general education schools, which were methodically and didactically prepared for children with hearing loss.

In the center of the methodical-didactical conception stood the musical practice, since active music-making in a group is about acquiring practical knowledge (procedural knowledge) by listening to the music produced by the group, recording musical structures and testing them by imitation (Gruhn 2003). The promotion and sensitization of auditory perception as well as the coordination of movements while playing music additionally supports the sensorimotor integration which is important for the entire development of a person (Jank 2010). The fields of experience of instrumental practice and vocal improvisation described in the following are to be introduced by whole-body sensorimotor processes in dance and movement exercises, so that through body movements in flow (proprioception) the prerequisites for the experience of a metrically bound sequence (beat) are internalized. Body experiences in the sense of sensory integration are the basis for the success of instrumental and voice improvisations.

8.3.3 Field of Experience: Instrumental Practice

Since the 1950s, the use of instrumental playing has been known from the education of the hearing impaired in the European language area (Uden van 1980). These teaching documentations show that the children who had played melodies on a wind organ (melodica) themselves learned melodies and kept them as a "single whole" better than other children without instrumental playing. It can be assumed that practical music making influences the memory capacity as well as the holistic thinking of these children (Mittmann 2009, 2013). Further research in the Anglo-American language area confirms that practical music-making has been successful in terms of pitch discrimination and exact intonation (Darrow 1990; Walczyk 1993; Hash 2003).

Based on these findings, the implementation of practice-oriented teaching lessons on keyboards and school guitars was designed. Ten school guitars and a keyboard studio with ten student keyboards were available for this purpose. It was planned that the children would vocally accompany the melodies played on the instrument (initially in a three-tone or five-tone space). It was assumed that playing on the instrument would positively support the audio-vocal learning process, since the motor areas in the brain responsible for vocal imitation are connected to the associative auditory cortex and thus cause cortical control of vocalization. What is meant here is a re-coding of the motor control of the muscles in the larynx through perceptively preserved acoustic perception (Gruhn 2010; Saß 2002; Jakubek 2009). Acoustic information can be neuronally consolidated and condensed by this auditory-motor coordination (phonological loop: "aural-oral-loop") (Gruhn 2010).

The methodical procedure is carried out in three steps: Orientation stage, elaboration of rhythmic patterns according to the method of class music-making with keyboards and finally the development of melodic contours (Yamaha Teamplay). Initially, basic questions on how to use the keyboard are explained and tested. Then simple rhythmic patterns are practiced in 4-bar time with body percussion and rhythmic language (Gordon) to train the metric-rhythmic skills necessary for the interaction. To enable rhythmic patterns to be incorporated into the body scheme, movement and dance actions or exercises with body percussion are fundamentally indispensable. The practiced patterns can then be better implemented on the instruments and accompanied vocally. Once the metric-rhythmic basis is given, melodies can be practiced with fingering. The melodies are first intoned without text parallel to the instrumental playing. By learning rhythmic sequences and melody contours, sensory stimulation takes place, which is central to language acquisition. Procedural knowledge is formed; an inner idea of music develops.

An image of the keyboard, which is projected onto the wall via overhead projector, serves as an aid to make the sounds to be played clearly visible to everyone.

To realize the instrumental playing on the guitar, the methodical steps are modified as follows: Orientation level (Posture of the guitar, striking exercises), elaboration of metric/rhythmic song accompaniment (changes on open strings) and development of melodic contours. Even when playing the guitar, the metric and rhythmic accompaniments as well as the melody contours are supported vocally with spoken verses and song lyrics. This promotes the automation of the playing technique of hand and finger movements. The combination of instrumental playing and language refers to the teaching concepts of Schatz and Ford in the 1990s; in particular, the methodological approaches of Theresa Ford, who used language as a medium for the appropriation of rhythmic patterns, should be mentioned here.

8.3.4 Field of Experience: Vocal Improvisation

"Canto—ergo sum." This formula goes back to Bjørkvold (1990), because for him, spontaneous children's singing is a natural expressive behavior that is "related to the dynamics of life existence" and serves "to express the experience of life" (cf. Spychiger 1997). According to Blank and Adamek (2010), singing promotes self-expression and community, because it causes "the experience of self-efficacy and successful community as a special activity of one's own" and makes one healthy and peaceful. Singing is generally associated with a positive emotional mood, as the activation of the reward system in the frontal cortex increases the production of dopamine and opioid. In addition, the hormone oxytocin is released, which lowers the concentration of the hormone testosterone and cortisol. Among all cultures, the biological principles of singing manifests itself (Wallin et al. 2000; Trehub 2000; Altenmüller and Grossbach 2003; Kreutz 2004) and singing transports communicative, social and religious functions (Xu et al. 2009). Since everyone is obviously predisposed to singing, it is a matter of developing the innate singing potential in hard of hearing children as well, so that they profit from the positive effects of singing and can thus increase their own quality of life. A particular advantage of experimenting with the voice is that it involves other perceptual systems that are involved in the process of singing. These include the visual system, somato-visceral sensitivity (tactile perception in vibration sensation) and depth sensitivity. All these complex modes of perception can be summarized under the term sensorimotor function (Stadler Elmer 2002). Singing represents "in its basic form an easier sensory and motor performance" than speaking (Altenmüller and Grossbach 2003) and is therefore considered as empowerment in hearing impaired children. For singing to be successful in the sense of empowerment and certain preconditions should be observed, because it is of immense importance to grant these children emotionally positive singing experiences and to prepare them sensitively.

Important Notes

1. Due to reduced hearing ability, these children have difficulty finding reference sounds because the audio-phonatory control is limited by the hearing loss.
2. When hard of hearing children sing, the sensory capacities of the skin act as a control system for musical pitch perception and differentiation and the combination of all sensory modalities leads to better results than one-sided stimuli (Obermüller 2008).
3. Additional limitations are given regarding the perception of tension in the vocal apparatus and mouth motor activity (Jakubek 2009).
4. Text-related singing can hinder correct pitch production, because concentration on correct speech articulation ties up too much attention (Penteker-Wolfheimer 1998; Haus 2002; Jakubek 2009).

The approach of text-free voice improvisation is best suited to pay attention to all these points, because it offers children the opportunity to discover and develop their voice sound in a playful way by exploring their own voice. When singing in or in front of the group, imitation learning always takes place: Students observe each other very closely. They register how individuals sing in front of and in the group and try to imitate this to some extent. Through this imitation learning, a voluntary tuning of the vocal fold muscles is initiated (Jakubek 2009). An "inner singing along" takes place, which influences the acoustic self-control of the voice. This can lead to complete glottis closure or even influence hyper functional dysphonia (whispered vocalizations), which are frequently found in hearing impaired children (Zimmermann 2000).

8.4 Findings

8.4.1 Musical Listening Skills

All participants showed an increase in musical listening skills over the course of the study period, both in the tonal and metric-rhythmic range. This can be determined independently of the respective hearing aid fitting, since the mean value comparisons of the sum differences show only marginal differences and apply equally to the subjects of the model group and control group (model group: difference sum value MG/CI = 13.58, difference sum value MG/HA = 13.66; control group: (difference sum value: CG/HA = 4.60; difference sum value: CG/CI = 5.40). The results of the subtests show that the children with CI significantly improved their performance in recognizing different rhythms (MG: M = 3.92; SD = 1.73; CG: 1.80; SD = 1.64; $p = 0.03$). Significant is also the progress in the subtests tone duration and rhythms as well as in the sum score; effect sizes: tone duration ($d = 1.2$), rhythm (d = 1.3), sum (d = 1). The children with hearing aids show significant group differences in the subtest metrum (MG: $M = 4.37$; SD = 2.82; CG: $M = 0.20$; SD = 1.64; $p = 0.03$); effect sizes can be detected in the categories tone duration ($d = 0.9$), metrum ($d = 1.8$) and sum difference ($d = 1.2$).

For the hearing aid of cochlear implantation (CI), significant differences in subtests between the model and control groups were found primarily in the tasks of processing temporal information: difference rhythms t1−t0 ($p = 0.03$), difference tone duration t2−t0 ($p = 0.01$), difference tempo t1−t0 ($p = 0.04$).

The positive development of musical listening skills in the model group of CI-supplied students is due to improved performance in frequency-related skills (especially melody interval recognition) and the differentiation of temporal information (tone durations, meters, and rhythmic figures). The students with Hearing Aids can also improve their overall musical listening skills, but the performance on the melody interval task remained unchanged.

The picture is different in the control group: Here, cochlear implant recipients improved their musical hearing in only three categories (pitch discrimination of large intervals, tone duration, rhythmic figures). No relevant differences between the children treated with CI were found in the comparison between the model group and the control group in the pitch discrimination tasks.

The results of the model and control group show a continuously growing ability to discriminate at large intervals, tone durations, tempi and rhythmic figures. They demonstrate an overall increase in the children's musical abilities and skills, which can be traced back to increases in temporal perception as well as in the ability to perceive large intervals of sound. However, the overall group of hard of hearing children with an average of six correct scores achieved in the subtests is at the level of normal hearing children without instrumental support (Figs. 8.1 and 8.2).

8.4.2 Cognitive Performance

In basic diagnostics, the subjects in the model group have significantly less intelligence; however, they can improve their cognitive performance over time. This is due to improved results in the tasks of Gestalt comprehension. Highly significant is the result of the standardized scale of holistic thinking (Std.SIM), (MG: $M = 8.43$; SD = 9.95; CG: $M = -2.6$; SD = 7; $p = 0.01$) (Fig. 8.3). In contrast to the subjects of the MG, the performance of the scale of detailed thinking (SEQ) improved in the control group.

The subjects in the model group who were fitted with hearing aids showed performance improvements in the subtests number repeat and word row. They were thus able to improve their performance in solving auditory memory problems. In contrast, students with cochlear implants lose performance on these subtests. Overall, the standardized test scores of hearing-aided students show improvement in both individual and holistic thinking. Students with cochlear implants have mainly improved in their ability to perform the holistic thinking tasks, especially the subtests shape recognition and triangles.

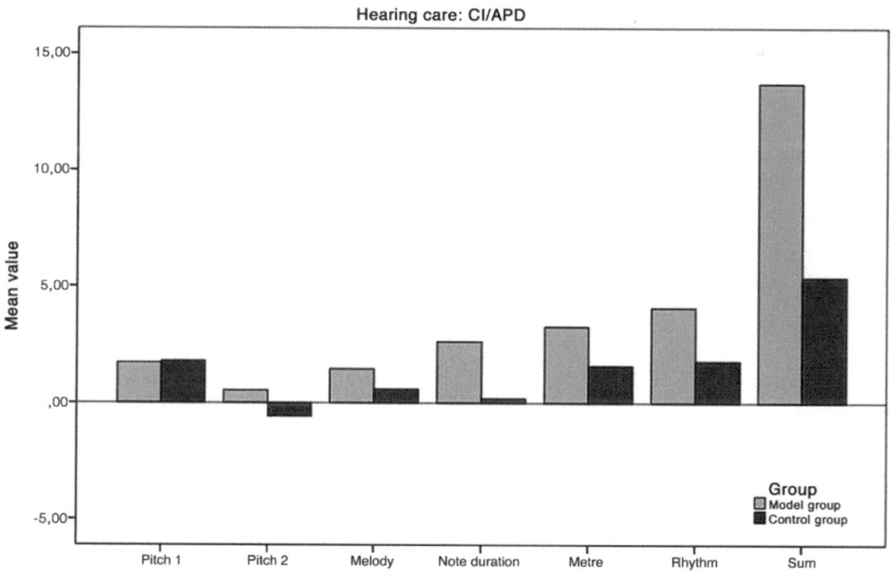

Fig. 8.1 Group comparisons of musical hearing abilities in relation to the hearing aid CI (difference t3-t0)

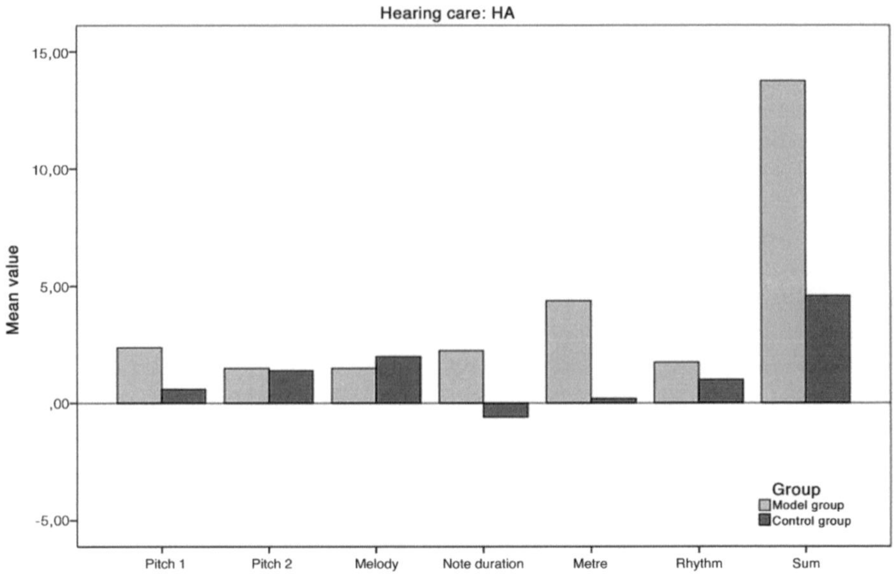

Fig. 8.2 Group comparisons of the musical hearing abilities in relation to the hearing care HA (difference t3-t0)

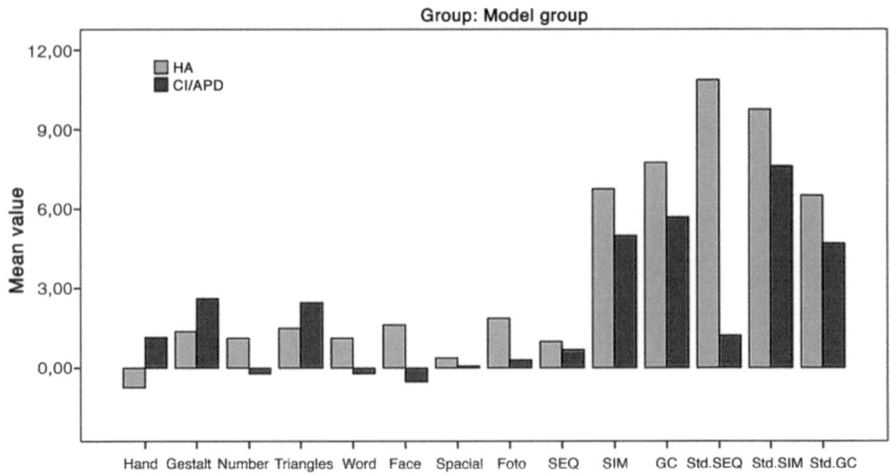

Fig. 8.3 Mean differences in cognitive abilities (K-ABC) of the model group 2003–2006 as a function of hearing aid fitting

Mean value comparisons of the control group of cochlear implant recipients revealed a drop in performance in the triangles, pictorial supplementation and spatial memory subtests. This leads to a drop in performance in the scale of holistic thinking (SIM). The subtests on detailed thinking show slight improvements. This resulted in an increase in the performance in the scale of individual thinking.

Marginal improvements in the tasks shape-closing and photo series are observed in subjects with HA of the control group. Otherwise, they showed a drop in performance, which leads to decreased overall test results (Fig. 8.4).

Effect sizes for CI hearing aid treatment can be observed in the tasks shape ($d = 1$) and triangles ($d = 1.1$). This led to an effect strength in the scale of holistic thinking ($d = 1.2$). Significant differences ($p \leq 0{,}05$) between the model and control group according to the Mann–Whitney U-Test are, however, only in the values of the standardized scale for holistic thinking = Std.SIM (MG: $M = 7{,}62$ (10,11), CG: $M = -3{,}40$ (7,13), $p = 0{,}05$) and in the standardized sum result = Std.GC (MG: $M = 4{,}69$ (7,53); CG: $M = 1{,}00$ (4,95); $p = 0{,}05$). Students fitted with hearing aids showed strong effects in the tasks triangles ($d = 0.8$) and photo ($d = 1$), which leads to strong effects in the scale of standardized holistic thinking ($d = 1.3$) and in the standardized cumulative result of intellectual abilities = GC ($d = 1.1$).

Correlations between the difference values of the musicality test and the difference values of the intelligence test are only given in weak linear form in the following categories:

$$\text{SEQ / pitch} : r = 0.4; \text{SIM / meters} : r = 0.4; \text{SIM / rhythms} : r = 0.4.$$

8.4.3 Voice Development

The participants of the model group can expand the difference frequencies of their voices by stimulating them with instrumental playing and singing, which leads to an improved modulation of the voices. Especially children with CI benefit significantly in their voice development (MG/CI: $p = 0.04$; $d = 1.2$) (Figs. 8.5 and 8.6).

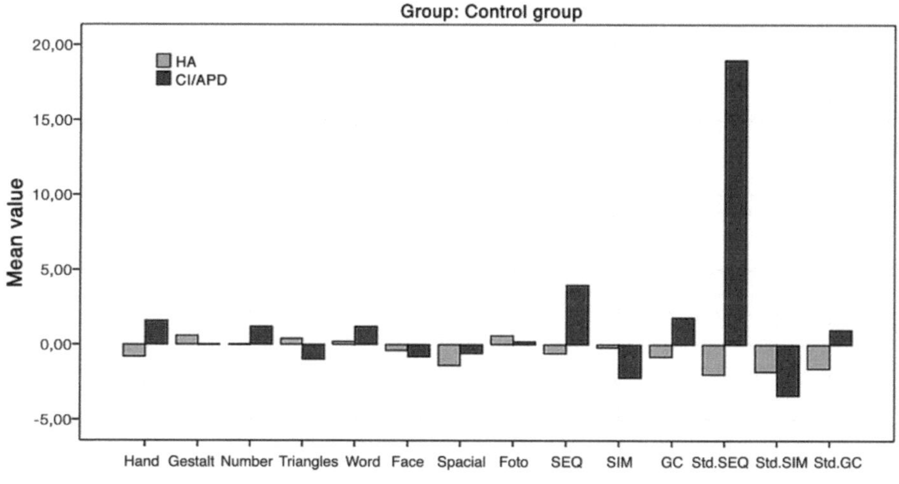

Fig. 8.4 Mean differences in cognitive abilities (K-ABC) of the control group 2003–2006 as a function of hearing aid fitting

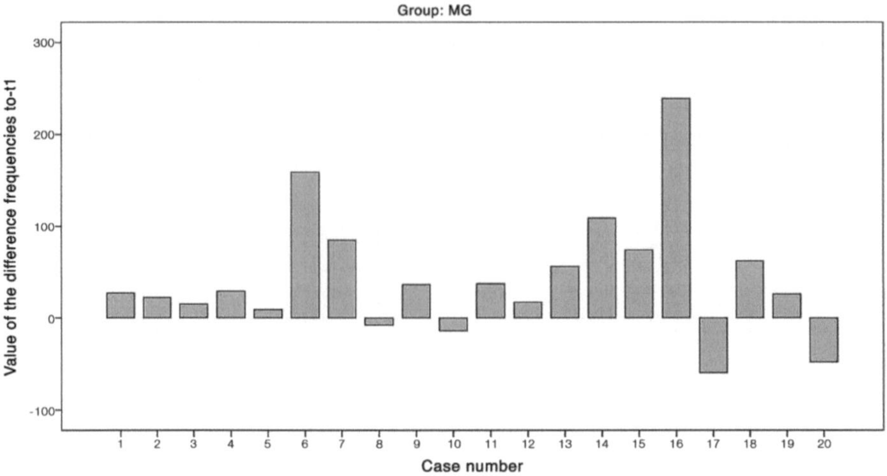

Fig. 8.5 Development of the difference frequencies of the model group

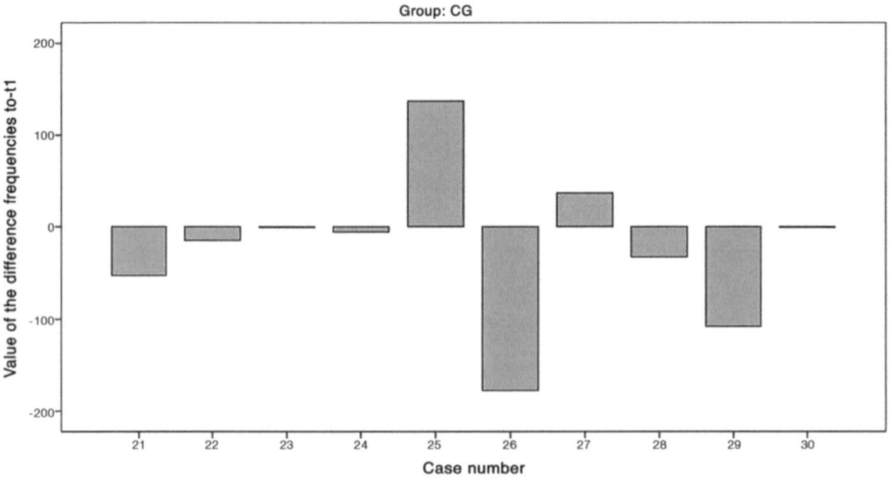

Fig. 8.6 Development of the difference frequencies of the control group

The individual case studies demonstrate the high inter-individual variance concerning the development of singing skills. However, it is noteworthy that only in four cases the modulation ability of the voice decreased resulting a positive score of 80% for the model group.

8.5 The Impact and Transfer Effects of Musical Practice with Children with Hearing Loss

Why is it so important making music together for people with hearing losses?

In course of the implementation of inclusion, special schools for hard of hearing children are mainly attended by those children for whom schooling in mainstream schools is not possible due to severe hearing impairment or the additional occurrence of partial performance disorders (e.g., in the social-emotional area). This remaining group of severely hearing losses up to partially deaf children requires a high degree of support to be able to use resources beyond the resulting disabilities.

Musical support proved to be an excellent means in this context: Beyond the development of basic musical skills, all the learning processes involved in instrumental playing in a group also support the development of personality and social skills of these children. This leads to an increase in self-esteem ("I am now able to do something I couldn't before.") and to increased empathy when listening to each other. In this way, relationship emotions (appreciation emotions) are positively influenced. Instrumental playing also has a positive influence on the development of fine motor skills since information on pitch and time can be recorded in perceptual-motor coupling (Mittmann and Kreutz 2005). The implementation of complex thought patterns can be successful, because instrumental practice helps to improve the comprehension of holistic structures, since practicing melodic contours and rhythmic sequences on the instrument requires storage capacity in the sense of holistic comprehension. The formation of groups and patterns is necessary to be able to recall and store what has been learned through practice. An improvement in the recognition of shapes is therefore possible based on increased instrumental instruction linked with corresponding movement experiences. The experience of auditory processes in music can also be excellently prepared through movement games and dance: melodic phrasing or different rhythmicity determine the choreography in dance; new phrases introduce, for example, different movement patterns. In this way, sound ideas can be formed as process forms, which are the first to be stored as experiences of form. On the basis of this pattern and group formation, the so-called, chunking, this "building block of cognition" creates holistic qualities (Harnischmacher 2008), which form a scheme as an organized knowledge structure that can be accessed again and again. Musical experiences are thus stored in the auditory memory as a "listening vocabulary" that can be called up (Mittmann 2013).

The development of listening patterns, a vocabulary of hearing, is of fundamental importance in general, and thus also for hard of hearing people, and can be excellently initiated by playing instruments together. Furthermore, the use of instrumental playing can not only improve the handling of musical instruments, but also the general hearing processing (Roden et al. 2012). The fact that listening to music and musical practice can also fundamentally prepare and support the language acquisition process is proven by the results of a research group of scientists from the Rice University of Maryland. On the basis of their research results, they argue that language can only develop on the basis of conscious perception of musical parameters: "We argue that music comes first and language arises from music" (Brandt et al.

2012). Accordingly, "speech is a concert of phonemes and syllables." Spoken language is thus interpreted as a specific kind of music: "Spoken language is a certain kind of music" (ibid.) Current research confirms this view in people with hearing impairment and supports the assumption of positive transfer effects of active music-making on their spoken language competence as well as on general language development (Torppa and Huotilainen 2019). We can therefore speak of a per se "natural" promotion of language through music, since the different sounds of all spoken languages are of a musical nature. This can be especially supportive for the German language acquisition of foreign-language hearing-impaired refugees, in order to prepare their language competence and expressiveness in the best possible way through targeted musical practice.

The use of instrumental playing combined with singing supports a successful linkage of the aural-oral loop and can thus influence the extension of vocal frequencies. Regarding the pedagogical concept, it makes sense in this respect to always prepare instrumental practice and voice work first of all through whole-body perception, since metric-rhythmic sensations provide the basal prerequisite for exact musical interaction and synchronization. The differentiation of hearing is thus in a larger context with the training of perception, especially for hard of hearing children.

It is a high priority to give these children opportunities to develop their own independent, strong and positive self-concept. Musical learning processes must therefore be initiated very sensitively so that the young people can later develop culture in their own way.

> Of course, I hope that they also have lives filled with music, but most of all, I want them to have dignity and respect. A.A. Darrow

8.6 Conclusions

In the previous remarks it was explained in detail that making music together offers a high potential of support for hard of hearing children. It could be shown that these children are able to positively develop their musical abilities, cognitive performance, and vocal abilities with appropriately modified methodological-didactic concepts for similar normal hearing children.

In conclusion, however, the question must be asked whether music lessons for hard of hearing children must first legitimize themselves, or is it not a human right per se? Does not every child have a fundamental right to the practice of music, the development of their musical abilities and musical knowledge to increase their well-being and enrich their lives? Where is the general right for everyone to experience music as a cultural asset ("music as an art")—to aesthetic experience that enriches life?

If we take heterogeneity and inclusion seriously, then new teaching concepts are required. Necessary conditions for making music together beyond handicaps must be created. In other words: To what extent can music making ultimately contribute to opening up better developmental opportunities for these children so that they can find their place in society? At the end—it is all about their right to self-realization.

References

Adamek MS, Darrow AA (2005) Music in special education. American Music Therapy Association
Altenmüller E, Grossbach M (2003) Singen—die Ursprache? Zur Hirnphysiologie des Gesanges. In: Üben und Musizieren, 2/2003. Schott, Mainz, pp 34–39
Bähr J (2001) Zur Entwicklung musikalischer Fähigkeiten von Zehn- bis Zwölfjährigen. Evaluation eines Modellversuchs zur Kooperation von Schule und Musikschule. Cuvillier, Göttingen
Bastian HG (2000) Musik(erziehung) und ihre Wirkung. Eine Langzeitstudie an Berliner Grundschulen, unter Mitarbeit von A Kormann, R Hafen, M Koch. Mainz Schott
Bjørkvold JR (1990) Canto - ergo sum. Musical child culture in the United States, the Soviet Union, and Norway. In: Wilson FR, Roehmann FL (eds) Music and child development. MMB Music, St Louis, pp 117–135
Blank T, Adamek K (2010) Singen in der Kindheit. Eine empirische Studie zur Gesundheit und Schulfähigkeit von Kindergartenkindern und das Canto-elementar-Konzept zum Praxistransfer. Waxmann, Münster
Brandt A, Gebrian M, Slevc LR (2012) Music and early language acquisition. Front Psychol 3. https://doi.org/10.3389/fpsyg.2012.00327
Brockmeier S (2005) Pilotstudie zur Musikwahrnehmung von CI-Trägern mit dem M.U.S.I.C. Test, 22. Wissenschaftliche Jahrestagung der Deutschen Gesellschaft für Phoniatrie und Pädaudiologie & 24. Kongress der Union Europäischer Phoniater, 16.-18.09.2005. Deutsche Gesellschaft für Phoniatrie und Pädaudiologie e. V, Berlin. http://www.egms.de/en/meetings/dgpp2005/05dgpp077.shtml
Chasin M, Russo FA (2004) Hearing aids and music. Trends Amplif 8(2):35–47
Chen JK, Chuang AY, McMahon C, Hsieh JC, Tung TH, Li LP (2010) Music training improves pitch perception in prelingually deafened children with cochlear implants. Pediatrics 125(4):e793–800. https://doi.org/10.1542/peds.2008-3620. Epub 2010 Mar 8. PMID: 20211951.
Ching TY, Incerti P, Hill M (2004) Binaural benefits for adults who use hearing aids and cochlear implants in opposite ears. Ear Hear 25(1):9–21
Darrow AA (1990) The effect of frequency adjustment on the vocal reproduction accuracy of hearing-impaired children. J Music Ther 27(1):24–33
Darrow AA (2013) Music therapy and special music education: interdisciplinary dialogues Alice-Ann Darrow interviewed by Giorgos Tsiris. http://approaches.gr/wp-content/uploads/2015/09/6-Approaches_512013_Darrow-Tsiris_Interview.pdf
Galvin J, Fu QJ, Nogaki G (2007) Melodic contour identification by Cochlear Im-plant listeners. Ear Hear 28 (3):302–319
Galvin J, Fu QJ, Oba S (2009) Effect of a competing instrument on melodic contour identification by cochlear implant users. J Acoust Soc Am 125(3):98–103
Gertner A, Schraer-Joiner L (2016) Music for children with hearing loss. In: VanderLinde Blair D, McCord KA (eds) Exceptional music pedagogy for children with exceptionalities: international perspectives. Print ISBN-13: 9780190234560, Published to Oxford Scholarship Online, pp 246–276
Gruhn W (2003) Lernziel Musik. Perspektiven einer neuen theoretischen Grundlegung des Musikunterrichts. Olms, Hildesheim [u. a.]
Gruhn W (2010) Anfänge des Musiklernens. Eine lerntheoretische und entwicklungspsychologische Einführung. Olms, Hildesheim [u. a.]
Harnischmacher C (2008) Subjektorientierte Musikerziehung. Eine Theorie des Lernens und Lehrens von Musik. Augsburg, Wißner
Hash P (2003) Teaching instrumental music to deaf and hard of hearing students. Res Issues Music Educ 1(1) http://www.stthomas.edu/rimeonline/vol1/hash1.htm
Hattie J, Beywl W, Zierer K (2013) Lernen sichtbar machen. Baltmannsweiler, Schneider Verlag

Haus R (2002) „Spiel noch mal…“ Musiktherapie als Hilfe, das Hören zu lernen bei Kindern mit Cochlea-Implantat. In: Musiktherapeutische Umschau 23 (1). Göttingen, Vandenhoeck & Ruprecht, pp 37–45

Jakubek E (2009) Fachbeitrag. Wenn CI-Kinder singen. In: HÖRPÄD 5/2009. Heidelberg, Median, pp 188–194

Jank W (2005) Plädoyer für Artenvielfalt. In: Schäfer-Lembeck HU (ed) Klassenmusizieren als Musikunterricht!? Theoretische Dimensionen unterrichtlicher Praxen, Beiträge des Münchner Symposions 2005, Musikpädagogische Schriften der Hochschule für Musik und Theater Bd. 1. Allitera, München, pp 109–117

Jank W (2010) Musik aufbauend lernen. In: Greuel T, Kranefeld U, Szczepaniak E (eds) Jedem Kind (s)ein Instrument, Die Musikschule in der Grundschule. Shaker, Aachen, pp 133–146

Kießling J, Kollmeier B, Diller G (2008, zweite Aufl.) Versorgung und Rehabilitation mit Hörgeräten. Stuttgart, Thieme

Klemm G (1987) Untersuchungen über den Zusammenhang musikalischer und sprachlicher Wahrnehmungsfähigkeiten. Europäische Hochschulschriften Bd. 27, Frankfurt/M., Peter Lang

Kreutz G (2004) Wirkungen und Bedeutungen des Chorsingens: Psychophysiologische und sozialpsychologische Aspekte. In: Kreutz G, Bähr J (eds) Anstöße—Musikalische Bildung fordern und fördern. Festschrift Hans Günther Bastian zum 60. Geburtstag. Wißner, Augsburg, pp 107–124

Limberger A et al (2005) “Bimodale Versorgung”—schon wieder etwas Neues? In: 8. Jahrestagung der Deutschen Gesellschaft für Audiologie, Deutsche Gesellschaft für Audiologie e.V, Kiel. http://www.uzh.ch/orl/dgaev/publikationen/tagungsbaende/tagungsbaende.html

Mittmann E (2009) Instrumentalspiel und Gesang als Mittel zur Stimm- und Sprachförderung hörgeschädigter Kinder im Grundschulalter. In: Gaul M (Hrsg.) Zukunftsmusik. Förderung musikalischer Potenziale in Kindergarten und Grundschule. Mainz [u.a.], Schott, 60-71

Mittmann E (2013) Musikalische Förderung hörgeschädigter Kinder—Eine empirische Studie im sonderpädagogischen Kontext. Die blaue Eule, Essen

Mittmann E, Kreutz G (2005) Musikalische Potenziale hörgeschädigter Kinder: Zwischenergebnisse einer Längsschnittstudie mit aktivem Musikunterricht. AMPF-Jahrestagung „Lehr-& Lernforschung in der Musikpädagogik“, Lingen

Obermüller A (2008) Musikpädagogisches Arbeiten mit Gehörlosen, Diplomarbeit, eingereicht und verteidigt an der Hochschule für. Musik Carl Maria von Weber, Dresden. http://www.taubenschlag.de/cms_pics/Diplomarbeit_OOo.pdf

Penteker-Wolfheimer U (1998): Rhythmisch-musikalischer Unterricht In: Diller G (Hrsg.) Hörgerichtetheit in der Praxis. Heidelberg, Ed. Schindele, pp 156–177

Pflug C (2011) Bimodale Musikhörfähigkeiten mit Cochlea Implantat und Hörgerät. Dissertation TU München, http://mediatum.ub.tum.de/doc/993315/993315.pdf

Prause MC (2001) Musik und Gehörlosigkeit. Dohr, Köln

Roden I, Kreutz G, Bongard S (2012) Effects of a school-based instrumental music program on verbal and visual memory in primary school children: a longitudinal study. Front Psychol 3:572. https://doi.org/10.3389/fpsyg.2012.00572

Rolle C (2010) Musikdidaktische Reflexionen: Was heißt musikalische Bildung durch Inszenierung ästhetischer Erfahrungsräume? In: Wallbaum C (ed) Perspektiven der Musikdidaktik. Olms, Hildesheim, pp 197–223

Rosa H *(2014)* Schule als Resonanzraum, *Vortrag TTS-Kongress—Archiv der Zukunft* „Nichts ist egal oder: die Kultivierung der Bildung“, München *14*–16. Februar 2014

Sammler D, Elmer S (2020) Advances in the neurocognition of music and language. Brain Sci 10(8):509. https://doi.org/10.3390/brainsci10080509

Saß A (2002) Dekodierung emotionaler Sprechweisen durch Patienten mit Innenohrprothese, Dresden: w.e.b. (Studientexte zur Sprachkommunikation Bd. 23)

Spitzer M (2002) Musik im Kopf. Schattauer, Stuttgart

Spychiger MB (1997) Aesthetic and praxial philosophies of music education compared: A semiotic consideration. Philosophy of music education review 33–41

Stadler-Elmer S (2000) Spiel und Nachahmung—Über die Entwicklung der elementaren musikalischen Aktivitäten. Nepomuk, Aarau

Stadler Elmer S (2002) Kinder singen Lieder—Über den Prozess der Kultivierung des vokalen Ausdrucks. Waxmann

Torppa R, Huotilainen M (2019) Why and how music can be used to rehabilitate and develop speech and language skills in hearing impaired children. Hear Res 380:108–121

Trehub SE (2000) Human processing predispositions and musical universals. In: Wallin NL, Merker B, Brown S (eds) The origins of music. MIT Press, Cambridge, MA, pp 427–448

Uden van A (1980) Das gehörlose Kind—Fragen seiner Entwicklung und Förderung. Groos, Heidelberg

Walczyk EB (1993) Music instruction and the hearing impaired. Music Educ J 80(1):42

Wallin NL, Merker B, Brown S (eds) (2000) The origins of music. MIT Press, Cambridge, MA

Wessel D, Fitz K, Battenberg E, Schmeder A, Edwards B (2007) Optimizing hearing aids for music listening, http://cnmat.berkeley.edu/publication/optimizing_hearing_aids_music_listening

Xu L et al (2009) Vocal singing by Prelingually deafened children with cochlea implants. Hear Res 255:129–134

Zimmermann S (2000) Hörübungen zur Stimmfunktion von Kindern. In: Lotzmann G (Hrsg.) Selbstwahrnehmung und Fremdwahrnehmung bei Sprach-, Sprech-, Stimm- und Hörstörungen. Störungen, Therapien, Manipulationen, Chancen. Würzburg, Ed. Bentheim (Sammelband der Inzigkofener Gespräche 18):154–159

Inclusion, Cultural Participation, and Music

9

Irmgard Merkt

In March 2009, the German Bundestag ratified the "Convention on the Rights of Persons with Disabilities." The UN Convention on the Rights of Persons with Disabilities—UNCRPD -thus came into force as the "Gesetz zu dem Übereinkommen der Vereinten Nationen vom 13. Dezember 2006 über die Rechte von Menschen mit Behinderungen" (Bundesgesetzblatt 2008, Part II, No. 35). What is new and special about this law, which has caused so many discussions and activities on the topics of disability and inclusion and actually has an impact on all areas of society?

The principles of the UNCRPD—in Germany UN-BRK—have a certain tradition in inclusively oriented initiatives and projects in some areas of music culture in Germany since the 1980s as outlined below. To this day, the UNCRPD is a motivation and a decisive argumentative aid in political, social, educational and artistic fields.

9.1 Inclusion

First of all: The UNCRPD itself defines neither "disability" nor "inclusion." It creates an image and understanding of persons with disabilities, "*Reaffirming* the universality, indivisibility, interdependence and interrelatedness of all human rights and fundamental freedoms and the need for persons with disabilities to be guaranteed their full enjoyment without discrimination" (UNCRPD Preamble, paragraph c). At the same time, it names and calls for measures to create a society that enables all persons to participate equally in community life "*Recognizing* the importance of accessibility to the physical, social, economic and cultural environment, to health and education and to information and communication, in enabling persons with

I. Merkt (✉)
Department of Rehabilitation Sciences, TU Dortmund University, Dortmund, Germany
e-mail: irmgard.merkt@tu-dortmund.de

G. Kreutz, G. Bernatzky (eds.), *Music and Medicine*, Neurocultural Health and Wellbeing, https://doi.org/10.1007/978-3-662-72175-9_9

disabilities to fully enjoy all human rights and fundamental freedoms" (ibid. paragraph v).

The question "What is inclusion?" is answered by societally, scientifically, educationally and politically relevant actors from various perspectives, but mostly with direct or indirect reference to human rights. However, a clear definition of inclusion seems unattainable: "So far, there is no generally accepted definition of inclusion that is clear-cut, logically consistent and free of contradictions" (Grosche 2015: 20).

However, numerous everyday definitions describe concrete levels of action and attitudes, such as that of the German Aktion Mensch:

> Inclusion means that everyone naturally belongs. Or in other words: inclusion is when everyone can take part. No matter what you look like, what language you speak or whether you have a disability. For example: children with and without disabilities learn together at school. When everyone can be involved everywhere, at work, at home or in their free time: that is inclusion. (Aktion Mensch 2024).

9.1.1 Inclusion: Education

In 50 articles, the UNCRPD outlines all ages, life topics and areas of life—it is, so to speak, a life-spanning text. The right to education and learning without discrimination in a common school system for all children is set out in Article 24. The political consequence is the gradual transformation of the still largely segregated school system in Germany into an inclusive one. The organization of an inclusive school system, desired by many parents of children with disabilities, favored by academics, and more or less decisively shaped by school policy, also affects the arts subjects. Music didactics are challenged to open up to the questions of teaching in which children with different abilities learn, research, and make music together (see Merkt 2019).

9.1.2 Inclusion: Culture

Article 30 of the UNCRPD deals with participation in cultural life outside the school context. The first two paragraphs of Article 30—the other paragraphs on recreation, leisure, and sport are not taken into account here—refer to two levels of activity: Paragraph 1 deals with access to culture at the level of reception, while paragraph 2 deals with the attribution of creative-artistic potential to people with disabilities at the level of production.

Article 30
Participation in cultural life, recreation, leisure and sport

1. States Parties recognize the right of persons with disabilities to take part on an equal basis with others in cultural life, and shall take all appropriate measures to ensure that persons with disabilities:
   (a) Enjoy access to cultural materials in accessible formats.
   (b) Enjoy access to television programs, films, theater, and other cultural activities, in accessible formats.
   (c) Enjoy access to places for cultural performances or services, such as theaters, museums, cinemas, libraries and tourism services, and, as far as possible, enjoy access to monuments and sites of national cultural importance.
2. States Parties shall take appropriate measures to enable persons with disabilities to have the opportunity to develop and utilize their creative, artistic and intellectual potential, not only for their own benefit, but also for the enrichment of society. (UNCRPD paragraph 30 (1) and (2).

9.1.3 Access to Culture: Barriers

Art. 30 Paragraph 1 requires persons with disabilities to have fundamental access to all levels and contents of cultural material, regardless of their existing interest: the possibility is the first prerequisite for actual use. On the "technical" level, it is about knowing and removing barriers. Barriers are not just steps for wheelchair users at the museum entrance or in the concert hall, barriers are also a lack of induction loops for persons who use hearing aids, a lack of tactile floor guidance systems for blind persons, a lack of information in "Plain Language" or "Easy Read" for persons with learning difficulties. Barriers are also websites without voice output or pages that cannot be read by certain programs and converted into Braille. A barrier-free or at least low-barrier website is nowadays a requirement for all cultural institutions.

Cultural events must address the issue of accessibility from three aspects: venue, information about the event and the event itself. Cinemas, concert halls, cultural centers, churches and castles, theaters and museums—they all have the issue of "accessibility." New houses have it easier. They can plan barrier-free access from the start. Exemplary: The Guggenheim Museum Bilbao (Guggenheim Bilbao 2024).

Traditional places don't always have it so easy, but they too have the task of solving the issue of access for everyone. A traditional house like the Bavarian State Opera—Bayerische Staatsoper—in Munich informs the audience comparatively briefly on the topic of accessibility on its own homepage under the following key points: Barrier-free access—places for wheelchair users—parking spaces for disabled people—hearing aids (Bayerische Staatsoper 2024) The page "Kultur barrierefrei München" provides more detailed information about the Bavarian State Opera as a cultural venue; It describes—only in German—the offers for persons in wheelchairs, persons with walking disabilities, deaf persons, persons with a hearing impairment, blind persons, persons with a visual impairment and persons with learning difficulties (Kultur barrierefrei München 2024).

The accessible Internet is the most important informant about cultural events. But print media are also required: A barrier-free poster, for example, is one that displays information about location, time and transport connections not only in writing, but also in symbols.

A visit to the theater becomes barrier-free or at least low-barrier for deaf persons if a sign language interpreter is available. The audio description—it describes the environment, atmosphere, facial expressions, and gestures of the actors in during the dialogue breaks—makes the film visit barrier-free for blind persons. A modern museum offers special guided, adapted tours. Tactile tours for visually impaired or blind persons or tours in Plain English for persons with a special need for explanations are offers that the cultural sector will have to adapt to in the future.

9.2 Cultural Education, Reception, and Production

Beyond the "technical" side of access to culture, equity in participation primarily means access to cultural content. At this point, society's education distribution processes are also repeated for persons with disabilities: the education of parents or other responsible persons is still decisive for participation in cultural life. Persons with disabilities are more dependent on their environment than others when choosing their cultural activities: the immediate environment largely determines cultural content and the way in which culture is used. An older study from 1998 on the subject of leisure and disability in Germany lists the leisure activities of persons with intellectual disabilities in this order: listening to music, doing nothing, watching TV, going on excursions, doing handicrafts and painting, disco/pubs and cinema/theater (Wilken and Pich 1998). Five of the activities are categorized as reception. The first three tend to take place at home. Excursions, disco/pub and cinema/theater, on the other hand, allow persons with disabilities to be present in public and require accessibility from the above-mentioned points of view.

9.2.1 Reception of Music

According to small surveys, the preferred content for listening to music is hits, especially evergreens. In North Rhine-Westphalia, the entertainment music station WDR 4 is the station of choice. It has been known since the Amrhein survey (1983) that children with disabilities are generally open to all styles of music: the children like what they get to know in an appropriate form. Classical, pop, rock, jazz, world music—basically no genre of music needs to be excluded. The age-appropriateness of the offer was and is particularly important for adults with intellectual disabilities. Braun rightly points out this problem:

> In many cultural programs, a methodically necessary elementarization is often confused with a kind of infantilization. It becomes particularly problematic when performances with

a repertoire that is in stark contrast to age-appropriate repertoire is presented to an audience (Braun, 2013 830).

Communicating the diversity of musical expressions is the task of all those who work with persons with disabilities—and also the task of all those who are involved in appropriate training courses and prepare the next generations for the field of cultural mediation work.

As a result of many years of inclusion efforts, access to cultural places is now better regulated than access to cultural content beyond listening to music, doing nothing, and watching television. The fact that persons with sensory impairments could become recipients, cultural tourists and critical event visitors was something that only a few planners thought of 20 years ago.

The "European Capitals of Culture" provide impetus here, and examples of inclusive cultural projects and festivals are "sicht:wechsel" in Linz/Austria 2009 (sicht:wechsel 2009) or "Europa InTakt" in Dortmund/Germany as part of RUHR.2010 (Europa InTakt 2010).

In many cities and regions, so-called "Kulturlogen" or "Kulturschlüssel" make an important contribution to the participation of persons with disabilities in cultural life. Persons with disabilities become "culture lovers" when "culture donors" give away unsold tickets to organizations, such as the Kulturschlüssel Saar (Kulturschlüssel Saar 2024) or the Lüneburger Kulturschlüssel (Lüneburger Kulturschlüssel 2024). Volunteer "cultural companions" visit events together with "culture connoisseurs" together and enable cultural participation that would otherwise not have taken place (cf. Seifert 2014: 42 ff.).

9.2.2 Production of Music

Exceptional musical artists such as Thomas Quasthoff and Felix Klieser draw society's respectful attention to the special and outstanding artistic possibilities of persons under special living conditions. The so-called musical savants, persons with autism and a special talent for music, also trigger a high level of admiration. Diametrically opposed to the admiration for the "top" is the skepticism regarding the musical and artistic competence of persons with disabilities without any obvious special talent. It is not without reason that the UNCRPD refers to the creative and artistic potential of all persons and calls for "appropriate measures" to develop it. There are currently no quantitative studies on the musical or other artistic talent of persons with disabilities. However, one can assume that the normal distribution curve of musical talent also applies to persons with disabilities. This is what the UNCRPD means: Those who can and want to develop their musical potential should have the opportunity to do so. To do this, however, they need competent support—in the form of methodically adapted lessons, sometimes in the form of assistance. In any case, it is necessary to train teachers—at universities or in further education.

9.3 Cultural Participation: The Bochum Model

Long before any discussion of inclusion, Werner Probst (1925–2007) introduced the principle of cultural participation through musical activity into music schools. Probst was head of the Bochum Music School from 1965 to 1969 and from 1969 to 1991, he was a lecturer and professor of music for the disabled at what was then the PH Ruhr and later the University of Dortmund. His credo: "Everyone is fundamentally capable of experiencing music and is in this sense musical" (Probst 1991, 23). And: "Skills and abilities can be developed, they can be trained" (ibid. 38). The model experiment "Instrumentalspiel mit Behinderten und von Behinderung Bedrohten" which Probst carried out with his team at the time, was already based on the awareness that the UNCRPD demands today. In the years 1979 to 1983, students from Bochum's special schools were successfully taught instruments of their choice and, as a matter of course, eventually became students at the Bochum Music School. Probst was convinced that the prerequisite for successful integration was the musical and pedagogical expertise of those who teach children with disabilities. He saw this competence in the teachers of music schools. Since they usually do not have experience in dealing with children with disabilities, they need additional qualifications in special education content. Following the model experiment, Probst, in conjunction with the Association of German Music Schools (Verband deutscher Musikschulen), founded the part-time course BLIMBAM, which trains music school teachers to teach children and young persons with disabilities at music schools. The BLIMBAM course is now in its 42nd year (BLIMBAM 2024). He qualified around 500 participants from all over Germany to work musically with children and young people at public music schools.

The model experiment continues to have an impact today: Today, around 11,700 children, young people and adults with disabilities are registered at around half of the 940 public music schools in Germany. In earlier years, there were only around 400.

What it means for children and adults with disabilities to be a member of an ensemble, play an instrument, and perform in public has not yet been researched in the sense of biographical research, but is described in many individual reports (Wagner 2014). What is highly relevant for the child—in addition to the joy of music—is experiencing their own learning skills. What is relevant for ensemble members is learning how to deal naturally and competently with children and adults with disabilities. Questions of teaching methodology as well as musical content are relevant for music teachers. A survey of music school teachers showed that, with a few exceptions, all of the music school teachers surveyed believe that, thanks to their work with children with disabilities, they have become better teachers for their non-disabled students (Wieczorek 2003). Parents of children with disabilities can experience their children being applauded in public through concert performances: a new and moving experience for them too.

The formation "just fun," a big band from the Bochum music school, has been inclusive since its founding more than 40 years ago: children and young people from schools between special schools and high schools in Bochum play pieces from musical areas such as rock, pop, jazz, ska, and rap and world music, which are arranged by the ensemble's leader, Claudia Schmidt, so that each voice corresponds to the skills of the players. The successful band performed several times at the German Federal President's summer party in Berlin and continues to set musical standards for demanding, inclusive work (just fun 2024).

Since the 1990s, numerous musical initiatives have emerged nationwide in facilities for disabled persons, sheltered workshops and music schools, often inspired by the Bochum Model of Music. In 2017, the Verband deutscher Musikschulen published a collection of basic articles and work aids entitled Spektrum Inklusion (2017). Regional and international festivals are increasingly being held. At the same time, more and more foundations are awarding prizes for various artistic disciplines. From 2004 to 2019, the Förderpreis InTakt honored almost 30 inclusive musical ensembles and individuals who developed innovative models for inclusive musical work (Förderpreis InTakt 2024).

9.4 Cultural Participation: The Dortmund Model

The Bochum model was a project for children and young people with the aim of sustainable musical education. In fact, until this day, some of the participants in the model experiment are still—long grown—members of inclusive ensembles at the Bochum Music School. In the spring of 2010, when the Ruhr area was the European Capital of Culture, the 3-year project Dortmunder Modell: Musik, DOMO for short, began in Dortmund, initiated by the Chair of Music in the Faculty of Rehabilitation Sciences at the TU Dortmund, financed by the Ministry of Labor, Integration and Social Affairs of the State of North Rhine -Westphalia (MAIS). In addition to and expanding the Bochum model BOMO, DOMO: Musik is a project of inclusive musical adult education (Merkt 2014).

Preliminary remarks on musical adult education for persons with disabilities: If a child's musical talent is recognized in a special school, this will ideally lead to private lessons or to a music school. With the end of school and the transition into the world of work, usually in sheltered workshops for persons with disabilities, there is no longer any adult education facility or training institution in which the musical competence of persons with disabilities would be promoted in a targeted and professional manner. The further development of musical potential remains a hobby and a private matter. The conservatory or the music college are available for persons without disabilities who are interested in musical training. However, most of these institutions do not yet feel responsible for the training of persons with disabilities—in case of doubt, they train music therapists for this clientele, but not the "clientele" themselves.

DOMO: Music has carried out inclusive musical adult education for persons with intellectual disabilities at three levels:

- Instrumental or singing lessons: Persons with disabilities receive individual lessons or lessons in small groups.

- Ensemble formation: Professional musicians from regional cultural life form inclusive ensembles with the DOMO musicians.
- Public performances: Concerts and artistic interdisciplinary projects become part of public cultural life. Persons with disabilities become visible in their musical competence as members of musical ensembles.

The path leads from the individual support or small group lessons to collaboration with professional musicians in an ensemble to the public. Learning processes take place on all sides: persons with disabilities experience their own learning ability and the increase in musical skills; they also develop stage presence. The instrumental teachers further develop their methodological skills. The professional musicians from the region also expand their social and methodological skills. Finally, the audience has the opportunity to experience persons with disabilities in new roles and in their musical competence. This is where the circle closes: Cultural education of persons with disabilities leads to a new perspective on persons with disabilities—not through moral appeals, but through musical action (Gerland 2022).

9.4.1 Project Levels Dortmund Model: Music

Project partners of DOMO were the three large Dortmund sheltered workshops with round 1700 workshop employees. The first phase of DOMO was about finding among these persons with musical potential and an interest in playing instruments or singing.

9.4.1.1 Introductory Phase: The Musical Interview

Almost all workshop employees answer the question "Do you want to learn to play a musical instrument?" with "yes." In order to clarify the actual willingness and also the individual competencies, the instrument of the "Musical Interview" was developed. It refers to two areas: On the one hand, musical interests and previous experiences are assessed via a guided interview, and on the other hand, rhythmic competence, movement competence and vocal competence are tested in a practical phase of around 10 min.

This "Musical Interview" was carried out with 679 workshop employees in an initial selection phase. This first look at the interests and the elementary musical abilities also revealed previously unknown musical skills of workshop employees. "I would have suggested completely different participants for DOMO," said the manager of one of the sheltered workshops, "I really learned something about our employees through the interviews."

9.4.1.2 Broad-Based Musical Education

300 interested people received three-month instrumental trial lessons in groups, which were mainly offered within the sheltered workshops during working hours.

At the same time, the choir called "Voices" was offered, which was open to everyone without prior knowledge: workshop employees, their friends and relatives, students from the Faculty of Rehabilitation Sciences and international students from the TU Dortmund, interested persons from the Behindertenpolitisches Netzwerk Dortmund—whoever wanted, could be there. Around 60 to 70 people sang in this choir, 25 of them came from the Dortmund sheltered workshops. The choir was defined as an offer of musical-cultural education, education understood as getting to know previously unknown music. The repertoire was consciously based on the range of musical cultures in the world, on high cultures and new music as well as on folk and popular cultures (Merkt 2012).

9.4.1.3 Talent Development

Eighty persons with disabilities qualified for further talent development in the form of individual or small group lessons: musical development, regular participation and participation in additional workshops were preconditions for further participation in the free instrumental lessons. Towards the end of the second DOMO year, 33 of the DOMO participants finally registered as students at the Dortmund Music School. An initial goal was achieved: the project provided the impetus, and the music school became a new and independently lived part of cultural leisure activities.

9.4.1.4 On the Way to Professionalism

Musical presence, stage presence, concentration and endurance were essential preconditions for further training and musical profiling. Around 15 DOMO musicians have been able to develop their artistic and creative potential to such an extent that they now perform in professional ensembles. In March 2013, the final concert "domo vision" saw 5 ensembles and 80 musicians on stage at the Freizeitzentrum West Dortmund. A half-hour film about the project DOMO: Music can be found online (domo vision 2014).

Some of the ensembles initiated by DOMO: Music are still on the path to professionalization. Above all, the ensemble "piano plus" under the direction of Claudia Schmidt (piano plus 2022), which went on a 2-week tour in October 2013 as part of the "Germany-Brazil Year," supported by the State Chancellery of North Rhine-Westphalia to Rio de Janeiro and Sao Paulo (domo brasil 2013). The "Tanzorchester Paschulke," now also founded by Claudia Schmidt, plays an inspiring brass sound with humorous scenic accompaniment and delights audiences in many cities throughout Germany (Tanzorchester Paschulke 2024).

9.5 Success Conditions for Inclusive Musical Processes

First of all, curiosity about people and openness to new, experimental and unusual things are essential for the success of inclusive processes at all levels and for all those involved.

This applies to the musical field as well as to all levels of the organization. The organizational effort involved in the context of inclusion is often underestimated.

9.5.1 Musical Creativity

The development of creativity in the context of inclusion is by no means the sole responsibility of persons with disabilities. The professional fields of music education and music mediation in particular have the task of dealing with the heterogeneity of learners of all ages in new and creative ways.

Understanding inclusion as the fact that all those who want to express themselves musically and develop further can do so results in new tasks at organizational and musical content levels.

Musical creativity lives in all forms of expression and genres. Creative things can be done in avant-garde music, in a mixture of classical and avant-garde, in music with sounds from nature, in the use of new electronic possibilities and instruments, in the alienation of classical sounds and also in the instrumentation of pieces of music from all cultures and genres based on the abilities of the players.

How do persons who cannot sing in tune become equal members of a choir? How does a sign language choir "work"? How is a choir with blind singers conducted? How do rhythmically insecure persons become interesting members of a drum group? How do string players who only play on open strings become part of an orchestra?

Questions like these show that learning and development processes are essential on all sides. In the artistic field, the development of new sound worlds and forms of presentation is unavoidable—if one does not want to remain in the so-called disability bonus and demand patience and generous listening from the audience instead of offering surprises and artistic quality.

9.5.2 Individualization

The individuality and musicality of persons with disabilities vary greatly. For example, persons with autism syndrome may be completely different in their musicality to persons with Down syndrome or persons with severe multiple impairments.

Some surprise with their reading skills and good memory, others with their perseverance. Some have language skills, and others have non-verbal expression skills that can be put to excellent use in a performance. Against the background of the extraordinary heterogeneity in appearance and musical-artistic expression, the idea of a "one" recipe for inclusive musical work is obsolete. The questions of if-then can only be answered by way of examples and general principles, but not by standardized rules or recipes.

However, the individuality of persons with disabilities is also a positive challenge for music education. If the teachers and artists accept the challenges of working with persons with disabilities, they seize the opportunity to experience themselves as individual and creative again and again.

In addition to the inevitable processes of doubt, these ever-surprising processes are also a constant source of enjoyment for the teachers' personal experience of expertise in the artistic fields. Only those who have developed the personal courage to work with persons with disabilities can report on the enjoyment of this experience. Courage lies particularly in leaving the role of the helper and thus the superior and actually meet at eye level.

9.5.3 Learning and Teaching

After the Second World War, Germany had to face up to the guilt of euthanasia, to which around 300,000 persons with disabilities fell victim. One of the responses—if you want to interpret it positively, an act of reparation—was the expansion of a "special" school system and the establishment and continuation of large and ultimately segregating institutions. Special education was a separate professional field. A few teachers specialized in music, and many repeatedly reported on the joy that music brings to persons with disabilities.

"Music with the disabled" was long a field of music therapy until, from the 1980s onwards, more and more educators referred the idea of musical learning ability to children with disabilities. As a result of the democratic "Culture for All" movement of the 1970s and 1980s, four music chairs for teacher training were established in West Germany—two in North Rhine-Westphalia, one in Baden-Württemberg and one in Hanover. The Bochum model outlined above showed the need for an intensified teacher training.

The most practical and methodological knowledge about pedagogical work has been acquired by those who have worked with children with disabilities with joy and courage. This knowledge has been incorporated into the teaching of committed university lecturers.

Universities cannot be forced to teach certain content—but they usually do react to social developments. "Music and inclusion" is still not a self-evident teaching content, even though more and more chairs have "... and inclusion" in their mandate. Some universities, such as Lübeck or Münster, are committed to the subject, while others do not consider it to be of great importance. The Culture and Inclusion Network has analyzed the situation, which, with a few exceptions, can still be greatly improved (Keuchel and Merkt 2019).

Beyond an "official" inclusion policy in the cultural sector, committed organizations are working intensively on the social mission of artistic education for persons with disabilities. First and foremost is the organization EUCREA, which has succeeded in organizing artistic training for persons with disabilities in cooperation with the Hamburg Conservatory, the Ottersberg University of the Arts and the Folkwang University in Essen (EUCREA 2024).

The Un-Label project is similarly committed, which, in addition to artistic projects, advises and qualifies cultural institutions of the performing arts as well as artists (Un-Label 2024).

9.5.4 Organization

It is not only the experience of the Dortmund project that the effort required to organize inclusive projects is underestimated. Typical organizational tasks include contact with families, carers, and daycare centers, organizing rooms and teaching dates, taking working hours into account, obtaining and borrowing instruments, and obtaining the rights for photo and film documentation—the list is incomplete.

The constructive cooperation of sheltered workshops is essential for all projects in which the working hours of adults with disabilities are affected. In this context, it should be borne in mind that many of the facilities for persons with disabilities are short-staffed and any request for exceptions and changes becomes an additional workload. In this respect, it is very important that everyone involved can experience the benefits that arise from musical and artistic activity.

Benefits can be: life satisfaction, balance, joy, experience of meaning, being focused on a goal, leisure activities experienced as meaningful, new contacts, external activities, etc. Music is never just music alone—it touches the entire environment of its participants.

9.5.5 Financing

Germany is a federal state with 16 federal states and city states. Each federal state has its own state budget and cultural sovereignty in its own area. The federal government in Berlin also has a budget for culture that finances projects of nationwide relevance. None of these budgets have their own position on culture and inclusion. This means that the many "music and inclusion" projects that are carried out outside of state schools and municipal music schools have to raise their own funds.

Numerous large and small public and private foundations promote and support inclusive projects. Nevertheless, it always remains a factor of uncertainty to have to continually raise new funds for what should be often long-term projects. In some cities and federal states, there are meanwhile responsible people in public institutions who support inclusive projects. Overall, however, it must be said that the development towards an inclusive musical and cultural life is still driven by the idealism of so many persons in artistic and educational fields, by parents and, not least, by persons with disabilities themselves.

9.6 Inclusive Music Culture

Inclusion means that what was separate comes together. Inclusive music means coming together on different levels—a coming together of institutions, of electronic with traditional means of production, of artistic disciplines and of artistic developments in countries around the world.

9.6.1 Cooperation

Inclusion demands new forms of coordination and cooperation, including from those involved in shaping culture. Musical theater and schools, orchestras and sheltered workshops, museums and associations for the disabled, choirs from different cultures and disability groups—the variety of cooperative projects is increasing. The Upper Bavarian government's "Zamma" project is an example of a successful cultural policy and, in particular, a successful funding policy: only initiatives and institutions that have not previously worked with each other are eligible to apply. (Zamma 2024) The targeted promotion of a culture of cooperation becomes a culture of social communication.

9.6.2 Digitality

Electronic and analogue music were and still are competitors: In recent years, however, new opportunities for participation in both fields have been opening up, particularly in the field of music-making. Creative inventors are constantly developing new instruments that are orientated towards the movement possibilities of persons with severe impairment. There are electronic musical instruments that turn the slightest breath into sound, such as The Magic Flute, which was created in Rotterdam (The Magic Flute 2007).

There are eye track programs that "understand" a person's gaze and trigger a sound or a chord when the eyes look at a point or field on a screen. Examples are EyePlayMusic (2024), also created in Rotterdam, or EyeHarp (Vamvakousis and Ramirez 2015), developed in Barcelona.

The Soundbeam, which works with ultrasonic sensors and converts movement into sound, was developed in Bristol/UK (Soundbeam 2024), while the Motion Composer, which uses different technology, was developed in Germany (Motion Composer 2024).

The new instruments also give rise to new music, often a mixture of digital and traditional instruments. Outstanding examples are the National Open Youth Orchestra, Bristol (National Open Youth Orchestra 2024), the tabula musica project, Bern (tabula musica 2024) and elefantora, Gothenburg. The German website "soundform—instrumente für alle" by the EUCREA.e.v. association (soundform 2019) provides an overview.

9.6.3 Interdisciplinarity

Inclusion itself is an interdisciplinary field of research. The interaction of different artistic disciplines has always led to new aesthetic and artistic forms of expression. Music and dance, music and theater, music and photography, music and painting, music and words—the multitude of combinations also applies to the field of inclusion.

An example. *Klassik mal anders: Beathoven* was a concert project by the WDR Funkhausorchester in 2020, which brought deaf, hearing-impaired and hearing students together in the Cologne Philharmonic for dance workshops and finally for the big concert evening with the deaf dancer Kassandra Wedel. The workshops for the 30 young people were not about the dance interpretation of Beethoven's music, but about what the music triggered in them (Klassik mal anders: BEAThoven 2020).

Another pioneering dance project was *Carmina—Es lebe der Unterschied*. The dance performance of Carl Orff's Carmina Burana was created in 3 weeks in 2014 by over 300 disabled and non-disabled performers—persons with and without disabilities, secondary school and special needs students, professional dancers and amateurs (CARMINA 2014).

The temporary large-scale projects are contrasted with long-term projects by small ensembles: The music theater ensemble *I can be your translator* combines music, language and scene in its now award-winning productions, which deal with themes ranging from the artistic reflection of the film icon Marilyn Monroe to Einstein and social justice. Currently *i can be your translator* and the Dortmund Theatre are co-production partners as part of the Program for Inclusive Cultural Practice PIK of the Federal Cultural Foundation (I can be your translator 2024).

9.6.4 Internationality

The exchange of artistic ideas not only within Germany but also beyond its borders is essential for the further development of the field of music and inclusion. There are innovative and inspiring inclusive projects in all European countries—and of course beyond—that can be traced back to the long-standing commitment of musicians and artists from all disciplines. Among other internationally orientated festivals such as Kultur vom Rande (Kultur vom Rande 2022), the event series "Europa InTakt" has brought ensembles from many European countries to Dortmund since its inception in 2003 (Europa InTakt 2022). From the Colour Sound Orchestra Parafonia from Hungary (Parafonia 2024) and body percussion with deaf people in Turkey (KeKeÇa 2024) to digitally oriented avant-garde from Switzerland (tabula musica 2024 and Sweden (elefantora 2024), the range and artistic aspirations of inclusive musical cultural work are clear to see.

One project from France and one from Italy are representative of many.

9.6.4.1 France: Les Percussions de Treffort

Les Percussions de Treffort have been in existence for more than 20 years. A small group of avant-garde musicians under the direction of Alain Goudard regularly work musically with adults with intellectual disabilities. Elements of new music are mixed with traditional musical forms, a mixture of composition and improvization creates a play with free and bound rhythms in a wide range of timbres through the use of newly developed instruments. Stage-filling, expansive and acoustically loud installations take place as well as quiet and intimate sound sequences. As the leader of the group, Alain Goudard does not orientate himself in any way to the presumed popular taste of the players or the audience: he offers quality that would be accepted at any festival of new music, and he demands curiosity about music beyond the mainstream, both from the players and the audience (Goudard and Mercier 1999).

9.6.4.2 Italy: Esagramma

The esagramma project in Milan is just as demanding and consistent. The three founding fathers and mothers insist on musical quality in the sense of classical symphonic music. After 3 years of training, people with intellectual disabilities are given the opportunity to play together with professional musicians in an orchestra. The classical pieces are rewritten in such a way that they retain their substance, often with the addition of atmospheric sounds. "esagramma" places an unmistakable educational demand on players and audiences in the spirit of European classical music (Esagramma 2024).

Internationality and inclusion also includes interculturality. In a society in which around a third of all citizens have immigrated from various countries in recent decades, "monocultural music education" in the sense of Western music culture is no longer conceivable. The first approaches to intercultural music education were developed in 1980 in connection with the Bochum model described above. Currently, there is an approach to linking intercultural and inclusive music education, which as a model combines research-based learning with practical music making and is based on the abilities of children and young people. The motto is: Around the world with one question. (Merkt 2019).

9.7 Cultural Policy Tasks

When looking at the developments of the last few years, one might get the impression that a lot has happened. For those who were and are involved, a lot has indeed happened—in more ways than one. The overarching view is different.

In August 2023, the UN Commission on the Implementation of the UNCRPD examined Germany's Second and Third State Report in Geneva. In response to the reports, the committee published the "Concluding Observations" on each article of the UNCRPD on 3 October 2023. These can certainly be read as criticism of the respective governments, even if they are formulated as recommendations.

The committee's recommendations on Article 30 relate to a total of five areas, all of them are of particular importance in the context of music.

The Committee recommends that the State party:

(a) Strengthen mechanisms to ensure that sporting, recreational, cultural and tourism venues are accessible for persons with disabilities.
(b) Ensure that persons with disabilities have access to personal assistance at no cost to practice sport and attend cultural and social activities.
(c) Promote the cultural and linguistic identity of deaf persons, with the participation of their representative organizations, in educational curricula, media and social events.

(d) In close consultation with and with the active involvement of persons with disabilities and their representative organizations, promote inclusion in and the accessibility of all creative arts studies.
(e) Promote cultural diversity in society and the contribution of refugees with disabilities to diversity. (CRPD 2023).

The task for politicians, cultural policy-makers, and society is clear: realization of accessibility, concrete support for participation in cultural life as recipients and producers, intensified support for deaf culture, opening up all creative art studies to students with disabilities and the topic of inclusion and, finally, inclusion of the cultures of people with disabilities who come to the country as refugees.

Not only music academies and conservatories but also all teacher training and social work programs have therefore been given clear homework by the committee in Geneva. Tasks that also include a new understanding of the social mission of their own institution. The central challenge is not the creation of new degree programs with new special situations, but rather the inclusion of the topic of inclusion in the existing system. This means new artistic and pedagogical paths.

9.7.1 Conclusion

What are the necessary next steps? First: The training of persons with disabilities in artistic fields must be further advanced. Artistic universities and teacher training programs in artistic subjects are called upon to open up to diversity and develop new training formats. Second: Cultural life must become more and more open to the artistic contributions of inclusive ensembles. Third: Inclusive ensembles— if they want to work professionally—must allow their artistic quality to be measured against the demands of cultural life. The creation of inclusive culture is both an opportunity and a challenge. The diversity of people corresponds with the diversity of the arts, with the diversity of music. It's a win–win situation in the long term, to shape this diversity artistically.

References

Amrhein F (1983) Die musikalische Realität des Sonderschülers—Situation und Perspektiven des Musikunterrichts an der Schule für Lernbehinderte. Bosse

Bayerische Staatsoper (2024) Service—your visit—accessibility. https://www.staatsoper.de/en/visit-accessibility. Accessed 29 June 2024

BLIMBAM (2024) Qualifizierung zur Musiklehrkraft für Menschen mit Behinderung. https://www.musikschulen.de/projekte/inklusion/menschen-mit-behinderung/blimbam/index.html. Accessed 29 June 2024

Braun E (2013) Kulturelle Bildung für Menschen mit Behinderung. In: Handbuch Kulturelle Bildung. Kopaed, pp 828–831. https://www.kubi-online.de/index.php/artikel/kulturelle-bildung-menschen-behinderung. Accessed 30 June 2024

CARMINA—Es lebe der Unterschied (2014). https://heinzelfilm.de/produkt/carmina-es-lebe-der-unterschied/?v=624007ebb72f. Accessed 30 June 2024

CRPD (2023) Concluding observations on the combined second and third periodic reports of Germany-advance unedited version CRPD/C/DEU/CO/2-3, 2023 (2023). https://tbinternet.ohchr.org/_layouts/15/treatybodyexternal/Download.aspx?symbolno=CRPD%2FC%2FDEU%2FCO%2F2-3&Lang=en. Accessed 30 June 2024

domo brasil (2013). https://domo-brasil.tumblr.com/. Accessed 30 June 2024

domo vision (2014). https://www.youtube.com/watch?v=BIqReCpsR-w. Accessed 29 June 2024

elefantora (2024). https://www.sharemusic.se/en/home. Accessed 30 June 2024

Esagramma (2024) Educazione Inclusiva e Orchestra. https://esagramma.net/educazione-inclusiva/. Accessed 30 June 2024

EUCREA (2024) art plus https://www.eucrea.de/artplus-ausbildung-2021-2024/was-wir-tun. Accessed 30 June 2024

Europa InTakt (2010). https://www.musik-inklusiv.de/europa-intakt/2010. Accessed 29 June 2024

Europa InTakt (2022) Classic goes digital. Dokumentation. https://www.musik-inklusiv.de/europa-intakt/2022. Accessed 29 June 2024

EyePlayMusic (2024). https://mybreathmymusic.com/en/eyeplaymusic. Accessed 29 June 2024

Förderpreis InTakt der miriam-stiftung (2024). https://www.musik-inklusiv.de/forderpreis-intakt. Accessed 29 June 2024

Gerland J (2022) Inklusive musikalische Bildung: Spielraum, Lebensraum, Arbeitsraum. Erfahrungen und Perspektiven aus dem Dortmunder Modell. In: Hiltner-Hennenberg, B. u

Gesetz zu dem Übereinkommen der Vereinten Nationen vom 13. Dezember 2006 uber die Rechte von Menschen mit Behinderungen (2008) In: Bundesgesetzblatt Jahrgang 2008 Teil II Nr. 35,ausgegeben zu Bonn am 31. Dezember 2008. http://www.un.org/Depts/german/uebereinkommen/ar61106-dbgbl.pdf. Accessed 30 June 2024

Goudard A, Mercier B (1999) Les Percussions de Treffort. 20 ans de creation. L'Harmattan; https://bfan.link/les-percussions-de-treffort-50-oeuvres-50-compositeurs. Accessed 30 June 2024

Grosche M (2015) Was ist Inklusion? In: Kuhl P, Stanat P, Lutje-Klose B, Gresch C, Pant H, Prenzel M (eds) Inklusion von Schülerinnen und Schülern mit sonderpädagogischemFörderbedarf in Schulleistungserhebungen. Springer VS. https://doi.org/10.1007/978-3-658-06604-8_1. Accessed 29 June 2024

Guggenheim Bilbao (2024) Guide to accessibility. http://cmsguggenheim-bilbaoeus/uploads/2023/02/Guide-to-accessibilitypdf, https://wwwguggenheim-bilbaoeus/en/useful-information/accessibility. Accessed 29 June 2024

I can be your translator (2024). https://www.icanbeyourtranslator.de/. Accessed 20 June 2024

Just fun (2024). http://justfunbigband.tumblr.com/. Accessed 29 June 2024

KeKeÇa (2024) KeKeÇa Bodypercussion. https://www.kekeca.net/. Accessed 30 June 2024

Keuchel S, Merkt I (2019) Inklusion und künstlerische Hochschulen Status quo und Zukunftsaufgaben. https://kultur-und-inklusionnet/netzwerktreffen/netzwerktreffen-2019/dokumentation-2019/. Accessed 30 June 2024

Klassik mal anders: BEAThoven (2020) Ein Konzert der Reihe WDR@Philharmonie. https://www1.wdr.de/orchester-und-chor/funkhausorchester/videos/video-klassik-mal-anders-beathoven-100.html. Accessed 29 June 2024

Kultur barrierefrei München (2024) Bayerische Staatsoper. https://www.kultur-barrierefrei-muenchen.de/bayerische-staatsoper/. Accessed 29 June 2024

Kultur vom Rande (2022) 8. Internationales inklusives Kulturfestival in Reutlingen. https://kulturvom-rande.de/2022/. Accessed 30 June 2024

Kulturschlüssel Saar (2024). https://www.kulturschluessel-saar.de/. Accessed 29 June 2024

Lüneburger Kulturschlüssel (2024). https://lueneburger-kulturschluessel.de/. Accessed 29 June 2024

Aktion Mensch (2024) Was ist Inklusion? aktion-mensch.de/dafuer-stehen-wir/was-ist-inklusion. Accessed 29 June 2024

Merkt I (2012) Voices. An inclusive choir in Dortmund, Germany. Music Ther Special Music Educ 4(2):93–100. https://approaches.gr/voices-an-inclusive-choir-in-dortmund-germany-irmgard-merkt/. Accessed 29 June 2024

Merkt I (2014) Dortmunder Modell: Musik. Eine Dokumentation. Mitarb. Lis Marie Diehl, Claudia Schmidt. http://docplayer.org/22702911-Dortmunder-modell-musik-eine-dokumentationirmgard-merkt-claudia-schmidt-lis-marie-diehl.html. Accessed 30 June 2024

Merkt I (2019) Musik—Vielfalt—Integration—Inklusion. ConBrio

Motion Composer (2024) https://motion. Accessed 29 June 2024

National Open Youth Orchestra (2024). https://noyo.org.uk/. Accessed 29 June 2024

Parafonia (2024). https://www.parafonia.hu/. Accessed 30 June 2024

piano plus (2022). https://pianoplus.tumblr.com/; https://www.musik-inklusiv.de/europa-intakt/2022. Accessed 29 June 2024

Probst W (1991) Instrumentalspiel mit Behinderten. Ein Modellversuch und seine Folgen. Schott

Seifert M (2014) Kulturelle Teilhabe von Menschen mit Behinderung. Ergebnisse einer Befragung von Gasten der Kulturloge Berlin mit Behinderung und Darstellung der Workshop-Diskussion. In: Mandel B, Renz Th. MIND THE GAP! (eds) Zugangsbarrieren zu kulturellen angeboten und Konzeptionen niedrigschwelliger Kulturvermittlung. Institut für, p 42

sicht:wechsel (2009) Internationale integrative Kunst. https://www.sicht-wechsel.at/archiv/festival-2009/. Accessed 29 June 2024

soundform (2019) Instrumente für alle: Die Zukunft der Musik ist inklusiv. https://www.eucrea.de/soundform Accessed 30 June 2024

Soundbeam (2024). https://www.soundbeam.co.uk/. Accessed 29 June 2024

Spektrum Inklusion (2017) Wir sind dabei! Wege zur Entwicklung inklusiver Musikschulen. Ed. Verband deutscher Musikschulen, Bonn https://www.musikschulen.de/projekte/inklusion/arbeitshilfe/. Accessed 29 June 2024

tabula musica (2024). https://www.tabulamusica.ch/en. Accessed 29 June 2024

Tanzorchester Paschulke (2024). https://tanzorchesterpaschulke.tumblr.com/. Accessed 29 June 2024

The Magic Flute (2007) The head sets the tone. https://mybreathmymusic.com/en/magic-flute. Accessed 29 June 2024

Un-Label (2024) Kunst. Kultur Inklusion https://un-label.eu/. Accessed 30 June 2024

Vamvakousis Z, Ramirez R (2015) The EyeHarp: an eye-tracking-based musical instrument. Proceedings of the 8th sound and music computing conference, SMC 2011. https://www.researchgate.net/publication/229038788_The_EyeHarp_An_eyetracking-based_musical_instrument. Accessed 30 June 2024

Wagner R (2014) „Selbst-verständlich" musizieren heißt selbstbestimmt Musik erleben. In: Merkt I (ed). *Musikkultur Inklusiv. 10 Jahre Förderpreis InTakt der miriam-stiftung* (S. 120–130). https://www.miriam-stiftung.de/forderpreis. Accessed 29 June 2024

Wieczorek M (2003) Menschen mit Behinderungen an Musikschulen. *Eine Untersuchung*. Unveroff.Manuskript TU Dortmund

Wilken U, Pich W (1998) Fernsehnutzungsverhalten von Menschen mit geistiger Behinderung.In: Spektrum Freizeit H 1–3. 112–123. https://duepublico2.uni-due.de/servlets/solr/find?condQuery=*&fq=mods.dateIssued:2010-12-09&owner=createdby:guest. Accessed 29 June 2024

ZAMMA (2024) Kulturfestival Oberbayern. https://www.bezirk-oberbayern.de/Service/Publikationen/Kultur/ZAMMA-Das-Festival-in-Oberbayern/. Accessed 29 June 2024

The Voice and Opera Doctor

10

Josef Schlömicher-Thier and Matthias Weikert

A special profile is expected and demanded from a professional singer, who as a freelance artist has to keep a tight schedule of performances in opera houses, concert halls, and at music festivals around the world. (Please note that in the following text the masculine form of address for the singers is used and thus addresses the ladies and gentlemen of the concert and opera business).

He is often only able to bridge the narrow time spans between rehearsals and concerts by plane. This requires a stable psychological and physical constitution. A good vocal and musical education with a clear assignment of vocal singing type must be successfully completed. The singer is expected to have a flexible ability to adapt to new directing situations with the ensemble members and the artistic director. The difficult roles with the corresponding melody and text passages require a study of roles and notes before rehearsals begin, which are often short, but nevertheless timely. However, professional singers are also subject to the same procedures and triggers for illnesses as the so-called normal population, and these are well known:

Acute viral and bacterial infections, allergies, dietary mistakes/preferences by nutritional problems, environmental influences at the working place stage, medication side effects, possible hormonal influences, especially by female singers, psychological stress due to family and social events, life crises, work overload and excessive demands during the working life (Sataloff 2005; Rubin et al. 2006).

J. Schlömicher-Thier (✉)
HNO-Stimmenzentrum Salzburg, International Voice Center Austria,
Neumarkt am Wallersee, Austria
e-mail: hno-stimmzentrum@sbg.at

M. Weikert
Specialist in Phoniatrics und Pediatric Audiology and Allergology, Consultant of HNOFORUM, Regensburg, Germany
e-mail: mweikert@bonvox.de

G. Kreutz, G. Bernatzky (eds.), *Music and Medicine*, Neurocultural Health and Wellbeing, https://doi.org/10.1007/978-3-662-72175-9_10

10.1 What Is Expected of the Doctor Who Takes Care of the Singers?

The voice specialist, usually an ear, nose, and throat specialist or a phoniatrist and pediatric audiologist, must be aware of the possible causes that can lead to vocal problems and impairment of the professional training of singers (Seidner and Wendler 2004; Richter 2013; Spahn et al. 2011; Schneider-Stickler and Bigenzahn 2013).

They has to know the high demands on the singer in terms of physical and mental strain with regard to their artistic and professional sensitivity, be aware of high individuality, and have empathy for the greatest possible expressiveness and vocal interpretation. He knows, and he has experienced it in the support of the singer as patient, with the increasing occupational achievements of the singers in the jet set world of the engagements and the special life circumstances of the singers, with its frequent change of place, fast journeys in air-conditioned airplanes, dry, noisy hotel rooms with various allergens, and exposure to unfavorable climatic influences on the stage by dust and heat and allergy-causing substances. All this can make the tuning apparatus of the singers susceptible to illness. Causes and diagnoses of the complaints of the indisposed singers require a quick, even emergency treatment of the artist. These are subject to a certain dynamic and time profile, which is very distinctive and unique in the field of vocal medicine (Richter 2013; Flach 1992; Spahn et al. 2011; Benninger et al. 2016; Schneider-Stickler and Bigenzahn 2013).

This special position of vocal medicine is explained in illustrations based on the data from a retrospective study of the Salzburg Festival's singer consultation hours over five seasons (Benninger et al. 2016). The vocal medicine data include 74 singers (37 women and 37 men) who had voice problems during the rehearsal and performance phases and were retrospectively evaluated during five festival summers of the years 2001–2005; they are explained in the current text and in the graphs.

10.2 The Situation of the Voice Doctor: For Example, How Should He React to a Vocal Emergency?

The medical history is most important, this occurs under extreme conditions and under time pressure, in terms of the general acute complaints, the vocal performance, and the vocal and physical demands in the performance piece at hand. The most important points to be asked are shown in Table 10.1.

The urgency of the questions of the singer anamnesis (Table 10.1) results, among other things, from the beginning of the illness, the requirement profile and the hormonal situation. Diagram 10.1 illustrates the staggering of the onset of the disease into a predominantly acute, intermediate and chronic time profiles, which leads to obtaining advice and treatment in the singers' consultation with the physician.

When looking at the voice types—soprano, alto, baritone, or bass, the study shows that female voices have a higher need for consultation and treatment than male voices, which leads to a higher danger of the female voice in the arts (Diagram 10.2), due to the special role of menstruation and the hormonal condition

Table 10.1 Singer anamnesis: what needs to be asked and examined

The start of the illness
Gradual or even chronic signs
Type and strength of the disease response with vocal involvement
Stress and demand profile
Medications being used
Personal disposition and stress estimate of the singer
Timepoint of the premenstrual/menstrual of women under singing strain
Stage and environmental influences, which could have led to acute vocal and also physical reactions/possible decompensation and thus indisposition.

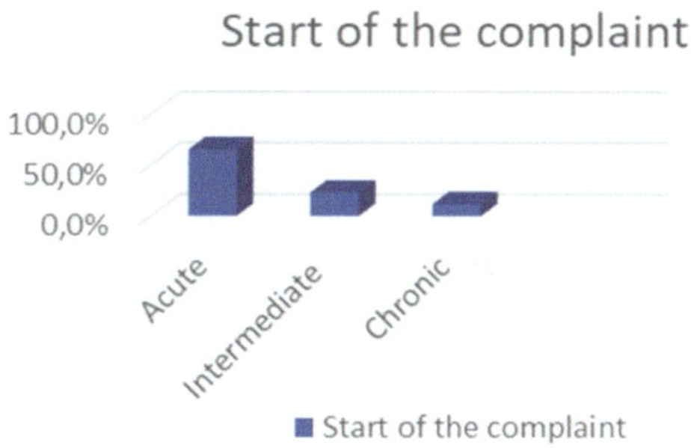

Diagram 10.1 (1)The beginning of the illness is divided into two parts: acute events that began 2–5 days before and (2) chronic problems that began more than a week before. Two-third of the illnesses are acute

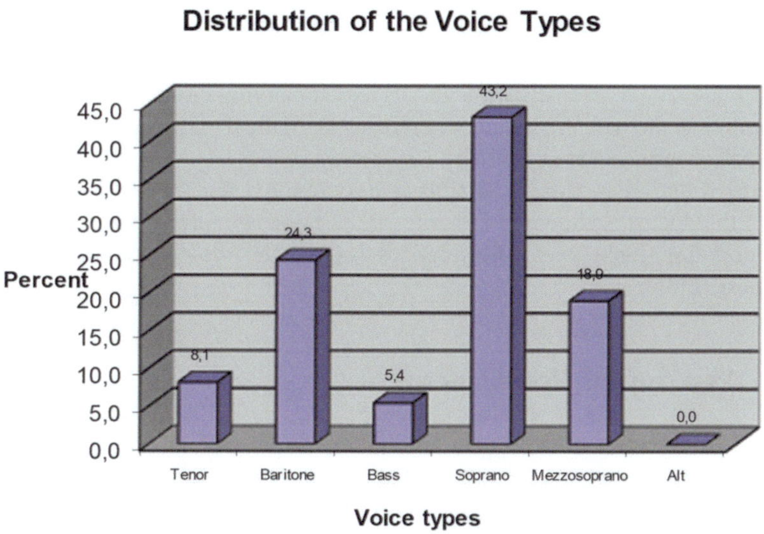

Diagram 10.2 Vocal type "Emergency treatment of the singer according to voice type" (soprano-alt, baritone bass; female voices seem more "vulnerable" than male voices)

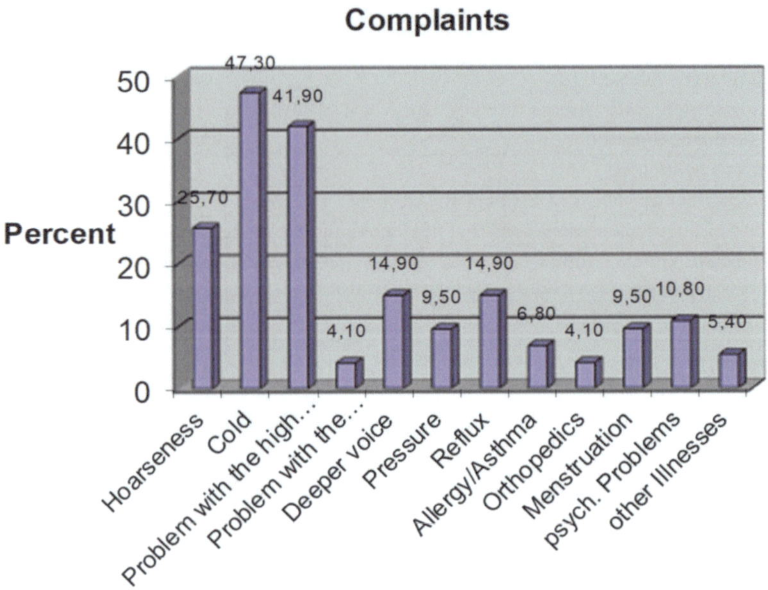

Diagram 10.3 Causes of illness and type of voice changes in percentage of frequency. Complaints were hoarseness, cold, problem with the high register, problem with the middle register, voice deeper, pressure, reflux, allergy/asthma, orthopedics, menstruation, psychological problems, and other illnesses. The majority of the singers had acute colds: 47%. 40% had problems in the upper register; up to 61% had functional vocal complaints; and 26% had hoarseness

of the female singer. Menstruation and its accompanying circumstances play a role by one-third of the women, which requires acute medical care (Sataloff 2005; Rubin et al. 2006; Benninger et al. 2016).

The distribution of the complaints and symptoms which results in the artists going to the doctor is shown in Diagram 10.3. These symptoms are acute infection (47%) and functional vocal disturbances (60%); the most frequent symptom is hoarseness (26%).

10.3 Tasks of the Voice Doctor

The tasks of the voice doctor begin with taking a thorough medical history (anamnesis). This often results in the differential diagnosis between a general disease and an isolated vocal dysfunction. The goal is therefore the rapid assessment of the singer's physical and psychological situation. The psychological situation may well require a longer period of attention, as shown above. The voice doctor should carry out an ENT and phoniatric diagnosis with a focus on ENT and phoniatrics with a rapid assessment of the vocal problem (Seidner and Wendler 2004; Flach 1992; Koufman and Isaacson 1991).

Table 10.2 Tasks of the voice doctor in the treatment of singer

Medical care on the stage/concert
ENT—medical—phoniatric examination (with the purpose of evaluation of the voice constitution and the suitability for the concrete performance)
Professional and competent application of the vocal physiology for the patient on the stage
No artistic judgment and influence of the singer, but most definitely guidance with much feeling in the medical emergency, when it must be decided if the performance will be continued or not.

The goal must be clear decisions for appropriate therapeutic measures adapted to the situation, meaningful, but not exaggerated therapeutic measures.

It is important to have good contact with those responsible in the opera and stage, such as the artistic director, management, evening management, conductor, technical staff, as well as singers and ensemble colleagues.

A very important question in this acute treatment of the singer is to find out reliably whether the singer has already had experiences of this kind:

Has he already sung in such a situation?
How did he cope with this situation?
Did the singer ever "fail" on the stage? (Table 10.2)

10.4 Psychological and Psychosomatic Background of the Endangered Artist

The robustness of the singer is not only endangered, for example, by an acute infection, but also by mental impairment.

Mental impairments can be stressful living conditions caused by frequent changes of location, with many often stressful journeys and separations from the family.

In addition, there are difficulties at the workplace concert and stage, such as conflicts with directors and partners on stage and in the ensemble.

A vocal overtaxing by closely spaced rehearsals or the difficulty of the repertoire can release mental impairments, which can show up then in concrete vocal difficulties in the acute performance or may have already existed for a longer time.

All in all, the psychophysical impairments described here are rather minor, but they can lead to uncertainty in the singer's self-assessment; how quickly the artist comes out of this performance deficit depends on his psychophysical reserves.

The most important initial question regarding the singer's psychophysical reserves is whether he is capable of activating his own physical and emotional reserves in such a way, that he feels confident enough to sing the performance, or whether he is sliding into mental insecurity, and thus also vocal underperformance, at the end of which indisposition threatens.

This case of imminent indisposition requires a voice doctor to intervene for emergency treatment (Fussi 2000; Sataloff 2005; Benninger et al. 2016).

The doctor must therefore be prepared for the singer himself to have doubts whether he will be able to perform; even a slight cold with the fear of indisposition can become a considerable stress situation and burden.

If we continue on this scale of stress before the performance, it is easy to imagine that the closer the performance gets to the performance, the more anxiety the singer feels. As a result, physical complaints, such as muscular tensions, can increase.

The voice, which is a highly sensitive indicator of emotional processes, threatens to fail. Pressure and tension increase.

The singer, possibly in a rash decision, comes to the realization that he cannot sing. The pressure is considerable: the audience is already somewhere in the opera house and the performance should begin soon. In this crisis, the singer shows signs of mental insecurity; he feels weakened, at the mercy of the situation, overwhelmed and threatened. He gets into a sort of helpless state and gives up his independence for a while.

He falls into a kind of regression. In regressive phases, the person—and in our case the singer—feels as if he is a child and is thus ready to accept help as he used to receive it from his mother; this is now the task of the doctor.

The singer seeks help, security and guidance in this situation; indeed, he demands it, without being able to say it. Recognizing this is the important task and also a chance for the voice doctor!

The more the singer gives up his independence in this situation, the more the physician takes over the control and the guidance. Empathy is especially necessary. In addition, the physician puts himself into the position of the threatened singer, who is inwardly asking himself: "Does the doctor see my weakness; does he recognize my latent fear? I am ashamed of myself, yes, I am afraid of embarrassing myself, before the others, before the audience."

In this psychological distress, the voice doctor must be unreservedly open, modest and humble, but also with a clear mandate to guide the singer.

The voice doctor shows the singer that he understands him in his helplessness, that he takes him seriously, that the singer has nothing to be ashamed of, that there is no laughing at the singer and that the singer's dignity is preserved even in this extreme situation where he needs medical help, which he does not really wish for in his innermost being. The singer must therefore feel the competence of the physician in this phase, under strict observance of discretion and medical secrecy.

If this psychological spell is broken, then one comes only to the actual medical examination, which must have the goal of a clear evaluation and the decision of whether the singer in this situation in the time remaining, can be strengthened and treated so that he can sing the role on the stage (Fussi 2000; Sataloff 2005; Spahn et al. 2011).

10.5 Lack of Time for Further Diagnostics

There is often not enough time for further diagnostics. The most important thing is to assess the vocal function and the performance of the voice in relation to the role to be sung. The physician must know that the faster and more differentiated he or she can detect the disorder, in the broadest sense, and not only the vocal component that has led to the singer's indisposition, the more reliably and specifically the therapy can be applied! For example, it may be sufficient to treat an inflammation of the eustachian tube or an acutely obstructed nasal breathing, in case of a largely normal voice function. This is not at all uncommon with jet set artists, both of which often have a devastating effect on the singer's sound, i.e., the vibrator—the larynx—the actual vocal organ is fine, but the resonating chambers are considerably impaired. However, these can very often be restored quickly and in a targeted manner.

After a short stabilization of the psychological situation described above, exercises in voice and breathing therapy can also be useful here. The voice therapist is not demanding and patronizing, but he is empathetic and is the one who provides the noble but specific support. He is the humble coach of the artist.

Here again the psychological guidance of the singer is important. Through skillful guidance and increased attention to the performance event, forces can be mobilized in the singer that counteract the indisposition.

At the same time, the voice doctor must also judge the difficulty of the role and the vocal capabilities of the singer.

If it is possible to change the conviction of the singer, that is, that he can sing his part in the performance, then the biological course in his body changes, muscular tension dissolves, vegetative processes are positively affected, the mood in the best sense improves and therefore the performance will be better. All of this takes place as a procedure of verbal intervention, embedded in manual medical examinations, which together are intended to support the singer and help him to release his psychological tension.

10.6 What Is the Situation of Voice Doctor at the Stage/Concert Hall (the Workplace)?

The vocal emergency treatment, as already briefly mentioned above, often takes place in the singer's dressing room, usually relatives, members of the ensemble or cloakroom attendants and make-up artists should not be present, but the voice doctor should develop a feeling for it, whether close relatives and confidants may be present. The ENT medical and vocal medical instruments are provided in an emergency "stage case," the components of which are summarized in Table 10.3.

In addition to the trained eye of the physician, the most important diagnostic tool for voice evaluation is the trained ear; however, simple manual manipulations, such as targeted sensitive neck and larynx manipulations can also be useful. Finally, the physician himself should be convincing in voice, breathing and posture, not a know-it-all, but projecting calmness and conveying a sense of security.

Table 10.3 Emergency "stage bag"

Head lamp (strong, small LED diodes), disposable instruments such as tongue blades, nasal specula, ear funnel, and tweezers
Laryngoscope in the form of endoscope with magnifying glass and mobile light source, possibly pocket stroboscope
Medication

10.7 The Problem of Medication Recently Taken at the Stage (Workplace)

It is 1 day or only a few hours before the actual performance. The voice doctor must know the influences of medication on the singing voice. Medication, but also environmental factors can influence the singer's very complex and highly sensitive balance between physical strain, maximum sensitivity and the greatest possible personal expression.

When prescribing drugs, the generally valid principles of pharmaco-dynamics and pharmaco-kinetics must be observed (Sataloff 2005; Rubin et al. 2006; Spahn et al. 2011). That means that the dose is to be individually determined. It is based on age, weight, organ function, life habits and from the type of application.

One should know or inquire about the singer's habits in the use of vocal aids as preparation before the performance (vocal initiation rites) (Richter 2013; Wendler et al. 2005).

In total, one has the impression, that illnesses of the upper airway have increased due to allergy, the increased mobility of the artist in international travel, triggered by crowded trains, airplanes with poor air-conditioning, shifting of the day/night rhythm, jet lag, and much more.

The purpose of these treatments and the verbal intervention is to avoid the cancellation of the singer's appearance. It is absolutely necessary to have absolute discretion and even the suggestion of an objective judgment of the singer is to be strictly avoided.

10.8 Cancellation: Is It Really Necessary?

The so-called cancellation policy, what should it accomplish? The voice doctor is the intermediary between the singer and the director of the opera or festival. However, due to his careful medical empathy, which is solely for the benefit of the singer, he needs the trust of both sides, the artist and the director. It is possible to avoid too much caution and timidness, e.g., by wrong and exaggerated protection of the singer, even in case of a small beginning infection, or by excessive safety announcements or advice like ... "stay at home for a week first, then we'll see," which causes both sides, artist and director, to become losers. The singer could lose his fee and the artistic director has to pay additionally for a replacement.

Only when both sides, the voice doctor and the artistic director, work together for the best benefit of the sick singer, is it possible to achieve an individual solution in an acute case that is also tailored to the stage as a workplace. For example, plans are changed, a standby singer is engaged, who then sings in the orchestra pit while the sick singer silently takes over the complicated directing tasks on stage (Richter 2013; Spahn et al. 2011; Benninger et al. 2016).

It is important that the voice doctor notifies the artistic director in good time, and this may well be at night, so that a replacement or standby can be organized as a precaution. In this way, the singer is relieved of his responsibility, pressure and stress are reduced and it saves and spares the nerves of the director.

10.8.1 Cancellation in the Performing Arts of the Opera: How Does One Handle This?

The indications can be seen in Tables 10.4 and 10.5.

In the event of acute Laryngitis a standby solution is possible, that means that the singer acts and the substitute sings, for example, in the orchestra pit or the side of the stage!

Experience shows that in the stage and singer medical care, the appearance of signs of illness resulting in cancellation that the singers can perform again within 4 days. This can be seen in Diagrams 10.4 and 10.5.

The recovering singer must be aware, that:

- He cannot force his voice
- He should not sing out to the maximum
- If he can perform with clear glissando, good messa de voce and safe passagio—and he feels safe—then he "can make it through the performance"

Table 10.4 Cancellations in the performance operation

Complete indication of a cancellation by acute events 1–2 days before the performance
1. Fulminating illness with high fever
2. Bleeding of the vocal cords
3. Laryngitis, tracheitis, and laryngitis
4. Pulmonary infection with strong cough
5. Gastroenteritis reflux with vomiting and gastroenteritis
6. Illnesses in the abdominal and urological area
7. Axis skeleton problems (disc problems), neurological problems
8. Acute cardiological/circulatory problems

Table 10.5 Relative indications of a possible cancellation/standby rule

1. Adequate relaxation time
2. Successful anti-allergic treatment, e.g., beginning vocal cord edema
3. Tonsillitis or pharyngitis without the involvement of the larynx, successfully treated with antibiotics and improving
4. Subacute reflux laryngitis that responds well to proton pump inhibitors
5. Soft discrete vocal cord thickenings, indicative of vocal stress symptom, e.g., "prenodal condition" occurring during pre-menstruation by existing glissando and messa di voce
6. Acute illnesses of the musculoskeletal system that can be compensated by aids (e.g., (1) knee injury of the "Devil" in "Jederman" (Salzburger Festspiele 2004) who used crutches or (2) the acute stretched ligament/tearing in the ankle joint of a tenor in Wozzek (Salzburger Festspiele 2011) who continued to perform in a wheelchair)
7. A situation when the roll can be sung with microport support.

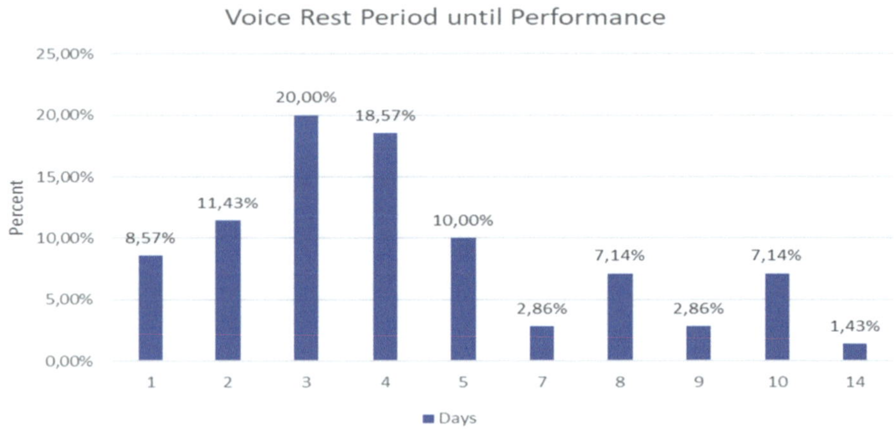

Diagram 10.4 Distribution of the voice resting time of the treated singers in a 2-week distribution. Two-third is within the first 5 days ready to perform, one-fourth still needs 4–5 additional days during the treatment by the voice doctor

Diagram 10.5 The singers need up to 5 days vocal rest before the performance and 10% can perform after 1 day

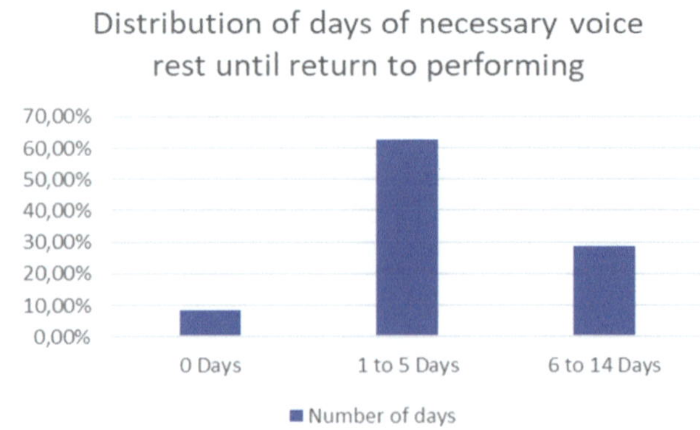

In today's economic pressure of the concert and festival operations, the motto can be:

The goal is to save the salary of the singer, but prevent damage to his health.

These are the general comments regarding the singer anamnesis and dealing with the singer at the workplace, concert or stage.

10.9 Summary

Special circumstances are existing if the decision is whether the singer can perform or not:

- The remaining time is limited.
- The vocal doctor must quickly recognize that a decision has to be made and the singer has to be helped.
- The examination is an emergency.

The response of the singer to the therapeutic intervention of the Phoniatrician (voice doctor) is often not predictable, because the singer is in a very stressful and special situation. The vocal doctor must send out quietness and security and the singer must be guided. This can only be achieved when he knows exactly the field of work of the singer.

- The voice doctor is well informed about opera and concert performances at the particular place of work, i.e., the stage/concert hall, or can inform himself quickly because he is familiar with the musical profession.
- The voice doctor can assess the difficulties of roles (ambitus, passagio, dynamics, special movements during vocal development).
- The voice doctor knows the effects of the drugs on the vocals.
- He has good contact to the singers and the persons responsible at the opera and the concert.

Responsible persons, in particular, the director, the conductor, the technician and the ensemble members must help and support the singer in his threatening indisposition.

This occurs when they show understanding in motivating the singer. This occurs in that they do excellent work in a stressful situation.

It is important to positively shape the field of work of the singer, especially of the so-called threatened singer, and also to bring the audience into a state of readiness, e.g., by a skillful, non-traumatizing announcement, to recommend the singer benevolently.

It is only possible when all involved work together, that the singer, who at the beginning is not quite disposed and who has received an emergency treatment, can find his voice and get through his part.

References

Benninger MS, Murray T, Johns MMIII (2016) The performer's voice, 2nd edn. Plural Publishing Inc

Flach M (1992) Indisposition und akute Dysphonie beim Berufssänge. Laryngo-Rhino-Otol 71:233–235

Fussi F (2000) La Voce del Cantante. Omega Edizioni, Torino

Koufman JA, Isaacson G (1991) The vocal usage classification system: the spectrum of vocal dysfunction. Otolaryngol Clin North Am 24(5):985–988

Richter B (2013) Die Stimme—Grundlagen, Künstlerische Praxis, Gesunderhaltung. Henschel Verlag

Rubin JS, Sataloff RT, Korovin GS (2006) Diagnosis and treatment of voice disorders, 3rd edn. Plural Publishing Inc

Sataloff RT (2005) Professional voice: the science and art of clinical care, 3rd edn. Plural Publishing, Inc, San Diego

Schneider-Stickler B, Bigenzahn W (2013) Stimmdiagnostik, 2nd edn. Springer Verlag

Seidner W, Wendler J (2004) Die Sängerstimme. Henschel, Berlin

Spahn C, Richter B, Altenmüller E (2011) MusikerMedizin—Diagnostik, Therapie und Prävention von musikerspezifischen Erkrankungen. Schattauer Verlag Ger

Wendler J, Seidner W, Kittel G, Eysholdt U (2005) Lehrbuch der Phoniatrie und Pädaudiologie, 4th edn. Thieme, Stuttgart

Part III

Music Therapy in Transition

Introduction to Neurologic Music Therapy

11

Michael H. Thaut, Volker Hömberg, and Stefan Mainka

With neurologic music therapy (NMT), for the first time in a long history of the idea of music as a therapeutic agent, a scientifically based and verifiable clinical system has emerged that can assign a clear role to music as a complex aesthetic-sensory language in neurological rehabilitation and therapy. In this context, neurobiological music research plays a crucial role in continuing to investigate the supportive effect of music on therapeutic learning, behavior, and neuroplasticity and to translate it clinically based on evidence. NMT relies both on experimental research and on the transfer of scientifically based motor and cognitive learning theories to therapeutic learning and practice. Therefore, the NMT methodology is well prepared for future developments in clinical applications. Meanwhile, NMT is practiced in over 60 countries and is increasingly playing a role in "Community Based Rehabilitation" in countries outside of the highly industrialized world.

The understanding of the role of music in therapy and rehabilitation has changed significantly in the last 20 years. Parallel to and guided by neuroscience research on the human brain, a new perspective on the biomedical potential effects of music as a

M. H. Thaut (✉)
Faculty of Medicine, Institute of Medical Sciences and Rehabilitation Science Institute, Director, Music and Health Science Research Collaborative and Graduate Programs, Collaborator Scientist CAMH Neuroimaging, Affiliate Scientist St. Michael's Hospital, Canada Research Chair Tier I in Music, Neuroscience and Health, University of Toronto, Toronto, Canada
e-mail: michael.thaut@utoronto.ca

V. Hömberg
Department of Neurology, Gesundheitszentrum Bad Wimpfen SRH-Group, Bad Wimpfen, Germany

S. Mainka
University of Arts Berlin, Berlin, Germany

Parkinsonklinik Beelitz-Heilstaetten, Beelitz, Germany
e-mail: Mainka@kliniken-beelitz.de

G. Kreutz, G. Bernatzky (eds.), *Music and Medicine*, Neurocultural Health and Wellbeing, https://doi.org/10.1007/978-3-662-72175-9_11

complex auditory biologically intrinsic "language" of the brain has opened up in the last decade of the twentieth century and in the first decade of the twenty-first century through clinical research and basic research. Driven by initial discovery studies on the influence of acoustic rhythms on motor control processes in the early 90s at Colorado State University (Thaut et al. 1993, 1996, 1997, 1998; Miller et al. 1996; McIntosh et al. 1997), NMT has developed as a standardized therapy methodology that is now not only scientifically but also clinically and educationally recognized. In this context, the musical structures and the corresponding perception processes play a crucial role in the rehabilitative effect. Of the 20 currently standardized techniques, 19 are based on musical-rhythmic perception processes, while only one method (music-supported psychosocial training, MPC) uses therapeutic exercises and role plays with emotional interpretation and with emotional expression exercises, when emotional dysfunctions are diagnostically a core function in rehabilitative training. The scientific basis of NMT is therefore based on clinical translations of neuroscientific mechanisms in music perception, music cognition, and music playing.

Three short examples may illustrate this conceptual "revolution." Rhythmic, melodic, and harmonic elements in music stimulate the motor nervous system and structure predictable time frames, which, as sensory information in the programming of motor planning and movement execution can significantly support and improve dysfunctional neurological control processes.

The complex acoustic composition architecture of music offers numerous ways to train auditory perception and attention, for example, through pattern recognition of musical elements in selective or sustained attention training. Rhythmic-melodic phrase patterns in music can be effectively used as mnemonic exercise units in memory training. Associative memory performance through music, for example in dementia, can stimulate still preserved long-term memory functions. Creative-rational task settings to stimulate executive functions can be used with patients through guided improvisation or elementary composition exercises, where in music the tasks can be solved in "real time": A concrete product emerges through a dynamic process that combines purely rational problem solving with creative and affective decision and evaluation elements, which are crucial for the restoration of the "global" executive function.

The overlaps and parallels between the processing, perception and production processes in music and in verbal language are so diverse that few explanations are needed for basic understanding. Music is another highly complex acoustic language with numerous common processes, but also important differentiations, which make it possible to stimulate and support language function when primary language centers are disturbed developmentally or due to illness or injury.

11.1 Music in Motor Therapy

Modern neurophysiology has shown that there is a close and complex networking between acoustics and motor skills in the human brain, which is laid out in parallel and hierarchically distributed neuronal levels from the brainstem and spinal area to the neocortex (Paltsev and Elner 1967; Rossignol and Melvill 1976; Ermolaeva and Borgest 1980). These networks provide a crucial neural basis for the use of music in motor therapy, especially the rhythm function as a temporal template, which plays a critical role as a timekeeper and drive stimulus ("Primer") in the movement control (Thaut et al. 1999a, b). Motor applications were not or only peripherally introduced in traditional music therapy. Interestingly, however, this field has developed over the last 20 years with the best evidence base in NMT following groundbreaking clinical research in gait rehabilitation with stroke (Thaut et al. 1993, 1997) and Parkinson's (Thaut et al. 1996; Miller et al. 1996; McIntosh et al. 1997). Clinical methods of music in motor therapy, such as Rhythmic Auditory Stimulation for gait training (RAS), are clinically established and recognized as state of the art.

Psychophysical and imaging studies have shown that motor timing coupling to acoustic rhythms occurs almost immediately, is achieved precisely and stably in the millisecond range, and that timing information also regulates movement below conscious perception (Stephan et al. 2002). It is important to understand that movement synchronization primarily occurs through coupling to the rhythmic stimulus period and not through phase coupling of movement to the "beat" (Thaut et al. 1998; Large et al. 2002). Acoustic rhythms sensorially form a stable and anticipatable time stretch, which allows the brain to program and implement control variables for movement, such as position, trajectory, speed, or acceleration, optimized in a continuous feedback-feedforward process. The time clamp of the rhythm, therefore, improves not only temporary stability and variability but also spatial and dynamic (force) movement control.

Research results for gait rehabilitation in stroke consistently show improvements in all basic gait parameters (speed, symmetry, stride length, and stride frequency), kinematic functions (e.g., knee and hip angle, center of mass trajectories), and improvement of EMG variability (Ford et al. 2007; Kenyon and Thaut 2000; Prassas et al. 1997; Roerdink et al. 2007, 2009; Schauer and Mauritz 2003; Schauer et al. 1996; Thaut et al. 1993, 2007). RAS is also used to optimize treadmill training for this clientele (Mainka et al. 2018). However, results for strokes in the thalamic region have shown mixed results, especially in improving the kinematics of gait symmetry, particularly for patients with severe sensory dysfunctions and increased paresis (Abiru et al. 2009; Nakano et al. 2009). Therefore, RAS applications must be individually adapted to the severity of the paresis and the presence of sensory dysfunctions.

Transfers of rhythmic-musical stimulation to arm and hand functions and coordination functions of the whole body follow the RAS model and have been well demonstrated by functional movement tests over the past 10 years (Altenmüller et al. 2009; Luft et al. 2004; Malcolm et al. 2009; McCombe et al. 2006; Rojo et al. 2011; Schneider et al. 2007, 2010; Senesac et al. 2010; Sharma et al. 2023; Whitall et al. 2000). Important additional aspects beyond rhythm in this area of motor therapy are the additional guiding signals of the music structure regarding spatial control (e.g., through different pitches) and muscle force control (e.g., through timbre, volume, tone density)—methodically established as Patterned Sensory Enhancement (PSE)—and in functional movement training on musical instruments the spatial movement guidance through the placement of the instruments and the feedback through the sound production when playing music. The latter applications are methodically summarized as Therapeutic Instrumental Music Playing (TIMP). New research findings not only underpin the functional effectiveness of TIMP in the chronic phase of hemiparetic arm rehabilitation (Haire et al. 2021) but also show through dynamic-kinematic measurements that the spatiotemporal structure of the TIMP exercises brings about improved mechanisms in speed control (acceleration, deceleration) of the paretic arm (Loria et al. 2022).

Furthermore, there is a more widely scattered number of studies for various patient groups, e.g., for Huntington's (Thaut et al. 1999a, b), Cerebral Palsy (Kwak 2007; Peng et al. 2011), Traumatic Brain Injury (Jones et al. 2021; Baram and Lenger 2012; Goldshtrom et al. 2010; Hurt 1998), Multiple Sclerosis (Baram and Miller 2007), Down Syndrome (Robertson et al. 2002), and Geriatrics (Clair and O'Konski 2006; Trombetti et al. 2011).

The evidence is particularly dense in the area of RAS for gait training in Parkinson's. A complete listing of all research work of the last 15 years would far exceed the scope of a review. The first discovery studies (Thaut et al. 1996; Miller et al. 1996; McIntosh et al. 1997) were followed by a multitude of studies that have confirmed and extended the significant gait improvements, e.g., on the improvement of akinetic states (Bernatzky et al. 2004; De Bruin et al. 2010; De Dreu et al. 2012; Del Olmo et al. 2006; Del Olmo and Cudeiro 2003, 2005; Freedland et al. 2002; Hausdorff et al. 2007; Howe et al. 2003; Lim et al. 2005; Ma et al. 2009; Morris et al. 2004; Nieuwboer et al. 2007; Rochester et al. 2005; Satoh and Kuzuhara 2008; Suteerawattanano et al. 2004; Van Wegen et al. 2006; Willems et al. 2006; Mainka et al. 2021). Significant reductions in falls through RAS were shown in a long-term study by Thaut et al. (2018).

In a 4-week TIMP study with patients with Parkinson's disease, significant improvements in arm movement control were demonstrated (Buard et al. 2019a, b). MEG measurements showed an increased neuronal signal synchronization between auditory and motor cortex.

Induced cortical plasticity through NMT-based methods of motor therapy for Parkinson's has been documented in three new research findings: changes in dopamine uptake in the striatum of the basal ganglia (Koshimori et al. 2019); activation of compensatory cortical-cerebellar networks to support dysfunctional basal ganglia activation (Braunlich et al. 2018); activation of significantly synchronized local field potentials in the Globus Pallidus Internus through rhythmically-acoustically controlled hand movements in intracranial measurements of deep brain stimulation electrodes during implantation (Sharma et al. 2023).

General assessments of rhythmically musical methods—particularly RAS—can be found in Jeffery and Good (1995), Hummelsheim (1999), and Hoemberg (2005).

In summary, the general evidence positions the rhythmically musical methods (RAS, PSE, TIMP) in motor therapy among the research-proven therapy forms (◉ Figs. 11.1 and ◉ 11.2). Therefore, these are part of the standard repertoire in neurorehabilitation. The methodology is standardized in NMT, but at the same time allows a broad patient-oriented interdisciplinary approach.

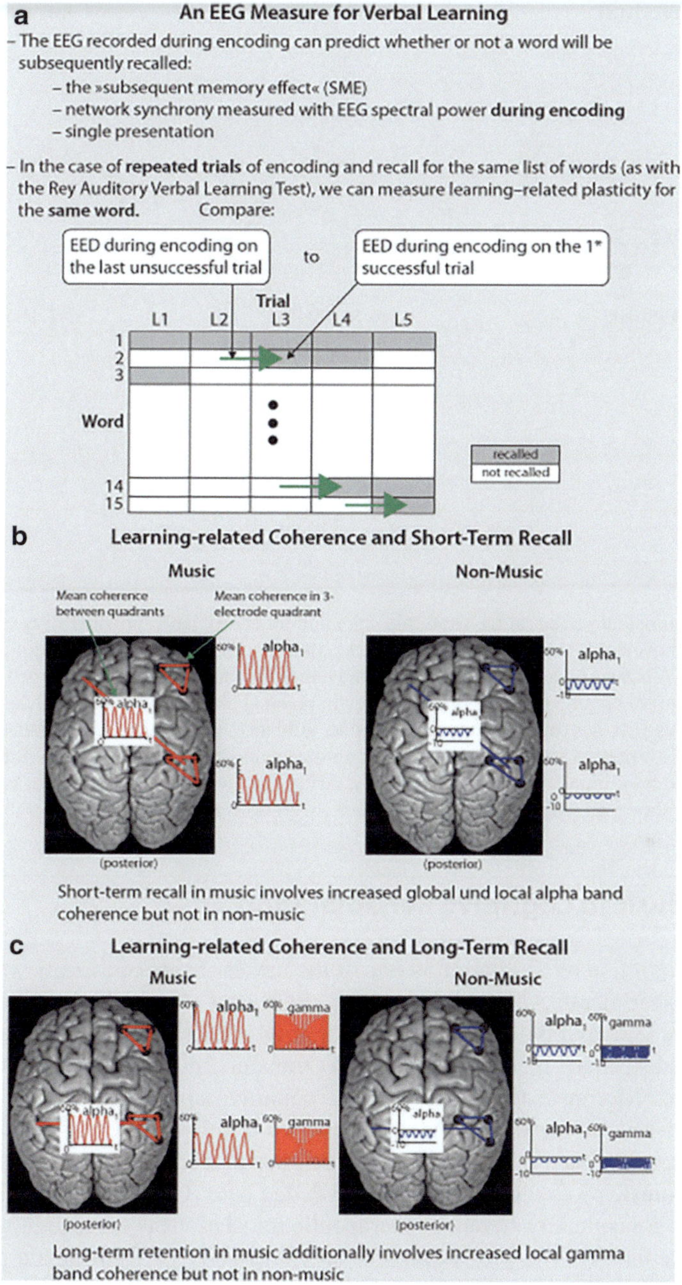

Fig. 11.1 (**a–c**) EEG measurements during verbal learning. (**a**) Measurement scheme to determine whether coherence measurements in the EEG during the first successful learning attempt of a word can predict later recovery in the memory post-test. (**b**) Successful learning in short-term memory involves global and local alpha band coherence in musically supported learning, but not in learning without music. (**c**) Long-term memory (20 min after the last learning session) in the music group additionally involves local gamma band coherence

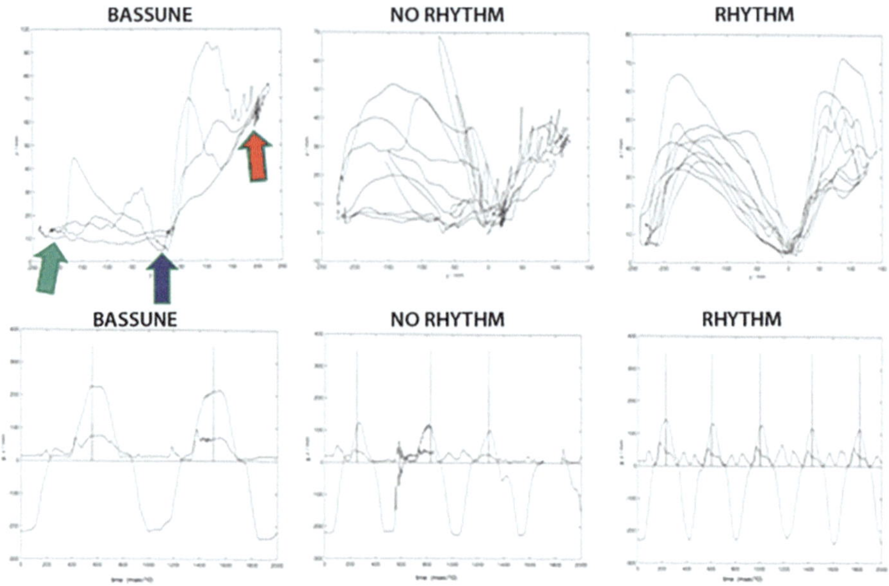

Fig. 11.2 Immediate effect of the rhythmic signal on trajectory path and variability of the paretic (right) arm movement of a CVA patient (4 weeks after insult). Upper image in sagittal alignment (side view, y/z space plane), cyclic reaching movement starts at target 1 (arrow left) to target 2 (arrow middle) to target 3 (arrow right). Movement reversal at target 3. Image 1: Baseline without practice. Image 2: Movement without rhythmic guidance after 3 min of practice. Image 3: Movement with metronome signal after 3 min with acoustic rhythm guidance; rhythm frequency is adjusted to baseline of movement frequency. Arrows show approximated target contacts. The lower image shows an arm movement in y/z plane, with time on the horizontal axis underneath

11.2 Music in Cognitive Rehabilitation

Music in cognitive rehabilitation is one of the newest fields of therapy where NMT has established itself. Although music cognition as a science in the connection of musicology and psychology has been a highly interesting research tradition for many decades, there were no concepts to transfer this research to rehabilitative applications. Moreover, in music therapy, cognitive applications were not in the primary scientific focus due to the dominance of psychotherapeutic models.

In the last 20 years, neuroscience research has placed the neurobiological foundations of music processing on a new knowledge base. One of the crucial discoveries that has conceptually advanced therapeutic translations is the realization that the neural systems in music processing do not exclusively perform music processing but are multifunctional or multimodal systems (shared systems) that are centrally involved in the control and processing of general nonmusical processes, e.g., for language, attention, memory, executive functions, and motor skills. These insights provide a new basis for how general cognitive and motor functions can be reached, driven, and regulated through music-based sensory stimulation. Music as a neurobiologically founded language of motor and cognitive stimulation of learning and re-learning has thus also made its way into cognitive rehabilitation. In NMT, nine clinical methods are coded.

Nine clinical methods in Neurologic Music Therapy

For attention training:
1. Musical Sensory Orientation Training (MSOT)
2. Musical Neglect Training (MNT)
3. Auditory Perception Training (APT)
4. Musical Attention Control Training (MACT)

For memory training:
5. Musical Echoic Memory Training (MEM)
6. Musical Mnemonics Training (MMT)
7. Associative Mood and Memory Training (AMMT)
8. Executive Function Training (MEFT)
9. Musical Psychosocial Training and Counseling (MPC)

The best-founded evidence base of clinical research lies in the area of music-based memory training. Two methodological approaches can be distinguished:

10. The mnemonic memory training (Musical Mnemonics Training, MMT), which aims at prospective learning and strengthening the working memory
11. The associative memory training to improve access to long-term memory and autobiographical memories (Associative Mood and Memory Training, AMMT)

The mnemonic training is based on a chunking model (Deutsch 1982; Hitch et al. 1996), in which the inherent time structure of music—communicated through its rhythmic-melodic patterns—represents a metric template or framework onto which nonmusical information is "loaded" and thereby sequenced into structured learning units with specific auditory sound patterns (container principle, "chunking principle"). The ABC song is the classic example. Examples of MMT research studies come from, among others, Wolfe and Hom (1993), Wallace (1994), Ho et al. (2003) and Chan et al. (1998), Kern et al. (2007) for autism, Gfeller (1983) and Claussen and Thaut (1997) for learning disabilities, Thaut et al. (2007, 2014) for multiple sclerosis and Moussard (2012) for dementia.

A multitude of research from the last 10–15 years shows that in neurological memory dysfunctions—such as dementia or Alzheimer's —functions of memory for music often remain preserved longer or the associated music memory opens access to nonmusical autobiographical memory performances (e.g., Baur et al. 2000; Cuddy and Duffin 2005; Foster and Valentine 2001; Halpern and O'Connor 2000; Haslam and Cook 2002; Irish et al. 2006; Samson et al. 2009; Son et al. 2002; Vanstone and Cuddy 2010; Vanstone et al. 2009). A study by Cowles et al. (2003) provides initial evidence that music-based memory processes may also be extended to prospective learning of new material. A violinist with an Alzheimer's diagnosis and profound retro- and anterograde memory deficits was not only able to continue playing music he knew but also to learn new unknown music.

Two imaging studies on neural memory networking in Alzheimer's disease (AD) interestingly showed that in Alzheimer's subjects, neural connections between the prefrontal cortex and amygdala were activated, while in healthy subjects the typical prefrontal-hippocampal networks were active (Grady et al. 2001; Rosenbaum et al. 2004). This may offer an explanatory model for thc mode of action of music: Music-based memory training enhances the activation of amygdala-based memory networks due to the prominent emotional character of music. The modulating influence of music on memory-oriented brain processing has also been investigated in research by Janata et al. (2002) and Peterson and Thaut (2007).

New insights as to why long-term music-based memories in the memory of people with AD often remain longer than other, newer memory imaging, were presented for the first time in a study by Thaut et al. (2020). Listening to long-known music (>25 years) with autobiographical relevance activated an extensive and strongly bilateral network of both cortical auditory and prefrontal as well as subcortical areas, some of which are not directly affected in the disease process (e.g., basal ganglia, cerebellum). This networking as a characteristic of neuronal "deep encoding" contrasted with mainly auditory-sensory activations by unknown music, which was played for the first time an hour before the fMRI measurements. In a follow-up study of 3 weeks of daily listening to long-known music, cognitive improvements in neuropsychological memory tests (MOCA) and increased connectivity in prefrontal areas and "White Matter Density" were found (Fischer et al. 2021).

In the field of attention training, there is solid basic research on how music stimuli and music training auditory attention functions, e.g., selective attention (Strait and Kraus 2011) can control and improve (e.g., Klein and Riess Jones 1996; Loui et al. 2005; Andrews and Dowling 1991). Research works, which investigate clinical transfers, are rarer. The best evidence is available for musical-acoustic neglect training. Two related explanatory approaches support the use of music in neglect training: the strong auditory arousal effect of music and the pronounced bilateral and tendentially right-dominant hemispheric activation of the brain by music perception. The successful use of acoustic stimulation as part of arousal-based techniques has been demonstrated by Robertson et al. 1998 and

Frassinetti et al. 2002a, b. Specifically for the use of music-based methods, there are research investigations, e.g., by Hommel et al. (1990), Soto et al. (2009) and Kang and Thaut (2019).

Practical Tip
One of the most effective active exercise protocols for neglect training in Neurologic Music Therapy is based on playing sound bars, whose spatial arrangement in front of the patient, starting in the central field of view, is increasingly set up into the neglect area.

In other areas of attention training, the development of a new research base for music-based methods can be observed. Three clinical areas can be distinguished:

12. The Auditory Perception Training (APT) (Amir and Schuchman 1985; Gfeller et al. 2002; Loui et al. 2008; Rochette and Bigand 2009)
13. The basic attention and arousal training (Musical Sensory Orientation Training, MSOT) for severe developmental disabilities, dementia, and consciousness disorders (Gregory 2002; Hammar et al. 2011; Magee 2007)
14. The focused training for sustained, selective, alternating, and divided attention (Musical Attention Control Training, MACT) (Barrow et al. 2006; Knox et al. 2003; Jones et al. 2021)

In these areas, a promising clinical practice and research direction is developing. However, the density of the evidence is still limited.

The newest area of NMT in cognitive rehabilitation is in the training of executive functions (MEFT). Here, through therapeutically structured improvisation, elementary composition, and musical learning exercises with the patients, attempts are made to target and specifically train executive processes. Initial research results show positive results (Bugos et al. 2007; Ceccato et al. 2006; Schweizer et al. 2011; Thaut et al. 2009). However, further research work is necessary to further substantiate this area scientifically and clinically.

The fourth traditional area of cognitive rehabilitation includes the rehabilitation of psychosocial processes (MPC). Traditional music therapy has always considered psychosocial therapy applications as a core area, e.g., in terms of concepts of well-being and social relationships. In NMT, this core area is preserved, but is functionally defined in coordination between diagnosis, assessment, and therapeutic goal. The traditional clinical literature in this area is diverse, the experimental research literature is limited but is beginning to develop more strongly under the functional approach (Carr et al. 2012; Cooke et al. 2010; Guetin et al. 2009; Kleinstauber and Gurr 2006; Nayak et al. 2000).

11.3 Music in Speech and Language Therapy

Music and language share the same acoustic foundations in perception and production. Singing and speaking have a common physical production apparatus. The neurobiological processing of language and music overlaps in cerebral areas, particularly in the Inferior Frontal Gyrus (IFG) of the dorsolateral prefrontal cortex and in the areas of the Superior Temporal Gyrus (STG, Auditory Cortex). However, there are also important distinguishing features. Here are four brief examples:

Singing involves bi-hemispheric regions, while language is mapped unilaterally (mainly left dominant) in the brain. Compared to speech acoustics, music has a temporally and spectrally richer, highly complex structured acoustic architecture. The singing voice has a richer acoustic profile (overtone presence) and an enhanced presence of the fundamental frequency compared to the speaking voice. Music has a rule-guided "grammar" of tone structure, which can be seen in analogy to language grammar, but which is also characterized by crucial differences in terms of rule function, communication function, and semantic meaning.

From these four examples, it can be relatively easily seen how methods can be derived in which music and rhythm can sustainably support language and speech training. The eight NMT methods for language and speech training can be summarized into three groups.

11.3.1 Methods That Operate on Neurobiological Foundations

The first group includes methods that operate on neurobiological foundations—mainly in aphasia therapy. Melodic Intonation Therapy (MIT) uses the translation of short speech units into sung, melodic-rhythmic phrases in Broca's aphasia to activate alternative language centers in the non-lesioned right hemisphere. This technique has now reached a well-founded basis in research (Wan et al. 2010). Musical Speech Stimulation uses overlearned musical forms (e.g., familiar song lyrics) to activate reflexive language centers and drive language production "automatically" (Basso et al. 1979).

11.3.2 Methods Based on Musically Rhythmic Exercises

The second group includes the three methods that improve speech mechanics through musically rhythmic exercises. This is firstly Rhythmic Speech Cuing (RSC), which regulates dysfunctions of speech flow through melodic and rhythmic-acoustic cues (Yorkston et al. 1990). This is secondly Vocal Intonation Therapy (VIT), which treats voice disorders or dysfunctions through vocal-based exercises to improve voice control, e.g., regarding pitch, volume, voice timbre, voice onset (Natke et al. 2003). The last method of this group (Oral Motor and Respiratory Exercises, OMREX) aims at improving oral-motor control (articulation, speech motor skills, dysarthria) and respiratory functions (e.g., Muscular Dystrophy).

11.3.3 Methods That Focus on Holistic Applications of Music-Based Exercises

The third group of methods focuses on global holistic applications of music-based exercises (Thaut 2005; Schon et al. 2007). An important method is the developmentally oriented stimulation of speech and language initiation (Developmental Speech and Language Training in Music, DSLM), especially in the neuropediatric area (early childhood brain damage or injuries), in early education (developmental disabilities) and with other development-related disorders (autism, developmental retardations). Music is used here as a holistic auditory language that promotes language concepts, pre-academic learning, and speech initiation through movement, singing, playing instruments, and other musical elements. Another method of music as a "language" is Symbolic Communication Training Through Music (SYCOM); it is intended for people who have never developed verbal language or lost it very early. In musical interaction on easily accessible instruments (percussion), pragmatic communication gestures and structures can be practiced nonverbally: dialogue forms, question-answer, approval-rejection, repetition-continuation/change. For SYCOM there are few direct research studies, although the structural analogy in group music-making between music and verbal language interaction offers itself as a translation of functional learning objectives and music is the only alternative auditory communication form that can translate verbal communication gestures analogously. The last method is Therapeutic Singing (TS), in which detail-focused aspects of the therapeutic methodology of NMT can be holistically brought together and practiced. In TS, the patient does not focus on technical aspects of speech/language therapy, but on singing a song, while simultaneously practicing all aspects, such as breath control, voice control, speech rhythm, prosody in a summarizing exercise structure. TS can also be used early on in nonmobile patients (bedridden) to start initial physical strength and endurance exercises.

11.4 Conclusion

Neurologic Music Therapy (NMT) is a new historical development for music-based interventions with a standardized and research-based clinical method system. The complete methodology is comprehensively described in the Oxford Handbook of Neurologic Music Therapy (Thaut and Hoemberg 2014). NMT has established itself in the last 20 years as an evidence-based therapy field and is medically recognized in neuroscience-based rehabilitation and in development-supporting interventions. Of great importance to understanding NMT is that the therapeutic methods were developed where "clusters" of clinical research data are available and insights continue to evolve. The NMT methodology is thus a clinical translation of research. The principles of NMT are integrable and transferable to other fields of application in neurological rehabilitation, which has led to rapid medical recognition. Furthermore, NMT has quickly positioned itself as an effective participant in initiatives for the global dissemination of Brain Health initiatives. These developments have finally led to the International NMT Academy (www.nmtacademy.co) being admitted into the World Federation of Neurorehabilitation (WFNR) as an institutional member in 2022.

Literature

Abiru M, Mihara B, Yoshii F (2009) Approach to therapy: neurologic disease and music therapy. Ann Rev Neurol 25:66–74

Altenmüller E, Marco-Pallares J, Munte TF, Schneider S (2009) Neural reorganization underlies improvement in stroke-induced motor dysfunction by music-supported therapy. Ann N Y Acad Sci 1169:395–405

Amir D, Schuchman G (1985) Auditory training through music with hearing-impaired preschool children. Volta Rev 87(7):333–343

Andrews MW, Dowling WJ (1991) The development of perception of interleaved melodies and control of auditory attention. Music Percept 8(4):349–368

Baram Y, Lenger R (2012) Gait improvement in patients with cerebral palsy by visual and auditory feedback. Neuromodulation 15(1):48–52

Baram Y, Miller A (2007) Auditory feedback control for improvement of gait in patients with multiple sclerosis. Neurol Sci 254:90–94

Barrow IM, Collins JN, Britt LD (2006) The influence of an auditory distraction on rapid naming after a mild traumatic brain injury: a longitudinal study. J Trauma Injury Infect Crit Care 61(5):1142–1149

Basso A, Capitani E, Vignolo LA (1979) Influence of rehabilitation on language skills in aphasic patients. Arch Neurol 36(4):190–196

Baur B, Uttner I, Ilmberger J, Fesl G, Mai N (2000) Music memory provides access to verbal knowledge in a patient with global amnesia. Neurocase 6:415–421

Bernatzky G, Bernatzky P, Hesse HP, Staffen W, Ladurner G (2004) Stimulating music increases motor coordination in patients afflicted by Morbus Parkinson. Neurosci Lett 361:4–8

Braunlich K, Seger CA, Jentink KG, Buard I, Kluger BM, Thaut MH (2018) Rhythmic auditory cues shape neural network recruitment in Parkinson's disease during repetitive motor behavior. Eur J Neurosci. https://doi.org/10.1111/EJN.1422

Buard I, Dewispelaere WD, Teale P, Rojas DC, Kronberg E, Thaut MH, Kluger BM (2019a) Auditory entrainment of motor responses in older adults with and without Parkinson's disease: an MEG study. Neurosci Lett. https://doi.org/10.1016/j.neulet.2019.134331

Buard I, Dewispelaere W, Thaut MH, Kluger B (2019b) Neurophysiological evidence for altered cortical activity and connectivity with neurologic music therapy in Parkinson's disease. Front Neurosci. https://doi.org/10.3389/fnins.2019.00105

Bugos JA, Perlstein WM, McCrae CS, Brophy TS, Bedenbaugh PH (2007) Individualized piano instruction enhances executive functioning and working memory in older adults. Aging Ment Health 11(4):464–471

Carr C et al (2012) Group music therapy for patients with persistent post-traumatic stress disorder—an exploratory randomized controlled trial with mixed methods evaluation. Psychol Psychother Theory Res Pract 85(2):179–202

Ceccato E, Caneva P, Lamonaca D (2006) Music therapy and cognitive rehabilitation in schizophrenic patients: a controlled study. Nord J Music Ther 15(2):111–120

Chan AS, Ho YC, Cheung MC (1998) Music training improves verbal memory. Nature 396:128

Clair AA, O'Konski M (2006) The effect of rhythmic auditory stimulation (RAS) on gait characteristics of cadence, velocity, and stride length in persons with late stage dementia. J Music Ther 43(2):154–163

Claussen D, Thaut MH (1997) Music as a mnemonic device for children with learning disabilities. Can J Music Ther 5:55–66

Cooke M et al (2010) A randomized controlled trial exploring the effect of music on agitated behaviors and anxiety in older people with dementia. Aging Ment Health 14(8):905–916

Cowles A, Beatty WW, Nixon SJ, Lutz LJ, Paulk J, Paulk K, Ross ED (2003) Musical skill in dementia: a violinist presumed to have Alzheimer's disease learns to play a new song. Neurocase 9:493–503

Cuddy LL, Duffin JM (2005) Music, memory, and Alzheimer's disease: is music recognition spared in dementia and how can it be assessed? Med Hypotheses 64:229–235

de Bruin N, Doan JB, Turnbull G, Suchowersky O, Bonfield S, Hu B, Brown LA (2010) Walking with music is a safe and viable tool for gait training in Parkinson's disease: the effect of a 13-week feasibility study on single and dual task walking. Parkinson's Disorders 13. https://doi.org/10.4061/2010/483530

de Dreu MJ, van der Wilk AS, Poppe E, Kwakkel G, van Wegen EE (2012) Rehabilitation, exercise therapy and music in patients with Parkinson's disease: a meta-analysis of the effects of music-based movement therapy on walking ability, balance and quality of life. Parkinsonism Relat Disord 18(Suppl 1):S114–S119

Del Olmo MF, Cudeiro J (2003) A simple procedure using auditory stimuli to improve movement in Parkinson's disease: a pilot study. Neurol Clin Neurophysiol 2:1–7

Del Olmo MF, Cudeiro J (2005) Temporal variability of gait in Parkinson disease: effects of a rehabilitation programme based on rhythmic sound cues. Parkinsonism Relat Disord 11:25–33

Del Olmo MF, Aria P, Furio M, Pozo M, Cudeiro J (2006) Evaluation of the effect of training using auditory stimulation on rhythmic movement in Parkinsonian patients—a combined motor and [18F]-FDG PET study. Parkinsonism Relat Disord 12:155–164

Deutsch D (1982) Organizational processes in music. In: Clynes M (ed) Music, mind and brain. Plenum Press, New York, pp 119–131

Ermolaeva VY, Borgest AN (1980) Intercortical connections of the auditory areas with the motor area. Neurosci Behav Physiol 10:210–215

Fischer CE, Churchill N, Leggieri M, Vuong V, Tau M, Fornazzari LR, Schweizer T, Thaut MH (2021) Long known music exposure effects on brain imaging and cognition in early-state cognitive decline. J Alzheimer's Dis. https://doi.org/10.3233/JAD-210610

Ford M, Wagenaar R, Newell K (2007) The effects of auditory rhythms and instruction on walking patterns in individuals post stroke. Gait Posture 26:150–155

Foster NA, Valentine ER (2001) The effect of auditory stimulation on autobiographical recall in dementia. Exp Aging Res 27:215–228

Frassinetti F, Bolognini N, Ladavos E (2002a) Enhancement of visual perception by crossmodal visual-auditory interaction. Exp Brain Res 147:332–343

Frassinetti F, Pavani F, Ladavos E (2002b) Acoustical vision of neglected stimuli: interaction among spatially convergent audio-visual inputs in neglect patients. J Cogn Neurosci 14:62–69

Freedland RL, Festa C, Sealy M, McBean A, Elghazaly P, Capan A, Brozycki L, Nelson AJ, Rothman J (2002) The effects of pulsed auditory stimulation on various gait measurements in persons with Parkinson's disease. NeuroRehabilitation 17:81–87

Gfeller KE (1983) Musical mnemonics as an aid to retention with normal and learning disabled students. J Music Ther 20:179–189

Gfeller K, Turner C, Woodworth G, Mehr M, Fearn R, Witt S, Stordahl J (2002) Recognition of familiar melodies by adult cochlear implant recipients and normal-hearing adults. Cochlear Implants Int 3:31–55

Goldshtrom Y, Knorr G, Goldshtrom I (2010) Rhythmic exercises in rehabilitation of TBI patients: a case report. J Bodyw Mov Ther 14(4):336–345

Grady CL, Furey ML, Pietrini P, Horwitz B, Rapoport SI (2001) Altered brain functional connectivity and impaired short-term memory in Alzheimer's disease. Brain 124:739–756

Gregory D (2002) Music listening for maintaining attention of older adults with cognitive impairments. J Music Ther 39(4):244–264

Guetin S, Soua B, Voiriot G, Picot MC, Herisson C (2009) The effect of music therapy on mood and anxiety-depression: an observational study in institutionalized patients with traumatic brain injury. Ann Phys Rehabil Med 52(1):30–40

Haire CM, Tremblay L, Vuong V, Patterson K, Chen J, Burdette JH, Schaffert N, Thaut MH (2021) Therapeutic instrumental music training and motor imagery in post stroke upper-extremity rehabilitation: a randomized controlled pilot study. Arch Rehabil Res Clin Transl. https://doi.org/10.1016/j.arrct.2021.1001162
Halpern AR, O'Connor M (2000) Implicit memory for music in Alzheimer's disease. Neuropsychology 14:391–397
Hammar L, Emami A, Engstroem G, Goetel E (2011) Communicating through caregiver singing during morning care situations in dementia care. Scand J Caring Sci 25(1):160–168
Haslam C, Cook M (2002) Striking a chord with amnesic patients: evidence that song facilitates memory. Neurocase 8:453–465
Hausdorff JM, Lowenthal J, Herman T, Gruendlinger L, Peretz C, Giladi N (2007) Rhythmic auditory stimulation modulates gait variability in Parkinson's disease. Eur J Neurosci 26(8):2369–2375
Hitch GJ, Burgess N, Towse JN, Culpin V (1996) Temporal grouping effects in immediate recall: a working memory analysis. Q J Exp Psychol A Hum Exp Psychol 49:116–139
Ho YC, Cheung MC, Chan AS (2003) Music training improves verbal but not visual memory: cross-sectional and longitudinal explorations in children. Neuropsychology 17:439–450
Hoemberg V (2005) Evidence based medicine in neurological rehabilitation—a critical review. In: von Wild K (ed) Re-engineering of the damaged brain and spinal cord. Springer, New York, pp 3–4
Hommel M, Peres B, Pollak P, Memin B (1990) Effects of passive tactile and auditory stimuli on left visual neglect. Arch Neurol 47:573–576
Howe TE, Lovgreen B, Cody FW, Ashton VJ, Oldham JA (2003) Auditory cues can modify the gait of persons with early-stage Parkinson's disease: a method for enhancing Parkinsonian walking performance. Clin Rehabil 17:363–367
Hummelsheim H (1999) Rationales for improving motor function. Curr Opin Neurol 12:697–701
Hurt CP (1998) Rhythmic auditory stimulation in gait training for patients with traumatic brain injury. J Music Ther 35:228–241
Irish M, Cunningham CJ, Walsh JB, Coakley D, Lawlor BA, Robertson IH, Coen RF (2006) Investigating the enhancing effect of music on autobiographical memory in mild Alzheimer's disease. Dement Geriatr Cogn Disord 22:108–118
Janata P, Tillmann B, Bharucha JJ (2002) Listening to polyphonic music recruits domain-general attention and working memory circuits. Cognit Affect Behav Neurosci 2:121–140
Jeffery DR, Good DC (1995) Rehabilitation of the stroke patient. Curr Opin Neurol 8:62–68
Jones C, Richard N, Thaut MH (2021) Investigating music-based cognitive rehabilitation for individuals with moderate to severe chronic acquired brain injury: a feasibility experiment. NeuroRehabilitation. https://doi.org/10.3233/NRE-208015
Kang K, Thaut MH (2019) Musical neglect training for chronic persistent unilateral visual neglect post-stroke. Front Neurol 10:474
Kenyon GP, Thaut MH (2000) A measure of kinematic limb instability modulation by rhythmic auditory stimulation. J Biomech 33:1313–1323
Kern P, Wolery M, Aldridge D (2007) Use of songs to promote independence in morning greeting routines for young children with autism. J Autism Dev Disord 37(7):1264–1271
Klein JM, Riess Jones M (1996) Effects of attentional set and rhythmic complexity on attending. Percept Psychophys 58(1):34–46
Kleinstauber M, Gurr B (2006) Music in brain injury rehabilitation. J Cognit Rehabil 24:4–14
Knox R, Yokota-Adachi H, Kershner J, Jutai J (2003) Musical attention training program and alternating attention in brain injury: an initial report. Music Ther Perspect 21(2):99–104
Koshimori Y, Strafella A, Valli M, Sharma V, Cho S, Houle S, Thaut MH (2019) Motor synchronization to rhythmic auditory stimulation (RAS) attenuates dopaminergic responses in ventral striatum in young healthy adults: a [11C]-(+)- PHNO PET study. Front Neurosci. https://doi.org/10.3389/fnins2019.00106
Kwak EE (2007) Effect of rhythmic auditory stimulation on gait performance in children with spastic cerebral palsy. J Music Ther 44(3):198–216

Large EW, Fink P, Kelso JA (2002) Tracking simple and complex sequences. Psychol Res 66:3–17

Lim I, Van Wegen E, de Goede C, Deutekom M, Nieuwboer A, Willems A, Jones D (2005) Effects of external rhythmical cueing on gait in patients with Parkinson's disease. Clin Rehabil 19:695–713

Loria T, De Grosbois JP, Haire C, Vuong V, Schaffert N, Tremblay L, Thaut MH (2022) Music-based intervention drives paretic limb acceleration into intentional movement frequencies in chronic stroke rehabilitation. Front Rehabil Sci. https://doi.org/10.3389/fresc.2022.989810

Loui P, Grent-'t-Jong T, Torpey D, Woldorff M (2005) Effects of attention on the neural processing of harmonic syntax in Western music. Cogn Brain Res 25(3):678–687

Loui P, Guenther FH, Mathys C, Schlaug G (2008) Action-perception mismatch in tone-deafness. Curr Trends Biol 18:331–332

Luft AR, McCombe-Waller S, Whitall J et al (2004) Repetitive bilateral arm training and motor cortex activation in chronic stroke: a randomized controlled trial. JAMA J Am Med Assoc 292:1853–1861

Ma HI, Hwang WJ, Lin KC (2009) The effects of two different auditory stimuli on functional arm movement in persons with Parkinson's disease: a dual-task paradigm. Clin Rehabil 23(3):229–237

Magee WL (2007) Music as a diagnostic tool in low awareness states: considering limbic responses. Brain Inj 21(6):593–599

Mainka S, Wissel J, Völler H, Evers S (2018) The use of rhythmic auditory stimulation to optimize treadmill training for stroke patients: a randomized controlled trial. Front Neurol 14(9):755

Mainka S, Schroll A, Warmerdam E, Gandor F, Maetzler W, Ebersbach G (2021) The power of musification: Sensor-based music feedback improves arm swing in Parkinson's disease. Mov Dis Clin Prac 8(8):1240–1247

Malcolm MP, Massie C, Thaut MH (2009) Rhythmic auditory—motor entrainment improves hemiparetic arm kinematics during reaching movements: a pilot study. Top Stroke Rehabil 16:69–79

McCombe WS, Harris-Love M, Liu W, Whitall J (2006) Temporal coordination of the arms during bilateral simultaneous and sequential movements in patients with chronic hemiparesis. Exp Brain Res 168(3):450–454

McIntosh GC, Brown SH, Rice RR, Thaut MH (1997) Rhythmic auditory—motor facilitation of gait patterns in patients with Parkinson's disease. J Neurol Neurosurg Psychiatry 62:22–26

Miller RA, Thaut MH, McInotsh GC, Rice RR (1996) Components of EMG symmetry and variability in parkinsonian and healthy elderly gait. Electroencephalogr Clin Neurophysiol 101:1–7

Morris GS, Suteerawattananon M, Entyre BR (2004) Effects of vosual and audirtory cues on gait in individuals with Parkinson's disease. J Neurol Sci 219:63–69

Moussard A (2012) Music as an aid to learn new verbal information in Alzheimer's disease. Music Percept 29(5):521–531

Nakano C, Abiru M, Kikuchi Y, Tokita K, Mihara Y, Fujimoto M, Mihara B (2009) The effects of RAS in gait disturbance caused by thalamic hemorrhage. Manuscript submitted for publication

Natke U, Donath TM, Kalveram KT (2003) Control of voice fundamental frequency in speaking versus singing. J Acoust Soc Am 113(3):1587–1593

Nayak S, Wheeler BL, Shiflett SC, Agostinelli S (2000) Effect of music therapy on mood and social interaction among individuals with acute traumatic brain injury and stroke. Rehabit Psychol 45:274–283

Nieuwboer A, Kwakkel G, Rochester L, Jones D, Van Wegen E, Willems AM, Chavret F, Hetherington V, Baker K, Lim I (2007) Cueing training in the home improves gait-related mobility in Parkinson's disease: the RESCUE trial. J Neurol Neurosurg Psychiatry 78:134–140

Paltsev YI, Elner AM (1967) Change in functional state of segmental apparatus of spinal cord under the influence of sound stimuli and its role in voluntary movement. Biophysics 12:1219–1226

Peng YC, Lu TW, Wang TH, Chen YL, Liao HF, Lin KH, Tang PF (2011) Immediate effects of therapeutic music on loaded sit-to-stand movement in children with spastic diplegia. Gait Posture 33(2):274–278

Peterson DA, Thaut MH (2007) Music increases frontal EEG coherence during verbal learning. Neurosci Lett 412(3):217–221
Prassas SG, Thaut MH, McIntosh GC, Rice RR (1997) Effect of auditory rhythmic cuing on gait kinematic parameters in stroke patients. Gait Posture 6:218–223
Robertson IH, Mattingley JM, Rorden C, Driver J (1998) Phasic alerting of neglect patients overcomes their spatial deficit in visual awareness. Nature 395:169–172
Robertson SD, Van Gemmert AW, Maraj BK (2002) Auditory information is beneficial for adults with downs syndrome in a continuous bimanual task. Acta Psychol 110(2/3):213–229
Rochester L, Hetherington W, Jones D, Nieuwboe A, Willems AM, Kwakkel G, Van Wegen E (2005) The effect of external rhythmic cues (auditory and visual) on walking during a functional task in homes of people with Parkinson's disease. Arch Phys Med Rehabil 86:999–1006
Rochette F, Bigand E (2009) Long-term effects of auditory training in severely or profoundly deaf children. Ann N Y Acad Sci 1169:195–198
Roerdink M, Lamoth CJC, Kwakkel G, van Wieringen PCW, Beek PJ (2007) Gait coordination after stroke: benefits of acoustically paced treadmill walking. Phys Ther 87(8):1009–1022
Roerdink M, Lamoth CJC, van Kordelaar J, Elich P, Konijnenbelt M, Kwakkel G, Beek PJ (2009) Rhythm perturbations in acoustically paced treadmill walking after stroke. Neurorehabil Neural Repair 23(7):668–678
Rojo N et al (2011) Music-supported therapy induces plasticity in the sensorimotor cortex in chronic stroke: a single-case study using multimodal imaging. Brain Inj 25(7/8):787–793
Rosenbaum RS, Furey ML, Horwitz CL, Grady CL (2004) Altered communication between emotion-related brain regions support short-term memory in Alzheimer's disease. Proc Soc Neurosci 203:8
Rossignol S, Melvill JG (1976) Audio-spinal influences in man studied by the H-reflex and its possible role in rhythmic movement synchronization to sound. Electroencephalogr Clin Neurophysiol 41:83–92
Samson S, Dellacherie D, Platel H (2009) Emotional power of music in patients with memory disorders: clinical implications of cognitive neuroscience. Ann N Y Acad Sci 1169:245–255
Satoh M, Kuzuhara S (2008) Training in mental singing while walking improves gait disturbance in Parkinson's disease patients. Eur Neurol 60(5):237–243
Schauer ML, Mauritz KH (2003) Musical motor feedback (MMF) in walking of hemiparetic stroke patients: randomized trials of gait improvement. Clin Rehabil 17:713–722
Schauer ML, Steingrueber W, Mauritz KH (1996) Die Wirkung von Musik auf die Symmetrie des Gehens von Schlaganfallpatienten auf dem Laufband. Biomed Tech 41:291–296
Schneider S, Scoenle PW, Altenmueller E, Muente TF (2007) Using musical instruments to improve motor skill recovery following stroke. J Neurol 254:1339–1346
Schneider S, Muente T, Rodriguez-Fornells Sailer M, Altenmueller E (2010) Music-supported training is more efficient than functional motor training for recovery of fine motor skills in stroke patients. Music Percept 27:271–280
Schon D, Boyer M, Moreno S, Besson M, Peretz I, Kolinsky R (2007) Songs as an aid for language acquisition. Cognition 106(2):975–983
Schweizer S, Hampshire A, Dalgleish T (2011) Extending brain-training to the affective domain: increasing cognitive and affective executive control through emotional working memory training. PLoS One 6(9):1–7
Senesac CR, Davis S, Richards L (2010) Generalization of a modified form of repetitive rhythmic bilateral training in stroke. Human Movement Science 29(1):137–148. https://doi.org/10.1016/j.humov.2009.05.004
Sharma V, Saha U, Saha J, Chen R, Thaut MH (2023) Intracranial basal ganglia LFP show increases in eventrelated beta synchrony during beat entrainment of finger movements in PD. Journal of Neurological Sciences 455:121076
Son GR, Therrien B, Whall A (2002) Implicit memory and familiarity among elders with dementia. J Nurs Scholarsh 34:263–267

Soto D, Funes MJ, Guzman-Garcia A, Warbick T, Rotshtein P, Humphreys GW (2009) Pleasant music overcomes the loss of awareness in patients with visual neglect. Proc Natl Acad Sci 106(14):6011–6016

Stephan KM, Thaut MH, Wunderlich G, Schicks W, Tian B, Tellmann L, Schmitz T et al (2002) Conscious and subconscious sensorimotor synchronization: prefrontal cortex and the influence of awareness. NeuroImage 15(2):345–352

Strait D, Kraus N (2011) Playing for a smarter ear: cognitive, perceptual and neurobiological evidence. Music Perxception 29:133–146

Suteerawattanano M, Morris GS, Etnyre BR, Jankovic J, Protas EJ (2004) Effects of visual and auditory cues on gait in individuals with Parkinson's disease. J Neurol Sci 950:2

Thaut MH, Hoemberg V (2014) Handbook of neurologic music therapy. Oxford University Press

Thaut MH, McIntosh GC, Rice RR, Prassas SG (1993) Effect of rhythmic cuing on temporal stride parameters and EMG patterns in hemiparetic gait of stroke patients. J Neurol Rehabil 7:9–16

Thaut MH, McIntosh GC, Rice RR, Miller RA, Rathbun J, Brault JA (1996) Rhythmic auditory stimulation in gait training with Parkinson's disease patients. Mov Disord 11:193–200

Thaut MH, McIntosh GC, Rice RR (1997) Rhythmic facilitation of gait training in hemiparetic stroke rehabilitation. J Neurol Sci 151:207–212

Thaut MH, Miller RA, Schauer LM (1998) Multiple synchronization strategies in rhythmic sensorimotor tasks: phase versus period adaptation. Biol Cybern 79:241–250

Thaut MH, Kenyon GP, Schauer ML, McIntosh GC (1999a) The connection between rhythmicity and brain function. IEEE Eng Med Biol Mag 18(2):101–108

Thaut MH, Miltner R, Lange HW et al (1999b) Velocity modulation and rhythmic synchronization of gait in Huntington's disease. Mov Disord 14:808–819

Thaut MH, Schicks W, McIntosh GC, Hömberg V (2002) The role of motor imagery and temporal cueing in hemiparetic arm rehabilitation. Neurorehabil Neural Repair 16:115

Thaut MH, Peterson DA, McIntosh GC (2005) Temporal entrainment of cognitive functions: musical mnemonics induce brain plasticity and oscillatory synchrony in neural networks underlying memory. Ann N Y Acad Sci 1060:243–254

Thaut MH, Leins AK, Rice RR, Argstatter H, Kenyon GP et al (2007) Rhythmic auditory stimulation improves gait more than NDT/Bobath training in near-ambulatory patients early poststroke: a single-blind, randomized trial. Neurorehabil Neural Repair 21:455–459

Thaut MH, Gardiner JC, Holmberg D, Horwitz J, Kent L, Andrews G et al (2009) Neurologic music therapy improves executive function and emotional adjustment in traumatic brain injury rehabilitation. Ann N Y Acad Sci 1169:406–416

Thaut MH, Schicks W, McIntosh GC, Hömberg V (2014) Musical mnemonics aid verbal memory and induce learning-related brain plasticity in multiple sclerosis. Front Hum Neurosci. https://doi.org/10.3389/fnhum.2014.00395

Thaut MH, Rice RR, Braun Janzen T, Hurt Thaut CP, McIntosh GC (2018) Rhythmic auditory stimulation for reduction of falls in Parkinson's disease: a randomized controlled study. Clin Rehabil. https://doi.org/10.1177/0269215518788615

Thaut MH, Fischer CE, Leggieri M, Vuong V, Churchill N, Fornazzari L, Schweizer T (2020) Neural basis of long-term musical memory in cognitively impaired older persons. Alzheimer Dis Assoc Disord 34(3):267–271. https://doi.org/10.1097/WAD.0000000000000382

Trombetti A, Hars M, Herrmann FR, Kressig RW, Ferrari S, Rizzoli R (2011) Effect of music-based multitask training on gait, balance, and fall risk in elderly people: a randomized controlled trial. Arch Int Med 171(6):525–533

Van Wegen W, Nieuwboer A, Rochester L, Jones D, Kwakkel G (2006) The effect of cueing therapy as measured by activity monitoring in the RESCUE trial. Proceedings of the 4th world congress for Neurorehabilitation, P1-061

Vanstone AD, Cuddy LL (2010) Musical memory in Alzheimer's disease. Aging Neuropsychol Cognit 17:108–128

Vanstone AD, Cuddy LL, Duffin JM, Alexander E (2009) Exceptional preservation of memory for tunes and lyrics: case studies in amusia, profound deafness, and Alzheimer's disease. Ann N Y Acad Sci 1169:291–294

Wallace WT (1994) Memory for music: effect of melody on recall of text. J Exp Psychol Learn Mem Cognit 20:1471–1485
Wan C et al (2010) The therapeutic effects of singing in neurological disorders. Music Percept 27(4):287–295
Whitall J, McCombe Waller S, Silver KH, Macko RF (2000) Repetitive bilateral arm training with rhythmic auditory cueing improves motor function in chronic hemiparetic stroke. Stroke 31:2390–2395
Willems AM, Nieuwboer A, Chavret F, Desloovere K, Dom R et al (2006) The use of rhythmic auditory cues to influence gait in patients with Parkinson's disease, the differential effect for freezers and non-freezers, an explorative study. Disabil Rehabil 28:721–728
Wolfe DE, Hom C (1993) Use of melodies as structural prompts for learning and retention of sequential verbal information by preschool students. J Music Ther 30:100–118
Yorkston KM, Hammen VL, Beukelman DR, Traynor CD (1990) The effect of rate control on the intelligibility and naturalness of dysarthric speech. J Speech Hear Disord 55(3):550–560

Music Therapy for Children and Young People with Mental Health Problems: An Overview

12

Thomas Stegemann and Hans Ulrich Schmidt

12.1 Introduction: Quality of Life and Well-Being in Children and Adolescents

> Creative therapeutic work with music in particular will gain in importance in the future given the increasing developmental disorders and behavioural problems in children. (Plahl and Koch-Temming 2005, p. 15)

According to the Federal Statistical Office (2020a), a total of 13.7 million children and young people under the age of 18 were living in Germany at the end of 2019. Thus, minors make up approx. 16.5% of the total population, which reflects the demographic change: "The falling number of people of younger age and the simultaneous increase in the number of elder people are shifting the demographic structure in an unprecedented way. Every second person in Germany is now older than 45 and every fifth person is older than 66" (Federal Statistical Office 2020b).

The Heidelberg child and adolescent psychiatrist Franz Resch (2012) cites the following factors for a real increase in mental disorders: Firstly, medical progress has improved the survival rate in childhood (e.g., after premature births). This increases somatopsychological risks. Secondly, a shift in overall morbidity can be observed in children and adolescents, especially from acute illnesses such as measles and other childhood diseases to chronic diseases such as asthma,

T. Stegemann (✉)
Department of Music Therapy, University of Music and Performing Arts Vienna, Vienna, Austria
e-mail: stegemann@mdw.ac.at

H. U. Schmidt
Outpatient Center für Psychosomatic Medicine, Clinic and Polyclinic for Psychosomatic Medicine and Psychotherapy, University Medical Center Hamburg-Eppendorf, Hamburg, Germany
e-mail: uschmidt@uke.uni-hamburg.de

G. Kreutz, G. Bernatzky (eds.), *Music and Medicine*, Neurocultural Health and Wellbeing, https://doi.org/10.1007/978-3-662-72175-9_12

neurodermatitis or obesity, which are often associated with psychosocial stress. Thirdly, social risks have increased, which should be seen in connection with economic factors (principally child poverty) and general social developments (including migration and the increasing complexity of interrelations in life contexts). However, there are arguments claiming the increase in mental health disorders can be explained by other factors: On the one hand, awareness of mental problems has increased, which means that mental disorders are recognized and diagnosed earlier. In addition, there is also a trend towards the "medicalization of social problems" (Resch 2012), an example of which is the increase in attention deficit/hyperactivity disorder (ADHD) and the associated prescription of psychostimulants (Ritalin). Shifts in norm values and changes in definitions and classifications of disorders also lead to increases in prevalence, as statistical artifacts, so to speak, as they are to be registered following the introduction of new classification systems such as the fifth edition of the *Diagnostic and Statistical Manual of Mental Disorders* (DSM-5) and the eleventh edition of the *International Classification of Diseases* (ICD-11).

Finally, however, an "epochal" change in symptoms can also be identified: While catatonia, for instance—as an expression of schizophrenic illnesses—or anorexia nervosa are less common today, self-harming behavior and suicidality have increased significantly in child and adolescent psychiatric populations. Headaches and psychosomatic disorders are also increasing in children and adolescents (Resch 2012). There is no doubt that the environment in which children and young people grow up in Germany is currently undergoing a change, and this is accompanied by an increase in the risks to the personal development of this age group.

Evidence of this can be found in studies on health-related quality of life (HRQoL) (Otto et al. 2021; Ravens-Sieberer et al. 2021). Although the living conditions of the majority of children and adolescents in the western industrialized countries can be considered as above average, several influencing factors can be identified that have a negative impact on certain groups. In German-speaking countries, in particular, there is a strong correlation between a lower socio-economic status and psychological abnormalities, which in turn are associated with an impairment of health-related quality of life (Klipker et al. 2018).

An earlier study by Erhart and Ravens-Sieberer (2009) also showed that the family background is a major influencing factor: On average, children of single parents reported a lower quality of life and well-being than children from typical nuclear families. In addition to mostly poorer economic conditions, this is likely to be related to increased psychosocial stress. Episodes of family breakdown and disharmony or loss of friendships due to a change in the living environment are examples. In addition, media aspects—use of the internet, smartphones, computers (games), television, etc.—seem to have significant effects on the health of children and adolescents. Erhart and Ravens-Sieberer (2009) were able to show that in a study of 1500 children and adolescents, the highest average quality of life and the best average well-being were found in the group of those 10% who used media least. In contrast, the 10% with the highest media usage reported the most significant impairments in the dimensions relevant to quality of life, namely physical well-being, moods and emotions, self-perception, relationship with parents, financial opportunities, and the school environment.

The authors of the study state that a lack of learning experiences in the social context due to excessive media use could result in deficits in social competence and problem-solving skills, which could in turn affect the quality of life and well-being. This is also relevant from a psychotherapeutic point of view. In this context, Hüther (2011) notes that real, multi-sensory experiences are far more effective than verbal (or "digital") representations of experiences:

> Only when people have new and first-hand experiences of self-efficacy, creative power and the joy of discovery involving activation of the emotional centres of their brains can these experiences be sustained in the form of corresponding neural interconnection patterns and therefore be anchored in their brains (Hüther 2011, p. 134).

The capacity of listening to music, making music, singing and dancing to contribute to a better quality of life and well-being is the subject of clinical-therapeutic and nonclinical discourses (MacDonald et al. 2012). Children and young people are particularly receptive to artistic media (music, dance, art, etc.) and can be touched emotionally by them.

With the help of sounds, movement and colors they can often express themselves better on a symbolic level than they can with words (Stegemann et al. 2012). This also (and especially) applies to those children and adolescents who suffer from psychological problems. According to Fegert, artistic therapies play a central role in the context of multimodal treatment concepts in child and adolescent psychiatry:

> Especially with children who have experienced neglect, mistreatment and sexual abuse in the past it is often these partly non-verbal approaches that contribute significantly to the success of the treatment. (...) Many children and adolescents whom we treated as inpatients subsequently say how important the creative therapies were to them (Fegert 2011, p. 287).

12.2 Historical Development

Plahl and Koch-Temming (2005) note that music therapy in childhood and adolescence emerged from practical experience in various disciplines. This development must be seen both in the context of the history of pediatrics and in the context of the history of special education and child psychotherapy. In his overview of the history of music therapy in pediatrics, Evers (2001) notes that "the music therapy used for children in earlier centuries always had to assume the position of an extreme outsider" (Evers 2001, p. 1). This is to be understood against the background of the historically subordinate importance of both pediatrics and music therapy in medicine. Pediatrics, for example, was only able to establish itself as an independent discipline at the end of the nineteenth century (Seidler 1991).

Furthermore, Evers' statement reflects the image of childhood, which was only recognized as a discrete phase of life in the last century. Only then were children not only seen as budding adults, but as "persons in their own right" (Grunert and Krüger 2006). Children's music therapy is based both historically and in terms of content on various neighboring specialized areas, although the static representation (Fig. 12.1) could hide the fact that it is really more of a flexible and nonlinear

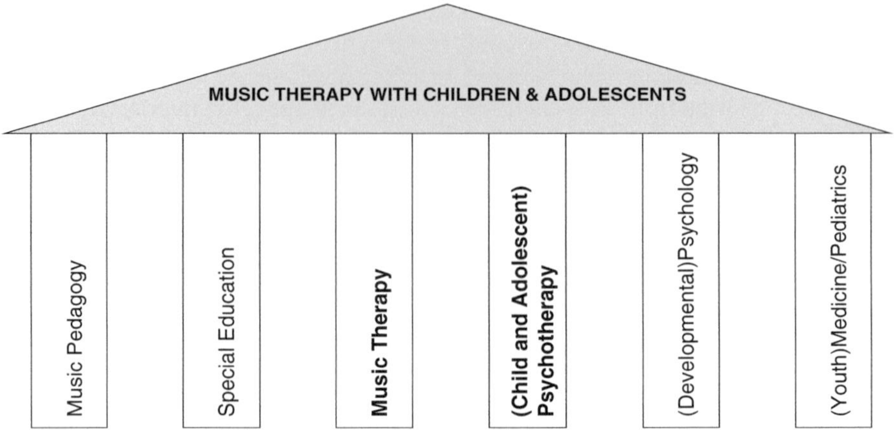

Fig. 12.1 Historical pillar model of child music therapy. (From Stegemann 2009; with kind permission)

development process. Nowadays, music therapy itself and child psychotherapy—as branches of child and adolescent psychiatry—can be considered some of the central pillars in this edifice.

12.2.1 Child and Society: The Cradle of Children's Music Therapy

The twentieth century was declared the "century of the child" (Key 1902). It was marked by experimental psychology and pedagogy, which went in search of scientific explanations for the world of children (Grunert and Krüger 2006). In particular, sociological, psychological and pedagogical studies on supportive development conditions for children contributed to a growing appreciation of children's play as an expression of creativity and a pronounced faculty of thought (Plahl and Koch-Temming 2005). The so-called reform movement also paved the way for a reassessment of fossilized forms of life and manners (Fitzthum 2003). Pioneering achievements in the field of child psychotherapy are associated with the names Hermine Hug-Hellmuth (1871–1924), Anna Freud (1895–1982), Melanie Klein (1882–1960) and Ada Müller-Braunschweig (1897–1959), who first introduced drawing, painting and modelling as means for children to express their conscious and unconscious impulses (Biermann 1988).

In the 1920s, under the influence of the anthroposophical teachings of Rudolf Steiner, music was increasingly used in curative education institutions. At the same time, influenced by Carl Orff (1895–1982), there were also far-reaching and lasting changes in the field of music education concerning the way children's musicality should be understood and promoted. In the period after the Second World War, the development of children's music therapy as an independent discipline was shaped by musicians and music educators. The approaches of Juliette Alvin (1897–1982), Paul Nordoff (1909–1977) and Gertrud Orff (1914–2000) are still of importance today.

There are currently ten state-approved institutions in German-speaking countries and seven additional private training and further education institutions in Switzerland and Germany. (See Schmidt and Stegemann 2020, p. 71 for a more detailed account). A total of around 250 music therapy study places per year can be assumed for the German-speaking countries (cf. Schmidt and Stegemann 2021, p. 47). Most of the training courses are part-time.

The "Studien- und Ausbildungslandschaft Musiktherapie," which is published by the German Music Therapy Association (DMtG) approximately every 2 years, offers current information on the range of courses (www.musiktherapie.de).

During the last five decades or so, various thought models and therapy directions have emerged in children's music therapy based on the developments described above and following schools of psychotherapy, which according to Ruud and Mahns (1992, cited in Schmidt 2002) can be classified as follows:

- Medical
- Behavioristic
- Anthroposophical
- Psychodynamic
- Humanistic
- Combined

As they emerged, "the first three followed a specific, sometimes highly mechanized conception of diagnosis and indication in an effect-oriented manner. The latter—process-oriented approaches—are concerned with growth, meaning and understanding" (Schmidt 2002, p. 83). Surveys that we conducted of employees in inpatient child and adolescent psychiatry (Stegemann et al. 2008) show that the majority of the music therapists surveyed feel obliged to have a background that is well-founded in psychoanalysis and depth psychology. This is followed by systemic and gestalt psychological approaches, which are often used in combination and according to the therapist's personal educational background. Regulatory music therapy according to Schwabe (ibid.) also seems to be influential for this professional group.

12.3 Overview of Functions of Music and Forms of Treatment in Music Therapy

The distinguishing features of music therapy with children and adolescents are, on the one hand, that it is very attractive for these age groups, and on the other hand, the high standards of professionalism expected of the therapist across a spectrum that spans music, pedagogy, developmental psychology, and psychotherapy (see Stegemann 2021). Today there are a large number of important and proven fields of treatment, which are discussed below. As an overview, we can first cite attentive listening to music and active music-making, accompanied and guided by trained music therapists in hospitals, practices, special schools, and many other facilities (e.g., music schools).

- Nonverbal activation of mental resources
- Promoting the development of children and young people (e.g., in special education and psychiatric facilities for children and adolescents)
- Strengthening personality and self-healing powers in life crises
- Help with overcoming illness and disability

Music therapy is currently an important and frequently used therapy component in the context of multimodal treatment approaches for severe mental health disorders in children and adolescents who require hospital treatment. In almost two thirds of child and adolescent psychiatric hospitals music therapy is used partly as an independent form of psychotherapy, partly as part of everyday inpatient care within the entire range of indications (Stegemann et al. 2008).

Music Therapy and Music Education

In recent years, music therapy elements have increasingly been integrated into the portfolio of schools and kindergartens from a preventive perspective (Timmermann and Schmidt 2007; Jordan et al. 2018). Collaboration between music educators and music therapists—especially on preventive aspects—has proven useful and fruitful in many areas. The prerequisite for this, however, is that each professional group knows and recognizes its specific mandate and its limits (ibid.). In this context, it is historically interesting that modern music therapy did not emerge primarily from psychotherapy. Rather, new paths in music education (especially improvisation) and the development of modern psychotherapy at times ran parallel, before common approaches led to music therapy (cf. Chap. 3).

Jacoby (1984) designed a modern music pedagogy that was strongly motivated by cultural therapy. He advocated a combination of instrumental expression and therapy. However, Timmermann and Schmidt (2007), and Schmidt and Timmermann (2012) point out that music therapy is primarily the treatment of ill persons. On the one hand, the pedagogical use of music can have a preventive effect, while on the other, there is a risk of pathologizing healthy children and young people, especially if the indication (pedagogical vs. therapeutic) remains unclear or a therapeutic offer is made too low-threshold.

Plahl refers to the important communicative significance of music. She believes that spontaneous singing by children may facilitate contact with their peers:

> Music therapy enables children to communicate without language or encourages verbal communication. In the music therapy situation, an environment is created that promotes the child's development, particularly in terms of communication. An essential part of this context of change is the therapeutic relationship that is created through specific music therapy techniques. The possibilities of expression and communication of music were and are used in a number of differently oriented approaches with children (Plahl 2000, p. 29).

For young people, music means the expression of their attitude towards life. Haffa-Schmidt says:

> If I ask young people to describe the music they enjoy listening to, utterances like, 'wicked', 'awesome', 'spacey', 'hot' are usually terms that give me no idea of the music. Or they automatically describe what music does to them: 'It really gets me goin', 'powerful', 'incredibly cool', 'I can forget all my problems'. (Haffa-Schmidt 1999, p. 27)

It should be borne in mind that listening to music is not always only beneficial for young people; music can also have negative effects on adolescents (see Sect. 12.6.3). Detrimental behavior patterns and depressive tendencies can be graded using the Healthy-Unhealthy Uses of Music Scale (HUMS) which is now also available in German (Riedl and Stegemann 2018). Other important issues that can be expressed in musical preferences of adolescents are desires for identity, individuality, authenticity and demarcation. (see Stegemann and Geipel 2018) Haffa-Schmidt et al. (1999) again:

> This balancing act between uniqueness and demarcation from the large crowd, also the simultaneous feeling of security as part of a group is a feeling that young people feel very strongly within themselves (...). In addition to these demarcation and role model functions of music within and also between the peer groups, (...) a whole range of development-specific factors play a role which causes young people to identify with certain music. Young people often change (music) scenes and seem to be able to tackle and cope with new development tasks. (ibid., p. 28)

Another important function of music and music therapy is the generation of processes of symbolization. This applies primarily to process-oriented treatment approaches. According to Mahns (2004), analytical music therapy, one such approach, uses

> the sensual-symbolic form of interaction of sound and music (...) to create awareness of unconscious experiences and the current transference relationship and to give it a name through verbal language (Mahns 2004, p. 75).

Furthermore, music in the therapeutic context is of great importance as a kind of "container" for dealing with aggression. Numerous authors address this topic. Degryse (2012) describes music therapy work with a traumatized young adult: By experiencing music therapy treatment as a safe space, it is gradually possible to build a stable relationship with the therapist. The rules of the game and the joint development of musical forms are important. "The development of a musical form is just as vulnerable a process that seems to follow a similar path as the process of individuation itself" (ibid., P. 53).

Free, active playing on easy-to-use musical instruments (e.g., drums), singing, listening, and moving to music in music therapy offer a space for play, sound and interaction, especially to ill people and young people with special needs. This potentially facilitates experiences of relationship, communication and self-awareness (Lutz Hochreutener 2009). Experiences of distress and general well-being become audible and open to empathetic understanding: wordlessly expressed in improvised and varying musical forms with the therapist they often result in possibilities for change and development, which can prove helpful and be experimented with.

Such an encounter, a contact within the shelter of music, is especially suitable for children with autism spectrum disorders (Schumacher et al. 2011).

Lutz Hochreutener describes the following music therapy methods and forms of treatment, which she groups within the concept of a "safe place" (Lutz Hochreutener 2009, p. 137). The methods can develop spontaneously out of a process of play and fluidly flow into one another, but can also be used as standalone activities (ibid., p. 138).

- Improvisation
- Songs
- Composing
- Handling instruments
- Body
- Language
- Role playing
- Imaginative music experience
- Silence

> The "via regia" of European, psychodynamically oriented music therapy is certainly improvisation with its various forms of play (e.g. free or thematic). In addition, listening to music together—and increasingly also songwriting—play an important role in working with adolescents (Gold et al. 2011).

Frohne-Hagemann and Pleß-Adamczyk (2005) work on a music therapy intervention theory for psychological problems in children and adolescents. The corresponding interventions are each related to the development and differentiation of relationship qualities. Unless it takes place in a relationship context, music therapeutic treatment makes little sense: "Therefore, every form of play in music therapy, every intervention and every music function is always a figure against the actual relationship background" (ibid., p. 104). They relate the music therapy interventions to the contact modes used by Schumacher et al. (2011) as part of a music therapy diagnostic instrument (AQR, Assessment of the Quality of Relationship):

Contact Modes of the AQR Tool
Mode 0: Contactlessness/defense
Mode 1: Sensory contact/contact reaction
Mode 2: Functionalizing contact
Mode 3: Contact with oneself/self-experience
Mode 4: Contact with the other/intersubjectivity
Mode 5: Relationship with others/interactivity
Mode 6: Encounter/inter-affectivity

Frohne-Hagemann and Pleß-Adamczyk (2005) name the following as global treatment goals for music therapy with children and adolescents:

- Recovery
- Coping with states of distress
- Emotional and social support
- Improvement of skills and abilities
- Fostering of potential and creative options
- Encouragement of autonomy and self-determination

In 2005, as a result of the multitude of clinical experiences, the two authors published an interdisciplinary and much-discussed manual (indication music therapy for psychological problems in children and adolescents: music therapy diagnostics and manual according to ICD-10). It also provides detailed music therapy diagnostics for doctors and psychologists and describes treatment options. Music therapy diagnostics and treatment approaches are integrated into common psychodiagnostic categories (e.g., OPD axes) and classifications (ICD-10).

12.4 Clinical and Other Uses of Music Therapy

Wormit et al. (2001) found that children under the age of 13 receive around a third of all outpatient music therapies. An unpublished telephone survey of members of the German Association for Music Therapy (DMtG) the following year showed that around 20% of those questioned work with children and young people (Plahl and Koch-Temming 2005). A large survey of arts therapies in Germany (Oster 2015) showed that over half of the music therapists (53.4%) work with children and adolescents. Children and adolescents with mental illness make up the largest proportion of this clientele.

An online survey in Austria carried out by the Music Therapy Research Centre Vienna finds that a total of 29.4% of the members questioned offer music therapy with children and adolescents with developmental/behavioral problems (22.5%) or with psychological (5.6%) or psychosomatic illnesses (1.3%). This field of work is now larger than that of music therapy with adults with mental illnesses (Phan Quoc et al. 2019).

Plahl and Koch-Temming (2005, p. 53) provide a profound summary of the clinical fields of application. This is mainly clinical-therapeutic, e.g., individual or group therapy, sometimes as part of project work. The fields are:

- Child and adolescent psychiatry
- Child and adolescent psychosomatics
- Pediatrics
- Social pediatrics
- Oncology
- Neurology

- Neonatology
- Internal medicine
- Cardiology

For somatic disorders (e.g., cancer or chronic diseases), music therapy treatment as psychosocial support has since become an essential component of therapy too. Institutions that focus chiefly on rehabilitation also work in individual and group settings, with special educational support or in the form of projects. Music therapy takes place in:

- Spa clinics
- Rehabilitation facilities
- Psychiatric aftercare facilities for children and adolescents
- Special and integrational day care centers (elementary and after-school care)
- Children's homes
- Institutions for early intervention
- Day groups
- Special schools
- Integration schools

The preventive use of music therapy is also playing an increasingly important role (cf. Jordan et al. 2018). Forms of application of music therapy are school lessons, workshops or projects such as "Drum power" (Wölfl 2021) or music therapy with refugees (Wiesmüller and Stegemann 2020).

Typical locations are health centers, schools, and institutions for cultural work with children and young people (e.g., music schools).

12.5 Indications and Contraindications

12.5.1 Indications

The indication—i.e., the determination of whether an intervention is to be chosen and, if so, which type (*indicare* [Lat.] = to show)—is the connecting factor between diagnosis and therapy within the framework of a treatment concept. All available information on the patient at the time is incorporated into the decision-making process, e.g., the disorder, environmental variables, etc. According to Mattejat (2008), the following questions should be taken into account when considering indications in children and adolescents:

Questions in the Context of Indications in Children and Adolescents (Based on Mattejat 2008)

- Is there an indication for treatment and how urgent is therapy or other interventions?
- Under what basic conditions and in which modality (inpatient, partial inpatient, outpatient) can a treatment be carried out?
- Which components should the treatment/assistance include (medication, functional exercise treatments, individual psychotherapy, parent, and family-related interventions, other school and environment-related measures, in particular youth and social welfare measures)?

Music therapy usually only comes into play when the second and third set of questions are addressed. The aim is to find a differential indication, i.e., the well-founded decision, "for whom and when which music therapy offer is best suited in which context" (Plahl and Koch-Temming 2005, p. 147). The careful clarification of these questions is an essential quality feature of evidence-based psychotherapeutic methods in general and music therapy in particular. Hegi-Protmann et al. (2006, p. 68) are referring to this when they point out that, "A scientific attitude cannot assume that music always somehow has an effect."

A survey regarding the practice of inpatient child and adolescent psychiatry (Stegemann et al. 2008) showed that today the entire spectrum of child and adolescent psychiatric disorders is treated with music therapy almost without restriction. In very few cases, however, is the indication made by the music therapist; it comes mostly from the case-leading doctors and psychologists (Stegemann and Schmidt 2010). This observation reflects the understanding expressed by Grawe et al. (1994) on the basis of the state of research and training of arts therapies at that time that the indication for music, art and dance therapy is seen as a merely secondary intervention: The indication should "only be provided by broadly trained therapists, and only after or in addition to the tried and tested therapeutic options," (Grawe et al. 1994, p. 735).

Today a more nuanced view is taken, at least in the literature on child and adolescent psychiatry. Mattejat (2008) explains that music therapy is particularly helpful for children "whose possibilities to express their inner experience or to communicate with other people are limited" (ibid., p. 91). He also states:

> In the field of child and adolescent health, the main indication for music therapy is for mental and physical disabilities and autism spectrum disorders or other pervasive developmental disorders. Secondarily, music therapy or other creative-therapeutic measures can also be used as a useful addition to medical-psychotherapeutic treatment for various mental illnesses in children and adolescents. (ibid.)

In this context, the authors regard the question of contraindications for music therapy treatment (cf. Stegemann and Schmidt 2010) and that of undesirable effects and treatment errors in music therapy (Schmidt and Stegemann 2019) as important.

These questions are still neglected both in the scientific field and in the practical application of music therapy.

Music therapy is only gradually and cautiously showing a readiness to discuss these issues, probably also due to concern that "addressing such questions too actively could result in music therapy being viewed critically both within the profession and outside it" (Schmidt and Stegemann 2019, p. 353). However, the discussion about possible negative aspects becomes more important with increasingly evidence-based references to the effectiveness of music therapy interventions. Reasons for the tendency to neglect or even exclude the contraindication question in music therapy could be bias in favor of one's own method, the idea that music stands for what is beautiful and good, and the consideration of music therapy as a noninvasive form of therapy (see also Schmidt and Stegemann 2019, p. 356). Most of the time, music therapy is certainly a relative contraindication.

According to Frohne-Hagemann and Pleß-Adamczyk (2005), the following main indications for music therapy for children and young people can be considered:

- Profound developmental disorders
- Circumscribed developmental disorders of speech and language
- Emotional disorders of childhood
- Combined disorders of social behavior and emotions
- Mutism
- Mental retardation
- Effects of traumatic brain injury

Koch-Temming (1998) also formulates the following indications:

- Aggressive symptoms with a tendency toward violence
- Depressive syndromes
- Difficulty concentrating
- Hyperactivity

However, in the music therapy literature the case is argued for not primarily taking diagnoses or the current symptoms of the patient as a guide. Instead "also their background, i.e. their emotional and communicative skills and needs, be these illness-related, acquired in the course of life or poorly developed" should be included (Haffa-Schmidt et al. 1999, p. 17) when deciding on a therapeutic method.

> Just as little should the young person's musicality or love of music be an indication criterion for music therapy – even if this still happens in practice out of ignorance, perplexity, well-intentioned care, at the request of parents and due to distorted ideas about music therapy. (ibid.)

Frohne-Hagemann and Pleß-Adamczyk (2005, p. 141) justify their scepticism about diagnosis-specific indications as follows:

> Since music therapy always refers to the catching up or corrective experience of self and identity-creating treatment qualities, the primary question that arises is not which disorders music therapy is indicated for, but rather in what context and how it is indicated: Music therapy does not address individual symptoms of a mental disorder, but the affective and interactional relationship qualities on a fundamental level. (ibid.)

In our study on indications and contraindications for music therapy (Stegemann and Schmidt 2010), we asked music therapists who work at child and adolescent psychiatric hospitals for their personal and professional assessment. Their answers to the question of which disorders music therapy works best for resulted in the following ranking:

- Depression (28%)
- Anxiety disorders (17%)
- Attachment disorders (11%)
- Social behavior disorders (11%)
- Eating disorders (9%)
- Disorders on the autistic spectrum (9%)
- Emotional disorders (7%)
- Addiction (4%)
- Self-esteem problems (4%)

It is noteworthy in this regard that this assessment from practice only partially coincides with the database from international research. It shows a discrepancy, which, in our opinion, is explained by the practice of diagnostics and the frequency of certain diagnoses, i.e., it is based more often on personal experiences of success with certain clinical phenomena. According to current data, the strongest evidence of the positive effects of music therapy is available for treatment in neonatology and for autism spectrum disorders (Stegemann et al. 2019).

There are hardly any studies on the effectiveness of music therapy for the treatment of depressive disorders, especially in children and adolescents. Plausible explanatory models for the modes of action of music therapy are available though, especially for affective disorders (Stegemann 2020). In a methodologically sound depression study (randomized controlled study, RCT) of adult patients, music therapy as an additional treatment method was found to be significantly superior to standard treatment in terms of depression symptoms, anxiety symptoms and general functioning (Erkkilä et al. 2011). A recent review by Geipel et al. (2018) was able to show that music-based interventions can reduce the severity of internalizing symptoms (e.g., anxiety).

12.5.2 Contraindications

Contraindications for the use of music therapy in child and adolescent psychiatry in the aforementioned questionnaire study (Stegemann and Schmidt 2010) were differentiated as follows: The majority of music therapists mentioned situations in which music therapy was not indicated or only indicated to a limited extent. With regard to particular disorders, acute psychoses and post-traumatic stress disorder (PTSD) come first for both absolute and relative contraindications. Only about a third of the respondents see no contraindications for certain situations or patient groups in music therapy.

Also according to Weiß (2008), there are no generally valid contraindications for music therapy with respect to a specific post-traumatic disorder, but caution is advised when "fear, stress and intrusions or potential retraumatizations may be intensified by music" (ibid., p. 15). These caveats apply in particular to nonmusic therapists who use music in their treatment setting, and to music therapists who have little or no experience of working with traumatized patients.

12.6 Empirical Research

The research landscape in music therapy has changed fundamentally over the past four decades. While in the past mainly individual case studies were carried out, the number of clinical studies especially has increased significantly since the turn of the last century. Overall, the number of published music therapy research papers increased from 534 articles in 1985 to around 6000 in 2018—a tenfold increase in publication output within 33 years (Riedl et al. 2020).

Thanks to these—increasingly interdisciplinary—research efforts, music therapy is on the way to becoming an evidence-based form of treatment that can substantiate its clinically evident benefit In a way that withstands scientific scrutiny.

Consequently, music therapy has now found its way into several medical guidelines. In a systematic literature search of the AWMF guidelines (Stegemann et al. 2021), 29 guidelines were identified in which music therapy is mentioned, including the guidelines on "dementia," "schizophrenia," and "psychosocial therapy for severe mental illnesses." Among citations with relevance for children and adolescents are the mention of music therapy in the guidelines on "Autism Spectrum Disorders," "Treatment of Depressive Disorders in Children and Adolescents," "Mental Retardation," and "Psychosocial Care in Pediatric Oncology and Haematology."

A meta-analysis by Pešek (2007) considered 125 music therapy studies (total number of subjects in all studies: $n = 4406$). On average, the effect size (Cohen's d) was 0.77. This corresponds to a medium effect size. The research that examined patients under the age of 18 shows, in comparison, above-average effect sizes (active music therapy: $d = 0.82$, receptive music therapy: $d = 0.78$ and receptive/active combined: $d = 0.95$). Since only 22 studies were included in the meta-analysis, the informative value must be classified as rather limited—also due to the different areas of application (affective disorders: 4 studies, psychosomatic medicine: 2, chronic pain: 1, cancer: 2, mental retardation: 6, neonatology: 7).

Another meta-analysis (Pelletier 2004) showed that the stress-reducing effects of music in combination with relaxation techniques were significantly greater in minors than in adults. Psychiatric disorders were not taken into account here. In a systematic review, Argstatter et al. (2007) come to the following conclusion:

> The comparison of the meta-analyses of music therapy with children and adolescents with psychotherapeutic methods shows that the treatment effectiveness of music therapy is particularly high for this clientele: While psychotherapeutic methods (irrespective of the therapy school) have an effect size of around d = 0.54, the meta-analyses examined here achieve values between d = 0.61 and d = 0.89 (Argstatter et al. 2007, p. 57).

In a meta-analysis, Gold et al. (2009) concluded that there is a dose-effect relationship in music therapy treatments. The study, which included data from 15 studies with a total of almost 700 adult patients with severe mental disorders, found that the number of therapy hours explained more than 70% of the variance in treatment success. Large effects are being achieved after 16–51 sessions. It can be assumed that this dose-effect relationship is also of similar relevance to the treatment of children and adolescents with mental health problems. In a current HTA report on the effectiveness of music therapy for selected indications, the following conclusion is drawn: "The findings of this update of reviews provide evidence that music therapy may help patients diagnosed with an autism spectrum disorder, dementia, depression, and insomnia. Music therapy improves physical, psychological and social aspects. It can be seen as an alternative or supplement to disease-specific therapies" (Gassner and Mayer-Ferbas 2020, p. 9).

In the following, exemplary music therapy research results for three disorders or symptom complexes will be presented, which are of great importance in child and adolescent psychiatry, and also represent classic fields of music therapy application.

12.6.1 Attention Deficit Hyperactivity Disorder (ADHD)

ADHD or hyperkinetic disorder (name according to ICD-10) is a disorder that is characterized by the triad of attention disorder, motor hyperactivity, and impulsivity. It is essential to consider age and time criteria when making a diagnosis: According to the definition, the disorder begins before the age of 6 and should last more than 6 months and occur in at least two areas of life/situations (e.g., at school, in the family, during examination). ADHD is one of the most frequently diagnosed disorders in childhood. The prevalence rates for 6–12-year-old boys are between 7% and 17%, for girls of the same age between 3.3% and 6% (Stegemann and Stellermann-Strehlow 2018).

Inattention, hyperactivity and disorders of social behavior are named as typical indications for music therapy work. No less than 60% of inpatients treated with music therapy in child and adolescent psychiatry have an F9 diagnosis (Stegemann et al. 2008). Despite this, few scientific studies have so far been carried out and relevant evidence-based literature on the subject is scarce. Schneider and Wilmers' (2004) first attempt at a systematic overview in the German-speaking area states that there are nine articles on the subject of music therapy and ADHD. The meta-analysis by Gold et al. (2004) on music therapy treatment of children and adolescents with psychopathological disorders showed a medium to large effect size (d = 0.61).

However, ADHD as a diagnosis (in combination with emotional disorders and learning disorders) is explicitly mentioned in only one of the 11 studies considered (Montello and Coons 1998). In summary, the authors of the meta-analysis interpret their results as showing that music therapy is particularly suitable for the treatment of clients with behavioral and developmental disorders (Gold et al. 2004).

In a separate review (Bosse et al. 2013), 18 original papers (including unpublished music therapy theses) were identified in which music therapy interventions with children with ADHD are described. Thus, there is a remarkable discrepancy between the importance of ADHD for everyday music therapy treatment and the amount of scientific research on this topic.

In a meta-analysis by Maloy and Peterson (2014) that included five studies, musical interventions in children and adolescents with ADHD led to slight improvements in the ability to cope with tasks (e.g., correct solving of maths problems, accuracy).

12.6.2 Autism Spectrum Disorders

Autism spectrum disorders (ASD) belong to the group of profound developmental disorders, which according to ICD-10 criteria, are characterized by qualitative impairments in mutual social interactions and communication patterns as well as by a restricted stereotypical, repetitive repertoire of interests and activities. The clinically most common and most significant autistic disorders are early childhood autism (Kanner syndrome) and Asperger's syndrome. Asperger's syndrome differs from Kanner syndrome in that language development initially proceeds normally.

Only later do these patients stand out due to a particularly elaborate, stilted and partly precocious-sounding language combined with difficulties adapting adequately to different social situations. The prevalence of ASD has increased in the last few decades and tends toward 1% overall. Boys are three to four times more likely to be affected by early childhood autism than girls; for Asperger's syndrome, the male:female ratio is approx. 8:1 (Stegemann and Stellermann-Strehlow 2018).

The treatment of ASD with music therapy probably goes back to the 1940s, when Kanner and Asperger first described the disorders named after them (Reschke-Hernandez 2011). The first empirical study to our knowledge was undertaken by Stevens and Clark (1969). Since then, numerous other studies with different target symptoms (communication, language skills, social skills, expressiveness, etc.) have been published (Reschke-Hernandez 2011).

In the HTA report by Gassner and Mayer-Ferbas (2020) the results from the Cochrane Review on music therapy for autism spectrum disorders (ASD) by Geretsegger et al. (2014; currently being revised) were summarized as follows: "In children with autism spectrum disorders, improvements in initiating behaviour, social-emotional reciprocity, verbal communication, and social interaction and adaptation were found, as well as [strengthening] the parent-child relationship (...).

Nonverbal communication, however, could not be improved by music therapy" (p. 8).

In addition to the studies included in Geretsegger et al., two more recent studies (Bieleninik et al. 2017; Sharda et al. 2018) were evaluated in the HTA report: "The update search revealed that music therapy in children with autism spectrum disorders improves behavior and social communication skills, as well as the quality of the parent-child relationship" (p. 8).

Bergmann and Geretsegger (2021) come to the following conclusion concerning the evidence of effectiveness: "There is evidence of the effectiveness of music therapy in ASD not only regarding changes within the therapy context but also for generalized skills. Findings on the action profiles of specific treatment characteristics for different groups of people with ASD are still pending" (p. 60).

12.6.3 Non-suicidal Self-Injury (NSSI)

Self-injurious behavior and suicidality represent the most common leading symptoms for acute treatment in child and adolescent psychiatry (Brunner and Resch 2008). Self-injurious behavior with non-suicidal intent is internationally known as "non-suicidal self-injury" (NSSI). The most common forms are cutting, intense scratching and hitting oneself.

Around 25–30% of young people in Germany report having injured themselves at least once in their lives (Plener et al. 2018). One in ten said they had done this repeatedly (more than four times). In a child and adolescent psychiatric population, these rates are significantly higher. According to our unpublished data from the basic documentation of a child and adolescent psychiatric clinic (2007–2008), over 50% of adolescents stated in a self-assessment tool that they had intentionally injured themselves.

In a questionnaire study (Stegemann et al. 2010) we investigated the role that music plays in connection with self-harming behavior. A total of 40 patients with an average age of 16 years, 36 of them female (90%), took part in the study. Most of them were in inpatient treatment for affective disorders (ICD-10: F3) as well as personality and behavioral disorders (ICD-10: F6 including in particular emotionally unstable personality disorders). The inclusion criteria for participation included self-harming behavior (NSSI) and/or suicidality during the previous 3 months.

The "Questionnaire on Music and Auto-Aggressiveness in Young People" (FMAJ) created by the authors recorded music preferences and the importance that music has for young people. In addition, questions were asked about NSSI and suicidality as well as specifically about the use of music in leisure time and in the context of psychological crises. The most important results of this study showed firstly that self-harming behavior and suicidality cannot be associated with certain music preferences.

Secondly, it found that music, which was rated as extremely important by almost all of the participants in the study, is mainly used to lighten the mood. This is remarkable since, according to other studies (Megert 2009), young people in particular tend to follow the so-called iso-principle, i.e., try to reinforce their current mood—regardless of whether it is positive or negative—with music.

The use of music to lighten the mood as found in our study could be seen as an expression of both a high level of suffering and a certain therapeutic experience that promotes the use of resources. Music was named twice as often as a suitable relaxation method in our study than reading, which was in second place. This finding is consistent with the aforementioned argument.

Thirdly, it should be noted that 19 of the 33 patients answered yes to the question of whether they had injured themselves while listening to music, but half of those with NSSI also answered the follow-up question ("Have you ever consciously used music to AVOID having to hurt yourself?") with a yes. This means that for young people music can, on the one hand, be part of the self-harm scenarios, but on the other hand, it is also consciously used as a coping mechanism, which can be interpreted as a protective factor.

The pieces of music cited by the young people were stylistically very different. In the qualitative evaluation, which can only be discussed in passing here, it was shown that the songs heard in order to avoid self-harm predominantly had a steady and energetic rhythm as well as positive lyrical content ("I don't give up"). On the other hand, there were also songs, such as "Narben" (German for "scars") by the German band Subway to Sally, which positively advocate NSSI but were also heard to prevent self-harming behavior.

A pilot study at the child and adolescent psychiatric hospital in Ulm has shown that music and music therapy can also be used specifically for the therapy of NSSI (Plener et al. 2010). Female adolescents (14–16 years) with predominantly depressive disorders and NSSI symptoms were treated with a combination of group music therapy (band workshop) and individual DBT-A (dialectical behavioral therapy for adolescents). The music therapy group sessions included receptive elements such as relaxation exercises with music and biography work ("soundtrack of my life"), as well as active music-making: selected songs were covered with vocals and instruments and then recorded in a studio. After 12 weeks, four of the five patients showed a significant improvement in their symptoms, which persisted until the check-up 2 months later.

In summary, these two studies show that in the treatment of adolescents with self-harming behavior (NSSI), music can be an important component of therapy. On the one hand, it can be used as a resource outside the therapy and, on the other hand, it seems suitable for improving compliance, which poses a major problem with this clientele. In a review article, Gold et al. (2009) showed that music therapy is generally suitable for promoting treatment motivation and compliance in patients with mental illness. Plener and Sukale (2020) provide a current overview of music therapy for NSSI.

12.6.4 Unresolved Issues

A basic problem of music therapy research oriented towards evidence-based practice is that the documentation and presentation of psychotherapeutic and musical processes are a highly complex challenge. There are still no gold standards, which often results in incomplete or insufficiently detailed descriptions of the music therapy procedure. Consequently, assessing the validity of research results, comparing studies with one another and identifying effective components are made considerably more difficult. Against this background, Robb and Carpenter (2009) created criteria in a review on the presentation of music-based interventions in pediatrics that can be used to assess the completeness of the information on treatment factors relevant to music therapy. These guidelines are based on the "Consolidated Standards of Reporting Trials" (CONSORT) and the "Transparent Reporting of Evaluations with Nonrandomized Designs" (TREND), which were developed to improve the quality of research reports and ensure complete reporting transparency to enable appropriate assessment and evaluation of research results (Altman et al. 2001; Des Jarlais et al. 2004). In their analysis of 22 selected publications from pediatrics in which music-based interventions were used, Robb and Carpenter (2009) come to the conclusion that none of the studies examined met all 11 criteria and that, among other things, there were gaps or inaccuracies in the following areas:

- Music Qualities: This means whether the title of the piece of music used is mentioned, whether there is information on the musical style, whether the tempo at which the piece was played is given, etc.
- Intervention Materials: A specific description of the musical (e.g., "acoustic guitar with nylon strings" vs. "guitar") and nonmusical materials used (e.g., "five plastic frogs" vs. "toys").
- Intervention Components: What type of intervention was used? For example, with active music therapy: What form of improvisation? Imagination or relaxation exercises with music support, listening to music together, songwriting? Etc.
- Interventionist: What qualification(s) does the practitioner have? How many practitioners with what professional background are involved? Etc.
- Setting: Where does the intervention take place? To what extent is it a screened/ protected area? How loud is the environment? Etc.

This excerpt from the criteria examined by Robb and Carpenter (2009) is enough to underline how extensive and difficult the influencing factors to be considered are and how crucial the accurate documentation of these parameters is for conveying a comprehensive and meaningful picture of the music therapy intervention. With regard to the latter aspect, in particular, it should be noted that music therapy interventions in group settings are often researched within an institution in which music therapy is one component of therapy alongside many others. Examination settings often do not do justice to this complex situation. In a field in which many different professions with different musical qualifications are involved in a research project it therefore appears that sensitivity to such factors is advisable as early as the research-planning phase.

12.7 Summary and Conclusion

> Music therapy with children and adolescents is defined as the targeted use of music and/or musical elements in the context of a therapeutic relationship to restore, maintain and promote mental and somatic health, as well as to correct and promote development. (Stegemann 2021, p. 418)

Music is of great importance—also in terms of developmental psychology—in childhood and adolescence. The special appeal and motivational character inherent in musical instruments and making music facilitate contact and communication with and within this age group. The experience-oriented and process-based approach in music therapy as a nonverbal procedure suits both the child who expresses himself in play and the adolescent who acts or stays silent.

Music therapy, which can look back on over 60 years of academic training in Europe, has now become an indispensable component of a multimodal treatment approach in child and adolescent psychiatry, psychosomatics and psychotherapy. There are now several meta-analyses and randomized controlled studies (RCTs) that prove the positive effects of music therapy in the treatment of mental disorders in children and adolescents.

Music-based interventions with children are therefore also an "effective approach in health care and education, as engaging with music also enables positive transfer effects to non-musical areas" (Kiese-Himmel 2012, p. 235). At the same time, further—ideally interdisciplinary—research efforts are required in order to further advance the evidence-based foundation of music therapy, i.e., more RCTs with larger case numbers and longitudinal studies in a naturalistic setting are necessary. Only in this way can music therapy benefit more children and adolescents with mental health problems by achieving recognition, especially by health insurance companies.

12.7.1 Conclusion

The developments presented in the introduction make it clear how important prevention and adequate psychotherapeutic care are for those who—as is often proclaimed in political soapbox oratory—represent the future of our society. As a conclusion, let's let a young person who was in inpatient treatment because of massive school problems have their say:

> On me, music therapy has the strongest effect. It is simply possible to change something through certain sounds that you either create or that the therapist creates – it's just crazy what happens sometimes! (Stiftung Musik hilft 2009)

References

Altman DG, Schulz KF, Moher D, Egger M, Davidoff F, Elbourne D et al (2001) The revised CONSORT statement for reporting randomized trials: explanation and elaboration. Ann Intern Med 134:663–694

Argstatter H, Hilleke TK, Bradt J, Dileo C (2007) Der Stand der Wirksamkeitsforschung—Ein systematisches Review musiktherapeutischer Meta-Analysen. Verhaltenstherapie & Verhaltensmedizin 28:39–61

Bergmann T, Geretsegger M (2021) Autismus-Spektrum-Störung. In: Decker-Voigt HH, Weymann E (Hrsg) Lexikon Musiktherapie (3. Aufl). Hogrefe, Göttingen, S 57–62

Bieleninik Ł, Geretsegger M, Mössler K et al (2017) Effects of improvisational music therapy vs enhanced standard care on symptom severity among children with autism spectrum disorder: the TIME-A randomized clinical trial. JAMA 318:525–535

Biermann G (1988) Zur Geschichte der analytischen Kinderpsychotherapie. In: Biermann G (Hrsg) Handbuch der Kinderpsychotherapie. Fischer, Frankfurt a. M., S 14–36

Bosse J, Stegemann T, Schmidt HU, Timmermann T (2013) Dem Aufmerksamkeitsdefizit mit Aufmerksamkeit begegnen—was die Musiktherapie Kindern und Jugendlichen mit einer ADHS-Diagnose bieten kann. Musikther Umsch 34(1):7–22

Brunner R, Resch F (2008) Borderline-Störungen und selbstverletzendes Verhalten bei Jugendlichen. Vandenhoeck & Ruprecht, Göttingen

Degryse M (2012) Ein geschützter Raum inmitten von Aggressionen. Musikther Umsch 33:46–54

Des Jarlais DC, Lyles C, Crepaz N (2004) Improving the reporting quality of nonrandomized evaluations of behavioral and public health interventions: the TREND statement. Am J Public Health 94:361–366

Erhart M, Ravens-Sieberer U (2009) Lebensqualität von Kindern in Deutschland. In: Resch F, Schulte-Markwort M (Hrsg.) Kindheit im digitalen Zeitalter. BeltzPVU, Weinheim, S 23–40

Erkkilä J, Punkanen M, Fachner J, Ala-Ruona E, Pöntiö I, Tervamiemi M, Vanhala M, Gold C (2011) Individual music therapy for depression: randomized controlled trial. Br J Psychiatry 199:132–139

Evers S (2001) Musiktherapie und Kinderheilkunde. G. Fischer, Stuttgart

Fegert JM (2011) Zum Standort der Künstlerischen Therapien an der Klinik. 5 Chefs, 5 Fragen, 5 Antworten. Musikther Umsch 32:338–343

Fitzthum E (2003) Von den Reformbewegungen zur Musiktherapie. Die Brückenfunktion der Vally Weigl. Wiener Beiträge zur Musiktherapie, Bd 5. Edition Praesens, Wien

Frohne-Hagemann I, Pleß-Adamczyk H (2005) Indikation Musiktherapie bei psychischen Problemen im Kindes- und Jugendalter. Vandenhoeck & Ruprecht, Göttingen

Gassner L, Mayer-Ferbas J (2020) Effectiveness of music therapy for autism spectrum disorder, dementia, depression, insomnia and schizophrenia. Update of systematic reviews, AIHTA Projektbericht No. 133. Austrian Institute for Health Technology Assessment GmbH, Vienna

Geipel J, Koenig J, Hillecke TK, Resch F, Kaess M (2018) Music-based interventions to reduce internalizing symptoms in children and adolescents: a meta-analysis. J Affect Disord 225:647–656

Geretsegger M, Elefant C, Mössler KA, Gold C (2014) Music therapy for people with autism spectrum disorder (review). Cochrane Datab Syst Rev Issue 6:Art. No.: CD004381. https://doi.org/10.1002/14651858.CD004381.pub3

Gold C, Voracek M, Wigram T (2004) Effects of music therapy for children and adolescents with psychopathology. A meta-analysis. J Child Psychol Psychiatry 45:1054–1063

Gold C, Solli HP, Krüger V, Lie SA (2009) Dose-response relationship in music therapy for people with serious mental disorders: systematic review and meta-analysis. Clin Psychol Rev 29:193–207

Gold C, Saarikallio SH, McFerran K (2011) Music therapy. In: Levesque RJR (ed) Encyclopedia of adolescence. Springer, New York, pp 1826–1834

Grawe K, Donati R, Vernauer F (1994) Psychotherapie im Wandel—Von der Konfession zur Profession. Hogrefe, Göttingen

Grunert C, Krüger HH (2006) Kindheit und Kindheitsforschung in Deutschland. Budrich, Opladen

Haffa-Schmidt U (1999) Musik und Identität—Die Bedeutung von Musik für Jugendliche. In: Haffa-Schmidt U, v. Moreau D, Wölfl A (Hrsg.) Musiktherapie mit psychisch kranken Jugendlichen. Vandenhoeck & Ruprecht, Göttingen, S 26–30

Haffa-Schmidt U, Moreau D, Wölfl A (1999) Musiktherapie mit Jugendlichen—Einführung in die Thematik. In: Haffa-Schmidt U, v. Moreau D, Wölfl A (Hrsg.) Musiktherapie mit psychisch kranken Jugendlichen. Vandenhoeck & Ruprecht, Göttingen, S 13–19

Hegi-Protmann F, Lutz Hochreutener S, Rüdisüli-Vorekel M (2006) Musiktherapie als Wissenschaft. Autorenverlag, Zürich

Hüther G (2011) Was wir sind und was wir sein könnten. Fischer, Frankfurt

Jacoby H (1984) Jenseits von „Musikalisch" und „Unmusikalisch". Christian, Hamburg

Jordan AK, Pfeifer E, Stegemann T, Lutz Hochreutener S (Hrsg) (2018) Musiktherapie in pädagogischen Settings. Impulse aus Praxis, Theorie und Forschung. Waxmann, Münster

Key E (1902) Das Jahrhundert des Kindes. S. Fischer, Berlin

Kiese-Himmel C (2012) Musikbasierte Intervention bei Kindern. Prax Kinderpsychol Kinderpsychiat 61:235–254

Klipker K, Baumgarten F, Göbel K, Lampert T, Hölling H (2018) Psychische Auffälligkeiten bei Kindern und Jugendlichen in Deutschland—Querschnittergebnisse aus KiGGS Welle 2 und Trends. J Health Monitor 3(3):37–45. https://doi.org/10.17886/RKI-GBE-2018-077

Koch-Temming H (1998) Musiktherapie in einem Sozialpädagogischen Zentrum. Musikther Umsch 19:226–230

Lutz Hochreutener S (2009) Spiel-Musik-Therapie. Methoden der Musiktherapie mit Kindern und Jugendlichen. Hogrefe, Göttingen

MacDonald R, Kreutz G, Mitchell L (2012) What is music, health, and wellbeing and why is it important? In: MacDonald R, Kreutz G, Mitchell L (eds) Music, health, & wellbeing. Oxford University Press, New York, pp 3–11

Mahns W (2004) Symbolbildung in der analytischen Kindermusiktherapie. Eine qualitative Studie über die Bedeutung der musikalischen Improvisation in der Musiktherapie mit Schulkindern. In: Tüpker R (Hrsg.) Materialien zur Musiktherapie (Buchreihe). Lit-Verlag, Münster

Maloy M, Peterson R (2014) A meta-analysis of the effectiveness of music interventions for children and adolescents with attention-deficit/hyperactivity disorder. Psychomusic Music Mind Brain 24:328–339

Mattejat F (2008) Fallkonzeptualisierung, Indikationsstellung und Therapieplanung. In: Remschmidt H, Mattejat F, Warnke A (Hrsg.) Therapie psychischer Störungen bei Kindern und Jugendlichen. Thieme, Stuttgart, S. 97–106

Megert C (2009) „Ohne meine Lieblingsmusik hätte ich es nicht geschafft..." Musikhören in der Initialphase der Musiktherapie mit Jugendlichen. Musikther Umsch 30:102–113

Montello L, Coons E (1998) Effects of active versus passive group music therapy on preadolescents with emotional, learning and behavioral disorders. J Music Ther 35:49–67

Oster J (2015) Berufsgruppenanalyse Künstlerische Therapeutinnen und Therapeuten. Ergebnisbericht zu den Fachbereichen Kunsttherapie, Musiktherapie, Tanztherapie, Eurythmietherapie, Theatertherapie, Sonstige. Hochschule für Kunsttherapie Nürtingen, Universitätsklinik für Psychosomatische Medizin und Psychotherapie Ulm

Otto C, Reiss F, Voss C, Wüstner A, Meyrose AK, Hölling H, Ravens-Sieberer U (2021) Mental health and well-being from childhood to adulthood: design, methods and results of the 11-year follow-up of the BELLA study. Eur Child Adolesc Psychiatry. https://doi.org/10.1007/s00787-020-01630-4

Pelletier CL (2004) The effect of music on decreasing arousal due to stress: a meta-analysis. J Music Ther 41:192–214

Pešek U (2007) Musiktherapiewirkung—eine Meta-Analyse. Musikther Umsch 28:110–135

Phan Quoc E, Riedl H, Smetana M, Stegemann T (2019) Zur beruflichen Situation von Musiktherapeut.innen in Österreich: Ergebnisse einer Online-Umfrage. [Music therapy in Austria: a national survey study on the professional situation of music therapists]. Musikther Umsch 40(3):236–248. https://doi.org/10.13109/muum.2019.40.3.236

Plahl C (2000) Entwicklung fördern durch Musik. Evaluation musiktherapeutischer Behandlung. Waxmann, Münster

Plahl C, Koch-Temming H (2005) Musiktherapie mit Kindern. Huber, Bern

Plener PL,, Sukale T (2020) Selbstverletzendes Verhalten. In: Schmidt HU, Stegemann T, Spitzer C (Hrsg) Musiktherapie bei psychischen und psychosomatischen Störungen. Elsevier, München, S 303–313

Plener P, Sukale T, Ludolph A, Stegemann T (2010) “Stop cutting-rock!”: a pilot study of a music therapeutic program for self-injuring adolescents. Music Med 2:59–65

Plener PL, Kaess M, Schmahl C, Pollak S, Fegert JM, Brown RC (2018) Nonsuicidal self-injury in adolescents. Dtsch Arztebl Int 115:23–30

Ravens-Sieberer U, Erhart M (2021) Die Beziehung zwischen sozialer Ungleichheit und Gesundheit im Kindes- und Jugendalter. In: Richter M, Hurrelmann K, Klocke A, Melzer W, Ravens-Sieberer U (Hrsg.) Gesundheit, Ungleichheit und jugendliche Lebenswelten. Juventa, Weinheim, S 39–66

Resch F (2012) Kindheit heute. Vorträge der 10. Psychotherapietage des Kindes- und Jugendalters, Langeoog (DVD). Auditorium Netzwerk, Müllheim/Baden

Reschke-Hernandez AE (2011) History of music therapy treatment interventions for children with autism. J Music Ther 48:169–207

Riedl H, Stegemann T (2018) Die Übersetzung der Healthy-Unhealthy Uses of Music Scale (HUMS) vom Englischen ins Deutsche. Musikther Umsch 39:229–240

Riedl H, Schmidt HU, Smetana M, Stegemann T (2020) Forschung in der Musiktherapie. In: Schmidt HU, Stegemann T, Spitzer C (Hrsg) Musiktherapie bei psychischen und psychosomatischen Störungen. Elsevier, München, S 81–90

Robb SL, Carpenter JS (2009) A review of music-based intervention reporting in pediatrics. J Health Psychol 14:490–501

Schmidt HU (2002) Forschung in der Kindermusiktherapie. Musikther Umsch 23:80–83

Schmidt HU, Stegemann T (2019) Kontraindikationen, unerwünschte Wirkungen und mögliche Behandlungsfehler in der Musiktherapie. Musikther Umsch 40(4):352–363

Schmidt HU, Stegemann T (2020) Ausbildungswege in der Musiktherapie. In: Schmidt HU, Stegemann T, Spitzer C (Hrsg) Musiktherapie bei psychischen und psychosomatischen Störungen. Elsevier, München, S 69–74

Schmidt HU, Stegemann T (2021) Ausbildung im deutschsprachigen Raum. In: Decker-Voigt HH, Weymann E (Hrsg) Lexikon Musiktherapie (3. Aufl). Hogrefe, Göttingen, S 45–52

Schmidt HU, Timmermann T (2012) Was kann Musiktherapie in der Schule leisten? Musik und Gesundsein 22:12–15

Schneider R, Wilmers C (2004) Aufmerksamkeits-Defizit-Syndrom mit Hyperaktivität. Zeitschrift für Musik-, Tanz- und Kunsttherapie 15:70–72

Schumacher K, Calvet C, Reimer S (2011) Das EBQ-Instrument und seine entwicklungspsychologischen Grundlagen. Vandenhoeck & Ruprecht, Göttingen

Seidler E (1991) Historische und ethische Aspekte der Kinderheilkunde. In: Betke K, Künzer W, Schaub J (Hrsg.) Lehrbuch der Kinderheilkunde. Thieme, Stuttgart

Sharda M, Tuerk C, Chowdhury R et al (2018) Music improves social communication and auditory-motor connectivity in children with autism. Transl Psychiatry 8:231

Statistisches Bundesamt (2020a) Kinder und Jugendliche nach Altersgruppen 2019. https://de.statista.com/statistik/daten/studie/1174053/umfrage/minderjaehrige-in-deutschland-nach-altersgruppen/ (zuletzt gesehen am 22.12.20)

Statistisches Bundesamt (2020b) Mitten im demografischen Wandel. https://www.destatis.de/DE/Themen/Querschnitt/Demografischer-Wandel/demografie-mitten-im-wandel.html (zuletzt gesehen am 22.12.20)

Stegemann T (2020). Was MusiktherapeutInnen über das Gehirn wissen sollten. Neurobiologie für die Praxis (2. Aufl). Reinhardt, München

Stegemann T (2021) Musiktherapie mit Kindern und Jugendlichen. In: Decker-Voigt HH, Weymann E (Hrsg.) Lexikon Musiktherapie (3. Aufl). Hogrefe, Göttingen, S. 418–424

Stegemann T, Geipel J (2018) Musiktherapie mit Jugendlichen. In: Stegemann T, Fitzthum E. (Hrsg.) Kurzlehrbuch Musiktherapie Teil 1. Wiener Ringvorlesung Musiktherapie—Grundlagen und Anwendungsfelder (2. Aufl). Praesens, Wien, S. 223–241

Stegemann T, Schmidt HU (2010) Zur Indikation und Kontraindikation in der Kinder- und Jugendpsychiatrie—eine Fragebogenuntersuchung. Musikther Umsch 31:87–101
Stegemann T, Stellermann-Strehlow K (2018) Kinder- und Jugendpsychiatrie. In: Leucht S, Förstl H (Hrsg.) Kurzlehrbuch Psychiatrie und Psychotherapie (2. Aufl). Thieme, Stuttgart
Stegemann T, Mauch C, Stein V, Romer G (2008) Zur Situation der Musiktherapie in der stationären Kinder- und Jugendpsychiatrie. Z Kinder Jugendpsychiatr Psychother 36:255–263
Stegemann T, Brüggemann-Etchart A, Badorrek-Hinkelmann A, Romer G (2010) Die Funktion von Musik im Zusammenhang mit selbstverletzendem Verhalten und Suizidalität bei Jugendlichen. Prax Kinderpsychol Kinderpsychiat 59:810–830
Stegemann T, Hitzeler M, Blotevogel M (2012) Künstlerische Therapien mit Kindern und Jugendlichen. Reinhardt, München
Stegemann T, Geretsegger M, Phan Quoc E, Riedl H, Smetana M (2019) Music therapy and other music-based interventions in pediatric health care: an overview. Medicine 6(1):25. https://doi.org/10.3390/medicines6010025
Stegemann T, Riedl H, Evers-Grewe B, Körber A (2021) Musiktherapie in Medizinischen Leitlinien—eine systematische Literaturrecherche der AWMF-Leitlinien
Stevens E, Clark F (1969) Music therapy in the treatment of autistic children. J Music Ther 6:98–104
Stiftung Musik hilft (2009) „Wo die Sprache aufhört“ (Film), Regie: Marcus Sternberg. Free the Dragon Filmproduktion GmbH
Timmermann T, Schmidt HU (2007) Unterstützung durch Musiktherapie. In: Menzel D, Wiater W (Hrsg.) Kinder und Jugendliche mit Förderbedarf in der Regelschule. Auer, Donauwörth, S 256–269
Weiß R (2008) Trauma und Musiktherapie—Ansätze und Wege in der musiktherapeutischen Behandlung psychisch traumatisierter Menschen. Musikther Umsch 29:5–25
Wiesmüller E, Stegemann T (2020) „The most relaxing place“. Eine Chronologie des Projekts „Musiktherapie mit Geflüchteten“. Musik und Gesundsein 38:18–23
Wölfl A (2021) TrommelPower—eine musiktherapeutische Projektmethode zur Gewaltprävention Musiktherapie mit Jugendlichen. In: Stegemann T, Fitzthum, E (Hrsg.) Kurzlehrbuch Musiktherapie Teil 2. Wiener Ringvorlesung Musiktherapie—Grundlagen und Anwendungsfelder. Praesens, Wien
Wormit AF, Hillecke TK, Flach SM, Bolay HV (2001) Ambulante Musiktherapie. Musik-, Tanz- und Kunsttherapie 12:166–170

The Role of Music in Patients with Traumatic Brain Injury

13

Elena Romana Gasenzer and Ayhan Kanat

Key Points Music interventions offers big chances for patients with mild or severe traumatic brain injury.

13.1 Introduction

In the history and the development of music and medicine, many relationships exist over a long period of time. Since the Neolithic age, early activities of medical treatment and cultural techniques such as music-making exist (Dastugue 2000a). Neolithic skull finds show signs of trepanations and healed skull fractures (Dastugue 2000b; Zhou et al. 2020). In that era, humans began with musical activities, and the first music instruments, like bone flutes, were developed (Tarasov 2005). Music and acoustic stimulation became an important part of ritual acts as well as medical treatment (Kirchner 1952). In present shamanistic cults, music is part of medical treatment (Brandl 1993). The function of music in shamanistic healing rituals is to have an analgesic and calming effect on the patient, and to inspire the healer. According to shamanistic conception, music empowers the healer and the patient (Timmermann 2009).

Because of that history, music interventions for patients with brain injuries or skull trauma have a long tradition. Since the middle of the twentieth century, music therapy gained in importance in different specialties in medicine, such like

E. R. Gasenzer (✉)
Department Physician Assistance, Carl Remigius Medical School,
Frankfurt am Main, Germany
e-mail: elena.gasenzer@carl-remigius.de

A. Kanat
Medical Faculty, Department of Neurosurgery, Recep Tayyip Erdogan University,
Rize, Turkey

G. Kreutz, G. Bernatzky (eds.), *Music and Medicine*, Neurocultural Health and Wellbeing, https://doi.org/10.1007/978-3-662-72175-9_13

anesthesiology, pediatrics, psychiatry, odontology, as well as in different surgical disciplines (Allred et al. 2010; Liu and Petrini 2015; Preti and Welch 2004; Spinthge 1997).

Because of the long history of music interventions on humans with different injuries of the brain or the skull, we will give an overview to the numerous applications of music interventions and music therapy, its´ effects and mechanism of action on patients with traumatic brain injury.

13.2 Neuronal Plasticity and the Effects of Music on the Injured Brain

Neuronal plasticity is the most important mechanism of the effects of music on an injured brain (Bernatzky et al. 2015; de Divitis 2010; Duffau 2006). In the last decades, the musicians´ brain became an object of much investigations, because in consequence of a long training of instrumental skills and music performance, the musicians brain shows the highest level of plasticity and changes of neuronal mapping (Elbert et al. 1995; Schlaug 2015). Every injury or loss of neuronal tissue requires a reorganization of the brain and its´ functional mapping. It requires some structural changes on different anatomic structures: on cellular structures, a remodeling of neuronosynaptic maps is necessary to reconstruct the function of cerebral networks (Särkämö et al. 2014). Some cases of musicians with neurosurgical diseases document the high ability of the musicians´ brains for remodeling (Galarza et al. 2014; Gasenzer et al. 2016a, b). Those results document the effects of different forms of music interventions and music making on the recovering brain. In patients with traumatic brain injury, the situations is different in some aspects. In the case of a brain tumor or an AVM, structural changes are made over a long time period, and the brain has time to connect new synaptic connections and reconstruct neuronal pathways. Modern techniques in neurosurgery offer the chance for a pre- or intraoperative brain mapping, to preserve important functional brain structures (Kanat and Epstein 2010). In case of TBI, the injury happens suddenly with damage to important structures. In most cases further complications like bleeding, edema, hypoxia, and increasing CPP or ICP occur (Vella et al. 2017). Because of the greater extent of injured brain tissue, more complications, and more injuries of grey and white matter structures, the neurorehabilitation of patients with TBI is long, and the patients have some special needs on therapy (Marklund et al. 2019).

13.3 The Role of Neurochemistry in Music-Related Neuronal Plasticity

Because of neuronal plasticity, the musicians´ brain shows some adaptations to music perception and instrumental playing (Pantev and Herholz 2011; Schlaug 2015). In violinists and string players the motor area of the left hand increases in size (Elbert et al. 1995), and in professional pianists, the size of the corpus collossum increases (Schlaug et al. 1995). The more years the instrumental training lasted, the greater were the changes of neuronal mapping and the increasing of functional areas (Vaquero et al. 2016). Because of the early beginning of music education and instrumental training in the lives of professional musicians, the musicians´ brains are more the brain is more flexible in its adaptability to the special requirements of music performance. Music making promotes brain plasticity along the live in young and older people as well as in patients after brain injury (Wan and Schlaug 2010). Music activates the neuronal plasticity by the activation of neurochemical pathways. Music enhances the production of neurotransmitters like dopamine, serotonin, and oxytocin and inhibits the pathways for stress reaction and its´ hormones like cortisol, CRH, and ACTH (Sutoo and Akiyama 2004).

Music also enhances the brain plasticity by activation of emotions and emotional pathways. The limbic system plays an important role in emotional perception, memory and cognition. These special structures of the brain work with the neurotransmitters serotonin, dopamine, and oxytocin. By the activation of the limbic pathways and its´ transmitters, music support the neuronal as well as the emotional function. Patients in a coma or vegetative state can be reached by emotional stimuli, such as a touch or by music (Okumura et al. 2014). The simple shape of communication is a touch or a sound!

Because of these results on musicians´ brains, some positive effects of music interventions on patients with traumatic brain injury are possible.

13.4 Different Types of Music Interventions on Patients with Brain Injury

Some different types of successful music interventions on patients with different types of brain injury or further neurosurgical treatments have been documented (Okumura et al. 2014; Särkämö et al. 2014). Specially hearing of a special program of classic music, which includes instrumental sounds, melody, rhythm, harmony, and language or voice perception, like opera airs or choir works, promotes the rehabilitation of patients after stroke (Särkämö et al. 2008, 2014, 2016). Music interventions for patients with awake craniotomy support the patients during surgery and influence mood, anxiety, and traumatic experiences. In cases of awake craniotomy, music supports the neuronal reorganization of the brain already during the operation, provides the opportunity of intraoperative neuronal mapping, and offers the chance for an early beginning of neuronal reorganization (Jadavji-Mithani et al. 2015). Most music interventions on neurosurgical patients were performed as passive music interventions or passive music therapy, which use passive forms of music use like music hearing, sound perception, or rhythmic stimuli. Usually passive music therapy is apply to patients, who are not able to make music actively. The reasons are different. Mostly the neurological state is worse, patients are not able to react actively to music, or they are paralyzed with motor deficits and loss of pyramidal functions. Another reason is that active music making such as instrumental playing needs specially trained instrumental techniques and some acquired skills like, fingering and bow technique, reading or understanding music skills. Because of that, active music making is only possible for patients, who learned instruments, or in rehabilitation programs which offers instrumental learning for patients after brain surgery (Cheung et al. 2019). Every form of music intervention, when patients take an active part in music-making called \active music therapy. Active music therapy are music interventions on an elementary level, like rhythmic movement activities, clapping hands, drumming on percussion instruments, playing Orff instruments, or singing. These forms of music activity are suitable for rehabilitations of elementary motor functions. Rhythmic structures support the initiation of movement sequences and the neuronal reorganization of motor pathways. Percussion and Orff instruments can be played without instrumental education and are suitable for people without special musical skills, or who are suffer by mental or movement disabilities. Such type of active music therapy are offer to patients with hemi or mild paresis, or cognitive deficits after brain damage, or for people with special needs (Formisano et al. 2001; Gooding et al. 2013) (Sihvonen et al. 2017).

13.5 The Neurologic Music Therapy

Neurologic music therapy uses the structures of music, rhythm, melody, and harmony to enhance pathways and functional areas and to support the reorganization of neuronal networks. Depending on the musical structure like melody or rhythm, the music enhances the functions of speech or motor pathways for body movement (Thaut 2014; Thaut and MHömberg 2015). Motor pathways, like pyramidal functions, can enhance by rhythm. Language or speech disabilities are well recovered by melody and speech patterns, such as singing in a choir. Practicing of movements and motor functions is easier, if the movement patterns are accompanied by the rhythm of music, whereas melody and harmony are good support for speech functions (Altenmüller and Schlaug 2013).

13.6 Music Interventions in Traumatic Brain Injuries

An amount of 29 controlled trials about music interventions on 775 patients with traumatic or further brain injury has documented by a Cochrane review (Magee et al. 2018). The aims of these studies and outcomes were walking speed, length of steps, and steps per minute, symmetry of body movements, fine motor skills of upper extremities, cognitive abilities, language, and quality of life. Communication abilities were investigated by naming, repetition, attention, and memory (Magee et al. 2018). Types of music interventions were passive music interventions or music hearing, as well as active music interventions, such as playing instruments and improvisation on instruments, instrumental musical performance, singing, and voice training to played music, aural and vocal intonation training, song writing, and moving to music. Included were patients up to 16 with traumatic brain injury, brain injury because of tumor or surgery, and patients after stroke or hemorrhage, infections, or inflammations, cerebral anoxia or metabolic insult. The problem is, studies about music interventions in different medical indications have a high risk of bias, because the conditions of patients are very different, and the methods, music styles, or instruments of the interventions are very different, too. Cultural imprint, music education, and music culture are very different, too.

Music intervention in case of traumatic brain injury leads to better cognitive rehabilitation. Music supports the improvement of speech production and understanding, it supports the rehabilitation of auditory and speech perception (Hegde et al. 2016). The effects are larger, if the music intervention starts in an acute state after injury, for example, passive music interventions during intensive care treatment (Bradt et al. 2010; Schlaug 2009). In the acute state after brain injury, the neuronal growth of the synaptic connections and the possibilities of a neuronal reorganization are bigger, because neuronal growth factors and activating transmitters such as serotonin and dopamine are released (Chanda and Levitin 2013). In coma patients with neurosurgical management after traumatic brain injury and a low score on GCS, music therapy affects the electric activity of the brain and supports the rehabilitation of neurons (Sun and Chen 2015). In patients with a mild cognitive state after TBI and craniotomy, music therapy and the perception of their preferred music increased the amplitudes of the EEG, the respiration rates, and the amounts of spontaneous body movements (O'Kelly et al. 2013).

In patients in coma rehabilitation after a coma longer than 15 days because of severe TBI, and with a GCS less than eight, active music therapy has been performed (Formisano et al. 2001). Depending on the neurological state, the cognitive abilities, and the severity of brain damage, an active music therapy is performed, three times per week in units of 20 or 40 min duration. The kind of music activities was depending on the patients´ physical and cognitive condition and the severe of function loss. Musical activities were voice activation like singing and vocalization, moving activities, and active music perception. The therapist accompanied the patients´ activities, by playing on piano, percussion or wind instruments. After the therapy, the patients show more interactive abilities and a reduction of psychomotor agitation (Formisano et al. 2001).

A study with 40 coma patients because of TBI with a GCS less than eight points, 20 patients receive music therapy (Sun and Chen 2015). Measurement of brain functions has been performed by EEG. The age of patients was between 18 and 55 years. The median value of GCS was 5.55 in the music group and 5.65 in the control group. After 1 month of treatment by music therapy the median GCS increased on 11.30 in the music group and on 9.45 in the control group (Sun and Chen 2015). These results document the large chances of music therapy and music-supported treatment in patients with severe TBI.

13.7 Effect of Active Instrumental Learning in Patients with Mild TBI

In patients with mild traumatic brain injury, different types of active music interventions or music therapy are possible. In nonmusician patients with mild traumatic brain injury, a daily (30 min) piano-playing training over a time period of 8 weeks, promotes the reorganization of neuronal networks and supports the rehabilitation of cognitive functions (Dykesteen Vik et al. 2018). After 8 weeks of piano training, the patients in the music group felt much better, had better abilities to concentrate, and had better results in neuropsychological testing (ANOVA, CVLT, Stroop Word/Colour test). The functional MRT imaging of the music group patients, showed large neuroplastic changes in the right medial orbitofrontal gyrus, the middle frontal gyrus, and the anterior insular cortex while hearing Dominant to Tonika cadenzas, and large changes in the supplementary motor area (Dykesteen Vik et al. 2018). The most traumatic brain injuries are mild, but patients suffer from headaches, memory disorders, or cognitive improvements over a long time after trauma. These patients have much benefit from an active musical training or from learning an instrument.

13.8 Applications to Other Areas of Neuroscience

The effects of music therapy in patients with traumatic TBI are similar in other areas of neuroscience of clinical neurology. One effect of music, called the Mozart effect, supports neuronal plasticity and reorganization as well as changes in the electrical activity of the brain (Hughes et al. 1998, 1999). Hearing music by W.A. Mozart and other composers suppresses epileptic patterns during an epileptic seizure (Coppola et al. 2015; Pietschnig et al. 2010). Studies on neurosurgical patients, who undergo awake craniotomy, report a better recovery of the injured brain and of neuronal functions as well as a reduction of pain, stress, and anxiety (Gasenzer et al. 2016a, b; Jadavji-Mithani et al. 2015; Piai et al. 2018).

Key Facts of the Role of Music for Patients with Traumatic Brain Injury

- Music has a long tradition in healing methods.
- Music enhances neuronal plasticity and supports the neuronal reorganization of an injured brain.
- Cases of musicians with neurosurgical diseases document the great effect of music making on the recovering of the brain.
- Music perception and music activities over a long period of time cause extensive changes in synaptic connection, the neuronal networks, and the functional area of the grey matter.
- Music enhances the secretion of the neurotransmitters serotonin, dopamine, and neuronal growth factors, which support the reconnection of synapses.
- Music causes changes in the electric activity of the brain and suppresses epileptogenic activities in the injured brain.

- Passive music therapy is available for patients with a low GCS, too.
- In patients with a low GCS passive music therapy improves the GCS by 5 points.
- In patients with mild TBI learning to play piano enhances the cognitive functions and shortened the duration of recovery.
- Music offers great changes for patients with mild or severe TBI.

13.9 Summary Points

In patients with mild or severe TBI, music supports the recovery and the neuronal reorganization of the injured brain. Music activated the secretion of neuronal growth factors and different neurotransmitters. Some different active and passive forms of music therapy are available. The neurologic music therapy enhances brain functions by melody, harmony, and rhythm. Passive music therapy is suitable for paralyzed patients, and for patients with a low GCS. Passive music therapy can increase the GSC by 5 points. Music offers a big chance for patients with TBI and should be used more often.

References

Allred K, Byers J, Sole M (2010) The effect of music on postoperative pain and anxiety. Pain Manag Nurs 11(1):15–25. https://doi.org/10.1016/j.pmn.2008.12.002

Altenmüller E, Schlaug G (2013) Neurobiological aspects of neurologic music therapy. Music Med 5(4):210–216. https://doi.org/10.1177/1943862113505328

Bernatzky G, Grebosz-Haring K, Wendtner F, Kreutz G (2015) Zerebrale Wirkungen von Musikhören. In: Bernatzky G, Kreutz G (eds) Musik und Medizin. Springer, Heidelberg, pp 86–87

Bradt J, Magee W, Dileo C, Wheeler B, McGilloway E (2010) Music therapy for acquired brain injury. Cochrane Database Syst Rev 7(7):CD006787. https://doi.org/10.1002/14651858.CD006787

Brandl R (1993) Musik und veränderte Bewußtseinszustände. 1. Ethologische und kulturhistorische Definitonen. 2. Schamanismus. In: Oerter R, Bruhn H, Rösing H (eds) Musikpsychologie. Rohwohlts Verlag, Reinbeck bei Hamburg, pp 599–605

Chanda M, Levitin D (2013) The neurochemistry of music. Trends Cogn Sci 17(4):179–193. https://doi.org/10.1016/j.tics.2013.02.007

Cheung A, Cheung Li W, Ho K, Ka Wai Lam K, Kwan Ho L, Chiu S et al (2019) Efficacy of musical training on psychological outcomes and quality of life in Chinese pediatric brain tumor survivors. Psychooncology 28(1):174–180. https://doi.org/10.1002/pon.4929

Coppola G, Toro A, Operto F, Ferrarioli G, Pisano S, A., V., & Verrotti, A. (2015) Mozart's music in children with drug-refractory epileptic encephalopathies. Epilepsy Behav 50:18–22

Dastugue J (2000a) Die Paläopathologie. In: T. R. (ed) Illustrierte Geschichte der Medizin, vol Band 1. Bechtermünz/Sonderauflage f. Weltbildverlag, Augsburg, pp 19–35

Dastugue J (2000b) Schädeltrepanationen. In: Toellner R (ed) Illustrierte Geschichte der Medizin, vol Band 1. Bechtermünz/Sonderauflage f. Weltbildverlag, Augsburg, pp 35–48

de Divitis E (2010) The magical power of music. World Neurosurg 73(5):454–455. https://doi.org/10.1016/j.wneu.2010.03.003

Duffau H (2006) Brain plasticity: from pathophysiological mechanisms to therapeutic applications. J Clin Neurosci 13:885–897

Dykesteen Vik B, Skeie G, Vikane E, Specht K (2018) Effects of music production on cortical plasticity within cognitive rehabilitation of patients with mild traumatic brain injury. Brain Inj 32(5):634–643. https://doi.org/10.1080/02699052.2018.1431842

Elbert T, Pantev C, Wienbruch C, Rockstroh B, Taub E (1995) Increased cortical representation of the fingers of the left hand in string players. Science 270(5234):305–307

Formisano R, Vinicola V, Penta F, Matteis M, Brunelli S, Weckel J (2001) Active music therapy in the rehabilitation of severe brain injured patients during coma recovery. Ann Ist Super Sanita 37(4)

Galarza M, Isaac C, Pellicer O, Mayes A, Broks P, Montaldi D et al (2014) Jazz, guitar, and neurosurgery: the Pat Martino case report. World Neurosurg 81(3–4):1–7. https://doi.org/10.1016/j.wneu.2013.09.042

Gasenzer E, Kanat A, Neugebauer EAM (2016a) First report of interesting awake craniotomy of a famous musician in history; The suprasellar tumor surgery of Pianist Clara Haskil in 1942 without general anaesthesia. J Neurol Surg A Cent Eur Neurosurg 78(03):260–268

Gasenzer E, Kanat A, Neugebauer E (2016b) The unforgettable neurosurgical operations of musicians in last century. World Neurosurg S1878-8750(16):31303–31301. https://doi.org/10.1016/j.wneu.2016.11.144. [Epub ahead of print]

Gooding L, Hudson M, Yinger O (2013) Students with special needs in the 21st century music classroom: practices and perceptions of Orff- and non-Orff trained educators. Music Ther Special Music Educ 5(2):166–174

Hegde S, Bharath R, Rao MB, Shiva K, Arimappamagan A, Sinha S et al (2016) Preservation of cognitive and musical abilities of a musician following surgery for chronic drug-resistant temporal lobe epilepsy: a case report. Neurocase 22(6):512–517. https://doi.org/10.1080/13554794.2016.1198815

Hughes J, Daabul Y, Fino J (1998) The Mozart effect on epileptiform activity. Cilin Electroencephalogr 29:109–119

Hughes J, Fino J, Melyn M (1999) Is there a chronic change of the "Mozart effect" on epileptiform activity? A case study. Clin Electroencephalogr 30(2):44–45

Jadavji-Mithani R, Venkatraghavan L, Bernstein M (2015) Music is beneficial for awake craniotomy patients: a qualitative study. Can J Neurol Sci 42(1):7–16. https://doi.org/10.1017/cjn.2014.127

Kanat A, Epstein C (2010) Challenges to neurosurgical professionalism. Clin Neurol Neurosurg:839–843. https://doi.org/10.1016/j.clineuro.2010.07.012

Kirchner H (1952) Ein archäologischer Beitrag zur Urgeschichte des Schamanismus. Anthropos 47(1, 2):244–286

Liu Y, Petrini M (2015) Effects of music therapy on pain, anxiety, and vital signs in patients after thoracic surgery. Complement Ther Med 23(5):714–718. https://doi.org/10.1016/j.ctim.2015.08.002

Magee W, Imogen C, Tamplin J, Bradt J (2018) Music interventions for acquired brain injury: findings from a Cochrane review. Arch Phys Med Rehabil 99(10):e109. https://doi.org/10.1016/j.apmr.2018.07.390

Marklund N, Bellander B, Godbolt A, Levin H, McCrory P, Thelin P (2019) Treatments and rehabilitation in the acute and chronic state of traumatic brain injury. Intern Med 285(6):608–623. https://doi.org/10.1111/joim.12900

O'Kelly J, James L, Palaniappan R, Taborin J, Fachner J, Magee WL (2013) Neurophysiological and behavioral responses to music therapy in vegetative and minimally conscious states. Front Hum Neurosci 7:884. https://doi.org/10.3389/fnhum.2013.00884

Okumura Y, Asano Y, Takenaka S, Fukuyama S, Yonezawa S, Kasuya Y, Shinoda J (2014) Brain activation by music in patients in a vegetative or minimally conscious state following diffuse brain injury. Brain Inj 28(7):944–950. https://doi.org/10.3109/02699052.2014.888477

Pantev C, Herholz S (2011) Plasticity of the human auditory cortex related to musical training. Biobehav Rev 35(10):2140–2154

Piai V, Vos S, Idelberger R, Gans P, Doorduin J, Ter Laan M (2018) Awake surgery for a violin player: monitoring motor and music performance, A case report. Arch Clin Neuropsychol 34(1):132–137. https://doi.org/10.1093/arclin/acy009
Pietschnig J, Voracek M, Formann A (2010) Mozart effect-Shmozart effect: a meta-analysis. Intelligence 38(3):314–323
Preti C, Welch G (2004) Music in a hospital setting: a multifaceted experience. Br J Music Educ 21(3):329–345. https://doi.org/10.1017/S0265051704005893
Särkämö T, Tervaniemi M, Laitinen S, Forsblom A, Soinila S, Mikkonen M et al (2008) Music listening enhances cognitive recovery and mood after middle cerebral artery stroke. Brain 131(Pt3):866–876. https://doi.org/10.1093/brain/awn013
Särkämö T, Ripollés P, Vepsäläinen H, Autti T, Silvennoinen H, Salli E, Laitinen S, Forsblom A, Soinila S, Rodríguez-Fornells A (2014) Structural changes induced by daily music listening in the recovering brain after middle cerebral artery stroke: a voxel-based morphometry study. Front Hum Neurosci 8. https://doi.org/10.3389/fnhum.2014.00245
Särkämö T, Altenmüller E, Rodríguez-Fornells A, Peretz I (2016) Editorial: music, brain, and rehabilitation: emerging therapeutic applications and potential neural mechanisms. Front Hum Neurosci 10:103. https://doi.org/10.3389/fnhum.2016.00103
Schlaug G (2009, 1169) Part VI introduction: listening to and making music facilitates brain recovery processes. Ann N Y Acad Sci:372–373. https://doi.org/10.1111/j.1749-6632.2009.04869.x
Schlaug G (2015) Musicians and music making as a model for the study of brain plasticity. Prog Brain Res 217:37–55
Schlaug G, Jancke L, Huang Y (1995) Increased corpus callosum size in musicians. Neuropsychologia 33:1047–1055
Sihvonen A, Särkämö T, Leo V, Tervaniemi M, Altenmüller E, Soinila S (2017) Music-based interventions in neurological rehabilitation. Lancet Neurol 16(8):648–660. https://doi.org/10.1016/S1474-4422(17)30168-0
Spinthge R (1997) Musik in der klinischen Medizin. In: Bruhn H, Oerter R, Rösing H (eds) Musikpsychologie, Ein Handbuch, 3rd edn. Rohwohlts, Reinbeck/Hamburg, pp 397–405
Sun J, Chen W (2015) Music therapy for coma patients: preliminary results. Eur Rev Med Pharmacol Sci 19(7):1209–1218
Sutoo D, Akiyama K (2004) Music improves dopaminergic neurotransmission: demonstration based on the effect of music on blood pressure regulation. Brain Res 1016(2):255–262
Tarasov N (2005) DIe ältesten Flöten der Welt. Windkanal Das Forum für die Blockflöte 1:6–11
Thaut M (2014) Neurologic music therapy in stroke rehabilitation. Curr Phys Med Rehabil Rep 2:106–113. https://doi.org/10.1007/s40141-014-0049-y
Thaut M, MHömberg V (2015) Einführung in die neurologische Musiktherapie. In: Bernatzky G, Kreutz G (eds) Musik und Medizin. Springer, Wien, pp 139–157
Timmermann T (ed) (2009) Lexikon Musiktherapie, 2nd edn. Hogrefe, Göttingen
Vaquero L, Hartmann K, Ripollés P, Rojo N, Sierpowska J, François C et al (2016) Structural neuroplasticity in expert pianists depends on the age of musical training onset. NeuroImage 126:106–119
Vella M, Crandall M, Patel M (2017) Acute management of traumatic brain injury. Surg Clin North Am 97(5):1015–1030. https://doi.org/10.1016/j.suc.2017.06.003
Wan C, Schlaug G (2010) Music making as a tool for promoting brain plasticity across the life span. Neuroscientist 16(5):566–577. https://doi.org/10.1177/1073858410377805
Zhou Y, Lin S, Gu W, He L, Zhang Q, Yeh H (2020) Early evidence of trepanation along the Yellow River Basin in Neolithic China. Archaeol Anthropol Sci 12(176):1–9

Music in the Treatment of Depression from the Perspective of Music Therapy and Music Psychology

14

Veronika Busch and Susanne Metzner

14.1 Premise

Many people find music uplifting and activating in their everyday lives. The positive expectations thus arising also play a role in the compliance of patients undergoing treatment for a mood disorder such as depression. This interdisciplinary study, rooted in music therapy and music psychology, examines the extent to which the therapeutic potential of music and/or making music transcends positive default settings, which influencing factors are involved, and which limitations must be considered.

Based on a clinical understanding of depression and the essential core statements on the field of music therapy, results from psychotherapy and music therapy research are discussed, devoting particular attention to their clinical validity. Subsequently, psychological, physiological, social and neuroscientific findings on the effect of music are presented, which appear to be substantial in connection with depressive disorders. They are examined with regard to their transferability to the clinical context. The aim of this approach is to determine the state of knowledge and research desiderata for the inclusion of music in the treatment of depression (including secondary prevention) from multiple perspectives and to propose upcoming research tasks.

V. Busch
Institute of Musicology and Music Education, University of Bremen, Bremen, Germany
e-mail: veronika.busch@uni-bremen.de

S. Metzner (✉)
Faculty of Philosophy and Social Sciences, Leopold Mozart College of Music, University of Augsburg, Augsburg, Germany
e-mail: susanne.metzner@uni-a.de

G. Kreutz, G. Bernatzky (eds.), *Music and Medicine*, Neurocultural Health and Wellbeing, https://doi.org/10.1007/978-3-662-72175-9_14

14.1.1 Depression

The term depression does not cover a homogeneous clinical picture. Rather, it comprises a group of depressive disorders categorised as affective disorders according to the International Classification of Disorders ICD-10 (DIMDI 2020). The clinical symptoms of a persistently depressed mood, lack of interest and reduced drive, sleep and concentration disorders, anxiety and self-doubt, feelings of shame and guilt, self-destructiveness and suicidal tendencies cause a high level of suffering among those affected. Depressive disorders are among the most common mental disorders worldwide, with one to two new cases per 100 people per year. The risk of developing depression in the course of a lifetime is 16–20% both nationally and internationally. According to epidemiological data in Germany (Bundesärztekammer et al. 2022, p.18ff), depression occurs at any age, women are more frequently affected than men, and single people affected than socially integrated people. Among the socio-economic factors, a higher level of education and secure employment correlate with lower rates of depression. A high prevalence of depressive disorders in patients with somatic diseases has been proven in many epidemiological studies and is associated with serious consequences such as increased mortality and morbidity as well as reduced quality of life (Bundesärztekammer et al. 2022, p. 26).

In this chapter, depression is understood as a psychosomatosis of emotion regulation (cf. Böker 2011, p. 66ff.), i.e. it is assumed that (neuro-)biological, psychological and social factors interact. The influence of genetic factors on serotonin metabolism has also been demonstrated (Northoff 2012), which corroborates the hypothesis of complex gene–environment and brain–environment interactions in the pathogenesis of major depression. From a psychodynamic perspective, vulnerability is seen in connection with early life experiences, i.e. interaction experiences that are characterised by a lack of emotional attunement, a lack of mirroring, insecure attachment, serious experiences of loss and separation anxiety or even overprotection. From this developmental psychological perspective, the core issues of depression lie in the areas of affect and impulse regulation as well as the regulation of self-esteem and self-worth.

Consequently, a variety of factors influence the choice of therapeutic approach, such as the onset of the disease, the severity and number of episodes, remissions, relapses, cycles and intervals, the different symptom manifestations, psychosocial risks, familial clustering and the often extensive comorbidity in depression, but ultimately also resources and coping strategies. The model of depression as a psychosomatosis disorder of emotion regulation can serve as a starting point for both pharmacological and psychotherapeutic treatment (psychodynamic psychotherapy, cognitive–behavioural therapy, interpersonal therapy). The German treatment guideline 'Unipolar Depression' (Bundesärztekammer et al. 2022, p. 25ff) uses an algorithm based on differential diagnostics for the staggering and staging of different treatment approaches. In the context of inpatient psychotherapeutic treatment, psychotherapeutic treatment methods, including artistic therapies, are also offered as part of a multimodal therapy concept (Bundesärztekammer et al. 2022, p. 169ff). In addition to symptom reduction and as complete a remission as possible, the general treatment goals are to reduce the risk of suicide and restore occupational and psychosocial performance. While improvements on depression scales are usually the decisive remission criterion in treatment studies, the German treatment guideline emphasises the subjective experience of those affected and names an affirmative attitude to life characterised by vitality, self-confidence and the will to live, a return to the usual level of psychosocial functioning, and improvements in coping with everyday life and the quality of relationships with close caregivers as specific treatment goals (ibid.).

14.1.2 Music Therapy

Music therapy is a scientifically based and practice-oriented psychotherapeutic discipline. On the basis of a biopsychosocial understanding of illness, psychological means are used to achieve therapeutic, rehabilitative and/or preventative goals. In the so-called Kasseler Theses (Kasseler Conference 1998, 232 f.), in Germany, a consensus was reached across schools, according to which music therapy forms intersections with neighbouring scientific fields, in particular medicine, psychology, social sciences and musicology. In contrast, the term 'music medicine' is used to describe the non-pharmacological use of music interventions with the aim of physiological and physical changes in (mostly somatic) medicine (e.g. Bradt et al. 2016).

Music therapy uses a broad definition of music and is linked to the development of a therapeutic relationship involving music. It is carried out in both individual and group settings, in the form of so-called active music therapy, in which instrumental and/or vocal music is played, especially improvisation, and so-called receptive music therapy, in which music is listened to live or from recordings. The concept includes the psychotherapeutic processing of the experiences triggered by music, so that intellectual competences of the clients are assumed, which is usually the case for people suffering from depression (see Lotter and van Staden 2019).

Music therapy for depression can be offered for outpatients, but usually is part of a multimodal inpatient treatment concept. Approximately 50–70% of inpatients suffer from recurring or chronic depressive disorders (DGPPN et al. 2009, p. 85). The German treatment guideline 'Unipolar Depression' (DGPPN et al. 2015) does not explicitly mention music therapy, and the 3rd edition (Bundesärztekammer et al. 2022) subsumes music therapy under 'artistic therapies' without making a recommendation. According to the German treatment guideline 'Psychosoziale Therapien bei schweren psychischen Erkrankungen' (Psychosocial Therapies in Severe Mental Illnesses) (DGPPN 2019, p. 42), artistic therapies should be offered to improve the psychopathological symptoms (recommendation grade B). Another reference source is the survey by Gühne et al. (2012), which concludes by noting that 'Artistic therapies should be offered within the framework of an overall treatment plan and adapted to the individual needs and preferences of the patients, especially in order to reduce negative symptoms' (ibid., p. 859; translated by V.B. and S.M.).

A number of institutions in the social and healthcare system provide music therapy for people who develop a depressive adjustment disorder in extreme life situations, for instance in connection with severe somatic illness (heart attack, cancer, burns injuries), traumatic experiences (natural disasters, train crashes), or the sudden loss of close relatives (the death of a child, disappearance). However, treating chronic symptoms of severe depressive disorder, music therapy, like all other therapeutic approaches, faces particular challenges, which is illustrated by a case study by Metzner (2016, pp. 459–464). As clinical experience indicates, improvisatory music therapy—in particular in comparison to receptive music therapy or music listening—appears to be well-suited to taking up the dissociation of thinking, feeling and acting, transformed experiences of time and feelings of alienation from the environment and the self, guiding the fine-tuning of contact and stimulating manifold synchronisation processes.

In view of the complexity of interrelated and mutually dependent processes, the therapeutic use of music does not follow a monocausal principle of action.

14.2 Psychotherapy and Music Therapy Research on Depressive Disorders

14.2.1 Research on Psychotherapy in the Treatment of Depression

The results of the extremely extensive control trials, meta-analyses and naturalistic studies on psychotherapy for depression are elaborated in the German treatment guideline 'Unipolar Depression' (DGPPN et al. 2015). All psychotherapeutic approaches outlined in the guideline are presented as evidence-based, but none of them receive a specific recommendation. 'For the treatment of depressive disorders, today psychotherapy has become extensively developed via a wide range of different procedures, in both out-patient and in-patient therapy. A plethora of studies demonstrate that psychotherapeutic treatment of depressive disorders is generally effective, its effectiveness varying according to the severity, chronicity and symptoms of depression' (DGPPN et al. 2015, p. 97; translated by V.B. and S.M.).

However, due to the frequent recurrence of depressive disorders in a large proportion of depressive patients, acute treatment only achieves partial rather than sustained recovery. Negative predictors of successful treatment must include the severity of the symptoms at the outset of therapy, the additional presence of a personality disorder and a reduced sense of coherence (cf. Antonovsky 1997, cit. Böker et al. 2010, p. 156). In their meta-analysis, Leichsenring and Rabung (2008) were able to demonstrate the advantage of psychodynamic long-term therapy in direct comparison with all kinds of short-term therapies with respect to their general effectiveness, changes in personality structure and the formulated therapeutic objectives, which also holds for the complex depressive disorders. Psychotherapeutic strategies that help preserve a treatment's success are of greater significance than long-term treatment with antidepressants in preserving therapeutic success and preventing recurrence (DGPPN et al. 2015, S. 117).

The field of long-term psychotherapy research is dominated by naturalist and follow-up studies on psychoanalytic therapy (DGPPN et al. 2015, p. 105; Böker 2011, pp. 206 ff.). Therapeutic success is defined as a reduction in symptoms and improved adaptation to life, and improved interpersonal interaction. Long-term behavioural therapy was shown to achieve similar levels of success. In both therapy groups, the relapse rate after 7 years stood at just 19% (Böker 2011, pp. 206 ff.).

14.2.2 Research on Music Therapy in the Treatment of Depression

Music therapy research covers all levels of the so-called evidence pyramid, from case studies to clinical trials, randomised controlled trials, systematic reviews and meta-analyses. Even if the available results have not yet led to music therapy being recommended in the treatment guidelines for unipolar depression, and further research efforts are necessary, it is worth taking a look at the findings to date on music therapy for depression as a main diagnosis.

14.2.2.1 Systematic Surveys

The Cochrane Systematic Review on music therapy for depression by Aalbers et al. (2017) included nine randomised controlled and controlled trials (RCT and CCT) under strict conditions ($N = 421$). Music therapy as an adjunct to standard therapy (TAU) is shown to have more effective short-term effects than TAU alone in terms of reducing symptoms of depression and anxiety and improving functioning level. The meta-analysis by Tang et al. (2020), which included 55 RCT ($N = 3954$) on the use of music therapy for depression, differentiated music therapy interventions (39 trials), and the functional use of music (music medicine). Significant symptom reductions were demonstrated for music therapy, whereas the effect size was larger for music medicine. The music therapy method and setting influence the effect; longer session duration can be a predictor of better outcome. The review by Zhao et al. (2016) included 19 randomised controlled trials of music therapy for geriatric depression. Positive effects may be assumed based on the data, but are not yet sufficiently consistent in terms of reliability and validity.

14.2.2.2 Controlled Effectiveness Studies

Looking at individual studies that included major depression (e.g. Albornoz 2011; Atiwannapat et al. 2016; Erkkilä et al. 2011), mostly the effects of music therapy in addition to TAU or in a waiting group design are investigated. While standardised measuring instruments are used in the studies to record changes in depressive symptoms, indicators for (neuro-)physiological processes such as heart rate variability have also been used recently (Schäfer 2023). Supplemented music therapy for adults with depression with home-based interim interventions showed enhanced symptom improvements (Castillo-Pérez et al. 2010; Erkkilä et al. (2021).

14.2.2.3 Adverse Effects

Adverse effects of music therapy for depression have yet to be researched. Erkkilä et al. (2011) merely reported isolated adverse events in the form of exacerbated symptoms or back pain. Aalbers et al. (2017), on the other hand, found adverse effects of music therapy interventions and TAU in equal measure.

14.2.2.4 The Dose–Response Relationship of Music Therapy in the Treatment of Depression

In their meta-analysis of 2009 (RCT, CCT, uncontrolled studies; $N = 691$), Gold et al. (2009) calculated the dose–response relationship in patients with severe mental disorders (including initial diagnosis of depression). With respect to the general condition, negative symptoms and the functioning level of patients undergoing music therapy, small effects could be observed after 3 to 10 sessions, moderate effects between 10 and 24 sessions and greater effects between 16 and 51 sessions. In their survey of various music interventions for depression (28 randomised control trials and longitudinal studies, including six music therapy studies; $N = 1.810$), Leubner and Hinterberger (2017) established an above-average effectiveness of (on average) 1.25 sessions per week, each at least 30 min in duration over a period of 4–6 weeks. At least in the younger and middle-aged groups, group therapy was more effective than an individual setting (ibid., p. 16). Only three of the studies (Hendricks et al. 1999; Choi et al. 2008; Esfandiari and Mansouri 2014) examined patients with severe depression.

14.2.2.5 Effective Factors of Music Therapy

With regard to the specific effective factors of music therapy for depression, (neuro-) biological, psychological and social processes are taken into consideration, which are included in the explanatory approaches for positive therapy results. Castillo-Pérez et al. (2010) explain the significant reduction in depressive symptoms and the increase in *joie de vivre* in the experimental group with the activation of neuronal reward systems and a possible increase in the neurotransmitter dopamine through music (ibid. p. 389), but without having verified this in their study.

Werner et al. (2017) attribute the significant reduction of depressive symptoms in nursing home residents ($n = 117$) during music therapy intervention compared to recreational singing led by a musician to the better quality of relationship in music therapy. In the specialist discipline, the low number of drop-outs after the start of treatment is always attributed to the professionally trained, interactive skills of music therapists and the positive relationship experience in music therapy. It is only recently that empirical studies have begun to investigate the effectiveness factors in music therapy. Aalbers et al. (2019) attach particular importance to interpersonal synchronisation in improvisational music therapy. They claim that it is suitable for stimulating the ability to regulate emotions in depressed adolescents and young adults. For empirical testing, they developed a 10-session treatment manual that is primarily intended for use in the field of prevention.

The importance of the group experience is reflected in the qualitative study by Windle et al. (2020). They analysed the subjective experiences, documented in interviews, of ten participants with long-term depression in the ongoing quantitative 'Synchrony Study' (Carr et al. 2017), in which group songwriting was used as an intervention. Three overarching themes were identified: 'the group as a happy and safe place', 'music stimulates new feelings and helps to express oneself in words when writing songs', and 'uncertainty, unfulfilled needs and the end were challenging' (Windle et al. 2020 pp. 3–6).

The fact that this may well be related to the music experience and not primarily to the group experience fits with the results of an experiment with healthy people by Schäfer et al. (2020). In their RCT study on active group music therapy with women, however, Gaebel et al. (2020) again focus on the intraindividual dynamics triggered by music-making. They investigate the correlations between symptom improvement and neurobiological stress regulation using the parameter of heart rate variability.

14.2.3 Discussion of the State of Research on Music Therapy in the Treatment of Depression

Overall, the state of research gives grounds for cautious optimism that music therapy interventions can help alleviate symptoms and improve coping with depression in a way that is easily accepted by patients. The high reliability and internal validity of the studies are essentially due to internationally established purely descriptive diagnostics in accordance with ICD-10 or DSM-IV, limited to a small selection of formal criteria (intensity, duration, oscillation with manic states). As stated in Bundesärztekammer et al. (2022 p.169), the evidence has improved compared to DGPPN (2019), but the validity of the evidence is still limited due to the high or unclear risk of bias, the small samples, and the high heterogeneity. The comparability of studies is restricted by the variety of music therapy interventions or even by the lack of detailed descriptions. As in psychotherapy, the existing studies on music therapy do not deliver sufficient proof of sustained effectiveness beyond the end of treatment.

Additionally, the overall evidence is limited due to the fact that the systematic overviews mostly include studies with patients suffering from mild or moderate depression. However, since a higher rate of spontaneous recovery can be expected here, it cannot be discounted that such cases may be due to unspecific effects, spontaneous recovery or placebo effects, as is also assumed for most antidepressant effects (DGPPN et al. 2009, p. 23). Critics of the consistently positive results of music therapy research might also argue that their homogeneity is an indication of insufficiently sensitive research methods or inadequate measurement criteria (cf. Böker et al. 2010, p. 166). For instance, the use of HDRS (Hamilton 1960), an instrument widely employed due to its simplicity (e.g. Albornoz 2011; Gaebel et al. 2020), is fundamentally questioned as a basis for assessing effectiveness (DGPPN et al. 2009, p. 23).

So far, it can essentially be assumed that music therapy follows the same unspecific effective factors that Wampold (2001) observes in various models of psychotherapy. Erkkilä et al. (2011) thought they had identified the independence of the therapeutic variable (ibid., p. 138) and sought to ascribe significance to music as the positive effective factor, even though the measuring instruments did not permit such conclusions. Their interpretation was also inconsistent with regard to the postulated proximity of the study design to naturalist conditions of a psychodynamic approach (Erkkilä et al. 2011, p. 134). Neither is this tenable in the context of psychotherapeutic meta-analyses (Wampold 2001; Norcross and Lambert 2006), according to which the effective factors 'therapist' and 'relationship' play a much larger role in successful treatment than 'methods' or 'techniques'. Nevertheless, a positive aspect that must be emphasised is that more recent and ongoing studies now pay greater attention to the significance of social processes mediated via music in group music therapy and to the regulation of the relationship between the patient and the therapist in improvised individual music therapy (e.g. Carr et al. 2017; Aalbers et al. 2019).

There remains, then, a lack of evidence concerning the specific effects of music therapy. Findings regarding which form of music therapy is best suited for the treatment of depression and which approach is recommended for which clients have yet to be subjected to empirical inquiry.

14.2.4 Interim Findings 1: Outcome Versus Research on Process and Effectiveness Factors

Research on depression in the field of both music therapy and psychotherapy performs a challenging balancing act; on the one hand, the prevailing paradigm in the current health policy conflict demands that effectiveness be proven via CCT or RCT studies, i.e. cause-and-effect relationships must be demonstrated irrespective of patient- or therapist-specific variables. On the other hand, clinical practice demands that knowledge be gained of the processes and variance within the different types of depression (Mentzos 2010, p. 126) and their causes in order to adapt music therapy's interventions to the specific requirements of patients as early as possible. Influential factors such as motivation, expectation or self-determination on the part of patients, theoretical convictions on the part of the therapist (known as the allegiance effect) and adaptation within the therapeutic relationship cannot be shown by highly standardised CCT or RCT studies. Hence, more care-oriented field research is required in order to increase the external validity of studies on music therapy.

While specific treatment planning is initially based on the ICD-10 diagnosis key, during treatment itself the aetiology, symptoms and interactions of different psychosocial factors influencing a given depressive disorder are taken into consideration, as outlined by the survey by Odell-Miller (2007) or individual case studies by Murphy (1991), Nolan (1991, 2003), Hannibal (2003) and Metzner (2013, 2016). Hence, in these pages, the authors privilege a dimensional perspective over a focus on diagnostic categories. While there is not sufficient space here to provide detailed comparative analysis of individual cases, a certain three-dimensionality can be observed in (severe) depression disorder:

1. Emotionality, i.e. from regulation of mood, emotions and stress to the ability to mentalise
2. Sociality, i.e. from the ability to find resonance and social coherence to the ability to establish contact and to deal with people
3. Sense of self, i.e. from a physical sense of self, motor skills/drive and a sense of authorship to self-esteem

If positive changes within these dimensions—which cannot be viewed in isolation—are to be connected not only with a reduction of depressive symptoms, but are also seen as a result of musical processes, the next step is to consult music-psychological findings on the effect of music or making music on both healthy people and people suffering from depression.

14.3 Multi-disciplinary Aspects on the Therapeutic Potential of Music in the Treatment of Depression

14.3.1 State of Research

Epidemiological, (social-)psychological and neuroscientific research findings indicate the therapeutic potential of music-related behaviours in the treatment of depression, but also highlight particular challenges (see Busch 2014).

14.3.1.1 Music and Well-Being

Specific indicators of a connection between increased receptive or creative cultural activity and reduced depressive and anxious affectivity are provided by Cuypers et al. (2012) in the HUNT study with $N = 50{,}797$ Swedish adults. In a questionnaire study, Clift et al. (2008) with $N = 1124$ choristers from three countries (England, Germany and Australia) reported positive effects of singing on stress reduction, reinforcement of positive feelings and a reduction in depression (cf. the survey in Clift 2012). In their systematic review ($N = 61$ studies), Daykin et al. (2018) observed reliable evidence that listening to music and singing had positive effects on adults' well-being, but reported that it was difficult to compare the findings due to the use of different instruments to measure subjective well-being.

The theory of so-called mood management (Zillmann 1988) assumes a hedonistic motivation to maximise pleasant moods and a (conscious or unconscious) media selection behaviour informed by experiences of effect. In this context, Batt-Rawden and DeNora (2005, p. 291) speak of 'lay-therapists'. This seems somewhat obvious, since music can be expected to have positive effects in both the everyday and the clinical context, at least as long as the initial diagnosis does not include severe affective disorder. McFerran (2016) observes increased use of media by young adults in phases of severe depression, especially with respect to listening to music. The selection of uplifting music has not been shown to be effective for people with depressive tendencies, however (Wilhelm et al. 2013; Hense et al. 2014); rather, a preference for music that reinforces the depressive mood has been observed (Garrido and

Schubert 2015a, b). Additionally, Stewart et al. (2019) note a discrepancy between the intention behind listening and the outcome for well-being and assume that intention and outcome are influenced by a mediator, namely the listener's degree of 'self-awareness' and knowledge of mood-regulating processes in listening to music. As a further problem, Garrido (2018) considers the discrepancy between subjectively perceived and objectively measured mood changes (cf. the review by McFerran 2016).

14.3.1.2 Music Preference and Affect Attunement

Punkanen et al. (2011) argue that in comparison to healthy individuals, depressive patients display an altered profile of musical preference, since they assess music classified as 'energetic', 'arousing' or 'angry' much more negatively. They interpret this psychodynamically as a defence mechanism against affect. From the authors' point of view, the problem is a reduced tolerance for stronger affects. While people suffering from depression can cognitively recognise vital, tense and contoured structures (including high tempo and high volume), they are unable to achieve the desired 'affect attunement' (see below) with this music. The negative connotation results from the painful experience of a discrepancy between subjective emotional numbing and external stimulus. Osuch et al. (2009) also report reduced neuronal activity in people suffering from severe depression with respect to their preferred music in comparison with healthy controls, although there were no differences in the degree of preference between the groups. This dysregulation is considered an 'anhedonic response to favourite music' (Lepping et al. 2016, p. 3). Decades ago, Ingram and Smith (1984) noted that people suffering from depression displayed a corresponding negativity bias, with negative hypersensitivity and positive hyposensitivity. Bodner et al. (2007) also observed that people suffering from depression show greater linguistic variety when describing music they experienced as negative. An extremely wide-ranging hypothesis interprets this heightened linguistic range of expression as indicative of an attempt to represent affective identification symbolically. This appears plausible as—according to Böker and Grimm (2012)– one of the characteristics of brain activity in people with depression is hyperactivity in the dorsolateral prefrontal cortex, which plays a large role in the processing of negative emotions.

If this is the case, then there would be a place in therapy not only for pleasant music, but for also music experienced as negative, since symbolisation offers the opportunity for (self-)distancing and affect regulation given that the therapeutic relationship provides the patient with sufficient attachment security to feel, tolerate and process what are ultimately his own vital impulses and tension-filled affective states. Here, too, however, it is important to differentiate between music-therapeutic approaches to the various degrees of depression.

14.3.1.3 Emotional Contagion Through Music

Preventive and, to a limited extent, therapeutic potential for the treatment of depression can be derived from intensive psycho-physical reactions to music (Gabrielsson 2011). Findings by Lundqvist et al. (2009) 'indicate a coherent manifestation in the experiential, expressive, and physiological components of the emotional response system, which supports the emotivist position in the debate on musical emotions' (Lundqvist et al. 2009, p. 73). Drawing on the concept of 'emotional contagion' (Hatfield et al. 1994), the authors assume that the participants perceive the emotion expressed via music and imitate its emotional expression, whereby afferent physiological feedback triggers analogous emotional induction (Lundqvist et al. 2009, S. 75, cf. Juslin 2001). According to Warren et al. (2006, p. 13072), an 'auditory-motor mirror network' triggers automatic neuronal activation in the premotor cortex via the perception of non-verbal emotional vocalisation, which also plays a role in controlling the facial muscles. Thus, in analogy to language and movement, the network of mirror neurons is assumed to exist for music too, supporting afferent responses and improving social interaction by representing a communicative (auditory) signal in the perceiver's brain, thereby allowing him to grasp the signal's meaning and intention (cf. the research review in Molnar-Szakacs and Overy 2006).

The authors consider it legitimate to assume that patients with mild depression experience emotional contagion via music and can thereby experience improvements in mood, at least in the short term. This might be the case because intensive emotional responses to music are presumably linked to evolutionary, very basal involuntary processes (Huron and Margulis 2010; Panksepp 1995, 1998). In turn, this would indicate potential therapeutic approaches—provided the depression is not so severe as to have fundamentally transformed the patient's processing mechanisms.

14.3.1.4 Music and Social Connectedness

Schäfer et al. (2020) observe a short-term significant increase in empathy and reduced loneliness in healthy participants ($N = 90$) when listening to self-selected music. Music might thus function as a social surrogate. The hormone oxytocin is considered a biomarker for this feeling of social bonding (cf. inter alia Gordon et al. 2011), but research has certainly not reached a consensus. Kreutz (2014) interprets the observed increase in oxytocin concentration in singers of amateur choirs as reinforcing the feeling of 'social bonding', while Schladt et al. (2017) find that both choral and solo singing increases perceived joy, reduces worry and sadness and is accompanied by a decrease in cortisol levels, but only choral singing involves a reduction in oxytocin too. They thus assume interactions between cortisol and oxytocin, claiming that stress reduction causes oxytocin levels to drop.

Despite the considerable need for further research, musical activities seem to be a social resilience factor—i.e. they appear to stimulate interpersonal cooperation and coherence. Particularly in view of social stigmatisation and exclusion faced by people suffering from depression and their negative impact on the course of the illness (Lasalvia et al. 2012), continuation of musical activities in singing groups following music therapy seems a promising approach.

14.3.1.5 Music and Interindividual Synchronisation

Further indications for the therapeutic potential of music in the treatment of depression can be found in synchronisation processes between individuals. In the 1980s, Daniel Stern described the interpersonal coordination of vocal, gestural, and mimic expression of affect as 'affect attunement' (Stern 2000, pp. 198 f.). Bunt and Pavlicevic (2001, p. 194) call this 'interactional synchrony', characterised in a mature relationship structure by a high level of flexibility and nuanced structuring with respect to temporal aspects of the observed behaviour and subjective experience. Merker (2003) advances the theory that rhythmic synchronising in interaction with others is a genuinely human ability of essential importance for the development of feelings of social cohesion (cf. also Wallin et al. 1999).

However, the development of stable structures of interaction are sensitive to disruption, as Robb (1999) has shown for mother–infant communication in a case study of a mother suffering from post-natal depression. She observed a decline in qualities of rhythmic attunement, reciprocity and overall satisfaction with the interaction. The mother's turn-taking behaviour was evidently disrupted. According to Robb, '[m]atching of pitch, low arousal, less "joining in" and negative mood states in the infant of the depressed mother suggested corresponding low affect in the baby' (Robb 1999, p. 123).

With the principle of resonance, Koelsch (2015) refers to aspects of emotional contagion via music produced by mirror neurons and can presumably be considered empathetic processes. Koelsch also postulates that mechanoreceptors (so-called Pacinian corpuscles) can be stimulated by music und suggest an affective response. Trost et al. (2017) consider rhythmic entrainment as an 'affect induction mechanism' (Trost et al. 2017, p. 106) and propose four levels of human entrainment (perceptual, autonomous, motor and social), all of which entail affective experience (Trost and Vuilleumier 2013).

14.3.1.6 Music and Time Experience

The authors regard the use of interpersonal rhythmic synchronisation as beneficial for the therapeutic context—especially as depression research indicates that depression can be linked to a transformed experience of time (cf. Mundt et al. 1998; Busch 2005, pp. 243ff.). Experimental studies by Münzel (1993) suggest corresponding changes in perception, assessment and experience that also correlate with the severity of depression. Experiencing time as expanded during depression is also confirmed by a controlled experimental study by Bschor et al. (2004). Mundt et al. (1998) interpret this transformed experience of time as the alienation of one's sense of time in the tradition of anthropological phenomenology. Other authors select metaphorical descriptive categories: for instance, Emrich (1994) describes depression as lacking the energy to cope with the past, while Theunissen (1992) considers it the inability to resist the rule of time with a sufficient amount of flexibility and creativity with respect to alternative ways of acting (cf. Hoffmann 2002, p. 108). The authors regard changes in the experience of time not only in connection with, but moreover in interaction with one of the main symptoms of depressive episodes according to ICD-10: reduced drive and mild fatigue. This is supported by clinical experiences of music therapists and a phenomenological music therapy study by Hoffmann (2002, 2003), who recognises in improvisation with depressive patients musical analogies to clinging to the past (Emrich 1994). Using musical material, Hoffmann demonstrates that at the beginning of music therapy, patients' activity is barely targeted and displays hardly any temporal organisation. Music therapy interventions, however, can markedly improve their capacity for rhythmic adjustment and phrasing (Hoffmann 2002, 2003).

The use of music in psychotherapy can be successful beyond the sessions themselves if the observed gain in what can be summarised as aesthetic skills (see above) does not remain limited to the musical activities and experiences of self-efficacy prompted and can be transferred to the bio-psycho-social shaping of one's life.

The author's argumentation is based on the abovementioned lifelong interactive regulation processes, although the severity or chronification of a depressive disorder undeniably represents a limiting factor. Depressive patients perceive encounters with both other people and their own bodies and their own cognition as alien. The self is experienced as detached from the outside world (Böker and Grimm 2012, pp. 329 f.). In order for therapy to help restore a positive feeling of the (physical) self and satisfactory relatedness to the world around oneself, special skills are required of the music therapist. Specifically, making music, as a physical and sensory, temporally structured and social activity in the treatment of severe depression, can only succeed if it does not ignore the condition of detachment and if this condition is not just contrasted with music. Rather, the therapist must be musically prepared for something that is difficult to realise during the therapeutic interaction, namely responsively reacting to asynchronous, amorphous and anachronistic expressions of life.

14.3.1.7 Music and Neurological Processes

According to neuroscientific findings, music-related behaviour can influence the release of the transmitter dopamine (among others, see Blood and Zatorre 2001; Salimpoor et al. 2011; Ferreri et al. 2019). Dopamine release is deduced from the activation of those (mesolimbic) structures of the brain responsible for the endogenous reward system (among others, the nucleus accumbens), and is thus considered an expression of well-being. Menon and Levitin (2005) also observe activation in the hypothalamus and the insula and assume they identified the autonomous and physiological reactions to satisfying and emotionally intense musical stimuli. The general effect is heightened functional and effective connectivity in brain regions responsible for endogenous reward; this, they argue, is why listening to music can produce such intense physical and emotionally satisfying responses. According to Koelsch and Stegemann (2012), musically evoked emotions intensify the activity in almost all the relevant brain structures (limbic/paralimbic) that generate emotion (amygdala, nucleus accumbens, hippocampus), and hence they also conclude that music is particularly well-suited to use in psychotherapeutic treatments.

However, with respect to depressive illnesses, music's potential to activate and regulate emotions requires more nuanced examination. For instance, in their assessment of neuroscientific and psychotherapeutic studies on emotion and cognition in depressive patients, Böker and Grimm (2012) observe disruption to the dopaminergic transmitter system and thus in the endogenous reward system. In the fMRT study by Aust et al. (2013), $N = 14$ patients with a severe depressive disorder displayed different neuronal activation to test subjects without a history of depression in response to pleasant and unpleasant audio-visual stimuli; this change in neuronal activity had no impact on subjective experience, however. Aust et al. (2013) interpret these findings as an indication of a neural marker (a vulnerability factor) of severe depression. Measurements of the anterior cingulate cortex (ACC) always show reduced volume in people with depression in comparison to healthy individuals (Lai 2013), and hence ACC volume is also considered to be a potential vulnerability factor for depression (Lepping et al. 2016). The ventral part of the ACC is regarded as essential for the processing of emotions and is also first reached by dopaminergic projections of the reward system (Bush et al. 2000).

Initial indications as to the extent to which these findings can apply to neuronal activity during acute depressive episodes are offered by an fMRI study by Lepping et al. (2016), who compare neuronal activity in the ACC and the striatum in $N = 19$ patients with major depression disorder (MDD) undergoing a depressive episode with $N = 20$ control subjects without depressive symptoms ('never depressed', ND). The subjects were exposed to a set of acoustic stimuli evoking either positive or negative emotions. These stimuli consisted of 36 musical, 24 non-musical and 9 neutral (pure tone) stimuli. It was revealed that MDDs process emotional acoustic stimuli differently than NDs: while NDs show the strongest neuronal activation in response to the positive emotional and the musical stimuli, MDDs responded more strongly to the negative emotional and the non-musical stimuli. Lepping et al. (2016) thereby emphasise the abovementioned negativity bias in people suffering from depression and conclude that music could play an important role in re-training the functions of the ACC and hence in the treatment of depression.

However, Böker and Grimm (2012, pp. 331 f.) refer to neuronal plasticity and associate changes in the functional interactions between different brain regions as a result of depression treatment in connection with clinical improvement. According to Mayberg's (1997, 2003, cit. Böker and Grimm 2012, pp. 318 ff.) network model, depression entails disruption to the functional interactions between the dorsolateral cortical and the ventromedial (paralimbic) structures. Depending on the severity of the depression disorder, changed patterns of neuronal activity can be observed, whereby limbic hyperactivity combined with frontal hypoactivity is associated with strong psychomotor and cognitive impairments (Böker and Grimm 2012, p. 319).

That therapeutic interventions with music-related activity can even induce neuroplastic restructuring was shown by an EEG study of $N = 32$ stroke patients (Altenmüller et al. 2009) and a specific MRT study of $N = 6$ aphasic patients (Schlaug et al. 2009). These studies are interesting for the present context in that they indicate that neuroplastic restructuring does not require years of playing music, but sets in after relatively short music-related therapeutic activities (21 and 75 days, respectively). Such indications are also provided by a study by Fachner et al. (2013) on music therapy in the treatment of patients with depressive disorders. Pre-post analysis of the EEG resting data for $N = 27$ depressive patients, most of whom displayed comorbid symptoms of anxiety, showed clear changes in cortical activity in the frontotemporal and temporoparietal areas after just 18 individual sessions of active music therapy adjunctive to standard treatment in comparison to a control group undergoing standard therapy. The authors interpret these neuronal changes as the influence of active music therapy on symptoms of anxiety, which are also significantly reduced along with depressive symptoms (cf. Erkkilä et al. 2011).

While pharmacological treatments of depression mainly function as bottom-up processes—from subcortical to cortical regions—psychotherapeutic interventions are more top-down—from cortical to para–/limbic regions. Despite all the uncertainty surrounding the interactions of neuronal processes and all the questions that remain open regarding changes in depressive patients' basic conditions, music therapy research is presented with a number of starting points. Both the neurophysiological bottom-up and the top-down processes would seem to be of relevance for the interdisciplinary discourse rooted in music psychology and music therapy, and hence the authors rather assume interactions than prioritisations.

14.3.2 Interim Findings 2: The Potential and Limitations of Music-Related Effects

The state of research on musical activities described above permits the following conclusions: musical activities (instrumental and vocal music making along with listening to music) have positive effects on both mentally healthy people and people with mild or short-term depression (for instance in mourning) in that slightly disrupted interactions of motor, sensory, emotional and cognitive processes are improved by the activation of specific brain regions. Although subjective and representational attitudes concerning music are a qualifying factor, it can be assumed that musical information can activate hormonal processes which, by circumventing the cortex, influence, among other things, how stress, happiness and social bonding are experienced.

The transferability of these findings to people suffering from severe depression is limited for instance by disruption to the dopaminergic transmitter system and what are presumed to be fundamental changes in the processing of musical information. While the current state of research would suggest that neuronal restructuring via musical intervention with more long-term effects is also plausible, short-term effects would also be beneficial, since musical activity's impulses for neurophysiological, emotional and psychosocial processes could have sustained effectiveness in combination with other therapeutic interventions with more long-term effects. To date, however, there is a lack of systematic research on therapeutic processes and follow-up studies confirming this interpretation or investigating the conditions in which such processes arise. On the level of pre-phenomenal, neurophysiological effects, this would depend on, among other things, successful synchronisation and regulation processes in the somato-auditory cortex. On the phenomenal level, from the perspective of music therapy, it may seem a little controversial that the effects of musical activity can also be understood as synchronisation processes in an imagined nexus between music, patient and therapist.

Since the ability to synchronise, per se, is perceived as something positive, this can certainly be achieved with music perceived to be emotionally negative. Against the background of the prefrontal asymmetry hypothesis, in persons suffering from depression, this kind of music can be assumed to be favoured by cortical processing (cit. Böker and Grimm 2012, pp. 314 ff.), which suggests that in individual cases, negatively connoted music has a therapeutic function via cognitive activation. Persons with depressive disorder have difficulties synchronising to music that they perceived as activating or aggressive however. From the perspective of music therapy this can not only be interpreted as experiences of alienation and negative projections, but, bearing in mind neurophysiological bottom-up processes, can also be considered as a defence mechanism against the heightened limbic hyperactivity triggered by the music. The affected person will perceive this (quite correctly) to be unpleasant and potentially regulate it with cognitive operations.

Due to the disparate results in the field of neurophysiological research—noted by Böker and Grimm in 2012 and still an issue to this day—and given the heterogeneous experiences in music-therapeutic practice, it is impossible to rule out the existence of potential fundamental changes between the different degrees of severity of depression affecting the entire system of interactions and hence also changes within the processing of musical information. This would suggest that future basic research on the effect of musical activities in the treatment of depressive disorders should place great emphasis on the homogeneity of samples in order to arrive at reliable results which are also valid for clinical practice.

Some researchers—drawing on, inter alia, Trost et al. (2017)—assume that synchronisation and regulation processes simultaneously take place on the psychophysical and neurophysiological emotional and social levels and are highly complex and individual. Certainly, music-psychological and music-therapeutic findings would support the somewhat bold hypothesis that both bottom-up and top-down processes are at play in music therapy. Accordingly, future research should synoptically combine both perspectives from the outset.

14.4 Conclusion: Summary and Research Outlook

On the premise that depression is a psychosomatic emotional regulation disorder with various aetiological symptoms, the authors have sought to examine the benefits of using music in the treatment of depression from an interdisciplinary perspective. In order to establish connections between music and musical experience and behaviour, the authors have chosen to focus on the dimensions of emotionality, sociality and self-perception instead of taking a perspective based on symptoms and diagnostic categories (cf. Sect. 14.2.4).

This survey of the research has taken into consideration the empirical findings of studies until 2020 from various disciplines (music therapy, psychotherapy, music psychology and neuroscience) and discussed them with respect to the clinical validity, transferability and the plausibility of explicative approaches. The authors have also focused on chronic and recurrent depression, since this presents the greatest challenge for therapeutic treatment. There was not sufficient space to deal with depression in comorbidity with dementia, chronic pain and severe somatic diseases, even if the use of music therapy is indicated and is the subject of extensive research.

All in all, the proof of effectiveness to date points to the therapeutic potential of music-related experience and behaviour in daily routine and therapy, whereby actively making music and singing in a group setting appears to be particularly beneficial. However, this primarily holds for people with mild and moderate depression. Besides positive effects such as improving mood, psychomotor and cognitive activation and improved affect regulation, the authors ascribe particular importance to social and temporal aspects of making music. The active use of music appears to stimulate self-regulatory and interactional synchronisation and structuring processes that contribute to successful social experiences, which in turn enhance emotional well-being and motivation to modify one's lifestyle.

Building on the findings of psychotherapeutic research, it can be assumed that due to the multiple emotional, cognitive, social and physical (inter-)actions induced by music, the effectiveness of music therapy unfolds on the neuronal level via both bottom-up and top-down processes, presumably offering a clinical advantage over pharmacological therapy or psychotherapy alone. For the treatment of acute depression, one must assume that music therapy utilising musical pieces has limitations. The changes in the mechanisms of neuronal processing may influence musical perception and experience, and hence it should not be assumed that the same psychophysical conditions exist as in healthy people or those with non-severe depression. Nevertheless, music therapy is indicated for severe depression, too, but for another reason. Individualised music therapy treatment seems to allow and reinforce significant experiences of basic contact and affective exchange. Psychotherapeutic research on severe depression suggests that expectations should remain modest, however. Nevertheless, it appears justified to hope for the utilisation of carry-over effects and for prophylaxis of relapse if musical everyday activities are initiated during inpatient treatment.

There is a need for further research in the fields of neuroscience and music psychology with respect to the processing of musical stimuli in various degrees of depression, especially with respect to the potential for using music to induce changes in the capacity for emotional experience. To further understanding of cause and effect in music therapy in the treatment of severe depression, however, there is a need for extensive field research combining the systematic descriptions and musical analyses, thereby isolating specific effectiveness factors. In the view of the authors, both lines of research should first place more importance on building sample groups as homogeneous as possible than on sample size, since the aim of fruitful interdisciplinary research is to enhance the precision or modification of both musical and music therapy treatments of depression.

Acknowledgements Our sincere gratitude goes to Professor Heinz Böker (Zurich) and Dr Michael Dümpelmann (Tiefenbrunn) for their helpful comments regarding the German edition of this chapter.

References

Aalbers S, Fusar-Poli L, Freeman RE, Spreen M, Ket JC, Vink AC, Gold C (2017) Music therapy for depression. Cochrane Database Syst Rev 11:CD004517

Aalbers S, Vink A, Freeman RE, Pattiselanno K, Spreen M, van Hooren S (2019) Development of an improvisational music therapy intervention for young adults with depressive symptoms: an intervention mapping study. Arts Psychother 65:101584

Albornoz Y (2011) The effects of group improvisational music therapy on depression in adolescents and adults with substance abuse: a randomized controlled trial. Nord J Music Ther 20(3):208–224

Altenmüller E, Marco-Pallares J, Munte TF, Schneider S (2009) Neural reorganization underlies improvement in stroke-in duced motor dysfunction by music-supported therapy. Ann N Y Acad Sci 1169:395–405

Antonovsky A (1997) Salutogenese. Zur Entmystifizierung der Gesundheit. Erweiterte deutsche Ausgabe von A. Franke, dgvt, Tübingen

Atiwannapat P, Thaipisuttikula P, Poopityastapornb P, Katekaewa W (2016) Active versus receptive group music therapy for major depressive disorder—a pilot study. Complement Ther Med 26:141–145

Aust S, Filip K, Koelsch S, Grimm S, Bajbouj M (2013) Music in depression: neural correlates of emotional experience in remitted depression. World J Psychiatry 3(2):8–17

Batt-Rawden KB, DeNora T (2005) Music and informal learning in everyday life. Music Educ Res 7(3):289–304

Blood AJ, Zatorre RJ (2001) Intensely pleasurable responses to music correlate with activity in brain regions implicated in reward and emotion. Proc Natl Adv Sci 98(2):11818–11823

Bodner E, Iancu I, Gilboa A, Sarel A, Mazor A, Amir D (2007) Finding words for emotions: the reactions of patients with major depressive disorder towards various musical excerpts. Arts Psychother 34:142–150

Böker H (2011) Psychotherapie der depression. Huber, Bern

Böker H, Grimm S (2012) Emotion und Kognition bei depressiv Erkrankten. In: Böker H, Seifritz E (eds) Psychotherapie und Neurowissenschaften. Integration—Kritik—Zukunftsaussichten. Huber, Bern, pp 309–351

Böker H, Himmighoffen H, Zahner J (2010) Zur empirischen Evidenz Psychodynamischer Psychotherapie bei depressiv Erkrankten. Oder: warum Eulen nach Athen tragen? In: Böker H (ed) Psychoanalyse im Dialog mit den Nachbarwissenschaften. Psychosozial, Gießen, pp 147–180

Bradt J, Dileo C, Magill L, Teague A (2016) Music interventions for improving psychological and physical outcomes in cancer patients. Cochrane Database Syst Rev:CD006911. https://doi.org/10.1002/14651858.CD006911.pub3

Bundesärztekammer (BÄK), Kassenärztliche Bundesvereinigung (KBV), Arbeitsgemeinschaft der Wissenschaftlichen Medizinischen Fachgesellschaften (AWMF) (2022) Nationale VersorgungsLeitlinie Unipolare Depression—Langfassung, Version 3.2.2022 [cited: 2022-02-20]. https://doi.org/10.6101/AZQ/000505

Bunt L, Pavlicevic M (2001) Music and emotion: perspectives from music therapy. In: Juslin PN, Sloboda JA (eds) Music and emotion: theory and research. Oxford University Press, Oxford, pp 181–201

Busch V (2005) Tempoperformance und Expressivität. Eine Studie zwischen Musikpsychologie und Musiktherapie. Peter Lang Verlag, Frankfurt/Main

Busch V (2014) Potenzial von Musiktherapie in der Behandlung von Depression aus musikpsychologischer Sicht. Musiktherapeutische Umschau 35(2):104–113

Bush G, Luu P, Posner MI (2000) Cognitive and emotional influences in anterior cingulate cortex. Trends Cogn Sci 4(6):215–222. PMID: 10827444

Bschor T, Ising M, Bauer M, Lewitzka U, Skerstupeit M, Müller-Oerlinghausen B, Baethge C (2004) Time experience and time judgment in major depression, mania and healthy subjects. A controlled study of 93 subjects. Acta Psychiatrica Scandinavica 109:222–229

Carr CE, O'Kelly J, Sandford S, Priebe S (2017) Feasibility and acceptability of group music therapy vs wait-list control for treatment of patients with long-term depression (the SYNCHRONY trial): study protocol for a randomised controlled trial. Trial 8(1). https://doi.org/10.1186/s13063-017-1893-8

Castillo-Pérez S, Gómez-Pérez V, Velasco MC, Pérez-Campos E, Mayoral MA (2010) Effects of music therapy on depression compared with psychotherapy. Arts Psychother 37:387–390. https://doi.org/10.1016/j.aip.2010.07.001

Choi AN, Lee MS, Lim HJ (2008) Effects of group music intervention on depression, anxiety, and relationships in psychiatric patients: a pilot study. J Altern Complement Med 14(5). https://doi.org/10.1089/acm.2008.0006

Clift S (2012) Singing, wellbeing and health. In: MacDonald R, Kreutz G, Mitchell L (eds) Music, health and wellbeing. Oxford University Press, Oxford, pp 113–124

Clift S, Hancox G, Morrison I, Hess B, Stewart D, Kreutz G (2008) Choral singing, wellbeing and health: findings from a cross-national survey. Sidney De Haan Reseach Cenre for Arts and Health, Canterbury Christ Church University

Cuypers K, Krokstad S, Lingaas Holmen T, Skjei Knudtsen M, Olov Bygren L, Holmen J (2012) Patterns of receptive and creative cultural activities and their association with perceived health, anxiety, depression and satisfaction with life among adults: the HUNT study, Norway. J Epidemiol Community Health 66(8):698–703

Daykin N, Mansfield L, Meads C, Julier G, Tomlinson A, Payne A, Grigsby Duffy L, Lane J, D'Innocenzo G, Burnett A, Kay T, Dolan P, Testoni S, Victor C (2018) What works for wellbeing? A systematic review of wellbeing outcomes for music and singing in adults. Perspect Public Health 138(1):39–46. https://doi.org/10.1177/1757913917740391

DGPPN (2019) S3-Leitlinie psychosoziale Therapien bei schweren psychischen Erkrankungen: S3-Praxisleitlinien in Psychiatrie und Psychotherapie, 2nd edn. Springer, Berlin, Heidelberg

DGPPN, BÄK, KBV, AWMF (eds) (2015) Unipolare Depression. S3-Leitlinie/Nationale VersorgungsLeitlinie Unipolare Depression—Langfassung, 2nd edition. Version 5. DOI: 10.6101/AZQ/000364. Accessed 2020-10-30

DGPPN—Deutsche Gesellschaft für Psychiatrie, Psychotherapie und Nervenheilkunde, Bundesausschuss der Ärzte und Krankenkassen BÄK, KBV, AWMF, AkdÄ, BPtK, BApK, DAGSHG, DEGAM, DGPM, DGPs, DGRW (eds) (2009) S3-Leitlinie/Nationale Versorgungs-Leitlinie „Unipolare Depression“, Langfassung, 1st edition. http://www.dgppn.de, http://www.versorgungsleitlinien.de, http://www.awmf-leitlinien.de. Accessed 2012-07-10

DIMDI: Deutsches Institut für medizinische Dokumentation und Information (eds) (2020) Internationale statistische Klassifikation der Krankheiten und verwandter Gesundheitsprobleme, 10. Revision, German Modification. https://www.dimdi.de/static/de/klassifikationen/icd/icd-10-gm/kode-suche/htmlgm2020/. Accessed 2020-09-05

Emrich HM (1994) Depression und “Herrschaft der Zeit”: Erklärungsansätze aus Sicht des Psychiaters. Aus Forschung und Medizin: Mensch und Zeit 9(1):39–52

Erkkilä J, Punkanen M, Fachner J, Ala-Ruona E, Pöntiö I, Tervaniemi M, Vanhala M, Gold C (2011) Individual music therapy for depression: randomised controlled trial. Br J Psychiatry 199:132–139. https://doi.org/10.1192/bjp.bp.110.085431

Erkkilä J, Brabant O, Hartmann M, Mavrolampados A, Ala-Ruona E, Snape N, Saarikallio S, Gold C (2021) Music therapy for depression enhanced with listening homework and slow paced breathing: a randomized controlled trial. Front Psychol 12:613821. https://doi.org/10.3389/fpsyg.2021.613821

Esfandiari N, Mansouri S (2014) The effect of listening to light and heavy music on reducing the symptoms of depression among female students. Arts Psychother 41:211–213. https://doi.org/10.1016/j.aip.2014.02.001

Fachner J, Gold C, Erkkilä J (2013) Music therapy modulates fronto-temporal activity in the rest-EEG in depressed clients. Brain Topogr 26(2):338–354

Ferreri L, Mas-Herrero E, Zatorre JR, Ripollés P, Gomez-Andres A, Alicart H, Olivé G, Marco-Pallarés J, Antonijoan RM, Valle M, Riba J, Rodriguez-Fornells A (2019) Dopamine modulates the reward experiences elicited by music. PNAS 116(9):3793–3798. https://doi.org/10.1073/pnas.1811878116

Gabrielsson A (2011) On strong experiences with music. Music is much more than just music. Oxford University Press, Oxford

Gaebel C, Rittner S, Stoffel M, Jarczok MN, Aguilar-Raab C, Ditzen B, Warth M (2020) Study protocol of the MUSED study: a randomized controlled trial to evaluate the psychobiological effects of group music therapy in women with depression. Nord J Music Ther. https://doi.org/10.1080/08098131.2020.1760921

Garrido S (2018) The influence of personality and coping style on the affective outcomes of nostalgia: is nostalgia a healthy coping mechanism or rumination? Pers Individ Differ 120:259–264. https://doi.org/10.1016/j.paid.2016.07.021

Garrido S, Schubert E (2015a) Moody melodies: do they cheer us up? A study of the effect of sad music on mood. Psychol Music 43:244–261. https://doi.org/10.1177/0305735613501938

Garrido S, Schubert E (2015b) Music and people with tendencies to depression. Music Percept 32:313–321. https://doi.org/10.1525/MP.2015.32.4.313

Gold C, Solli HP, Kruger V, Lie SA (2009) Dose-response relationship in music therapy for people with serious mental disorders: systematic review and meta-analysis. Clin Psychol Rev 29:193–207

Gordon I, Martin C, Feldman R, Leckman JF (2011) Oxytocin and social motivation. Dev Cogn Neuro Sci 1(4):471–493. https://doi.org/10.1016/j.dcn.2011.07.007

Gühne U, Weinmann S, Arnold K, Ay E-S, Becker T, Riedel-Heller S (2012) Künstlerische Therapien bei schweren psychischen Störungen. Sind sie wirksam? Nervenarzt 83:855–860

Hannibal N (2003) A woman's change from being nobody to somebody: music therapy with a middle-aged, speechless, and self-sestructive woman. In: Hadley S (ed) Psychodynamic music therapy: case tudies. Barcelona Publishers, Gilsum, pp 403–414

Hamilton M (1960) A rating scale for depression. Journal of Neurology, Neurosurgery and Psychiatry 23:56–62

Hatfield E, Cacioppo JT, Rapson RL (1994) Emotional contagion. Cambridge University Press, Cambridge

Hendricks CB, Robinson B, Bradley LJ, Davis K (1999) Using Hendricks CB, Robinson B, Bradley B, Davis K. Using music techniques to treat adolescent depression. J Hum Counsel Educ Dev 1999(38):39–46. https://doi.org/10.1002/j.2164-490X.1999.tb00160.x

Hense C, McFerran K, McGorry P (2014) Constructing a grounded theory of young people's recovery of musical identity in mental illness. Arts Psychother 41:594–603

Hoffmann P (2002) „Zur (Wieder-)Entdeckung der Zeit". Die Bedeutung des Phrasierens in Improvisationen der Musiktherapie—eine Untersuchung an Improvisationen von Patienten der Erwachsenenpsychiatrie. Dissertation Universität Witten-Herdecke, Bereich Medizin

Hoffmann P (2003) Phrasing as expression of time and timing in improvised music therapy. In: Kopiez R, Lehmann AC, Wolther I, Wolf C (eds) Proceedings of the fifth triennial ESCOM conference. Hanover University of Music and Drama, Hanover, pp 50–54

Huron D, Margulis EH (2010) Musical expectancy and thrills. In: Juslin PN, Sloboda JA (eds) Handbook of music and emotion: theory, research, applications. Oxford University Press, Oxford, pp 575–604

Ingram RE, Smith TW (1984) Depression and internal versus external focus of attention. Cogn Ther Res 8(2):139–151. https://doi.org/10.1007/Bf01173040

Juslin PN (2001) Communicating emotion in music performance: a review and a theoretical framework. In: Juslin PN, Sloboda JA (eds) Music and emotion: theory and research. Oxford University Press, New York, pp 309–337

Kasseler Konferenz (1998) Thesen der Kasseler Konferenz. Musikther Umsch 19:232–235

Koelsch S (2015) Music-evoked emotions: principles, brain correlates, and implications for therapy. Ann N Y Acad Sci 1337:193–201. https://doi.org/10.1111/nyas.12684

Koelsch S, Stegemann T (2012) The brain and positive biological effects in health and clinical populations. In: MacDonald RAR, Kreutz G, Mitchell L (eds) Music, health, and wellbeing. Oxford University Press, Oxford, pp 436–456

Kreutz G (2014) Does singing facilitate social bonding? Music Med 6(2):51–60

Lai C-H (2013) Gray matter volume in major depressive disorder: a meta-analysis of voxel-based morphometry studies. Psychiatry Res 211(1):37–46. https://doi.org/10.1016/j.pscychresns.2012.06.006

Lasalvia A, Zoppei S, Van Bortel T et al (2012) Global pattern of experienced and anticipated discrimination reported by people with major depressive disorder: A cross-sectional survey. Lancet. https://doi.org/10.1016/S01406736(12)613798

Leichsenring F, Rabung S (2008) Effectiveness of long-term psychodynamic psychotherapy: a meta-analysis. JAMA 300:1551–1565

Lepping RJ, Atchley RA, Chrysikou E, Martin LE, Clair AA, Ingram RE, Simmons WK, Savage CR (2016) Neural processing of emotional musical and nonmusical stimuli in depression. PLoS One 11(6):e0156859. https://doi.org/10.1371/journal.pone.0156859

Leubner D, Hinterberger T (2017) Reviewing the effectiveness of musical interventions in treating depression. Front Psychol 8:1109. https://doi.org/10.3389/fpsyg.2017.01109

Lotter C, van Staden W (2019) Verbal affordances of active and receptive music therapy methods in major depressive disorder and schizophrenia-spectrum disorder. Arts Psychother 64(1):59–68

Lundqvist LO, Carlsson F, Hilmersson P, Juslin PN (2009) Emotional responses to music: experience, expression, and physiology. Psychol Music 37(1):61–90

Mayberg HS (1997) Limbic-cortical dysregulation: a proposed model of depression. J Neuropsychiatry Clin Neurosci 9:471–481

Mayberg HS (2003) Modulating dysfunctional limbic-cortical circuits in depression: towards development of brain-based algorithms for diagnosis and optimised treatment. Br Med Bull 65:193–207

McFerran K (2016) Contextualising the relationship between music, emotions and the well-being of young people: a critical interpretive synthesis. Music Sci 20:103–121

Menon V, Levitin DJ (2005) The rewards of music listening: response and physiological connectivity of the mesolimbic system. NeuroImage 28:175–184

Mentzos S (2010) Lehrbuch der Psychodynamik. Die Funktion der Dysfunktionalität psychischer Störungen. Vandenhoeck & Ruprecht, Göttingen

Merker B (2003) Musik an der Wurzel des Menschseins. In: Bastian HG, Kreutz G (eds) Musik und Humanität. Interdisziplinäre Grundlagen für (musikalische) Erziehung und Bildung. Schott, Mainz, pp 108–119

Metzner S (2013) From cliff to cliff, year after year, down into the unknown. Music therapy and depression. In: Metzner S (ed) Reflected sounds. Case studies from psychodynamic music therapy. English EPUB edition of the German original edition. Psychosozialverlag, Giessen, pp 55–79

Metzner S (2016) Psychodynamic music therapy. In: Edwards J (ed) The Oxford handbook of music therapy. Oxford University Press, Oxford, pp 448–471

Molnar-Szakacs I, Overy K (2006) Music and mirror neuros: from motion to 'e'motion. Soc Cogn Affect Neurosci 1(3):235–241

Mundt C, Richter P, van Hess H, Stumpf T (1998) Zeiterleben und Zeitschätzung depressiver Patienten. Nervenarzt 69:38–45

Münzel K (1993) Depression und das Erleben von Dauer: Zeitpsychologische Grundlagen und Ergebnisse klinischer Studien. Springer, Berlin

Murphy M (1991) Group music therapy in acute psychiatric care: the treatment of a depressed woman followong neurological trauma. In: Bruscia K (ed) Case studies in music therapy. Barcelona Publishers, Gilsum, pp 465–478

Nolan P (1991) Group improvisation therapy for a resistant woman with bipolar disorder-manic. In: Bruscia K (ed) Case studies in music therapy. Barcelona Publishers, Gilsum, pp 451–464

Nolan P (2003) Through to therapeutic attachment: psychodynamic music psychotherapy with a musician with dysthymic disorder. In: Hadley S (ed) Psychodynamic music therapy: case studies. Barcelona Publishers, Gilsum, pp 319–338

Norcross JC, Lambert MJ (2006) The therapy relationship. In: Norcross JC, Beutler LB, Levant RF (eds) Evidence-based practices in mental health. Debate and dialogue on the fundamental questions. American Psychological Association, Washington, DC, pp 208–218

Northoff G (2012) Gene, brains, and environment-genetic neuroimaging of depression. Curr Opin Neurobiol 4388(12):00137–7. pii: S0959. https://doi.org/10.1016/j.conb.2012.08.004
Odell-Miller H (2007) The practice of music therapy for adults with mental health problems: the relationship between diagnosis and clinical method. PHD-dissertation. Aalborg University. http://old.musikterapi.aau.dk/forskerskolen_2006/helen_odell-miller.htm. Accessed 11.7.2012
Osuch EA, Bluhm RL, Williamson PC, Theberge J, Densmore M, Neufeld RW (2009) Brain activation to favorite music in healthy controls and depressed patients. Neuroreport 20(13):1204–1208. https://doi.org/10.1097/WNR.0b013e32832f4da3. PMID: 19617860
Panksepp J (1995) The emotional source of 'chills' induced by music. Music Percept 13:171–207
Panksepp J (1998) Affective neuroscience: the foundations of human and animal emotions. Oxford University Press, Oxford
Punkanen M, Eerola T, Erkkilä J (2011) Biased emotional recognition in depression: perception of emotions in music by depressed patients. J Affect Disord 130:118–126
Robb L (1999) Emotional musicality in mother-infant vocal affect, and an acoustic study of postnatal depression. Music Sci Special Issue 1999–2000:123–154
Salimpoor VN, Benovoy M, Larcher K, Dagher A, Zatorre RJ (2011) Anatomically distinct dopamine release during anticipation and experience of peak emotion to music. Nat Neurosci 14(2):257–262. https://doi.org/10.1038/nn.2726. PMID: 21217764
Schäfer A (2023) Achtsamkeitsbasierte rezeptive Musiktherapie bei Menschen bei Menschen mit Depression. Eine randomisiert kontrollierte Pilotstudie zur Evaluation der Herzratenvariabilität und Achtsamkeit. In: Glawischnig- Goschnik M, Münzberg C (eds) Kunst und Wissen der Musiktherapie. Reichert Verlag, Wiesbaden, pp 89–122
Schäfer K, Saarikallio S, Eerola T (2020) Music may reduce loneliness and act as social surrogate for a friend: evidence from an experimental listening study. Music Sci 3:1–16
Schladt TM, Nordmann GC, Emilius R, Kudielka BM, de Jong TR, Neumann ID (2017) Choir versus solo singing: effects on mood, and salivary oxytocin and cortisol concentrations. Front Human Neurosci 11:430. https://doi.org/10.3389/fnhum.2017.00430
Schlaug G, Marchina S, Norton A (2009) Evidence for plasticity in white-matter tracts of patients with chronic Broca's aphasia undergoing intense intonation-based speech therapy. Ann N Y Acad Sci 1169:385–394
Stern DN (2000) The interpersonal world of the infant. Basic Books, New York
Stewart J, Garrido S, Hense C, McFerran K (2019) Music use for mood regulation: self-awareness and conscious listening choices in young people with tendencies to depression. Front Psychol 10:1199. https://doi.org/10.3389/fpsyg.2019.01199
Tang Q, Huang Z, Zhou H, Ye P (2020) Effects of music therapy on depression: a meta- analysis of randomized controlled trials. PLoS One 15(11):e0240862. https://doi.org/10.1371/journal.pone.0240862
Theunissen M (1992) Negative Theologie der Zeit. Suhrkamp, Frankfurt/Main
Trost W, Vuilleumier P (2013) 'Rhythmic entrainment' as a mechanism for emotion induction and contagion by music: a neurophysiological perspective. In: Cochrane T, Fantini B, Scherer KR (eds) The emotional power of music. Oxford University Press, New York, pp 213–225
Trost W, Labbé C, Grandjean D (2017) Rhythmic entrainment as a musical affect induction mechanism. Neuropsychologia 96:96–110
Wallin NL, Merker B, Brown S (eds) (1999) The origins of music. MIT Press, Cambridge, MA
Wampold BE (2001) The great psychotherapy debate: model, methods, and findings. Erlbaum, Mahwah
Warren JE, Sauter DA, Eisner F, Wiland J, Dresner MA, Wise RJS, Rosen S, Scott SK (2006) Positive emotions preferentially engage an auditory–motor "mirror" system. J Neurosci 26(50):13067–13075
Werner J, Wosch T, Gold C (2017) Effectiveness of group music therapy versus recreational group singing for depressive symptoms of elderly nursing home residents: pragmatic trial. Aging Ment Health 21(2):147–155. https://doi.org/10.1080/13607863.2015.1093599
Wilhelm K, Gillis I, Schubert E, Whittle EL (2013) On a blue note: depressed people's reasons for listening to music. Music Med 5:76–83

Windle E, Hickling LM, Jayacodi S, Carr C (2020) The experiences of patients in the synchrony group music therapy trial for long-term depression. Arts Psychother 67:101580. https://doi.org/10.1016/j.aip.2019.101580

Zhao K, Bai Z, Bo GA, Chi I (2016) A systematic review and meta-analysis of musictherapy for the older adults with depression. Int J Geriatr Psychiatry 31(11):1188–1198

Zillmann D (1988) Mood management through communication choices. Am Behav Sci 31(3):327–341

Part IV

Listening to Music, Amateur Singing and Dancing

Music Listening in Everyday Life

15

Anja C. Feneberg, Stefanie Hirsch, Ricarda Mewes, and Urs M. Nater

A. C. Feneberg (✉)
Institute of Clinical and Health Psychology, Faculty of Psychology, University of Vienna, Vienna, Austria

University Research Platform "The Stress of Life (SOLE) – Processes and Mechanisms underlying Everyday Life Stress", University of Vienna, Vienna, Austria

Clinical Psychology and Psychotherapy for Children and Adolescents, Department of Psychology, University of Münster, Münster, Germany
e-mail: anja.feneberg@uni-muenster.de

S. Hirsch
Institute of Clinical and Health Psychology, Faculty of Psychology, University of Vienna, Vienna, Austria

University Research Platform "The Stress of Life (SOLE) – Processes and Mechanisms underlying Everyday Life Stress", University of Vienna, Vienna, Austria

Psychological Research, Teaching and Practice Outpatient Clinic, Faculty of Psychology, University of Vienna, Vienna, Austria
e-mail: s.hirsch@univie.ac.at

R. Mewes
University Research Platform "The Stress of Life (SOLE) – Processes and Mechanisms underlying Everyday Life Stress", University of Vienna, Vienna, Austria

Psychological Research, Teaching and Practice Outpatient Clinic, Faculty of Psychology, University of Vienna, Vienna, Austria
e-mail: ricarda.nater-mewes@univie.ac.at

U. M. Nater
Institute of Clinical and Health Psychology, Faculty of Psychology, University of Vienna, Vienna, Austria

University Research Platform "The Stress of Life (SOLE) – Processes and Mechanisms underlying Everyday Life Stress", University of Vienna, Vienna, Austria
e-mail: urs.nater@univie.ac.at

G. Kreutz, G. Bernatzky (eds.), *Music and Medicine*, Neurocultural Health and Wellbeing, https://doi.org/10.1007/978-3-662-72175-9_15

15.1 Introduction

Music has been used across cultures for thousands of years to treat illnesses and promote health. For example, music already played a central role in ritual healing ceremonies of the Babylonians and in Ancient Egypt (Thaut 2015). While mankind relied exclusively on analog music performances for special occasions for many eras, technological progress in recent decades has contributed to considerable changes in the performance and use of music. According to a representative online survey in 2019 that asked people in 19 countries about their music listening habits, the average person spent 2.6 h a day listening to music (International Federation of the Phonographic Industry 2019). Furthermore, on-demand music streaming services are becoming increasingly important across all age groups. According to the survey, this may be due to the possibility of selecting preferred music pieces from an enormous collection and listening to them anytime and anywhere with mobile devices (e.g., smartphones).

This easy availability creates potential for scientific research into the links between music and health. Systematic reviews and meta-analyses suggest that music can be used to improve depressive symptoms (Chan et al. 2011), reduce anxiety (Panteleeva et al. 2017), and relieve acute and chronic pain (Garza-Villarreal et al. 2017; Kühlmann et al. 2018), among other things. As a readily available intervention with few—if any—side effects, listening to music is therefore suitable for a wide range of applications, although the underlying affective, cognitive, and neurobiological mechanisms of action have not been completely understood (Chanda and Levitin 2013; Fancourt et al. 2014). Most of the available findings originate from experimental laboratory studies or clinical–therapeutic studies, which are characterized by highly standardized and controlled settings or the need for medical or therapeutic personnel. As a result, it remains unclear to what extent the reported health-promoting effects of music listening can be transferred to everyday life. In this context, the aforementioned technical developments open up interesting possibilities for researching the connections between listening to music and health directly in everyday life. Building on this, music-based interventions for health promotion that are suitable for everyday use can be developed and evaluated. The aim of this chapter is to provide an overview of the current state of research in this field, to explain the underlying methodology and to illustrate the far-reaching health potentials of music listening in everyday life.

15.2 Music Listening in Everyday Life: Current State of Research

A sound understanding of *for whom, under what conditions,* and *how* listening to music in everyday life has health-promoting effects is essential in order to provide personalized recommendations for effective music-based interventions. The technical progress of recent decades regarding mobile devices and applications ("apps") has greatly facilitated the ecologically valid assessment of situational, psychological, behavioral, and biological parameters in everyday life. "Electronic diaries" are widely used today to assess fluctuating psychological phenomena such as stress levels in people's everyday lives. The procedure can also be supplemented by the use of saliva samples to assess biomarkers (e.g., cortisol, alpha-amylase) and sensors to record heart rate and skin conductance, for example (Trull and Ebner-Priemer 2013). These so-called ecological momentary assessment (EMA) methods are therefore ideally suited to researching relationships between listening to music and subjective and biological health-related variables in an ecologically valid manner, over longer periods of time and in real time. Key findings from this field of research are summarized below.

Ecological Momentary Assessment

"Ecological momentary assessment"(EMA) refers to the collection of subjective, biological, behavioral, and/or environmental data in (almost) real time in everyday life (Trull and Ebner-Priemer 2013). Among other things, experiences, behavior, and biological parameters are thus repeatedly recorded in the natural environment of individuals across various everyday situations. Field and (analog) diary studies have been conducted in psychological research since the 1980s (Pawlik and Buse 1982). However, it is only in recent years that the use and further development of the method has been so advanced that EMA methods are now increasingly being integrated into the methodological research repertoire of clinical psychology and behavioral medicine. Data acquisition is usually achieved through the use of mobile devices (e.g., smartphones) with pre-installed apps and, if necessary, portable sensors (e.g., for measuring heart rate and/or movement).

In addition to the high ecological validity, a further advantage of this method is the minimization of recall bias, which is one frequently criticized drawback of traditional retrospective questionnaires and interview methods (Schwarz 2007). In addition, EMA enables the depiction of time-varying psychological, biological, and behavioral processes and their interactions with a high temporal resolution. Moreover, the investigation of whether and how individuals differ with regard to these (micro)processes can be examined. In addition to the term "ecological momentary assessment," the terms "ambulatory assessment" (AA) and "experience sampling method" (ESM) are also frequently used in the literature, whereby ESM studies, in contrast to EMA and AA studies, exclusively involve the collection of subjective data (Mehl and Conner 2014).

15.2.1 Music Listening and Health Parameters

"Health" is a broad construct that cannot be defined solely by the absence of illness, but rather as comprehensive well-being on a physical, mental, and social level (Grad 2002). Consequently, somatic complaints such as exhaustion or pain, but also depressive mood or sleep problems, can be regarded as health parameters. These complaints can occur temporarily in the everyday lives of healthy people and are also persistent symptoms of certain stress-related illnesses, such as chronic fatigue syndrome, chronic pain disorders, or depression, which have a lasting impact on the everyday lives of those affected.

Most of the existing findings on the correlation between music listening in everyday life and health parameters come from studies with healthy people. For example, young, healthy adults reported less fatigue and a better mood the longer they had listened to music during the day (Strahler et al. 2019). Furthermore, several studies suggest that listening to music can be used specifically to regulate affective states in everyday life depending on the initial mood, the characteristics of the music, and the characteristics of the person (Greasley and Lamont 2011; Juslin et al. 2008; Randall and Rickard 2017). For example, the study by Randall and Rickard (2017) showed that negative affective states were associated with listening to music for the specific purpose of emotion regulation (e.g., to express feelings, to think about feelings). Interestingly, this, in turn, was associated with a higher level of music enjoyment and a simultaneous (short-term) worsening of affect. One possible explanation for these findings is that people in negative moods tend to choose *mood-congruent* music to "share their misery," which can be associated with a certain satisfaction, but does not seem to support an immediate improvement of negative affect (Randall and Rickard 2017). However, people who initially reported rather negative emotions benefited particularly from *happy* music in the form of improved mood (Randall and Rickard 2017). Personal characteristics also play a role (albeit possibly a subordinate one compared to situational characteristics; Juslin et al. 2008). For example, there is evidence that people with high scores for the personality traits "extraversion" and "openness to experience" are more likely to listen to music in everyday life with the aim of mood regulation (Randall and Rickard 2017).

Initial EMA studies also indicate positive effects of listening to music in patients suffering from long-term somatic complaints. For example, music listening in everyday life was associated with increased feelings of control over one's own pain in patients with fibromyalgia, a chronic pain disorder (Linnemann et al. 2015b). This effect was particularly strong in those who generally listened to music more frequently in everyday life, which indicates a possible dose–response relationship. In addition, listening to music for the reasons of *activation* and *relaxation* was associated with greater feelings of pain control. Music characteristics also play a modulating role in this regard: listening to *happy* music was associated with lower somatic complaints in everyday life (Feneberg et al. 2021; Linnemann et al. 2015b). This is consistent with experimental laboratory studies (Roy et al. 2008) and can be explained by the fact that music-induced positive emotions, mediated via the central nervous system, can contribute to a reduced perception of pain (see Bernatzky et al. 2011).

15.2.2 Music Listening and Stress

Initial studies from our research group show that music listening in everyday life can also impact stress experience and biological stress levels (e.g., Linnemann et al. 2015a, 2016, 2018; Wuttke-Linnemann et al. 2019). In these studies, the participants were asked several times a day about their current perception of stress and indicated whether they had listened to music since the last data entry. If the answer was yes, participants were also asked to indicate perceived music characteristics and reasons for listening to music. With each data entry, saliva samples were provided for the analysis of biological stress parameters to assess "stress"on multiple dimensions (i.e., subjective and biological; Nater 2018). The stress hormone cortisol was measured as an indicator for the activation of the hypothalamic–pituitary–adrenal axis (HPA axis) and the activity of the salivary enzyme alpha-amylase as an indicator for the activation of the autonomic nervous system (ANS). Overall, the results of these studies suggest that (1) the stress-reducing effects of listening to music in everyday life depend on a complex interplay of characteristics of the music, the situation, and the person and (2) the stress systems react differentially to these characteristics.

The relationship between listening to music and subjective stress in everyday life has been studied most frequently to date. Listening to music was associated with lower subjective stress levels in some studies (Feneberg et al. 2021, 2023; Linnemann et al. 2015a, 2018) but not in others (Linnemann et al. 2016; Wuttke-Linnemann et al. 2019). This heterogeneity indicates moderating factors, which were examined in further studies. For example, it was shown that music listening was associated with lower levels of subjective stress, especially when the music was listened to for the reasons of *relaxation* or *activation* (Linnemann et al. 2015a, b, 2016). In addition, evidence suggests that music listening seems to contribute to lower subjective stress, especially when experiencing high and chronic stress levels (Feneberg et al. 2023) and when listening to music for a duration of at least 20 min (Linnemann et al. 2018).

With regard to the ANS, the degree of how arousing the music is seems to exert a significant modulating influence, whereby *energizing* music was associated with an upregulation of the ANS (indicated via increased salivary alpha-amylase activity) and *calming* music with a downregulation of the ANS (Feneberg et al. 2021; Linnemann et al. 2015a, 2016).

The HPA axis, on the other hand, seems to respond primarily to characteristics of the music listening context (i.e., the situation), whereby the reasons *relaxation* and *activation* could be particularly relevant here (as with subjective stress levels). Listening to music for the reason of *relaxation* was associated with lower (Linnemann et al. 2015a) and for the reason of *activation* with higher (Linnemann et al. 2016) cortisol levels in everyday life. In addition, the *presence of other people* while listening to music might influence an individual's selection of music and reasons for music listening, which in turn has displayed differential associations to the stress-responsive systems (Linnemann et al. 2016).

The abovementioned findings on music listening in everyday life and stress parameters originate from studies with healthy participants and have, in part, not been replicated in studies with patients suffering from stress-associated illnesses such as fibromyalgia, depression, and somatic symptom disorder (Feneberg et al. 2021; Linnemann et al. 2015b). In addition to physical complaints, these illnesses are usually characterized by a dysregulation of the biological stress systems. This leads to the assumption that more intensive music-based activities in everyday life may be necessary for individuals with stress-related disorders to regulate the activity of the HPA axis and/or ANS (e.g., prolonged listening to music or singing). This assumption needs to be investigated in future studies.

15.2.3 Integration of Previous Findings

How is it possible that simply listening to music in everyday life can modulate the activity of biological stress systems (HPA axis, ANS) and exert positive effects on health parameters (e.g., mood, exhaustion, pain experience)?

The processing of music in the brain involves numerous areas in addition to the auditory cortex. These include the amygdala, the hippocampus, and the hypothalamus as parts of the limbic system, which are responsible for emotional processing and exert important functions in the control of the HPA axis and the ANS. Moreover, the early processing of acoustic features in the brain stem may contribute to the modulation of autonomic processes such as heart rate and breathing (Chanda and Levitin 2013; Koelsch 2014).

In addition to the everyday findings described above, numerous laboratory and clinical studies have already pointed to the stress-reducing effects of music listening (see Fancourt et al. 2014; Kreutz et al. 2013; Thoma and Nater 2011; de Witte et al. 2019). The HPA axis and ANS play a central role in the regulation of vital bodily functions (e.g., metabolism, cardiovascular functions) and interact closely with the immune system (Charmandari et al. 2005; Dhabhar 2014). Extreme and/or prolonged psychologically and/or physically stressful situations (and the associated excessive activation of the stress systems) can contribute to dysregulation of the HPA axis, the ANS, and the immune system. This can be measured, for example, by permanently high or low cortisol concentrations and/or inflammation levels. An imbalance in the complex interplay of these biological systems can thus contribute to an increased risk for the development and/or maintenance of mental and physical illnesses such as depression, chronic fatigue, and/or chronic pain (McEwen 1998).

The *biopsychological mediation model of music listening* (see Fig. 15.1; Thoma and Nater 2011; Wuttke-Linnemann et al. 2020) illustrates the relationships between music listening, stress, and health. The model assumes that listening to music can regulate the stress systems, which in turn has positive effects on health-related parameters. Mental and physical complaints such as pain, exhaustion, and depressive symptoms could therefore be countered by music listening as a complementary intervention or prevention strategy, mediated by the regulation of the stress systems.

In summary, previous EMA studies suggest that listening to music in everyday life, when applied appropriately, has positive effects on stress and health in both healthy people and those suffering from health problems. Characteristics of the music play an important role. For example, in line with previous laboratory studies, studies set in everyday life showed that the valence (sad–happy) and the arousal (calming–energizing) of the music can modulate biological stress levels, mood, and physical complaints. Situational factors (e.g., reasons for music listening, current mood, presence of others) and personal characteristics (e.g., health status, chronic

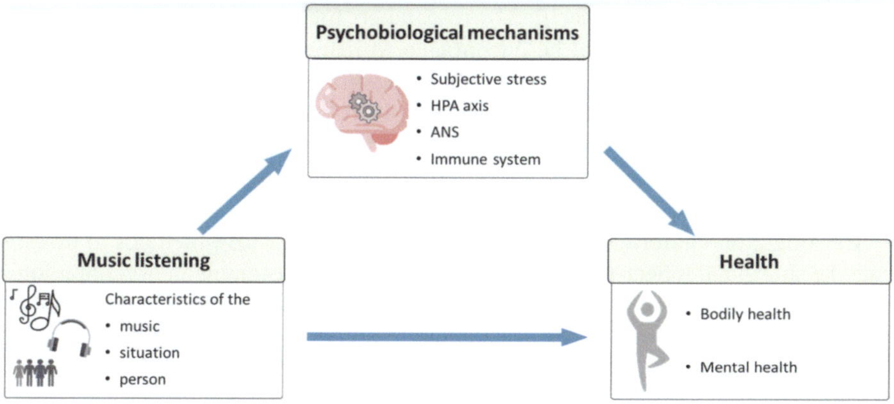

Fig. 15.1 Biopsychological mediation model of music listening. *Note*. The model assumes that the health-promoting effects of music listening are mediated, among other things, by psychobiological stress systems. In addition, the stress-reducing and health-promoting effects of music listening in everyday life are based on a complex interplay between the characteristics of the music, the situation, and the person. (Icons in this figure created by www.flaticon.com) *HPA* axis: Hypothalamic-pituitary-adrenal axis; ANS: Autonomic nervous system

stress) also take on modulating functions regarding the music selection and the effects of music listening on bodily and mental health.

As research in the field of music listening in everyday life is still relatively new, further studies are needed to replicate and expand on previous findings. It should be noted that the findings described above are mostly based on observational studies focusing on *naturally occurring* music listening in everyday life. Accordingly, this research focused on conscious music listening (compared to no music listening) and examined its prospective associations with subjective and biological parameters that were recorded a certain time after music listening. It should be emphasized that these observational studies do not imply causality, since, for example, there was no randomization to conditions (music listening vs. control). This would require studies that randomly offer music listening as a targeted intervention in everyday life and investigate its effectiveness in terms of stress reduction and health promotion in comparison to alternative activities.

15.3 Music Listening Interventions in Everyday Life

The EMA studies described above suggest that listening to music in everyday life can have positive health effects. These findings should be used for the development and evaluation of music-based interventions in everyday life, realized via "ecological momentary interventions" (EMIs). EMIs are characterized by the fact that people are offered help in the form of a mostly digitally mediated intervention while they go about their everyday lives (Heron and Smyth 2010). This can be implemented in a more or less formalized way. For example, people could be encouraged to listen to a music playlist specified by researchers for 30 min at a certain time each day. Alternatively, they could be encouraged to listen to music via an app at the precise moments of increased stress (or increased somatic complaints, negative mood, etc.). The latter "just-in-time" intervention approach appears to be a particularly promising and effective, albeit technically challenging, way of using personalized and context-sensitive music listening interventions to promote health (Smyth and Heron 2016).

Existing interventions applied more or less context-sensitive methods to investigate the short- and longer-term effects of targeted music listening on psychobiological stress markers and health-related parameters. For example, in the study by Helsing et al. (2016), the effects of listening to relaxing vs. energizing music were investigated regarding stress experience, emotions, and salivary cortisol in everyday life. For this purpose, the participants were instructed to select their own relaxing or energizing pieces of music, which were then used during the study. The relaxing and activating playlists were to be listened to for 30 min every evening at home after work for a duration of 1 week, respectively. The research team examined differences between the 2 weeks (week with relaxing vs. week with activating playlist). In addition, differences in an initial control week in which the participants were asked to relax for 30 min each evening with alternative activities (e.g., reading, crafting, meditating, etc.) were examined. Subjective stress and cortisol levels decreased over the study period and positive emotions were experienced more intensely. Furthermore, lower subjective stress levels were reported in the week in which relaxing music was listened to compared to the week with activating music.

Other studies investigated changes in ANS activity in relation to music-based interventions applied in everyday life (Carissoli et al. 2015; Kappert et al. 2019; Kirk and Axelsen 2020). In these studies, participants could freely choose when they wanted to listen to music (i.e., carry out the intervention) in their everyday lives. For example, in the study by Carissoli et al. (2015), the participants were encouraged to listen to music twice a day for 15 min at a time, although the time of day and place were not specified. In all three studies, the researchers provided playlists from which the participants could select their preferred songs, and listening to music was compared with the effects of meditation exercises (or voice-based instructions for relaxation/activation in Kappert et al. 2019). There was an increase in heart rate variability compared to a baseline phase (Kirk and Axelsen 2020) and a decrease in heart rate from immediately before to immediately after listening to music (Carissoli et al. 2015), both of which suggest a physical relaxation effect. Kappert et al. (2019), on the other hand, report increased ANS activity as measured by skin conductance, which suggests a state of physical activation. In addition, increased subjective activation and relaxation, as well as reduced stress levels, were reported from before to after listening to music. The different findings regarding the activity of the ANS in Kappert et al. (2019) compared to the other two studies can possibly be explained by differences in the examined population and by differences in the music. It should also be taken into account that intense positive emotions can also lead to increased sympathetic activation, which may have played a role in the study by Kappert and colleagues.

The intervention approaches described so far included more or less restrictive guidelines on when exactly music should be listened to in everyday life (e.g., every day after work or at self-selected times but for a predefined duration). In contrast, the research group led by Neal-Barnett et al. (2019) implemented a more context-sensitive intervention approach in everyday life. As part of an initial exploratory evaluation study, young people were asked via an app to listen to their personal favorite song whenever they reported particularly high subjective stress levels. Overall, stress levels decreased from before to after study participation, and the young people reported a high level of perceived effectiveness, for example, in the form of inner calm and clear thoughts in stressful situations within the family, when they had used the situation-specific music offer.

Numerous other studies have documented the health-promoting effects of music listening in healthy and clinical samples (e.g., with regard to improvements in sleep quality, chronic pain, mood and emotion regulation, cognitive functions in dementia, and psychiatric symptoms). In most cases, participants were instructed to listen to music during a stay in a clinical-medical facility and/or at home for a certain period of time over several weeks. It should be noted that often only changes in health parameters from before to after the entire intervention period were examined using retrospective questionnaires in a control group design (for an overview, see Dingle et al. 2021; Golden et al. 2021). In contrast to this, the EMA/EMI approaches described above recorded *direct* effects of music listening in everyday life. Future studies could benefit from adding an EMA/EMI component to the assessment of traditional baseline-post effects. This would enable researchers to examine direct psycho(bio)logical effects and thus relevant change mechanisms of the music listening interventions in everyday life.

Overall, previous music listening EMIs have produced promising preliminary evidence in the areas of stress reduction and health promotion. Targeted music listening directly modulated stress experience, emotions, and biological stress indicators across different forms of intervention (with regard to frequency, duration, and timing of the intervention). Compared to established forms of relaxation (e.g., meditation), listening to music achieved comparable effects on subjective and/or biological stress markers. Interestingly, Carissoli et al. (2015) also pointed out that listening to music at the end of the intervention period was associated with reduced self-reported pain and physical discomfort (compared to meditating). Listening to music was also the most frequently chosen form of intervention when subjects were free to choose and was associated with higher usage rates compared to non-musical means of relaxation (Carissoli et al. 2015; Kappert et al. 2019; Kirk and Axelsen 2020). As previous studies are exploratory in nature, further and larger-scale studies are needed to enable solid statements about the effectiveness of music-based EMIs and the differential effects compared to alternative relaxation methods. Nevertheless, the current literature offers many indications that listening to music can indeed be an appropriate and popular tool for prevention and intervention programs to reduce stress and promote health in everyday life. Context-sensitive interventions, which offer music precisely when it is needed most, represent interesting and novel possibilities for future research thanks to technological advances (Feneberg and Nater 2022).

In the following, methodological features for the planning and implementation of EMA studies with a focus on music listening in everyday life are first described. Section 15.5 concludes with an exemplary description of a music-based EMI that pursues the goal of stress reduction in everyday life.

15.4 Methodological Features of EMA Studies

EMA studies for the ecologically valid assessment of stress-related and health-related effects of music listening should be carefully planned. Depending on the research question(s) and target population, considerations should be made in advance regarding (1) the survey protocol, (2) the selection of participants, (3) the operationalization of constructs of interest and software/hardware components used, and (4) the statistical analyses methods. In addition to these considerations in the planning and evaluation phase, corresponding recommendations should be taken into account when reporting the study (see Linnemann et al. 2017; Shiffman et al. 2008; Trull and Ebner-Priemer 2020).

15.4.1 Assessment Protocol

The assessment protocol includes the duration of the study as well as the number and type of measurement points per day. A duration of several days to several weeks is recommended in order to capture a representative section of an individual's everyday life.

In principle, a distinction can be made between time-contingent and event-contingent data assessment. Time-contingent assessment means the repeated collection of subjective or other parameters over a certain period of time. Measurements can be taken either at predefined times (e.g., every day at 10:00, 12:00, 14:00, 16:00, 18:00), at random times within predefined time windows ("semi-randomly"; e.g., every day between 10:00 and 12:00, 12:00 and 14:00, 14:00 and 16:00, 16:00 and 18:00) or at completely random times. At the corresponding measurement times, participants usually receive an auditory signal from a preprogrammed app, often with the option of postponing the respective data entry for a certain time if an immediate response is not possible. In addition, so-called event-contingent assessment is used to record data when certain events occur. This procedure is recommended if a behavior or phenomenon of interest occurs rather rarely and has a specific starting point. In addition, a combination of time-contingent and event-contingent assessment is possible in order to record occurrences and experiences throughout the day, as well as distinctively occurring events. For example, people could be asked several times throughout the day whether they have listened to music since the last measurement time point or are currently listening to music (= time-contingent). Alternatively, or additionally, participants could be asked to start a data entry each time immediately before, during, and/or after listening to music (= event-contingent). Depending on which approach is chosen, more or less immediate temporal observations of the relationship between music listening and other recorded parameters (e.g., stress, mood, fatigue, etc.) are possible.

The frequency and distribution of measurement time points per day in the context of time-contingent measurement determine the temporal resolution of the recorded phenomena of interest. It should be based on the everyday dynamics of the phenomenon, if these are already known (Myin-Germeys et al. 2009). In addition to the scientific interest, participant burden must be considered. It should also be borne in mind that participants should not adapt their everyday life routines because of participating in the study, as this biases the assessment of "natural" experience and behavior. It is advisable to familiarize the participants with the procedure, the content, and the materials (e.g., frequency and meaning of the questions, handling of the app, and, if necessary, saliva samples, see below) in a detailed training session before the start of the study.

15.4.2 Selection and Number of Participants

We highly recommend defining inclusion/exclusion criteria regarding the participants in advance. If biological parameters are collected, it is particularly advisable to check for certain health and lifestyle-related conditions (Strahler et al. 2017). If specific populations are of interest (e.g., patient populations, professional musicians), the inclusion criteria must be expanded accordingly. Especially when listening to music in everyday life is of primary interest, it is important to consider that previous experience with music, absolute pitch or hearing impairment can systematically influence the findings. These aspects should therefore be defined as exclusion criteria where appropriate or assessed and then statistically controlled for. Due to the nested data structure and correspondingly complex statistical analysis procedures, sample size planning for everyday studies should be carried out with the help of simulations that take these particularities into account (see e.g., Arend and Schäfer 2019).

15.4.3 Operationalization

The first step is to ask about the occurrence of music listening using a filter item in the context of time-contingent data collection protocols (see Fig. 15.2, note: this initial question is omitted in the case of event-contingent measurement). It should be clearly communicated to the participants before study commencement what exactly is meant by "music listening": for instance, whether music listening implies active music listening (e.g., music is the focus of attention) or passive music listening (e.g., background music in a shopping center). If the filter item is answered with *yes*, further questions should be asked to characterize the music, the music listening context, and the perceived experiences of music listening. These include, for example, the perceived music characteristics valence (can be recorded on a visual analogue scale from *sad* to *happy*) and arousal (can be recorded on a visual analogue

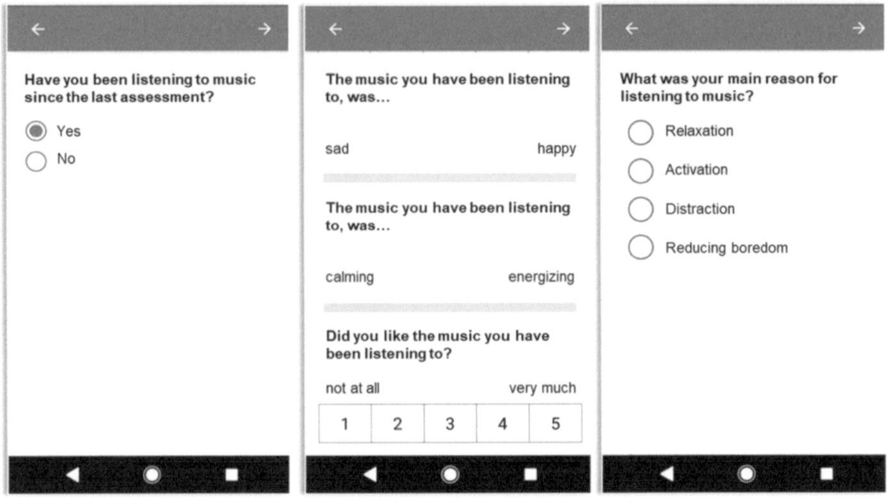

Fig. 15.2 Example screenshots of a smartphone-based research app with music listening questions*Note*. Participants can be examined regarding their music listening behavior and its correlation with psychobiological parameters while they go about their regular everyday lives

scale from *calming* to *energizing*). In addition, the reasons for listening to music should be asked. The most common reasons for listening to music, based on previous research, are *relaxation* (e.g., due to a previous stressful event or a general need for relaxation), *activation* (e.g., to move to the music or to energize), *distraction* (e.g., to distract oneself from certain thoughts), and *against boredom* (e.g., to pass time). Depending on the question, other reasons may be presented (e.g., aesthetic pleasure, concentration). If the participant finds it difficult to decide on a particular answer (e.g., if both happy and sad songs were listened to or if several reasons apply), the participant should choose the option that corresponds to their predominant impression. In addition to the main reason for music listening, further reasons can also be asked for. Furthermore, the liking of the music and other important characteristics of the music listening situation can be asked. These include, for example, the presence of others while listening to music (e.g., friends, acquaintances, strangers; multiple selection possible) and the duration of listening to music (see relevant literature: Greasley and Lamont 2011; Greb et al. 2019; Juslin et al. 2008; Krause et al. 2015; Linnemann et al. 2017; Randall and Rickard 2017; Sloboda et al. 2001).

For the further assessment of self-reports (e.g., levels of stress experience, mood, fatigue, etc.), it should be taken into account that the measurement should take as little time as possible and be practicable to carry out in everyday life. As a rule, each data entry should be limited to a few items, which should nevertheless represent the target construct reliably and validly (Cranford et al. 2006; Lesage et al. 2012). If salivary stress markers are of interest (e.g., cortisol as an indicator of HPA axis activity and/or alpha-amylase as an indicator of ANS activity), specially manufactured plastic containers that are clearly labeled for the respective measurement time points are suitable, into which the saliva can be transferred using a straw (Schlotz 2014; Strahler et al. 2017).

15.4.4 Software and Hardware

With regard to software and hardware components, a range of commercial and freely accessible apps are available that can be used for the self-report data to be recorded. Typically, the data is provided with a time stamp, which makes subsequent data processing and analysis much easier. When selecting the software solution, it is important to check which operating systems the app runs on (e.g., Android and/or iOS), whether certain programming skills need to be acquired, whether the app developers offer customer support, what financial options are available, and whether data protection guidelines regarding data storage and processing are implemented by the developers. Finally, it is important to consider whether smartphones should be provided for participants or whether it is practical and technically feasible to allow participants to use their private smartphones for study participation. In addition, there are various sensors, for example, for measuring movement, heart rate (variability), and electrodermal activity. Numerous other applications can be used to record location, communication behavior (calls, text messages, chat apps), ambient noise, and volume, as well as objective music listening behavior (title, artist, time), depending on the research questions.

15.4.5 Statistical Analysis Methods

EMA studies usually involve several measurement points per day over several days per participant and consequently produce a large amount of data with a complex structure. These are longitudinal data, whereby the data points collected over time from the same person are more closely related to each other than the data points from different persons. For this reason, multilevel models (also known as mixed-effects modeling or hierarchical linear models) are usually the statistical analysis method of choice, as they can take into account the dependencies of the data. These are extended regression analyses. Depending on the issue at hand, structural equation models can also be useful (multilevel structural equation modeling). In general, with the analysis methods presented, the relationships between variables can be examined simultaneously at several levels, for example at the level of measurement time points (from moment to moment), at the day level (from day to day), and at the person level (from person to person) (Enders and Tofighi 2007; de Haan-Rietdijk et al. 2016). The investigation of moderation and mediation effects and the modeling of nonlinear relationships are also possible. For a detailed introduction to the basics and application of multilevel models, we recommend the relevant literature (e.g., Bolger and Laurenceau 2013; Finch and Bolin 2017).

15.5 Music Listening During Stress and Discrimination in Everyday Life

The EMI described here was developed by the authors of the book chapter and refers to the health-relevant, specific stressor of ethnic discrimination. *Ethnic discrimination* refers to unjustified disadvantage or degradation based on an individual's ethnicity (Contrada et al. 2000). It is a stressor that can provoke immediate psychobiological stress reactions (Brondolo et al. 2009). If ethnic discrimination occurs chronically, it can lead to health impairments (Sempértegui et al. 2019). Suitable interventions that can mitigate the immediate stress reactions and their negative effects are therefore urgently needed. Due to its flexibility and direct application in the everyday lives of those affected, an EMI is a particularly suitable form of intervention here. Against this background, a music-based EMI was developed to reduce psychological and biological stress parameters in moments of increased stress and/or after perceived discrimination. The EMI is aimed at Turkish immigrant women, who belong to one of the largest immigrant groups in many European countries (e.g., Statistics Austria 2019). Women might be particularly targeted, as they are often exposed to both gender- and ethnic-related discrimination (Seaton and Tyson 2019). The following is an example of the study protocol of an initial pilot study used to investigate the feasibility and effectiveness of the music-based EMI.

15.5.1 Selection and Number of Participants

The pilot study is intended to allow conclusions regarding a healthy female sample aged between 18 and 65 years. The women are Turkish immigrants or direct descendants of Turkish immigrants. Only women who report chronic ethnic discrimination in their everyday lives are included. As the study described here is an initial pilot study, the sample size is limited to $N = 20$ people.

15.5.2 Assessment Protocol

The 35-day study period is divided into a 7-day baseline phase, a 21-day intervention phase, and a final 7-day post-intervention phase. Over the entire study period, individual stress levels and perceived discrimination are recorded using a smartphone-based app. For this purpose, the subjective stress experience and perceived discrimination are recorded three times a day using semi-random, time-contingent prompts (between 08:00 and 12:00, 12:00 and 16:00, 16:00 and 20:00). In addition, event-contingent data entries in moments of subjectively increased stress and/or perceived discrimination should be self-initiated by the participants. In order to record the course of these parameters in such situations, the app automatically prompts participants to answer further questions 20 and 35 min after event-contingent data entries. For the multidimensional assessment of "stress," the participants also provide saliva samples at each of the described data entries. These

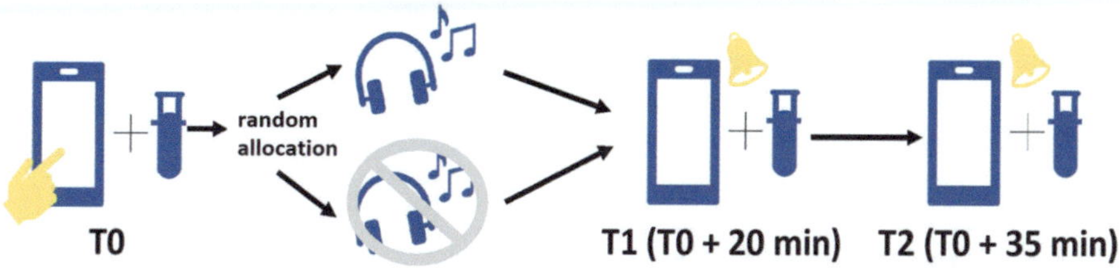

Fig. 15.3 Procedure after event-contingent data entries during the intervention phase*Notes*. After each event-contingent data entry during the intervention phase (T0), random allocation to the intervention or control condition takes place. The first automatic prompt takes place 20 min after T0 (T1), the second 35 min after T0 (T2)

can be used to analyze the biological stress markers cortisol and alpha-amylase. Every evening, participants self-initiate a data entry before going to sleep, which the study participants are automatically reminded of by the app at 21:00.

The music listening intervention is carried out as an individualized and situation-sensitive EMI in the intervention phase. An intraindividual randomized design was chosen for this purpose. After each event-contingent data entry, i.e., in the case of increased stress and/or perceived discrimination, random allocation to the intervention condition (listening to a self-created study playlist for 20 min) or the control condition (no music listening for 20 min) takes place via a 50:50 ratio. Immediately after listening to music or not listening to music, and 15 min later, the app automatically prompts participants to answer questions and provide a saliva sample (Fig. 15.3).

15.5.3 Operationalization

In the present study, the momentary subjective experience of stress is assessed using the single-item *How stressed do you feel at the moment?*, which is answered on a visual analogue scale (0 *not at all*—100 *very much*). Further items for a more precise assessment of the current subjective experience of stress are only presented if the subsequent filter item *Do you feel stressed at the moment?* Is answered with *yes*. Perceived discrimination is recorded with the single item *How discriminated do you feel at the moment?*, which can also be answered on a visual analogue scale from 0 *not at all* to 100 *very much*. If the filter item, *Do you feel discriminated against at the moment?* is answered with *yes*, further items are presented to ask for details of the discriminatory event.

15.5.4 Statistical Evaluation

As part of the EMI described above, repeated measurement data are collected for each participant, which allows the investigation of intra-individual trajectories between the measurement time points using multilevel models. By comparing the strength of the changes in the subjective and biological stress parameters between the intervention and control conditions, the immediate effect of the music-based EMI on the experience of stress and discrimination can be determined. The intermediate effect can be examined by comparing the aforementioned stress parameters in the baseline phase vs. the post-intervention phase.

15.5.5 Concluding Remarks

In the study described here, the possibility of combining time- and event-contingent data entries is implemented. The study was designed in such a way that participant burden was reduced to a minimum. Alarms for daily measurements can therefore be postponed by a maximum of 1 h. To reduce the time required for responding to prompts, the number of items recorded was kept to a minimum, and only the (individual) items necessary to achieve the study objective were used.

The advantages of EMIs already mentioned in this chapter also apply to the presented study. These include the multidimensional recording of "stress," both subjectively and biologically. In addition, the provision of EMIs on the study participants' smartphones increases the flexibility of the intervention and ensures good integration into the natural environment. This enables the provision of low-threshold, easily accessible, and individually tailored support.

15.6 Conclusion

For many people, music is an accessible means of reducing stress and evoking positive moods. Music listening in everyday life is also associated with fewer somatic complaints, such as pain or fatigue. EMA methods offer the opportunity to investigate the underlying psychobiological mechanisms of the health-promoting effects of music listening in everyday life. Important characteristics of the music, the situation, and the person that modulate the stress-reducing and health-promoting effects of listening to music have already been identified. Based on these findings, music listening interventions for stress reduction and health promotion can be developed that offer support tailored to the person and situation and thus can be used in a targeted and flexible manner in everyday life.

References

Arend MG, Schäfer T (2019) Statistical power in two-level models: a tutorial based on Monte Carlo simulation. Psychol Methods 24(1):1–19. https://doi.org/10.1037/met0000195

Bernatzky G, Presch M, Anderson M, Panksepp J (2011) Emotional foundations of music as a non-pharmacological pain management tool in modern medicine. Neurosci Biobehav Rev 35(9):1989–1999. https://doi.org/10.1016/j.neubiorev.2011.06.005

Bolger N, Laurenceau J-P (2013) Intensive longitudinal methods: an introduction to diary and experience sampling research. Guilford Press. http://site.ebrary.com/lib/alltitles/docDetail.action?docID=10649558

Brondolo E, Brady Ver Halen N, Pencille M, Beatty D, Contrada RJ (2009) Coping with racism: a selective review of the literature and a theoretical and methodological critique. J Behav Med 32(1):64–88. https://doi.org/10.1007/s10865-008-9193-0

Carissoli C, Villani D, Riva G (2015) Does a meditation protocol supported by a mobile application help people reduce stress? Suggestions from a controlled pragmatic trial. Cyberpsychol Behav Soc Netw 18(1):46–53. https://doi.org/10.1089/cyber.2014.0062

Chan MF, Wong ZY, Thayala NV (2011) The effectiveness of music listening in reducing depressive symptoms in adults: a systematic review. Complement Ther Med 19(6):332–348. https://doi.org/10.1016/j.ctim.2011.08.003

Chanda ML, Levitin DJ (2013) The neurochemistry of music. Trends Cogn Sci 17(4):179–193. https://doi.org/10.1016/j.tics.2013.02.007

Charmandari E, Tsigos C, Chrousos G (2005) Endocrinology of the stress response. Annu Rev Physiol 67:259–284. https://doi.org/10.1146/annurev.physiol.67.040403.120816

Contrada RJ, Ashmore RD, Gary ML, Coups E, Egeth JD, Sewell A, Ewell K, Goyal TM, Chasse V (2000) Ethnicity-related sources of stress and their effects on well-being. Curr Dir Psychol Sci 9:136–139. https://doi.org/10.1111/1467-8721.00078

Cranford JA, Shrout PE, Iida M, Rafaeli E, Yip T, Bolger N (2006) A procedure for evaluating sensitivity to within-person change: can mood measures in diary studies detect change reliably? Personal Soc Psychol Bull 32(7):917–929. https://doi.org/10.1177/0146167206287721

de Haan-Rietdijk S, Kuppens P, Hamaker EL (2016) What's in a day? A guide to decomposing the variance in intensive longitudinal data. Front Psychol 7:891. https://doi.org/10.3389/fpsyg.2016.00891

de Witte M, Spruit A, van Hooren S, Moonen X, Stams G-J (2019) Effects of music interventions on stress-related outcomes: a systematic review and two meta-analyses. Health Psychol Rev 1–31. https://doi.org/10.1080/17437199.2019.1627897

Dhabhar FS (2014) Effects of stress on immune function: the good, the bad, and the beautiful. Immunol Res 58(2–3):193–210. https://doi.org/10.1007/s12026-014-8517-0

Dingle GA, Sharman LS, Bauer Z, Beckman E, Broughton M, Bunzli E, Davidson R, Draper G, Fairley S, Farrell C, Flynn LM, Gomersall S, Hong M, Larwood J, Lee C, Lee J, Nitschinsk L, Peluso N, Reedman SE, Vidas D et al (2021) How do music activities affect health and well-being? A scoping review of studies examining psychosocial mechanisms. Front Psychol 12:713818. https://doi.org/10.3389/fpsyg.2021.713818

Enders CK, Tofighi D (2007) Centering predictor variables in cross-sectional multilevel models: a new look at an old issue. Psychol Methods 12(2):121–138. https://doi.org/10.1037/1082-989X.12.2.121

Fancourt D, Ockelford A, Belai A (2014) The psychoneuroimmunological effects of music: a systematic review and a new model. Brain Behav Immun 36:15–26. https://doi.org/10.1016/j.bbi.2013.10.014

Feneberg AC, Nater UM (2022) An ecological momentary music intervention for the reduction of acute stress in daily life: a mixed methods feasibility study. Front Psychol 13:927705. https://doi.org/10.3389/fpsyg.2022.927705

Feneberg AC, Mewes R, Doerr JM, Nater UM (2021) The effects of music listening on somatic symptoms and stress markers in the everyday life of women with somatic complaints and depression. Sci Rep 11(1):24062. https://doi.org/10.1038/s41598-021-03374-w

Feneberg AC, Stijovic A, Forbes PAG, Lamm C, Piperno G, Pronizius E, Silani G, Nater UM (2023) Perceptions of stress and mood associated with listening to music in daily life during the COVID-19 lockdown. JAMA Netw Open 6(1):e2250382. https://doi.org/10.1001/jamanetworkopen.2022.50382

Finch WH, Bolin JE (2017) Multilevel modeling using Mplus. Chapman & Hall/CRC statistics in the social and behavioral sciences series. CRC Press

Garza-Villarreal EA, Pando V, Vuust P, Parsons C (2017) Music-induced analgesia in chronic pain conditions: a systematic review and meta-analysis. Pain Physician 20(7):597–610

Golden TL, Springs S, Kimmel HJ, Gupta S, Tiedemann A, Sandu CC, Magsamen S (2021) The use of music in the treatment and Management of Serious Mental Illness: a global scoping review of the literature. Front Psychol 12:649840. https://doi.org/10.3389/fpsyg.2021.649840

Grad FP (2002) The preamble of the constitution of the world health organization. Bull World Health Organ 80(12):981–984

Greasley AE, Lamont A (2011) Exploring engagement with music in everyday life using experience sampling methodology. Music Sci 15(1):45–71. https://doi.org/10.1177/1029864910393417

Greb F, Steffens J, Schlotz W (2019) Modeling music-selection behavior in everyday life: a multilevel statistical learning approach and mediation analysis of experience sampling data. Front Psychol 10:390. https://doi.org/10.3389/fpsyg.2019.00390

Helsing M, Västfjäll D, Bjälkebring P, Juslin P, Hartig T (2016) An experimental field study of the effects of listening to self-selected music on emotions, stress, and cortisol levels. Music Med 8(4):187–198. https://doi.org/10.47513/MMD.V8I4.442

Heron KE, Smyth JM (2010) Ecological momentary interventions: incorporating mobile technology into psychosocial and health behaviour treatments. Br J Health Psychol 15(Pt 1):1–39. https://doi.org/10.1348/135910709X466063

International Federation of the Phonographic Industry (2019) Music listening 2019. https://www.ifpi.org/wp-content/uploads/2020/07/Music-Listening-2019-1.pdf. abgerufen am 13.10.2021

Juslin PN, Liljeström S, Västfjäll D, Barradas G, Silva A (2008) An experience sampling study of emotional reactions to music: listener, music, and situation. Emotion 8(5):668–683. https://doi.org/10.1037/a0013505

Kappert MB, Wuttke-Linnemann A, Schlotz W, Nater UM (2019) The aim justifies the means-differences among musical and nonmusical means of relaxation or activation induction in daily life. Front Hum Neurosci 13:36. https://doi.org/10.3389/fnhum.2019.00036

Kirk U, Axelsen JL (2020) Heart rate variability is enhanced during mindfulness practice: a randomized controlled trial involving a 10-day online-based mindfulness intervention. PLoS One 15(12):e0243488. https://doi.org/10.1371/journal.pone.0243488

Koelsch S (2014) Brain correlates of music-evoked emotions. Nat Rev Neurosci 15(3):170–180. https://doi.org/10.1038/nrn3666

Krause AE, North AC, Hewitt LY (2015) Music-listening in everyday life: devices and choice. Psychol Music 43(2):155–170. https://doi.org/10.1177/0305735613496860

Kreutz G, Quiroga Murcia C, Bongard S (2013) Psychoneuroendocrine research on music and health: an overview. In: MacDonald RAR, Kreutz G, Mitchell L (eds) Music, health, and wellbeing. Oxford University Press, pp 458–476. https://doi.org/10.1093/acprof:oso/9780199586974.003.0030

Kühlmann AYR, de Rooij A, Kroese LF, van Dijk M, Hunink MGM, Jeekel J (2018) Meta-analysis evaluating music interventions for anxiety and pain in surgery. Br J Surg 105(7):773–783. https://doi.org/10.1002/bjs.10853

Lesage F-X, Berjot S, Deschamps F (2012) Clinical stress assessment using a visual analogue scale. Occup Med 62(8):600–605. https://doi.org/10.1093/occmed/kqs140

Linnemann A, Ditzen B, Strahler J, Doerr JM, Nater UM (2015a) Music listening as a means of stress reduction in daily life. Psychoneuroendocrinology 60:82–90. https://doi.org/10.1016/j.psyneuen.2015.06.008

Linnemann A, Kappert MB, Fischer S, Doerr JM, Strahler J, Nater UM (2015b) The effects of music listening on pain and stress in the daily life of patients with fibromyalgia syndrome. Front Hum Neurosci 9:434. https://doi.org/10.3389/fnhum.2015.00434

Linnemann A, Strahler J, Nater UM (2016) The stress-reducing effect of music listening varies depending on the social context. Psychoneuroendocrinology 72:97–105. https://doi.org/10.1016/j.psyneuen.2016.06.003

Linnemann A, Strahler J, Nater UM (2017) Assessing the effects of music listening on psychobiological stress in daily life. J Visual Exp. https://doi.org/10.3791/54920

Linnemann A, Wenzel M, Grammes J, Kubiak T, Nater UM (2018) Music listening and stress in daily life—a matter of timing. Int J Behav Med 25(2):223–230. https://doi.org/10.1007/s12529-017-9697-5

McEwen BS (1998) Stress, adaptation, and disease: Allostasis and allostatic load. Ann N Y Acad Sci 840(1):33–44. https://doi.org/10.1111/j.1749-6632.1998.tb09546.x
Mehl MR, Conner TS (eds) (2014) Handbook of research methods for studying daily life. Guilford
Myin-Germeys I, Oorschot M, Collip D, Lataster J, Delespaul P, van Os J (2009) Experience sampling research in psychopathology: opening the black box of daily life. Psychol Med 39(9):1533–1547. https://doi.org/10.1017/S0033291708004947
Nater UM (2018) The multidimensionality of stress and its assessment. Brain Behav Immun 73:159–160. https://doi.org/10.1016/j.bbi.2018.07.018
Neal-Barnett A, Stadulis R, Ellzey D, Jean E, Rowell T, Somerville K, Petitti K, Siglow B, Ruttan A, Hogue M (2019) Evaluation of the effectiveness of a musical cognitive restructuring app for black inner-city girls: survey, usage, and focus group evaluation. JMIR Mhealth Uhealth 7(6):e11310. https://doi.org/10.2196/11310
Panteleeva Y, Ceschi G, Glowinski D, Courvoisier DS, Grandjean D (2017) Music for anxiety? Meta-analysis of anxiety reduction in non-clinical samples. Psychol Music 46(4):473–487. https://doi.org/10.1177/0305735617712424
Pawlik K, Buse L (1982) Rechnergestützte verhaltensregistrierung im feld: Beschreibung und erste psychometrische überprüfung einer neuen erhebungsmethode [computer-based behavior registration in the field: description and first psychometric evaluation of a new recording method]. Zeitschrift für Differentielle und Diagnostische Psychologie 3(2):101–118
Randall WM, Rickard NS (2017) Personal music listening. Music Percept 34(5):501–514. https://doi.org/10.1525/mp.2017.34.5.501
Roy M, Peretz I, Rainville P (2008) Emotional valence contributes to music-induced analgesia. Pain 134(1–2):140–147. https://doi.org/10.1016/j.pain.2007.04.003
Schlotz W (2014) Ambulatory psychoneuroendocrinology: assessing salivary cortisol and other hormones in daily life. In: Mehl MR, Conner TS (eds) Handbook of research methods for studying daily life. Guilford, pp 193–209
Schwarz N (2007) Cognitive aspects of survey methodology. Appl Cogn Psychol 21(2):277–287. https://doi.org/10.1002/acp.1340
Seaton EK, Tyson K (2019) The intersection of race and gender among black American adolescents. Child Dev 90(1):62–70. https://doi.org/10.1111/cdev.13093
Sempértegui GA, Knipscheer JW, Baliatsas C, Bekker MHJ (2019) Symptom manifestation and treatment effectiveness, -obstacles and -facilitators in Turkish and Moroccan groups with depression in European countries: a systematic review. J Affect Disord 247:134–155. https://doi.org/10.1016/j.jad.2018.12.060
Shiffman S, Stone AA, Hufford MR (2008) Ecological momentary assessment. Annu Rev Clin Psychol 4(1):1–32. https://doi.org/10.1146/annurev.clinpsy.3.022806.091415
Sloboda JA, O'Neill SA, Ivaldi A (2001) Functions of music in everyday life: an exploratory study using the experience sampling method. Music Sci 5(1):9–32. https://doi.org/10.1177/102986490100500102
Smyth JM, Heron KE (2016) Is providing mobile interventions "just-in-time" helpful? An experimental proof of concept study of just-in-time intervention for stress management. IEEE Wireless Health (WH) 2016:1–7
Statistik Austria (2019) Migration und Integration. Zahlen, Daten, Indikatoren 2019. https://www.integrationsfonds.at/mediathek/mediathek-publikationen/publikation/migration-und-integration-zahlen-daten-indikatoren-4265. abgerufen am 27.09.2021
Strahler J, Skoluda N, Kappert MB, Nater UM (2017) Simultaneous measurement of salivary cortisol and alpha-amylase: application and recommendations. Neurosci Biobehav Rev 83:657–677. https://doi.org/10.1016/j.neubiorev.2017.08.015
Strahler J, Nater UM, Skoluda N (2019) Associations between health behaviors and factors on markers of healthy psychological and physiological functioning: a daily diary study. Ann Behav Med. https://doi.org/10.1093/abm/kaz018
Thaut MH (2015) Music as therapy in early history. Prog Brain Res 217:143–158. https://doi.org/10.1016/bs.pbr.2014.11.025

Thoma MV, Nater UM (2011) The psychoneuroendocrinology of music effects in health. In: Costa A, Villalba E (eds) Horizons in neuroscience research. Nova Science Publishers, Inc

Trull TJ, Ebner-Priemer U (2013) Ambulatory assessment. Annu Rev Clin Psychol 9:151–176. https://doi.org/10.1146/annurev-clinpsy-050212-185510

Trull TJ, Ebner-Priemer UW (2020) Ambulatory assessment in psychopathology research: a review of recommended reporting guidelines and current practices. J Abnorm Psychol 129(1):56–63. https://doi.org/10.1037/abn0000473

Wuttke-Linnemann A, Nater UM, Ehlert U, Ditzen B (2019) Sex-specific effects of music listening on couples' stress in everyday life. Sci Rep 9(1):4880. https://doi.org/10.1038/s41598-019-40056-0

Wuttke-Linnemann A, Feneberg AC, Nater UM (2020) Music and health. In: Gellman MD, Turner JR (eds) Encyclopedia of behavioral medicine. Springer, New York, pp 1–5. https://doi.org/10.1007/978-1-4614-6439-6_101901-1

Music for Socio-emotional Coping During the COVID-19 Pandemic

16

Claire Howlin and Niels C. Hansen

16.1 Introduction

In March 2020, the World Health Organization (WHO) announced the first global pandemic officially caused by a coronavirus (World Health Organization 2020). COVID-19 was identified as a new respiratory illness resulting from infection with the novel coronavirus SARS-CoV-2, with the potential to spread across the globe. Public health measures (e.g., increased handwashing, reducing social contacts) were introduced to reduce the rate of transmission (Ayouni et al. 2021). These measures also included the closure of spaces and events that encourage high levels of social interaction, along with 'lockdowns' confining people to the vicinity of their homes. Throughout the world, gatherings were banned, cultural and sporting events were cancelled, curfews were brought into effect, travel and commuting were restricted, and bars, restaurants, schools and businesses were forced to close (Hale et al., 2021; Porcher 2020). The scale of the disruption caused by the considerable number of cases and the implementation of lockdowns led to widespread social and emotional disruption. Uncertainty and financial insecurity arising from these measures cascaded into widespread increases in stress, fear, anxiety, panic attacks, depression, anger and sleep disorders (Hossain et al. 2020). This created a unique situation where music-related behaviours and music therapy played an important role.

The current chapter will review how music was used in a range of contexts and settings to support the social, emotional and physical needs that developed because

C. Howlin (✉)
School of Psychology, Trinity College Dublin, Dublin, Ireland
e-mail: howlincl@tcd.ie

N. C. Hansen
Interacting Minds Centre, Aarhus University, Denmark and Centre of Excellence in Music, Mind, Body & Brain, University of Jyväskylä, Jyväskylä, Finland

G. Kreutz, G. Bernatzky (eds.), *Music and Medicine*, Neurocultural Health and Wellbeing, https://doi.org/10.1007/978-3-662-72175-9_16

of the coronavirus pandemic and resulting lockdowns. We highlight the rapid changes that occurred in relation to music use in the general population and music therapy practices as the world adjusted to the new challenges posed by the unprecedented circumstances.

16.2 Everyday Music Use in Lockdown to Promote Socio-emotional Coping

16.2.1 The Need for Rapid, Individualised, User-Driven Coping Strategies

The use of music for managing stress and promoting well-being in the general population during the novel coronavirus pandemic occurred in the context of pervasive mental health challenges resulting from the forceful societal lockdowns described above. While some travel constraints were already adopted during early 2020, the vast majority of restrictions on personal mobility, liberty and social life were introduced extremely rapidly around the time of the pandemic declaration on 11th March 2020 (Hale et al., 2021; Porcher 2020). In need of urgent health crisis management, governments, understandably, at first, did not prioritise the well-being needs of their citizens, who consequently had to swiftly pursue and develop safe, accessible and affordable coping strategies on their own (Hansen 2022a, in 2022b).

Following the announcement of the pandemic and the rapid onset of public health measures, many people may have experienced a decline in their mental health and wellbeing (Torales et al. 2020), particularly at the initial stages of lockdown (Fancourt et al. 2021). At the population level, people were more likely to report symptoms of mild depression (Fancourt et al. 2021) compared to representative data collected in 2003 and 2008 (Kocalevent et al. 2013). Importantly, however, some groups were more susceptible to developing symptoms of depression than others (Fancourt et al. 2021; Young et al. 2022). Those who were female (Torales et al. 2020; Wang et al. 2020a; Young et al. 2022), young (Kiernan et al. 2021; Wang et al. 2020b; Young et al. 2022), single, separated or divorced (Ribeiro et al. 2021), unemployed (Young et al. 2022), possessed lower education levels (Mazza et al. 2020), worked in the healthcare sector (Benfante et al. 2020), had limited access to personal protective equipment (Wang et al. 2020a), or had received prior chronic or mental health diagnoses (Young et al. 2022), for example, suffered more severely.

These risk groups did, however, only partly overlap with the young, highly educated, socially supported, but infection-worried people who were more likely than average to adopt creative, artistic activities such as digital arts and writing, crafts, reading for pleasure and music during lockdown (Mak et al. 2021). Some of these may indeed have belonged to the sizeable minority who experienced occasional positive effects of reduced social pressure and work burden (Pan et al. 2021). Lockdown-induced changes in musical consumption and creation patterns, which will be reviewed here, served psychological needs both for effective coping and for filling up additional leisure time and fighting boredom and social hypo-stimulation arising from home confinement.

In factor analysis on demographically representative, large-scale survey data collected during the early months of lockdown (April–May 2020) in France, Germany, India, Italy, the United Kingdom and USA ($n = 5113$), Fink et al. (2021) found support for a bifurcation between those primarily experiencing negative and positive emotions. Whereas negative-experiencers chiefly listened to music and danced solitarily to regulate their own emotions and stress levels, positive-experiencers tended to sing, play and listen with others at home and via the Internet as a proxy for the social interactions and aesthetic experiences that they were deprived of. Relatedly, Henry et al. (2021) found that positive reframing and active coping strategies were associated with using music for entertainment, revival, achieving strong sensations, diversion and mental work.

Despite some indications that negative-experiencers may have relied more on nostalgic music, whereas corona-themed music was important to both groups (Fink et al. 2021), evidence on music selection behaviour during lockdown remains tentative. Between a quarter and half of respondents discovered new styles and artists (Cabedo-Mas et al. 2021; Ferreri et al. 2021; Fink et al. 2021), and between one and two-thirds consumed nostalgic music (Fink et al. 2021; Gibbs and Egermann 2021), resulting in a quantitatively measurable increase compared to previous years (Yeung 2020). Nostalgically themed Spotify playlists did, however, not generally gain followers (Sim et al. 2020), which could be suggestive of individualised rather than consensus-based nostalgia consumption. On the other hand, Tim Burgess' 750+ listening parties with interactive live commentary and sharing of concert memories and memorabilia on Twitter have indeed been associated with collective nostalgia (Lee & Kao, 2020).

Other survey studies found increased happy-music and decreased sad-music listening (Ferreri et al. 2021). Hansen et al.'s (2021) Coronamusic Database certainly contains a multitude of humorous and positively biased music videos, and these sentiments have been claimed to constitute defining traits of coronamusic (Hansen 2022b). Conversely, negatively valenced music was prominently consumed by younger age groups (Vidas et al. 2021) who, as previously mentioned, generally experienced greater well-being impediments (Kiernan et al. 2021; Wang et al. 2020b). Positive (66%), negative (11%) and mixed (19%) emotions were all featured amongst university students' reasons for selecting specific signature songs as typical for their lockdown life (Hurwitz and Krumhansl 2021). Future research should investigate how these diverse music selection behaviours may relate to the divergent coping strategies, identified by Fink et al. (2021), aimed towards fulfilling emotional and social needs, respectively. Although many musical activities achieved these two goals concurrently, we will attempt to highlight behaviours most typical of either type.

16.2.2 Musical Engagement for Emotional Needs

The motivations for musical engagement that increased the most during lockdown were enjoyment, mood enhancement, relaxation and energisation (Fink et al. 2021). Mothers who used music to regulate their children's emotions in home confinement, for example, reported higher well-being and satisfaction with their parental role (Cho and Ilari 2021). Indeed, many rated music the most effective creative activity for enhancing mental well-being goals such as enjoyment, maintaining a good mood and venting negative emotions (Granot et al. 2021; Kiernan et al. 2021). Others have found that the coping effectiveness of musical engagement at least matched or outperformed competitors such as exercise, sleep and changing location (Vidas et al. 2021). While pandemic social media usage and TV watching were negatively associated with life satisfaction, music listening showed the opposite relationship (Krause et al. 2021) and was also negatively associated with depression scores (Ribeiro et al. 2021). Interestingly, psychological distress only correlated negatively with music listening during—but *not* before—lockdown (Mas-Herrero et al. 2020).

Engaging with music thus became the potentially most frequent solitary leisure activity during lockdown (Finnerty et al. 2021). Various self-report studies suggest it was adopted for coping purposes by more than 50% of the general population (Cabedo-Mas et al. 2021; Fink et al. 2021; Kiernan et al. 2021), providing benefits especially for younger people and those to whom music already held great importance (Fink et al. 2021; Granot et al. 2021; Henry et al. 2021; Martínez-Castilla et al. 2021).

Even though many people reported increased music listening during lockdown when asked directly (Cabedo-Mas et al. 2021; Carlson et al. 2021; Ferreri et al. 2021; Fink et al. 2021; Hurwitz and Krumhansl 2021; Ziv and Hollander-Shabtai 2021; see, however, Krause et al. 2021), consumer-based user statistics from streaming platforms tell the opposite story (cf. Hansen 2022a). Analysis of aggregated weekly streaming counts on Spotify of top-200 songs in 60 countries, for example, showed that consumption decreased quantitatively as opportunities for everyday listening during commuting and public exercising disappeared (Sim et al. 2020). Since playlist followership exhibited similar declines, the authors argue these changes could not merely be explained by migration towards a more specialised niche repertoire. Subjective and objective reports, however, agree that many consumers replaced audio-based platforms with video-based alternatives such as YouTube (Carlson et al. 2021; Sim et al. 2020). Hence, to fulfil emotional coping goals, engagement with music may have become more attentive, immersive, multimodal and active, manifesting in greater perceived consumption despite fewer measurable listening hours (Hansen 2022a, b).

16.2.3 Musical Engagement for Social Needs

The migration of music consumers from audio- to video-based streaming services may reflect that, platforms in the latter category—such as YouTube—afford substantially greater degrees of active participation than is traditionally possible on Spotify and Pandora. Granot et al. (2021) applied multilevel regression models to demonstrate that when it came to reducing loneliness and creating a sense of togetherness, music-related activities outperformed news watching, movies and games, eating and cooking, physical exercise, housework, reading, hobbies and spiritual practice, but not actual socialising with others. Music also provided diversion from the crisis more effectively than other activities—including socialising—whereas movies and games worked just as well towards this end. Deprived of opportunities for face-to-face encounters, individuals like the positive-experiencers identified by Fink et al. (2021) may thus proactively have pursued dynamic user interaction and co-creation online to compensate for lockdown-induced social isolation.

Greater rates of pandemic music making were observed in people with high openness to experience (Finnerty et al. 2021), and those scoring high on the Social Reward factor from the Barcelona Music Reward Questionnaire more frequently attended concerts remotely and played and composed music during lockdown (Ferreri et al. 2021). People who regularly went to concerts before lockdown were also more likely to make music to cope once live music had ceased (Fink et al. 2021).

Such music making for social coping took multifarious forms. Key examples from the Coronamusic Database (Hansen et al. 2021) and other sources include various formats of joint, remote singing and playing by choirs and ensembles (Draper and Dingle 2021; Morgan-Ellis 2021), live-streamed concerts (Swarbrick et al. 2021), digital raves (Palamar and Acosta 2020), online listening parties (Lee and Kao 2020) and daily rituals of clapping for healthcare workers (Imber-Black 2020) and making music from balconies (Calvo and Bejarano 2020).

Calvo and Bejarano's (2020) interviews with participants engaging in balcony singing and playing revealed that their motivations were dominated by social and identity-based themes such as battling loneliness, connecting with neighbours, celebrating birthdays, solidifying cultural or national identities, commemorating the dead, and fulfilling one's duty as an artist. Entertainment, affect expression and stress relief were, however, also mentioned. Although participation varied widely from 4% in Mexico to 36% in Spain, music-making from balconies was generally associated with strong feelings of togetherness (Granot et al. 2021).

Substantial proportions of dancing groups (86%), choirs (83%), and instrumental ensembles (60%) adopted remote formats rather than fully ceasing activities during lockdown (Draper and Dingle 2021). Although many such initiatives were severely troubled by technological challenges and lower ratings of group identification and psychological needs satisfaction in remote compared to in-person formats (Draper and Dingle 2021), they generally succeeded in maintaining identity, sense of purpose, empowerment and social anchoring during difficult times (Morgan-Ellis 2021).

Despite predating the COVID-19 pandemic, live-streamed concerts experienced a notable upsurge during this time. While the well-being implications of new remote concert setups remain to be thoroughly investigated, emerging empirical studies suggest that performances delivered remotely in real time can elicit higher levels of perceived social connection than pre-recorded concerts or originally live-streamed concerts that were watched after the fact (Swarbrick et al. 2021). Wearing virtual reality headsets may further increase feelings of physical presence and connection with the artist (Onderdijk et al. 2021). Intriguingly, felt social connection with performers and fellow audience members increases with the salience of the coronavirus crisis in virtual concert contexts (Swarbrick et al. 2021).

This last finding, in particular, contributes to a growing research literature alluding to the purportedly exceptional coping potential of topically tailored musical repertoires. Specifically in the context of the COVID-19 pandemic, Fink et al. (2021) applied light gradient-boosted regressor models to show that interest in other people's corona-related music was the by far strongest predictor of successful coping through making and listening to music during lockdown. In other words, those who actively engaged with corona-themed repertoires benefited most noticeably from music as a socio-emotional coping tool. This finding emphasises the significance of achieving a scientific understanding of what has been termed the corona-music phenomenon (Hansen 2022b; Hansen et al. 2021). Google search trends for 'music AND corona' in 2020 suggest that interest in this phenomenon increased dramatically in mid-February, peaked in mid-March, and had levelled off by June (Hansen 2022a). Early survey studies from April and May show that 57% developed a moderate-to-extreme interest in coronamusic in France, Germany, India, Italy, the United Kingdom and USA (Fink et al. 2021), and 87.5% of Israelis had been exposed to coronamusic video clips (Ziv and Hollander-Shabtai 2021). Additionally, more than half of Spaniards resided in neighbourhoods with balcony singing, and a quarter of them actively took part (Cabedo-Mas et al. 2021). Some also increased their attendance of live-streamed concerts (Carlson et al. 2021), which was significantly associated with overcoming social isolation (Ferreri et al. 2021).

16.3 Impact of COVID-19 on Music Therapy Approaches

Adapting music therapy for remote delivery.

In addition to everyday coping in the general population, the coronavirus pandemic had a direct effect on music therapy services, which effectively changed overnight. Physical distancing measures coupled with safety concerns for vulnerable clients and low supplies of personal protective equipment meant that music therapists rapidly pivoted to online delivery formats. Remote technologies such as Zoom, Microsoft Teams, Skype, Google Hangouts, WhatsApp and the humble telephone were all used to implement music therapy delivery via video call software (Cole et al. 2021; Knott and Block 2020). An international survey of music therapists in Asia, Europe and the USA indicated that 32.1% of music therapy services were forced to stop globally due to restricted access to suitable software (Agres et al. 2021). Agres et al. (2021) identified that even after the lockdowns ended, many music therapists were no longer allowed to use musical instruments during face-to-face sessions, and many were forbidden from singing. These changes meant that therapists had to adapt how they delivered music therapy in order to maintain a therapeutic relationship with their clients. The proportion of music therapists using technology to deliver their practice has increased from 30% in 2006 to 85.7% during the coronavirus pandemic (Agres et al. 2021).

To support the rapid uptake of remote music therapy, the American Music Therapy Association (AMTA) produced formal guidelines and considerations for remote practice (AMTA 2020). However, many music therapists started implementing remote music therapy before official guidelines were released and documented their experiences to inform future practice. For example, the North London Music Therapy Phone Service had pivoted to a remote service as early as the 19th of March 2020, and was nominated for an award for the speed with which they were able to transform their service (Rizkallah 2020). Additionally, during the COVID-19 pandemic, numerous resources for developing remote music therapy services rapidly emerged on the Internet, such as audio, videos and music-making instructions (Knott and Block 2020). Music therapists now have a wider array of resources to draw from to help them to curate asynchronous sessions (i.e., the music therapist directs people to pre-recorded material that they can engage with at a time that is convenient for them) alongside or instead of synchronous sessions (Knott and Block 2020; Kantorová et al. 2021).

Several case studies and cross-sectional surveys indicate that a range of music therapy practices, including those for dementia, paediatric patients, rehabilitative and palliative care, were able to offer remote options from the early stages of the pandemic. Remote music therapy involves using video call or other types of software to facilitate music therapy sessions with a music therapists, so that the client and therapist are no longer required to physically be in the same room (Note the use of the term 'remote' rather than 'virtual', this is to emphasise the fact that the therapist and music therapy are real and are not part of a 'virtual reality' which tends to involve virtual reality headsets). Remote music therapy is now being used in solo and group contexts (Knott and Block 2020; Kantorová et al. 2021). For example, a joint music-making and listening programme for people with dementia and their caretakers was moved to an online format (Molyneux et al. 2020). Rather than meeting in person, group music therapy sessions were held using Zoom video call software, with a similar structure to in-person sessions. However, given that singing or playing with synchronous feedback was not possible via this platform, a series of activities that required turn-taking were developed. Molyneux et al. (2020) highlighted key learnings that helped to facilitate the sessions more smoothly. The resulting advice included: (i) Provide clear verbal instructions to ensure participants can follow the structure, because more subtle physical gestures may not be easy to understand in a remote setting; (ii) look into the camera rather than at the screen to facilitate more direct engagement from participants; and (iii) manage each participants' microphone during turn-taking activities using the mute function to minimise disruption. It is important to recognise that while opportunities for music-making are limited, continuing online provided continuity and social interactions for participants who may have otherwise become completely isolated due to physical distancing restrictions (Molyneux et al. 2020).

In one mental health setting, co-improvisation approaches were replaced with receptive approaches that involved playing improvised and pre-composed music (Eugster 2021). Active listening approaches were used to help people living in a psychiatric in-patient setting to manage high levels of acute stress during the COVID-19 pandemic. Due to safety protocols, it was not possible for all of the inpatients to engage in active music making. Instead, the music therapist moved to a larger room to facilitate distancing and engaged in thorough before- and after-cleaning protocols. The music therapist reported that this approach led to spontaneous musical interactions including vocalisations, dancing and body movements, which supported further dialogue.

Paediatric patients have also benefitted from remote music therapy during the coronavirus pandemic. In a series of case studies, Goicoechea and Lahue (2021) outlines how remote music therapy delivered using video call software was successfully adopted for children with a range of health conditions, including a 5–year-old that needed a heart transplant, an 11-year-old receiving dialysis and a 16-year-old experiencing grief. Individualised approaches to music therapy were used that followed in-person models of care as closely as possible. Songwriting, music listening and music discussions were all successfully facilitated using video call software. The flexibility of remote music therapy was beneficial because it allowed people to attend music therapy sessions from the comfort of their own homes. This helped to provide patients with an additional avenue of support when they later transitioned out of the hospital environment. However, direct comparisons between in-person and remote singing sessions for children indicate that there are greater benefits from in-person sessions (Grebosz-Haring et al. 2021). A very small study that was conducted before and during the pandemic indicated that both in-person and remote weekly singing sessions may lead to improvements in mood. In-person sessions were also associated with significant decreases in levels of salivary cortisol, whereas remote sessions were associated with increases. The cortisol decreases for in-person sessions was mirrored by a decrease in self-reported stress levels and an increase in self-reported calmness (Grebosz-Haring et al. 2021). This finding suggests that even though remote music therapy can be beneficial, in-person sessions may lead to enhanced efficacy. However, it is not possible to be conclusive with this comparison given that the in-person sessions were conducted in a completely different context (i.e., pre-pandemic), compared to the remote sessions (i.e., during the pandemic). It is also possible that the reported differences in cortisol and stress levels may be related to the acutely stressful nature of the pandemic itself. Future research comparing the efficacy of remote sessions compared to in-person sessions should ensure adequate control for the broader context, perhaps by running different types of sessions at the same time, or by using cross-over trial designs.

16.3.1 Music Therapists' Perspective on Remote Approaches Compared to In-Person Approaches

The opportunity to transition to a remote format was broadly welcomed by music therapists (Kantorová et al. 2021). However, music therapists also highlighted the limitations of technology-based approaches and inherent challenges that arise from not being in the same room (Agres et al. 2021; Cole et al. 2021). Technological issues that disrupted the flow of communication between client and therapist included poor and unreliable Internet speeds, difficulty in achieving dual sound (i.e., two or more simultaneous audio streams) and poor sound quality (Agres et al. 2021). For example, some music therapists report difficulties with using video call software for synchronous music playing between the therapist and client, due to time delays and acoustic feedback issues (Cole et al. 2021; Molyneux et al. 2020; Goicoechea and Lahue 2021). Time delays can be minimised when the therapist and client both use Ethernet cables rather than relying on Wi-Fi connections. However, it seems that the future success of remote music therapy may depend on software improvements or on introducing specialised music-making software that can facilitate synchronous music playing, to music therapy settings (Goicoechea and Lahue 2021). Greater access to software that allows for better real-time music making, including simultaneous instrument-playing and singing, will vastly improve the quality and variety of remote music therapy interactions (Goicoechea and Lahue 2021).

Another technological challenge is that video call and music-making software is not typically adapted for the needs of people with limited physical mobility or intellectual disabilities (Agres et al. 2021). This is particularly challenging for remote music therapy intended to support physical rehabilitation. Future attempts to deliver music therapy using video call or other types of software will need to consider the accessibility and reliability of the technology used to ensure that they meet the needs of specific client groups.

Although some technological limitations may be possible to address in the future, remote interactions will always be more limited when the client and therapist are not in the same room. In a large, cross-sectional survey of music therapists in Asia, the USA and Europe, 38% reported that 'not being in the same room' reduced their capacity to know the right timing for interventions. Reduced physical proximity and limited visual access limit the degree to which therapists can attune to and empathise with the client (Agres et al. 2021). In these scenarios, therapists and clients are required to take turns to play music, which potentially limits the vitality and richness of the interaction and eliminates the possibility of achieving musical resonance (Kantorová et al. 2021). The reduced richness in the interactions may also lead to reduced levels of engagement and attention with the therapeutic sessions, evidenced by clients who are more easily distracted and more easily exhausted (Agres et al. 2021). Not being in the same room also makes it more difficult for the therapist to maintain healthy boundaries in the client-therapist relationship (Kantorová et al. 2021). This may be part of the reason that 48–60% of music therapists across two studies felt that remote sessions were not as effective as in-person sessions (Agres et al. 2021; Cole et al. 2021). Similarly, neurologic music therapists reported that not being in the same room limited the degree to which they could deliver some sensorimotor approaches (Cole et al. 2021).

Although most aspects of neurologic music therapy could be delivered, therapists reported specific difficulties with gait training. Gait training requires physical supports and, therefore, cannot be delivered in a remote environment (Cole et al. 2021). Although it is clear from the case studies above that remote music therapy is better than no music therapy, there may be additional benefits from physical in-person music therapy that cannot be readily replaced with technology. Hybrid approaches to music therapy, which use a mix of both in-person and remote sessions to provide a more flexible and accessible service while maintaining the full clinical benefits of music therapy, should be considered.

16.4 Emergence of COVID-19-Specific Music Therapy Practices

Along with the transition of longstanding music therapy services into remote formats, entirely new music therapy practices were also developed during the novel coronavirus pandemic. Safety procedures meant that hospital patients had less physical contact and human interactions with healthcare staff. Visors, bodysuits, facemasks and extensive hygiene procedures across hospital and care home settings reduced the degree to which healthcare staff could effectively interact with and reassure patients. Music therapy was identified as a strategy to overcome the barriers posed by physical distancing measures in a range of settings, including (i) in high-risk settings (e.g., intensive care units); (ii) to support rehabilitation of long-term COVID-19 symptoms; and (iii) for mental health management for patients and healthcare staff.

16.4.1 Intensive Care Units

Music was used in intensive care units to overcome the barriers of social isolation and re-humanise the experience of intensive care (Ettenberger et al. 2021; Rivi et al. 2021; Reidy and MacDonald 2021; Silva Junior et al. 2021). A meta-analysis based on 14 randomised controlled trials indicates that music listening can help to reduce anxiety in mechanically ventilated patients (Bradt and Dileo 2014) and provides support for using music with COVID-19 patients who are mechanically ventilated. Similarly, music was introduced for COVID-19 patients to reduce the burden from extended isolation (Rivi et al. 2021). Patients with COVID-19 who were admitted to intensive care units would not be able to see their friends and family until they were discharged, and restricted visitation schedules may have been particularly traumatic for patients and their loved ones, given the high mortality rate (Rivi et al. 2021).

Despite the challenges of physical restrictions, some music therapists found ways to deliver music therapy in the most restricted parts of intensive care units

(Reidy and MacDonald 2021). Wireless speakers were used to bring music into isolation rooms, and music therapy sessions were able to continue through screens (Reidy and MacDonald 2021), and nursing staff played live music in intensive care (Silva Junior et al. 2021). An initial qualitative study from Paraíba in Brazil identified that live music playing in intensive care units was beneficial to patients because it was associated with reduced stress and improved mood (Silva Junior et al. 2021). Qualitative reports from seven nurses who were working clinically at the time identified that some patients' sad facial expressions transformed into happy faces, and they noticed several members of staff also became emotional. These findings are broadly consistent with formal evaluations of music therapy in intensive care units that identify that music listening can help to reduce anxiety (Bradt and Dileo 2014), stabilise stress levels, attenuate stress and reduce caregiver anxiety (Yue et al. 2021). Further evaluations will help to identify specific strategies required to tailor music interventions to meet the needs of patients in the context of COVID-19.

16.4.2 Supporting Rehabilitation of Long-Term COVID-19 Symptoms

Music may be useful to help with long-term rehabilitation of long COVID-19 symptoms. Typical long-term effects of COVID-19 include anxiety, breathlessness, pain and difficulty sleeping (Del Rio et al. 2020), and there is strong evidence to suggest that music can be used to manage these symptoms. Numerous randomised controlled trials, systematic reviews and meta-analyses demonstrate the clinical benefits of music for pain management (Lee 2016), insomnia (Jespersen et al. 2015) and pulmonary obstructive disorder (McNamara et al. 2017). Although these previous studies do not look directly at COVID-19, their approaches could be adapted for COVID-19. Current rehabilitation programmes for COVID-19 tend to focus on the core issues related to breathlessness and respiratory function by using progressive exercise programmes and multicomponent interventions (Goodwin et al. 2021). Preliminary studies suggest that there may be an added benefit of including music in psychological interventions. For example, one study with 70 participants incorporated soothing music listening to a series of pulmonary exercises and psychological group interventions and found that this combination of interventions reduced symptoms of anxiety and improved insomnia for people with COVID-19 (Ying et al. 2021). Unfortunately, the study did not isolate the relative contributions from each component of the interventions, so the degree to which music contributes to the added benefits is not clear from this study. Nonetheless, given the evidence that demonstrates the role of music in reducing pain (Lee 2016), insomnia (Jespersen et al. 2015), and improving physical function in the context of respiratory disease (McNamara et al. 2017), there is good reason to think that music could also be beneficial in the context of long-COVID-19 symptom management.

Based on these findings, practitioners have tailored music activities to rehabilitate lung function. Initiatives such as the ENO Breathe program developed by the English National Opera use vocal training techniques and breathing exercises developed and used by opera singers to support breathing control and reduce associated anxiety (Brunjes 2021). Over the course of a six-week programme, participants learn breathing exercises (e.g., blowing bubbles in a glass of water using a straw, singing the shape of their names if written in the air in cursive, and gently stretching their neck) and are given access to supportive online resources between sessions. Using a single blind randomised controlled trial with 150 participants, Philip et al. (2022) identified that participation in the operatic breathing exercises led to significant reductions in breathlessness and improvements in mental health scores. Regional health trusts across the United Kingdom are now beginning to adopt the ENO approach to help long-COVID-19 survivors (Brunjes 2021).

16.4.3 Mental Health Management for Patients and Healthcare Staff

The COVID-19 pandemic placed an enormous emotional burden on healthcare staff (Benfante et al. 2020). Longer working hours and an increased risk of contracting COVID-19 made healthcare workers vulnerable to acute stress and mental health concerns such as anxiety or depression (Rivi et al. 2021). In acknowledgement of the intense acute levels of stress experienced by hospital workers during the first pandemic wave, new music therapy phone lines were established to support hospital workers (Rizkallah 2020). In the United Kingdom, this was initially done on an ad-hoc basis by local charity groups and was eventually replaced by a national music therapy service for staff supported by the National Health Service (NHS). Given the sense of emergency during the early stages of the pandemic, music therapy in this context was delivered on a short-term basis. Psychological first-aid techniques were used as the basis of care rather than cognitive behavioural or psychotherapeutic approaches. This means that the music therapist put a greater emphasis on actively listening to the stress being experienced by the client in the present moment, without encouraging them to reflect on previous experiences or perceived associations. Rizkallah (2020) identified that healthcare staff needed a place to talk and offload on a short-term basis, to cope with the daily stress that they were experiencing. Clients were given the opportunity to engage in music-making, playlist-building and music listening; however, none of the 22 service users opted to participate in the music aspects of the service and relied wholly on talking to their music therapist. Further evaluation is required to determine why healthcare staff would opt in for music therapy sessions voluntarily and then decline to participate in music-related activities. Nonetheless, this case report demonstrates a clear role for music therapists in an emergency response.

16.5 Concluding Remarks and Recommendations

Just as the emergence of music therapy can be traced to the global trauma of the Second World War, it seems the second wave of music therapy may have started in the COVID-19 pandemic. Faced with sudden societal lockdowns and enforced social isolation during the early months of the novel coronavirus pandemic, the general population developed a wide range of lockdown-compatible psychological coping strategies. Music played an exceptionally prominent role amongst these strategies, showing superior coping potential compared to many other available pastime activities. Depending on individual predispositions and the severity with which people were affected by the pandemic, musical coping behaviours served to regulate emotions and stress levels, compensate for social hypo-stimulation and/or fight boredom with much-needed entertainment and diversion. Consequently, music selection was exceptionally diverse with concurrent elements of sad and happy emotions and exploratory alongside nostalgic repertoires. However, findings that interest in corona-themed music was especially popular and constituted the strongest predictor of how much music helped people regulate emotions and feel connected to others suggest that contextually tailored musical innovations could have been particularly adaptive for managing past and future societal crises.

Unique adaptations were made to music therapy approaches to support and rehabilitate people with coronavirus. Physical distancing measures such as masks, visors, aprons and time limits reduced the degree to which medical staff and visitors could interact with coronavirus-infected patients. To bridge the isolation created by physical distancing measures in hospitals and intensive care units, music was introduced to help COVID-19 patients feel emotionally connected to people. Music therapists adapted their practice almost overnight using video call software, so that they could continue to provide treatment services to their patients when they needed it most. New initiatives, such as the English National Opera Breathe programme, which used operatic breathing and singing exercises to improve breathlessness and mental health, were introduced. Overall, the emerging research literature on the use of music during lockdown converges on the conclusion that music has been instrumental in the fight against the novel coronavirus pandemic and its associated effects, to support the social, emotional and physical needs of a range of populations, including healthy people in lockdown, patients in intensive care units, long-term survivors and healthcare workers in hospital settings.

References

Agres KR, Foubert K, Sridhar S (2021) Music therapy during COVID-19: changes to the practice, use of technology, and what to carry forward in the future. Front Psychol 12:1317

American Music Therapy Association (AMTA) (2020) AMTA telehealth/therapy statement. Retrieved from https://www.musictherapy.org/music_therapy_in_telehealth. Accessed 5 Jan 2022

Ayouni I, Maatoug J, Dhouib W, Zammit N, Fredj SB, Ghammam R, Ghannem H (2021) Effective public health measures to mitigate the spread of COVID-19: a systematic review. BMC Pub Health 21(1):1–14

Benfante A, Di Tella M, Romeo A, Castelli L (2020) Traumatic stress in healthcare workers during COVID-19 pandemic: a review of the immediate impact. Front Psychol 11:2816. https://doi.org/10.3389/fpsyg.2020.569935

Bradt J, Dileo C (2014) Music interventions for mechanically ventilated patients. Cochrane Database Syst Rev 12:CD006902. https://doi.org/10.1002/14651858.CD006902.pub3

Brunjes HO (2021) ENO Breathe: 'The art of medicine and the science of the arts'. J R Soc Med 114(5):246–249

Cabedo-Mas A, Arriaga-Sanz C, Moliner-Miravet L (2021) Uses and perceptions of music in times of COVID-19: a Spanish population survey. Front Psychol 11:606180. https://doi.org/10.3389/fpsyg.2020.606180

Calvo K, Bejarano E (2020) Music, solidarities and balconies in Spain. Interface 12(1):326–332

Carlson E, Wilson J, Baltazar M, Duman D, Peltola H-R, Toiviainen P, Saarikallio SH (2021) The role of music in everyday life during the first wave of the COVID-19 pandemic: a mixed-methods exploratory study. Front Psychol 12:647756. https://doi.org/10.3389/fpsyg.2021.647756

Cho E, Ilari BS (2021) Mothers as home DJs: recorded music and young children's well-being during the COVID-19 pandemic. Front Psychol 12:637569. https://doi.org/10.3389/fpsyg.2021.637569

Cole LP, Henechowicz TL, Kang K, Pranjić M, Richard NM, Tian GL, Hurt-Thaut C (2021) Neurologic music therapy via telehealth: a survey of clinician experiences, trends, and recommendations during the COVID-19 pandemic. Front Neurosci 15:347

Del Rio C, Collins LF, Malani P (2020) Long-term health consequences of COVID-19. JAMA 324(17):1723–1724

Draper G, Dingle GA (2021) It's not the same: a comparison of the psychological needs satisfied by musical group activities in face to face and virtual modes. Front Psychol 12:646292. https://doi.org/10.3389/fpsyg.2021.646292

Ettenberger M, Sgobbi B, Eguchi R, Ardila YMB, Serrano SAT, Bolis ME, Agosti M (2021) COVID-19: implications and considerations for NICU music therapy in Italy, Japan and Colombia. Music Med 13(2):112–123

Eugster M (2021) Adaptations of music therapy practice in an acute mental health setting during the COVID-19 pandemic. J Music Health Wellbeing:1–12

Fancourt D, Steptoe A, Bu F (2021) Trajectories of anxiety and depressive symptoms during enforced isolation due to COVID-19 in England: a longitudinal observational study. Lancet Psychiat 8(2):141–149. https://doi.org/10.1016/S2215-0366(20)30482-X

Ferreri L, Singer N, McPhee M, Ripollés P, Zatorre RJ, Mas-Herrero E (2021) Engagement in music-related activities during the COVID-19 pandemic as a mirror of individual differences in musical reward and coping strategies. Front Psychol 12:673772. https://doi.org/10.3389/fpsyg.2021.673772

Fink L, Warrenburg LA, Howlin C, Randall WM, Hansen NC, Wald-Fuhrmann M (2021) Viral tunes: changes in musical behaviours and interest in coronamusic predict socio-emotional coping during COVID-19 lockdown. Hum Soc Sci Commun 8(180). https://doi.org/10.1057/s41599-021-00858-y

Finnerty R, Marshall S, Imbault C, Trainor LJ (2021) Extra-curricular activities and well-being: results from a survey of undergraduate university students during COVID-19 lockdown restrictions. Front Psychol 12:647402. https://doi.org/10.3389/fpsyg.2021.647402

Gibbs H, Egermann H (2021) Music-evoked nostalgia and wellbeing during the United Kingdom COVID-19 pandemic: content, subjective effects, and function. Front Psychol 12:647891. https://doi.org/10.3389/fpsyg.2021.647891

Goicoechea T, Lahue K (2021) Case studies in pediatric music therapy during COVID-19. Music Ther Perspect 39(2):126–132. https://doi.org/10.1093/mtp/miab009

Goodwin VA, Allan L, Bethel A, Cowley A, Cross JL, Day J et al (2021) Rehabilitation to enable recovery from COVID-19: a rapid systematic review. Physiotherapy 111:4–22

Granot R, Spitz D, Cherki B, Loui P, Timmers R, Schaefer R, Vuoskoski J, Cárdenas-Soler R-N, Soares-Quadros JF Jr et al (2021) Help! I need somebody: music as a global resource for

obtaining wellbeing goals in times of crisis. Front Psychol 12:648013. https://doi.org/10.3389/fpsyg.2021.648013
Grebosz-Haring KA, Schuchter-Wiegand AK, Feneberg AC, Skoluda N, Nater UM, Sebastian S, Leonhard TH (2021) The psychological and biological impact of "in-person" vs. "virtual" choir singing in children and adolescents: a pilot study before and after the acute phase of the COVID-19 outbreak in Austria. Front Psychol:5999
Hale, T., Angrist, N., Goldszmidt, R., Kira, B., Petherick, A., Phillips, T., ... & Tatlow, H. (2021). A global panel database of pandemic policies (Oxford COVID-19 Government Response Tracker). Nature human behaviour, 5(4), 529–538.
Hansen NC (2022a) Music for hedonia and eudaimonia during pandemic social isolation. In: Chemi T, Brattico E, Fjorback LO, Harmat L (eds) Arts and mindfulness education for human flourishing. Routledge, pp 89–105. https://doi.org/10.4324/9781003158790-8
Hansen NC (2022b) Coping with crisis through coronamusic. In: Agamennone M, Palma D, Sarno G (eds) Sounds of the pandemic: accounts, experiences, reflections, perspectives in times of Covid-19, New York, Routledge, pp 272–284. https://doi.org/10.4324/9781003200369-25
Hansen NC, Treider JMG, Swarbrick D, Bamford JS, Wilson J, Vuoskoski JK (2021) A crowd-sourced database of coronamusic: documenting online making and sharing of music during the COVID-19 pandemic. Front Psychol 12:684083. https://doi.org/10.3389/fpsyg.2021.684083
Henry N, Egermann H, Kayser D (2021) Music in mood regulation and coping orientations in response to COVID-19 lockdown measures within the United Kingdom. Front Psychol 12:647879. https://doi.org/10.3389/fpsyg.2021.647879
Hossain MM, Tasnim S, Sultana A, Faizah F, Mazumder H, Zou L, Lisako E, McKyer J, Ahmed HU, Ma P (2020) Epidemiology of mental health problems in COVID-19: a review. F1000Research 9:636. https://doi.org/10.12688/f1000research.24457.1
Hurwitz ER, Krumhansl CL (2021) Shifting listening niches: effects of the COVID-19 pandemic. Front Psychol 12:648413. https://doi.org/10.3389/fpsyg.2021.648413
Imber-Black E (2020) Rituals in the time of COVID-19: imagination, responsiveness, and the human spirit. Fam Process 59(3):912–921. https://doi.org/10.1111/famp.12581
Jespersen KV, Koenig J, Jennum P, Vuust P (2015) Music for insomnia in adults. Cochrane Database Syst Rev 8:CD010459. https://doi.org/10.1002/14651858.CD010459.pub2
Kantorová L, Kantor J, Hořejší B, Gilboa A, Svobodová Z, Lipský M et al (2021) Adaptation of music therapists' practice to the outset of the COVID-19 pandemic—Going virtual: A scoping review. Int J Environ Res Public Health 18(10):5138
Kiernan F, Chmiel A, Garrido S, Hickey M, Davidson JW (2021) The role of artistic creative activities in navigating the COVID-19 pandemic in Australia. Front Psychol 12:696202. https://doi.org/10.3389/fpsyg.2021.696202
Knott D, Block S (2020) Virtual music therapy: developing new approaches to service delivery. Music Ther Perspect 38(2):151–156
Kocalevent RD, Hinz A, Brähler E (2013) Standardization of the depression screener patient health questionnaire (PHQ-9) in the general population. Gen Hosp Psychiatry 35(5):551–555
Krause AE, Dimmock J, Rebar AL, Jackson B (2021) Music listening predicted improved life satisfaction in university students during early stages of the COVID-19 pandemic. Front Psychol 11:631033. https://doi.org/10.3389/fpsyg.2020.631033
Lee JH (2016) The effects of music on pain: a meta-analysis. J Music Ther 53(4):430–477
Lee W, Kao G (2020) You know you're missing out on something: collective nostalgia and community in Tim's Twitter Listening Party during COVID-19. Rock Music Studies 8(1):36–52. https://doi.org/10.1080/19401159.2020.1852772
Mak HW, Fluharty M, Fancourt D (2021) Predictors and impact of arts engagement during the COVID-19 pandemic: analyses of data from 19,384 adults in the COVID-19 social study. Front Psychol 12:626263. https://doi.org/10.3389/fpsyg.2021.626263
Martínez-Castilla P, Gutiérrez-Blasco I, Spitz DH, Granot R (2021) The efficacy of music for emotional wellbeing during the COVID-19 lockdown in Spain: an analysis of personal and context-related variables. Front Psychol 12:647837. https://doi.org/10.3389/fpsyg.2021.647837

Mas-Herrero E, Singer N, Ferreri L, McPhee M, Zatorre R, Ripolles P (2020) Rock'n'roll but not sex or drugs: music is negatively correlated to depressive symptoms during the COVID-19 pandemic via reward-related mechanisms. PsyArXiv. https://doi.org/10.31234/osf.io/x5upn

Mazza C, Ricci E, Biondi S, Colasanti M, Ferracuti S, Napoli C, Roma P (2020) A nationwide survey of psychological distress among Italian people during the COVID-19 pandemic: immediate psychological responses and associated factors. Int J Environ Res Public Health 17(9):3165. https://doi.org/10.3390/ijerph17093165

McNamara RJ, Epsley C, Coren E, McKeough ZJ (2017) Singing for adults with chronic obstructive pulmonary disease. Cochrane Database Syst Rev 12:CD012296. https://doi.org/10.1002/14651858.CD012296.pub2

Molyneux C, Hardy T, Lin YTC, McKinnon K, Odell-Miller H (2020) Together in sound: music therapy groups for people with dementia and their companions–moving online in response to a pandemic. Approaches:1–17. ISSN 2459-3338

Morgan-Ellis EM (2021) Like pieces in a puzzle: online sacred harp singing during the COVID-19 pandemic. Front Psychol 12:627038. https://doi.org/10.3389/fpsyg.2021.627038

Onderdijk KE, Swarbrick D, Van Kerrebroeck B, Mantei M, Vuoskoski JK, Maes PJ, Leman M (2021) Livestream experiments: the role of COVID-19, agency, presence, and social context in facilitating social connectedness. Front Psychol 12:647929. https://doi.org/10.3389/fpsyg.2021.647929

Palamar JJ, Acosta P (2020) Virtual raves and happy hours during COVID-19: new drug use contexts for electronic dance music partygoers. Int J Drug Policy 93:102904. https://doi.org/10.1016/j.drugpo.2020.102904

Pan K-Y, Kok AAL, Eikelenboom M, Horsfall M, Jörg F, Luteijn RA, Rhebergen D, van Oppen P, Giltay EJ, Penninx BWJH (2021) The mental health impact of the COVID-19 pandemic on people with and without depressive, anxiety, or obsessive-compulsive disorders: a longitudinal study of three Dutch case-control cohorts. Lancet Psychiatry 8(2):121–129. https://doi.org/10.1016/S2215-0366(20)30491-0

Philip KE, Owles H, McVey S, Pagnuco T, Bruce K, Brunjes H et al (2022) An online breathing and wellbeing programme (ENO breathe) for people with persistent symptoms following COVID-19: a parallel-group, single-blind, randomised controlled trial. Lancet Respir Med 10(9):851–862

Porcher S (2020) Response2covid19, a dataset of governments' responses to COVID-19 all around the world. Sci Data 7(1):1–9. https://doi.org/10.1038/s41597-020-00757-y

Reidy J, MacDonald MC (2021) Use of palliative care music therapy in a hospital setting during COVID-19. J Palliat Med 4(11):1603–1605

Ribeiro FS, Lessa JPA, Delmolin G, Santos FH (2021) Music listening in times of COVID-19 outbreak: a Brazilian study. Front Psychol 12:647473. https://doi.org/10.3389/fpsyg.2021.647473

Rivi V, Melegari G, Blom JM (2021) How to humanise the COVID-19 intensive care units. BMJ Evid Based Med. https://doi.org/10.1136/bmjebm-2020-111513

Rizkallah M (2020) The North London music therapy phone support service for NHS staff during the COVID-19 pandemic: A report about the service and its relevance for the music therapy profession. Approaches:1–9

Silva Junior SV, Machado AG, Alves AMRS, Cordeiro KJS, Barbosa MB, Teodozio GC et al (2021) Humanizing intensive nursing care for people with COVID-19. Rev Rene 22:e62584. https://doi.org/10.15253/2175-6783.20212262584

Sim J, Cho D, Hwang Y, Telang R (2020) Virus shook the streaming star: estimating the COVID-19 impact on music consumption. SSRN Electron J. https://doi.org/10.2139/ssrn.3649085

Swarbrick D, Seibt B, Grinspun N, Vuoskoski JK (2021) Corona concerts: the effect of virtual concert characteristics on social connection and Kama muta. Front Psychol 12:648448. https://doi.org/10.3389/fpsyg.2021.648448

Torales J, O'Higgins M, Castaldelli-Maia JM, Ventriglio A (2020) The outbreak of COVID-19 coronavirus and its impact on global mental health. Int J Soc Psychiatry 66(4):317–320. https://doi.org/10.1177/0020764020915212

Vidas D, Larwood JL, Nelson NL, Dingle GA (2021) Music listening as a strategy for managing COVID-19 stress in first-year university students. Front Psychol 12:647065. https://doi.org/10.3389/fpsyg.2021.647065

Wang C, Pan R, Wan X, Tan Y, Xu L, McIntyre RS, Choo FN et al (2020a) A longitudinal study on the mental health of general population during the COVID-19 epidemic in China. Brain Behav Immun 87:40–48. https://doi.org/10.1016/j.bbi.2020.04.028

Wang H, Xia Q, Xiong Z, Li Z, Xiang W, Yuan Y, Liu Y, Li Z (2020b) The psychological distress and coping styles in the early stages of the 2019 coronavirus disease (COVID-19) epidemic in the general mainland Chinese population: a web-based survey. PLoS One 15(5):e0233410. https://doi.org/10.1371/journal.pone.0233410

World Health Organization (2020) Director-General's opening remarks at the media briefing on COVID-19—11 March 2020. World Health Organization (WHO) (Press release). 11 March 2020. Archived from the original on 11 March 2020. Retrieved 15 Feb 2022

Yeung TYC (2020) Did the COVID-19 pandemic trigger nostalgia? Evidence of music consumption on Spotify. SSRN Electron J. https://doi.org/10.2139/ssrn.3678606

Ying L, Yan-Qing Y, Yan L, Sheng-Li P, Hui-Hui Y, Jia-Jia W, Cai-Kui L (2021) Effects of group psychological intervention combined with pulmonary rehabilitation exercises on anxiety and sleep disorders in patients with mild coronavirus disease 2019 (COVID-19) infections in a Fangcang hospital. Psychol Health Wellbeing. https://doi.org/10.1080/13548506.2021.1916956

Young KS, Purves KL, Hübel C, Davies MR, Thompson KN, Bristow S et al (2022) Depression, anxiety and PTSD symptoms before and during the COVID-19 pandemic in the UK. Psychol Med 1-14. https://doi.org/10.1017/S0033291722002501

Yue W, Han X, Luo J, Zeng Z, Yang M (2021) Effect of music therapy on preterm infants in neonatal intensive care unit: systematic review and meta-analysis of randomized controlled trials. J Adv Nurs 77(2):635–652

Ziv N, Hollander-Shabtai R (2021) Music and COVID-19: changes in uses and emotional reaction to music under stay-at-home restrictions. Psychol Music. https://doi.org/10.1177/03057356211003326

17 Listening to Music and Emotion Regulation in Adulthood

Tim Loepthien and Bernhard Leipold

One of the most fascinating aspects of *experiencing* music is the dynamic in feelings that arises, i.e., how music plays with emotions. Arousal moods and self-forgetfulness are not rare experiences felt by only a few experts. Music is used widely as a relaxation method, not only for its emotion-regulating function but also for educational demands that can be involved. This has been documented throughout history many times. In the introduction to his music theory (circa sixth century BC), Boetius reports Plato's view that minds suffer from immoral music and agrees with Cicero that the frenzied exuberance of drunken young men can be calmed down by a change in the way the flute is played (Boetius 1985). Descriptions of music such as *the language of feeling* (Ludwig Feuerbach), *of passion* (Richard Wagner), and as having *the deepest influence on the mind of all arts* (Napoleon Bonaparte) are quotes that are still widely used in everyday language.

As plausible as these examples that illustrate the connection between music and emotions may still seem today, regarding their influence by music, on closer inspection they are not self-evident but are rather in need of explanation. They are opposed to scientific studies that have investigated the effects of music on emotions when listening or making music, thereby highlighting the enormous complexity of this interaction (Eerola and Vuoskoski 2013; Juslin and Laukka 2004; Panksepp and Bernatzky 2002). In the following, the phenomenon of emotion regulation through music will be considered in more detail, especially in adulthood. We focus on some aspects, e.g., what it means to regulate not only one's emotions but also one's own development (i.e., the psychological processes involved, the extent of their control or intentional inducibility). The lifespan perspective (Baltes et al. 1999) has played an increasing role in the consideration of musical activities in recent decades

T. Loepthien (✉) · B. Leipold
Universität der Bundeswehr München, Institut für Psychologie, Neubiberg, Germany
e-mail: tim.loepthien@unibw.de; bernhard.leipold@unibw.de

G. Kreutz, G. Bernatzky (eds.), *Music and Medicine*, Neurocultural Health and Wellbeing, https://doi.org/10.1007/978-3-662-72175-9_17

(Gembris 2012, 2018). It has also led to studies showing age-related changes in emotion regulation.

17.1 Basics

17.1.1 Emotion Regulation, Coping, and Self-Regulation

Emotion regulation refers to the issue of how to control one's feelings. This issue is of broad interest; corresponding needs are addressed by the music industry (cf. relaxation music, entertaining music) and are the subject of consultant books. However, techniques for coping with negative emotions are also applied in psychotherapy. General and comprehensive process models of emotion regulation (Gross 1998; Koole and Aldao 2016) refer to the regulation of specific emotional responses and global moods and include short-term changes as well as chronic, persistent emotional states. Gross defines emotion regulation as "the processes by which individuals influence which emotions they have, when they have them, and how they experience and express these emotions." (Gross 1998, S. 275). He distinguishes between *antecedent-focused emotion regulation* and *response-focused emotion regulation*. The former includes regulation by manipulating the input to the system through which one avoids situations or modifies an environment to alter its emotional impact (see also attentional deployment and cognitive reinterpretation), while processes of response modulation relate to the regulation of intensity, expression, and experience of already triggered emotions. In contrast to process models, (Gross 1998) in which emotion regulation itself is the subject of interest, there are mediation models (Karreman and Vingerhoets 2012), which focus on how emotion regulation is associated with other constructs and, for example, mediates the connection with general well-being.

The construct of *self-regulation* is closely related to that of emotion regulation and is also treated jointly with it (Brandtstädter 2007; Carver 2015; Saarikallio 2011). Whereas in emotion regulation, efforts focus on controlling or changing emotions; in the case of self-regulation, it is the goals of actions in general which contribute to a person's identity development that are the focus of change. The intention to learn an instrument in retirement can become an identity project, the implementation of which is one form of positive ageing.

Another construct that overlaps with emotion regulation is *coping*, i.e., adaptation to stressful or traumatizing situations. Coping refers to strategies and responses (Carver 2011) that people use to solve problems, e.g., problem-oriented, emotion-oriented, and meaning-oriented coping. If listening to music helps alleviate depressive feelings in difficult life situations, then coping and emotion regulation overlap.

A common function of the processes described (emotion regulation, self-regulation, coping), which will be discussed in more detail in the course of the current chapter, is the compensation of the discrepancies between actual states and desired or ought states. If a person notices a discrepancy between their current and desired state, then regulatory processes set in. Thus, actions can be taken to achieve the desired state (the personal goal), or one's own standards can be changed (Brandtstädter 2007; Leipold 2020). Discrepancies are accompanied by emotions, (Carver 2015) such as anger over blocked personal goals, joy at achieving such goals, or sadness that these goals can no longer be achieved. Emotions are not by-products of self-regulatory processes; however, some of them, insofar as they motivate people to initiate actions or regulate certain cognitive states (e.g., attention) that are functional for the achievement of goals (Carver 2015; Fredrickson 2001; Karnaze and Levine 2018). In this sense, emotion regulation is also related to the pursuit of personal goals (Tamir 2016), self-regulating processes, and coping.

Emotion regulation, self-regulation, and coping are characterized by planning and strategic efforts; in the purposeful listening of relaxing music after a strenuous day, these efforts are consciously initiated and intentionally controlled. In particular, strategies were used to refer to planned action steps (Saarikallio 2011). However, this also includes psychological and physiological processes that take place automatically and are not subject to wilful control (Koole and Rothermund 2011) For example, the positive reinterpretation of a rejection (e.g., after an audition with a renowned big band) presupposes the processing of cognition (e.g., being part of a renowned, international touring ensemble), which then results in a plausible, non-constructed view ("It is not bad that I did not get the place in the big band. Now I can spend more time with my family"). However, the emotion regulation strategies that are necessary for attentional deployment and cognitive reinterpretation (Gross 1998) are often not subject to intentional control (Brandtstädter 2007; Koole and Rothermund 2011), which is also valid for many processes that are involved in musical emotion regulation. We will return to this topic later.

In the following, we refer to musical settings (e.g., listening to and making music, musical interventions) in relation to emotion regulation, self-regulation, and coping. The focus is on adulthood, i.e., what role listening to music and making music plays against the background of ageing (changes in physical and mental resources). The psychology of the lifespan provides the conceptual framework.

17.1.2 Lifespan Psychology

The division of the human lifespan into life phases can be traced back to antiquity and has been the subject of novels and pieces of art (e.g., the motif of life stairs). Friedrich August Carus (1808) differentiated general mental characteristics of childhood, adolescence, adulthood, and old age, while Charlotte Bühler (1933) relied on 50 anamnesis and approximately 200 biographies to generalize the structures of the life course. Influential works that have taken into account the entire lifespan have been related to *developmental tasks* (Havighurst 1948) and *psychosocial crises* (Erikson 1959). Nevertheless, it should be noted that in developmental psychological research, interest in childhood and growth dominated for a long time; it was not until the 1960s and the beginning of the field of lifespan psychology that interest in adulthood and old age increased, and methodological standards (e.g., the limitations of longitudinal and cross-sectional studies) came to be discussed. Both

Erikson's and Havighurst's models can be used to derive life paths that the authors evaluate as either successful or socially desirable. The current models of lifespan psychology do not formulate normative standards. Rather, a specific adaptation can be considered "successful" if personal and social resources and skills are expanded or maintained; thus, it remains possible to deal with future challenges and losses (Baltes et al. 1999; Greve and Thomsen 2019).

In particular, developmental regulation theories have described psychological processes that allow the individual to adapt to demands and changed circumstances (the *two-process model of assimilation and accommodation*, Brandtstädter 2007; the *model of selection, optimization and compensation* (SOC), Baltes et al. 1999; *the lifespan theory of control*, Heckhausen and Schulz 1995). These theories have formulated assumptions about the change in motivational and emotional processes in adulthood, which are also important for understanding musical emotion regulation. When dealing with demands in adolescence and young adulthood, the development of personal resources and competencies is crucial to overcome obstacles and achieve personal goals (Baltes et al. 1999). If a new piano piece or a particularly challenging passage confronts a young pianist with enormous challenges, she can deal with by increasing practice and reducing distractions. However, the adaptation processes change due to increasing age and the associated physical and cognitive losses. Maintaining the current level of functionality and minimizing losses become more important, and resources are less invested in growth.

To explain the *SOC model,* Paul Baltes liked to quote the advanced-aged yet still-concerting pianist Arthur Rubinstein, who described in a television interview how he was able to give concerts despite his age-related losses. He plays fewer pieces (selection), practises them more frequently (optimization), and introduces a ritardando before fast passages, which makes them appear faster (compensation; Baltes et al. 1999). These strategies are also observable in younger adults, and people differ in the concrete means by which they implement them. The motivation to use resources, however, is more focused on developmental gains in younger adulthood (Freund and Nikitin 2018). According to the *two-process model* (Brandtstädter 2007), people have two methods of adaptation when their goals are blocked. One method tenaciously holds on to them (assimilation), increases the effort and, for example, continues to pursue a soloist career despite an accident-related handicap. It is possible that one's own demands are fulfilled and positive emotions are triggered. In the second method (accommodation), one comes to terms with the circumstances and shifts one's plans to composing music, music education, management, or other alternatives, depending on one's interests and abilities. By adjusting one's own standards, well-being can be maintained despite restrictions in certain areas of one's life. In the first half of life, the focus is on adaptation processes that tend to be more focused on adhering to personal goals, while in old age, processes that are aimed at adapting personal goals to changing circumstances and resource losses gain more relevance (Baltes et al. 1999; Brandtstädter et al. 1993).

The development regulatory models have in common an action-theoretical perspective that sees goal setting, commitment, and disengagement processes as central to development despite declining action resources. These processes are also involved in coping, emotion, and self-regulation and play an important role in the individual's adaptation to challenges and losses. There is empirical evidence that emotional experience changes over the lifespan. Older people report more positive emotional well-being, are more emotionally stable, and experience more complex emotional states, i.e., the co-occurrence of positive and negative emotions, compared to their counterparts (Carstensen et al. 2011). Since emotion regulation requires resources, it is also subject to age-related adaptation processes. Based on the SOC model, the SOC-ER model (selection, optimization, and compensation with emotion regulation, Opitz et al. 2014; Urry and Gross 2010) assumes that resource-intensive regulatory processes (e.g., cognitive reinterpretation) decrease due to age. Instead, older adults should experience an increase in the less resource-intensive process of situation selection. The growing importance of situation selection as a regulatory strategy in old age has already been shown in various studies. The decrease in cognitive reinterpretation processes in old age, on the other hand, is less evident (Allen and Windsor 2017; Opitz et al. 2014). Instead, there is evidence to the contrary, i.e., that these processes even gain importance in old age (Brandtstädter 2007; Heckhausen and Schulz 1995).

Emotions play an important regulatory function both in the pursuit of personal goals and in dealing with challenges or losses. They can be a source of information about the current status of goal achievement; i.e., joy shows progress, while anger indicates obstacles (Tamir 2016). Emotions can also influence information processing, thus facilitating adaptation to a specific challenge. For example, anger narrows the focus of attention, thus making it easier to target obstacles and minimizing distractions (Lench et al. 2015). Positive emotions, on the other hand, broaden the field of attention and thus facilitate creative and flexible thinking, which in turn makes the adaptation of personal goals more flexible (Fredrickson 2001; Isen 1990).

17.2 Music and Emotion Regulation Across the Lifespan

The relationship between emotion regulation and goals is relevant to music psychology in many ways. On the one hand, there are efforts made to influence emotions in a targeted manner, i.e., by turning on the radio or using an instrument (planned emotion regulation). On the other hand, goals (e.g., career goals of musicians) change over the course of life and, in turn, contribute to changes in one's emotional experience. Musical activities such as playing in an orchestra are subject to age-related losses that can be recognized by older musicians (Gembris 2012). The fact that this is not directly expressed in the perceived quality of one's own performance is an indication that older people can adapt to age-related changes (Krampe 2006). In a survey of more than 2500 orchestral musicians, Gembris and Heye (2014) found that older musicians were more likely to notice age-related performance losses and difficulties compared to their counterparts. More than 60% of the total sample pointed out practising (optimization) and paying attention to one's health as strategies for dealing with age-related challenges. Gembris and Heye interpreted the findings of the study as showing that the SOC model is only applicable to a limited extent to orchestral musicians who do not decide on the repertoire and can thus only compensate to a limited extent. On the other hand, most participants agreed with the statement that they could use their previous experience as compensation for the age reduction in instrumental playing. The high level of professional satisfaction of the sample and the finding that the perceived age was even more below the actual age, the older the respondents were may be surprising outcomes. However, these findings can be explained by accommodative processes (e.g., positive reinterpretation, adaptation of aspirations, downwards social comparison), which contribute to the stabilization of well-being and gain in importance during the second half of life (Brandtstädter 2007).

17.2.1 Emotion Regulation Through Listening to and Making Music

Studies on emotion regulation can be distinguished in terms of whether music is listened to or actively played. One focus of research on emotion regulation through listening to music is on changes in music preferences (Bonneville-Roussy et al. 2017; North and Hargreaves 2008). In a study of adults aged 18–65 years (Bonneville-Roussy and Eerola 2018), age was found to be related to preferences for musical attributes such as *less energetic, intense, complex,* or *simple.* From young to middle adulthood (40–65 years), the preference for music clips could increasingly be predicted by sound parameters such as timbre, dynamics and tonal clarity. It was also found (Cohrdes et al. 2017) that older adults (60–75 years) preferred music with positive valence and low arousal, while younger adults preferred music with more arousal and more negative valence. After listening, significant changes in the participants' current mood could be found. In another study, the valence and arousal of songs were assessed (Cohrdes et al. 2020). On average, adolescents and older adults rated the song stimuli as more positive and less exciting than did people in young and middle adulthood. The assessment of the affective quality of the music pieces was significantly associated with musical characteristics. Older people, on average, attributed a more positive valence to music with a faster tempo and lower timbre qualities (perceived roughness, intensity). In addition, a mood-incongruent perception of affective qualities in music was found at older ages; i.e., the more negative the valence of the current mood was, the more positive their perceptions of music were. How can these findings be explained? The authors interpreted the findings on the pro-hedonic processing motivation of older people (Carstensen et al. 2011) to mean that arousal is more likely to be experienced aversively and thus causes difficulty when recovering from it. Labouvie-Vief (2015, 131f.) provided a compensatory interpretation; older people report more positive emotions due to their declining cognitive abilities, while negative emotions are cognitively more difficult to process and integrate into the cognitive–emotional system.

Experimental studies have repeatedly shown that music can be effectively used to induce moods and emotions (Kreutz et al. 2007; Panksepp and Bernatzky 2002; Västfjäll 2002). Here, positive and basic emotions are most often experienced, and more complex emotional states such as guilt, shame, and jealousy are rare (Juslin and Laukka 2004). However, the question arises as to how long the induced states last. Panksepp and Bernatzky (2002) found a decrease in music-induced joy and sadness after 10 min and a complete decrease after 20 min. Anger and tension were also reduced by listening to music, but the effect was no longer noticeable after 10 min. Especially with regard to possible therapeutic interventions, studies are necessary that investigate longer-term effects, also with regard to cumulative effects of positive emotions, supported by musical activities (cf. the resource-building effect of positive emotions, Fredrickson 2001). Based on studies that suggest age-related differences in the regulation of emotions (Carstensen et al. 2011), it remains an interesting question to what extent age-related changes influence the inducibility of emotions through music.

Further insight into age-related differences in musical emotion regulation is provided by studies that investigate functions and reasons for listening to music. In a study examining younger adults, Schäfer et al. (2013) distinguished three pivotal functions of listening to music: self-awareness, social connectedness, and mood and arousal regulation. The latter function was the most frequently mentioned, followed by self-perception and social connectedness. A comparative study with a sample of older adults yielded two interesting results: (1) older adults did not experience a loss of the importance of music over the course of their lives and (2) they showed a pattern consistent with younger adults in terms of functions, in which the most important function of listening to music is the regulation of mood and arousal in old age (Schäfer and Riedel 2018). In a questionnaire study of music listening functions, an age-heterogeneous sample was asked about the tendencies to concentrate on the pieces when listening to music (attentive listening) or to react emotionally to music (emotional listening) (Leipold and Loepthien 2015). Neither facet correlated with the age variable. Thus, music is also important in old age, and its relative importance is comparable to that of young adults. However, there are significant correlations with different forms of coping and emotion regulation. Emotional listening is associated with rumination, and attentive-analytical listening with accommodation (flexible goal adjustment, reorientation).

To date, numerous studies on strategies of emotion regulation through music have been published, which have contributed to a differentiation of motivation. In two interview studies, Saarikallio und Erkkilä (2007) and Saarikallio (2011) investigated emotion regulation through music in adolescents and adults. Seven strategies of emotion regulation by listening to music were extracted from the statements of the young people as follows:

1. *Entertainment*: Music to accompany everyday tasks, which are then perceived as more positive and less boring.
2. *Revival*: Listening to music for relaxation and energization.
3. *Strong Sensation*: Experiencing intense emotions while listening to music.
4. *Diversion*: Distraction from negative emotions by listening to music.

5. *Discharge*: Letting out negative emotions through listening to music.
6. *Mental Work*: Music providing a background for contemplation and stimulating reflection on one's experiences.
7. *Solace*: Music is perceived as a friend who shows understanding and with whom difficulties can be shared (Saarikallio and Erkkilä 2007; see also Saarikallio 2008).

This list gives an overview of different strategies used to regulate emotions with music. Based on this information, Saarikallio (2011) examined 21 adults (21–70 years) in a follow-up interview study and found strategies that were consistent with those applied by young people. She further identified age differences and summarized the main causes of changes in the emotion-regulating use of music (Saarikallio 2011, S. 316 ff.):

1. *Change by age:* Music is related to one's personal life history. Due to older age, older people have been able to gain more experience with the possibilities of using music for emotion regulation.
2. *Event-related fluctuations:* Emotion regulation through music is subject to fluctuations over the lifespan. Music can become particularly important in times of personal crisis, and this importance subsides with the resolution of the crisis.
3. *Retirement transition:* With the elimination of professional obligations after retirement, there is more time for intense engagement with music.

Interview techniques can be used to indicate idiosyncratic differences between people. The extent to which these age differences or changes can be generalized requires clarification in longitudinal studies. In a recent work, a distinction was made (Baltazar and Saarikallio 2019) between five main categories of emotion regulation and different combinations thereof. These categories were associated with different mechanisms (e.g., preferences, emotions, aesthetic judgments). Whether the variety of fine nuances identified in adolescents and young adults can also be observed in old age needs to be examined in more detail. To what extent the strategies actually lead to the desired affects has to do with the confirmation or nonconfirmation of expectations; however, emotional reactions often occur even when expectations are not met (Sloboda and Juslin 2005).

Emotion-regulating effects can be found not only when listening to music but also during musical activities. With regard to active music-making, a study with 126 musicians (Antonini Philippe et al. 2019) found overall high values in subjective well-being in this group (see also Weinberg and Joseph 2017). However, it was not clear whether this outcome was due to playing music or factors such as social interaction. Positive effects of singing were more evident in a study conducted with people older than 60 years (Coulton et al. 2015). Here, singing increased mental well-being more within 6 months than in a comparative sample that pursued other activities during this period. Similar effects of active music-making can be found in further studies (e.g., Lord et al. 2012; Williams et al. 2019). Numerous studies have shown that the experience of flow during active music-making, i.e., a state of complete absorption in the activity performed that is combined with the experience of positive emotions (Nakamura and Csikszentmihalyi 2002), is related to well-being (e.g., Heller et al. 2015; Loepthien and Leipold 2022). Flow-following musical activities can also be a source of well-being in adulthood and old age. This is also supported by the fact that there is currently no empirical evidence of age differences in experiencing flow over the lifespan (see, e.g., Konradt et al. 2003; Loepthien and Leipold 2022). An additional connection between flow and individual development over the lifespan (also with regard to musical development) can be seen in the motivational effect of flow, which causes the search for increasingly complex situations and thus promotes the development of one's own abilities (Csikszentmihalyi and Rathunde 1998).

In summary, empirical studies have provided evidence for the emotion-regulating function of listening to and making music in adulthood. The findings regarding age differences provide no homogeneous picture. On the one hand, there are indications that are consistent with the positivity effect of emotion in old age (Carstensen et al. 2011); on the other hand, there are many partly method-related nuances of emotion regulation through music, and many findings have not yet been replicated. The facets of emotion regulation also have to be examined with regard to age-related (e.g., cognitive and neuronal) changes.

17.2.2 Music, Stress, and Coping with Crisis

As already described in the first section, stress management by means of music can be understood as a specific form of emotion regulation. Research on music psychology shows that the influence of musical activities, especially listening to music, on the experience of stress has often been examined. A stress-regulating effect can be found in experimental studies, in which participants are exposed to a stress-generating situation (e.g., a social evaluation situation) and either listen to music or receive a control treatment (for an overview, see de Witte et al. 2020) In addition, numerous studies investigate the influence of musical activities on the stress experience in everyday life or during particularly stressful situations (e.g., medical treatments) (Bernatzky et al. 2011; Västfjäll et al. 2012).

Studies on the influence of listening to music on stress differ in whether the participants themselves choose the music to be listened to or whether music is presented that was previously classified as relaxing (e.g., Mitchell and MacDonald 2012; Västfjäll 2002). In an experimental study, Labbé et al. (2007) examined the influence of self-selected relaxation compared with classical music selected by the instructor on the stress response after a stress-inducing task. The authors found that both self-chosen and classical music had positive effects on subjective stress. In terms of physiological stress responses, participants who chose music themselves showed a decrease in heart rate, while classical music led to a lower breathing rate. In general, listening to self-selected relaxing music led to changes in indicators of relaxation most often, as compared to listening to classical or Heavy Metal music, or no music at all. Thoma et al. (2013) conducted a study that differed from the one just reported in two respects; they examined the effects of listening to music *before* a stressor was presented and focused exclusively on the effects of music classified as relaxing by the researchers (Allegri's "Miserere"). The results of the study show that previous listening to relaxing music caused cortisol levels to rise more than did listening to the sound of water as a reaction to a stressful situation. In addition, there was also a faster recovery period after the stress reaction (measured by the enzyme alpha-amylase) when listening to music before. In general, there are only a few differences in the efficiency of self-selected music and music chosen by researchers (de Witte et al. 2020).

Neither of these two studies specifically investigated the role of age with regard to the stress-reducing effect of listening to music. Peck et al. (2020), however, compared the effects of previous music listening on the stress response of young and older adults in a study similar to that of Thoma et al. (2013) (with self-selected music). This study showed no clear effects of listening to music on the subsequent stress experience induced by stressors. Notably, the study did not show any different reactions between young adults and older adults. This result converges with the results of a meta-analysis (de Witte et al. 2020) in which no age differences in the effectiveness of music-related interventions on stress were identified.

It is difficult to discuss to what extent music supports coping with crises, as the number of studies dealing with this question is still quite low. In a first attempt, findings from studies that have examined the effectiveness of music therapeutic interventions on coping with traumatic events can be used here. Bensimon et al. (2008) investigated the effects of active music-making in soldiers suffering from posttraumatic stress disorder. After 16 weekly music therapy sessions, participants reported a strong group feeling during the sessions and that they were able to use drums to find a way to vent their anger, which is a typical symptom of posttraumatic stress disorder. Furthermore, interview statements by the soldiers involved in the study suggest that although the drumbeats reminded them of traumatic experiences, these associative connections diminished over time, which may suggest a less stressful handling of the traumatic events. The COVID-19 pandemic, with all its consequences, also posed a challenge to the coping skills and resources of each individual. Recent studies have shown music listening can be a means to regulate negative emotions following the COVID-19 pandemic (Fink et al. 2021; Hennessy et al. 2021; Martín et al. 2021; Vidas et al. 2021; Ziv and Hollander-Shabtai 2022). Martín et al. (2021) investigated age-related differences in using music to regulate one's emotions during COVID-19-related lockdown. The results, however, do not show a clear picture. Younger adults (18–40 years) indicated listening less frequently to music to regulate their emotions during a lockdown than did middle-aged and older adults (>41 years). However, younger adults used music more frequently than older adults to cope with loneliness and more frequently reported experiencing well-being through music listening. In a study on the influence of listening to music, Giordano et al. (2020) found positive effects of a music therapeutic intervention in terms of the stress experienced by hospital employees during the pandemic. After listening to music, these employees reported less fatigue, sadness, anxiety, and worry. However, possible age differences have not been studied in this regard.

In Sect. 17.1, we pointed out that coping and regulation processes of flexible goal adjustment (e.g., reinterpretation of negative situations or events) are sometimes not subject to intentional control. This entails difficulties for the development of interventions aimed at promoting these adaptive processes. Cognitive factors such as attention and divergent and creative thought processes also need to be taken into account (Fredrickson 2001; Isen 1990). Listening to music is related to affective and cognitive processes that possibly trigger emotion-regulating coping (reinterpretation and reorientation processes, i.e., a flexible structure of personal goals) (Campion and Levita 2014; Loepthien 2015). To what extent this mechanism leads to a palliative effect in real-life stressful situations remains a question for future research.

In summary, the current findings indicate positive effects of listening to music on coping with stress, whereby the difference in the effects of self-selected vs. music previously classified as relaxing is small. If the focus is on everyday music listening, then the use of self-selected music is appropriate; however, if the influence of structural music features is to be investigated, then experimental variation should be used. The extent to which musical activities support cognitive processes that have a positive effect on regulation processes that cannot be controlled intentionally is a relevant question that will have to be addressed more intensively in future research. There are only a few empirical studies that explicitly deal with age-related changes in coping with stress through music listening and making. However, the results of these studies do not show any significant changes over the lifespan. Further studies are needed that do not merely examine age as a control variable.

17.3 Fields of Application: Health and Education

An essential part of research on musical emotion regulation in adulthood deals with the maintenance or restoration of health. Musical interventions in this field are concerned with a variety of psychological and physical symptoms. The healing power of music was mentioned as early as the *Old Testament* (1st Book of Samuel, chapters 10 and 16). In a more recently developed model, Hillecke and Wilker (2007) specified factors that are assumed to mediate the therapeutic effects. The authors argue that a modulation takes place in the domains of attention, emotion, cognition, motor skills/behavior, and communication. Musical interventions are also used to reduce symptoms of depression in adulthood. Important functions can be seen in the release of dopamine in the reward system of the brain or in the flexibilization of emotions, in which music can contribute to both their relaxation as well as activation. We concentrate on a few domains in which emotional regulation is of crucial importance in middle and older adulthood.

17.3.1 Musical Interventions in Practice

With a significant number of people reaching advanced age, dementia (Alzheimer's disease, multi-infarction dementia) has become a major challenge for society.

Because the most common forms of dementia cannot be cured, the primary goals of therapeutic efforts are currently symptomatic alleviation of cognitive performance losses and an improvement in emotional well-being and quality of life. To date, there is also a broad body of studies documenting the effects of musical and music therapeutic interventions. Review articles and meta-analyses in recent years (Chang et al. 2015; Leggieri et al. 2019; Lou 2001; Moreno-Morales et al. 2020) show that music therapy can improve cognitive performance and mood, and reduce tension and behavioral disorders experienced by dementia patients. Even if the progression of age-related dementiacannot be stalled, and positive long-term effects are difficult to achieve, the findings are promising and have led to an upswing in the practice of therapeutic musical interventions. Songs from childhood and adolescence are often retrievable for a long time and associated with emotional valence. Singing and listening to music together is communication, rhythm can stimulate coordination exercises (Wosch 2011). The promotion of subjective quality of life is visible in many domains and is the goal of intervention in the last lifetime. Gembris (2018) reports studies with positive findings in which active music-making in old age was investigated to prevent cognitive decline and dementia.

Intervention effects have also been found for adjustments in well-being in cancer patients. In a study with 84 cancer patients receiving palliative treatment (Warth et al. 2015), one group received a musical therapeutic intervention over two sessions, in which a music therapist played a monochord and sang for 15 min. In the control group, a mindfulness-based relaxation was conducted for the same amount of time. After completion of the study, subjective well-being was more pronounced in the music therapy intervention group.

The effectiveness of music-psychological interventions for the treatment of depression in different age groups was the subject of a review article by Leubner and Hinterberger (2017). One result was that older people benefited in particular, however, the authors also described the very limited data in controlled studies and identified some difficulties. They pointed out standards that should be used in assessing the effectiveness of treating symptoms of clinical disorders. Only 28 original papers with an experimental control group design met the scientific criteria.

Some of the difficulties that arise in assessing many music therapeutic studies should be mentioned here because they are relevant not only to the treatment of depression. There are a variety of implementation and combination options. In *receptive* therapy, music is heard (by individuals or in groups). In *active* therapy, people make music (e.g., playing with simple instruments such as drums, singing bowls, Orff instruments, or by using the voice to sing). It is about experimenting and experiencing, sometimes in very different settings. A consistent separation of both modalities is often not possible in practice and many studies provide inaccurate information on the implementation. Complicating the interpretation of the findings is the fact that music therapy is offered in clinics as part of a therapy concept, e.g., in combination with standard therapy. In clinical efficacy studies, different comorbidities must be considered. Other factors making a comparison of the studies difficult are the different degrees of professionalization of the instructors and therapists, and the generous use of the term music therapy for very different intervention qualities. The issues that Leubner and Hinterberger (2017) point out are symptomatic not only of the treatment of depression with music but also affect the entire field of therapy research. The idea of wanting to (or having to) measure *effect sizes* at all is alien to many music educators, sociologists, or gerontologists. Music therapy is a field in which empirical research ranges from numerous, case-based, qualitative impressionisms to randomized control group designs.

One of the peculiarities of music is how it appeals to people emotionally, binds their attention, and triggers or accompanies human action in this way. The fact that music is used in grief work points to its protective effect on experiences of loss. Even Plato saw the manifold function of music, and in the second book of *Nomoi* discussed its contribution to the education of youth as it relates to movement (gymnastics, dance, singing) (Platon 2009, S. 189–218). He recalls the ease of youth in celebrating, in sport and music competitions; the reminiscence of the older generation and its role as a jury; the enchantment of the soul, the healing of the sick, the virtue, in short: the Dionysian and Apollonian. In addition, what can we learn today with regard to emotion regulation?

17.3.2 Emotion Regulation Through Music, Education, and Lifelong Learning

If emotion regulation is understood to be an intentional skill, following ones respective needs, it is obvious that one could attempt to refine the strategies of musical emotion regulation (Baltazar and Saarikallio 2019) and to train the processes of emotion regulation (situation selection and modification, attention control, cognitive reinterpretation, emotional up- and down-regulation, Gross 1998; Mallory and Rupp 2018). This includes observation of one's own emotions, the screening of one's own evaluation system, one's own thought patterns, and the development of meaningful alternatives. This is a process in which learning does not end, even in old age. Self-management techniques can help regulate feelings—at least to some extent. However, emotional states are known to be characterized by volatility so that a conscious intentionality can often not be claimed. There are non-intentional automatisms or processes of counter-regulation. When one considers the mechanisms discussed in the generation of emotions through music (see Egermann and Kreutz 2018, S. 627), it is not surprising that a strategic emotion induction does not necessarily have the desired effect, and one is disappointed by the music in a radio broadcast from which one had expected a lot. Brainstem reflexes, conditioning processes, or musical expectations cannot be planned according to a recipe, but are rather subject to processes that are largely beyond our control. Even with familiar music, expectation discrepancies can arise on a nonconscious level (Sloboda and Juslin 2005). Perhaps it is advisable to reflect on one's own goals, and to distinguish between goals that one associates, pursues, and wants to realize with music (music as an identity project), and the emotions that result from unfulfilled life plans (e.g., professional or family crises), which require action steps that lie outside the musical regulation.

In our opinion, apart from the desire to be able to induce emotions in a planned way, one of the strengths of music lies in its training to learn to distinguish emotional nuances, in listening to and actively making music. Beethoven's 32 piano sonatas have often been characterized with landscapes, natural events, times of day, and seasons to characterize their soul statements. To give an example, the pianist Edwin Fischer (1958, S. 13) said that Beethoven appeals to man's will to build. Beethoven achieved his musical expressiveness through the highest spiritual discipline, though the extent to which discipline is necessary can here remain open. Self-cultivation approaches (Schmid 2016) and action-theoretical development perspectives (Brandtstädter 2007) examine how feelings are formed or affect is handled. Both have analyzed the relationship between emotions and goals and see the planned regulation of feelings not only as change in a symptom (i.e., Make me happy, instantaneously), but regard feelings as reactions that can motivate actions, although not necessarily the object of one's own desires.

Decisive for the motivation to learn here is not that it must be Beethoven, who may or may not go against one's grain emotionally because he presupposes certain demands on musical education and cannot simply be played. Emotional attachment to music is present across genre and class differences: It depends on the respective preferences and motivational structures that refine one's taste. The term *lifelong learning* has a negative connotation for some emancipated adults who associate it with negative memories of school learning. *Self-directed learning* emphasizes a person's contribution, their competencies, intentions, interests, plans, and psychological processes, which help explain why amateur musicians form a growing group in adulthood. Noteworthy is the increase that music schools are seeing in the enrollment of adult students who are 60 years and older (Gembris 2018). Against the background of declining learning and performance competencies in the second half of life, music can be seen as an important source of motivation, which also helps to define workload and make progress oneself.

17.4 Outlook

In this article, emotion regulation through music was introduced from an *action* development standpoint (Brandtstädter 2007; Greve and Thomsen 2019; Leipold 2020). Regulation describes an adaptive process that includes intentions, planning, and control, on the one hand, but also the accommodation of developmental goals, which presupposes non-intentional processes of development regulation. Undoubtedly people are motivated to listen to or make music, either for professional reasons or out of passion, to distract themselves, to experience feelings, to induce emotions or perhaps also a desired positive development. In this respect, one can speak of a self-design that has biological or cultural limits, but that at least makes people co-producers of their development by regulating obstacles.

It seems too one-sided to treat the topic of emotion regulation through music from a perspective of minimizing or maximizing a hedonic balance or under the premise that the controllability of emotions is a decisive developmental goal. In general research on emotion regulation, the question of motives has established itself in research (Tamir 2011). Motives can refer to the intensification of positive or the reduction of negative emotions (*hedonic* motives), but also to the achievement of further, overarching goals (*instrumental* motives). For example, a person could specifically intensify anger in order to be more athletically motivated. An increase in sadness could aim at social support or create a framework for thinking about blocked life paths. The model of *instrumental emotion regulation* (Tamir 2016) assumes that emotions have specific functions and affect motivation and cognition. The intensification of certain emotional states thus affects the achievement of goals by establishing a favorable motivation and cognitive state. Hence, this model touches on the question of the adaptivity of certain episodes of emotion regulation. With the inclusion of instrumental motives, the intensification of negative emotions through music can therefore also be adaptive, provided this supports the achievement of personal goals. In music-psychological research on emotion regulation, little attention has been paid to instrumental emotion regulation. An exception is the experimental study by Tahlier et al. (2012) in which the influence of higher-order goals on situational music preference was shown.

In summary, music is an object of intentional self-development and individuals can contribute to the cultivation of musical experiences through their actions. Planning one's own development is a strategic event that includes long-term goals and is changed by the impairments of aging. Emotions, however, have a spontaneous nature; the fluctuations of the emotional experience are not easy to capture strategically, but are also subject to developmental processes over the lifespan. In Richard Strauss' *Rosenkavalier,* Octavian sings: *The honor is presented to me.* This sentence does not express control, but rather an experience, a feeling which, like other feelings, can be intensified in happy moments by music.

References

Allen VC, Windsor TD (2017) Age differences in the use of emotion regulation strategies derived from the process model of emotion regulation. A systematic review. Aging Ment Health:1–14. https://doi.org/10.1080/13607863.2017.1396575

Antonini Philippe R, Kosirnik C, Vuichoud N, Williamon A, von Roten FC (2019) Understanding wellbeing among college music students and amateur musicians in western Switzerland. Front Psychol 10:820. https://doi.org/10.3389/fpsyg.2019.00820

Baltazar M, Saarikallio S (2019) Strategies and mechanisms in musical affect self-regulation. A new model. Music Sci 2(23):177–195. https://doi.org/10.1177/1029864917715061

Baltes PB, Staudinger UM, Lindenberger U (1999) Lifespan psychology. Theory and application to intellectual functioning. Annu Rev Psychol 50:471–501

Bensimon M, Amir D, Wolf Y (2008) Drumming through trauma: music therapy with post-traumatic soldiers. Arts Psychother 35(1):34–48. https://doi.org/10.1016/j.aip.2007.09.002

Bernatzky G [Guenther], Presch M, Anderson M, Panksepp J (2011) Emotional foundations of music as a non-pharmacological pain management tool in modern medicine. Neurosci Biobehav Rev 35(9):1989–1999. https://doi.org/10.1016/j.neubiorev.2011.06.005

Boetius AMS (1985) Buch 1: Vorrede. In: Paul O (Hrsg) Boetius: Fünf Bücher über die Musik. 2. Nachdruck der Ausgabe von 1872. Georg Olms Verlag, S 1–37

Bonneville-Roussy A, Eerola T (2018) Age trends in musical preferences in adulthood: 3. Perceived musical attributes as intrinsic determinants of preferences. Music Sci 22(3):394–414. https://doi.org/10.1177/1029864917718606

Bonneville-Roussy A, Stillwell D, Kosinski M, Rust J (2017) Age trends in musical preferences in adulthood: 1. Conceptualization and empirical investigation. Music Sci 21(4):369–389. https://doi.org/10.1177/1029864917691571
Brandtstädter J (2007) Das flexible Selbst. Selbstentwicklung zwischen Zielbindung und Ablösung [The flexible self: self-development between goal-commitment and detachment]. Spektrum Akademischer Verlag, München
Brandtstädter J, Wentura D, Greve W (1993) Adaptive resources of the aging self. Outlines of an emergent perspective. Int J Behav Dev 16(2):323–349
Bühler C (1933) Der menschliche Lebenslauf als psychologisches Problem [The human lifespan as a psychological problem]. Hirzel, Leipzig
Campion M, Levita L (2014) Enhancing positive affect and divergent thinking abilities. Play some music and dance. J Posit Psychol 9(2):137–145. https://doi.org/10.1080/17439760.2013.848376
Carstensen LL, Turan B, Scheibe S, Ram N, Ersner-Hershfield H, Samanez-Larkin GR et al (2011) Emotional experience improves with age. Evidence based on over 10 years of experience sampling. Psychol Aging 26(1):21–33. https://doi.org/10.1037/a0021285
Carus FA (1808) Psychologie [Psychology]. Ambrosius Barth, Leipzig
Carver CS (2011) Coping. In: Contrada RJ, Baum A (eds) The handbook of stress science. Biology, psychology, and health. Springer, New York, pp 221–229
Carver CS (2015) Control processes, priority management, and affective dynamics. Emot Rev 7(4):301–307. https://doi.org/10.1177/1754073915590616
Chang Y-S, Chu H, Yang C-Y, Tsai J-C, Chung M-H, Liao Y-M et al (2015) The efficacy of music therapy for people with dementia: a meta-analysis of randomised controlled trials. J Clin Nurs 24(23–24):3425–3440. https://doi.org/10.1111/jocn.12976
Cohrdes C, Wrzus C, Frisch S, Riediger M (2017) Tune yourself in: valence and arousal preferences in music-listening choices from adolescence to old age. Dev Psychol 53(9):1777–1794. https://doi.org/10.1037/dev0000362
Cohrdes C, Wrzus C, Wald-Fuhrmann M, Riediger M (2020) "The sound of affect": age differences in perceiving valence and arousal in music and their relation to music characteristics and momentary mood. Music Sci 24(1):21–43. https://doi.org/10.1177/1029864918765613
Coulton S, Clift S, Skingley A, Rodriguez J (2015) Effectiveness and cost-effectiveness of community singing on mental health-related quality of life of older people: randomised controlled trial. Br J Psychiatry 207(3):250–255. https://doi.org/10.1192/bjp.bp.113.129908
Csikszentmihalyi M, Rathunde K (1998) The development of the person. An experiential perspective on the ontogenesis of psychological complexity. In: Damon W, Lerner RM (Hrsg) Handbook of child psychology. Theoretical models of human development, Bd. 1, 5. Aufl. John Riley & Sons, New York, S 635–684
de Witte M, Spruit A, van Hooren S, Moonen X, Stams G-J (2020) Effects of music interventions on stress-related outcomes. A systematic review and two meta-analyses. Health Psychol Rev 14(2):294–324. https://doi.org/10.1080/17437199.2019.1627897
Eerola T, Vuoskoski JK (2013) A review of music and emotion studies: approaches, emotion models, and stimuli. Music Percept 30(3):307–340. https://doi.org/10.1525/MP.2012.30.3.307
Egermann H, Kreutz G [Gunter] (2018) Emotionen und ästhetische Gefühle [Emotions and aesthetic feelings]. In: Lehmann AC, Kopiez R (Hrsg) Handbuch Musikpsychologie [Handbook psychology of music], 1. Auflage. Hogrefe, Bern, S 617–640
Erikson EH (1959) Identity and the life cycle. International University Press, New York
Fink LK, Warrenburg LA, Howlin C, Randall WM, Hansen NC, Wald-Fuhrmann M (2021) Viral tunes. Changes in musical behaviours and interest in coronamusic predict socio-emotional coping during COVID-19 lockdown. Humanit Soc Sci Commun 8(1). https://doi.org/10.1057/s41599-021-00858-y
Fischer E (1958) Ludwig van Beethovens Klaviersonaten [Ludwig van Beethoven's Piano Sonatas]. Insel Verlag, Leipzig
Fredrickson BL (2001) The role of positive emotions in positive psychology. The broaden-and-built theory of positive emotions. Am Psychol 56(3):218–226. https://doi.org/10.1037/0003-66X.56.3.218

Freund AM, Nikitin J (2018) Entwicklung im jungen und mittleren Erwachsenenalter. In: Schneider W, Lindenberger U (Hrsg) Entwicklungspsychologie, 8. Auflage. Beltz, Weinheim/Basel, S 265–290

Gembris H (2012) Musik-making as a lifelong development and resource for health. In: MacDonald RAR, Kreutz G, Mitchell L (eds) Music, health, and wellbeing. Oxford University Press, Oxford, pp 367–382

Gembris H (2018) Musikalische Entwicklung im Erwachsenenalter [Musical development in adulthood]. In: Lehmann AC, Kopiez R (Hrsg) Handbuch Musikpsychologie [Handbook psychology of music], 1. Auflage. Hogrefe, Bern, S 217–246

Gembris H, Heye A (2014) Growing older in a symphony orchestra: the development of the age-related self-concept and the self-estimated performance of professional musicians in a lifespan perspective. Music Sci 18(4):371–391. https://doi.org/10.1177/1029864914548912

Giordano F, Scarlata E, Baroni M, Gentile E, Puntillo F, Brienza N et al (2020) Receptive music therapy to reduce stress and improve wellbeing in Italian clinical staff involved in COVID-19 pandemic: a preliminary study. Arts Psychother 70:101688. https://doi.org/10.1016/j.aip.2020.101688

Greve W, Thomsen T (2019) Entwicklungspsychologie. Eine Einführung in die Erklärung menschlicher Entwicklung [Developmental psychology. An introduction to the explanation of human development]. Springer, Wiesbaden. https://doi.org/10.1007/978-3-531-93432-7

Gross JJ (1998) The emerging field of emotion regulation. An integrative review. Rev Gen Psychol 2(3):271–299. https://doi.org/10.1037/1089-2680.2.3.271

Havighurst RJ (1948) Developmental tasks and education. McKay, New York

Heckhausen J, Schulz R (1995) A life-span theory of control. Psychol Rev 102(2):284–304

Heller K, Bullerjahn C, von Georgi R (2015) The relationship between personality traits, flow-experience, and different aspects of practice behavior of amateur vocal students. Front Psychol 6:1901. https://doi.org/10.3389/fpsyg.2015.01901

Hennessy S, Sachs M, Kaplan J, Habibi A (2021) Music and mood regulation during the early stages of the COVID-19 pandemic. PLoS One 16(10):e0258027. https://doi.org/10.1371/journal.pone.0258027

Hillecke TK, Wilker, FW (2007) Ein heuristisches Wirkfaktorenmodell der Musiktherapie. [Heuristic working factors or music therapy]. Verhaltenstherapie & Verhaltensmedizin, 28:62–85

Isen AM (1990) The influence of positive and negative affect on cognitive organization. Some implications for development. In: Stein N, Leventhal B, Trabasso T (eds) Psychological and biological approaches to emotion. Erlbaum, Hillsdale, pp 75–94

Juslin PN, Laukka P (2004) Expression, perception, and induction of musical emotions. A review and a questionnaire study of everyday listening. J New Music Res 33(3):217–238. https://doi.org/10.1080/0929821042000317813

Karnaze MM, Levine LJ (2018) Sadness, the architect of cognitive change. In: Lench HC (ed) The function of emotions. When and why emotions help us. Springer, New York, pp 45–58

Karreman A, Vingerhoets AJ (2012) Attachment and well-being. The mediating role of emotion regulation and resilience. Personal Individ Differ 53(7):821–826. https://doi.org/10.1016/j.paid.2012.06.014

Konradt U, Filip R, Hoffmann S (2003) Flow experience and positive affect during hypermedia learning. Br J Educ Technol 34(3):309–327

Koole SL, Aldao A (2016) The self-regulation of emotion. Theoretical and empirical advances. In: Vohs KD, Baumeister RF (eds) Handbook of self-regulation: research, theory, and applications, 3rd edn. The Guilford Press, New York, pp 24–41

Koole SL, Rothermund K (2011) "I feel better but I don't know why". The psychology of implicit emotion regulation. Cognit Emot 25(3):389–399. https://doi.org/10.1080/02699931.2010.550505

Krampe RT (2006) Musical expertise from a lifespan perspective. In: Gembris H (ed) Musical development from a lifespan perspective. Peter Lang, Frankfurt am Main, pp 91–106

Kreutz G [G], Ott U, Teichmann D, Osawa P, Vaitl D (2007) Using music to induce emotions. Influences of musical preference and absorption. Psychol Music 36(1):101–126. https://doi.org/10.1177/0305735607082623

Labbé E, Schmidt N, Babin J, Pharr M (2007) Coping with stress. The effectiveness of different types of music. Appl Psychophysiol Biofeedback 32(3–4):163–168. https://doi.org/10.1007/s10484-007-9043-9

Labouvie-Vief G (2015) Integrating emotions and cognition throughout the lifespan. Springer, Heidelberg

Leggieri M, Thaut MH, Fornazzari L, Schweizer TA, Barfett J, Munoz DG et al (2019) Music intervention approaches for Alzheimer's disease. A review of the literature. Front Neurosci 13:132. https://doi.org/10.3389/fnins.2019.00132

Leipold B (2020) Intentional self-development and positive ageing. How individuals select and pursue life goals. Routledge, Abingdon

Leipold B, Loepthien T (2015) Music reception and emotional regulation in adolescence and adulthood. Music Sci 19:111–128. https://doi.org/10.1177/1029864915570354

Lench HC, Bench SW, Darbor KE, Moore M (2015) A functionalist manifesto. Goal-related emotions from an evolutionary perspective. Emot Rev 7(1):90–98. https://doi.org/10.1177/1754073914553001

Leubner D, Hinterberger T (2017) Reviewing the effectiveness of music interventions in treating depression. Front Psychol 8:1109. https://doi.org/10.3389/fpsyg.2017.01109

Loepthien T (2015) Musikhören und der Umgang mit persönlichen Zielen. Der Zusammenhang zwischen aufmerksam-analytischer Musikrezeption und akkommodativen Prozessen [Listening to music and dealing with personal goals. The relationship between attentive-analytical music reception and accommodative processes]. Tectum Verlag, Marburg

Loepthien T, Leipold B (2022) Flow in music performance and music-listening. Differences in intensity, predictors, and the relationship between flow and subjective well-being. Psychol Music 50(1):111–126. https://doi.org/10.3389/fpsyg.2017.01109

Lord VM, Hume VJ, Kelly JL, Cave P, Silver J, Waldman M et al (2012) Singing classes for chronic obstructive pulmonary disease. A randomized controlled trial. BMC Pulm Med 12:69. https://doi.org/10.1186/1471-2466-12-69

Lou M-F (2001) The use of music to decrease agitated behaviour of the demented elderly: the state of the science. Scand J Caring Sci 15(2):165–173. https://doi.org/10.1046/j.1471-6712.2001.00021.x

Mallory DB, Rupp DE (2018) Focusing in on the emotion laborer. Emotion regulation at work. In: Vohs KD, Baumeister RF (eds) Handbook of self-regulation. Research, theory, and applications. The Guilford Press, New York, pp 323–342

Martín JC, Ortega-Sánchez D, Miguel IN, Gil Martín GM (2021) Music as a factor associated with emotional self-regulation: a study on its relationship to age during COVID-19 lockdown in Spain. Heliyon 7(2):e06274. https://doi.org/10.1016/j.heliyon.2021.e06274

Mitchell L, MacDonald R (2012) Music and pain. Evidence from experimental perspectives. In: MacDonald RAR, Kreutz G, Mitchell L (eds) Music, health, and wellbeing. Oxford University Press, Oxford, pp 230–238

Moreno-Morales C, Calero R, Moreno-Morales P, Pintado C (2020) Music therapy in the treatment of dementia. A systematic review and meta-analysis. Front Med 7:160. https://doi.org/10.3389/fmed.2020.00160

Nakamura J, Csikszentmihalyi M (2002) The concept of flow. In: Csikszentmihalyi M, Csikszentmihalyi IS (eds) A life worth living. Contributions to positive psychology. Oxford University Press, Oxford/New York, pp 89–105

North AC, Hargreaves DJ (2008) The social and applied psychology of music. University Press, Oxford

Opitz PC, Lee IA, Gross JJ, Urry HL (2014) Fluid cognitive ability is a resource for successful emotion regulation in older and younger adults. Front Psychol 5:609. https://doi.org/10.3389/fpsyg.2014.00609

Panksepp J, Bernatzky G [Günther] (2002) Emotional sounds and the brain. The neuro-affective foundations of musical appreciation. Behav Process 60:133–155

Peck K, Totosy de Zepetnek J, Fiocco AJ (2020) Music listening does not inoculate the stress response in young and older adults. Int J Stress Manag. https://doi.org/10.1037/str0000217
Platon. (2009) Timaios, Kritias, Minos, Nomoi. Rowohlt, Reinbek
Saarikallio S (2008) Music in mood regulation. Initial scale development. Music Sci 12(2):291–309
Saarikallio S (2011) Music as emotional self-regulation throughout adulthood. Psychol Music 39(3):307–327. https://doi.org/10.1177/0305735610374894
Saarikallio S, Erkkilä J (2007) The role of music in adolescents' mood regulation. Psychol Music 35(1):88–109. https://doi.org/10.1177/0305735607068889
Schäfer T, Riedel J (2018) Musikhören im Alter. Untersuchung der Nutzungsweisen und psychosozialen Ressourcen [Listening to music in older age. Examination of uses and psychosocial resources]. Z Gerontol Geriatr 51(6):682–690. https://doi.org/10.1007/s00391-017-1229-z
Schäfer T, Sedlmeier P, Stadtler C, Huron D (2013) The psychological functions of music listening. Front Psychol 4:511. https://doi.org/10.3389/fpsyg.2013.00511
Schmid W (2016) Philosophie der Lebenskunst. Eine Grundlegung [Philosophy of the art of living. A fundament]. Suhrkamp, Franfurt am Main
Sloboda JA, Juslin PN (2005) Affektive Prozess. Emotionale und ästhetische Aspekte musikalischen Verhaltens [Affective processes. Emotional and aesthetic aspects of musical behaviour]. In: Stoffer TH, Oerter R (Hrsg) Allgemeine Musikpsychologie [General psychology of music]. Enzyklopädie der Psychologie, Themenbereich D, Serie VII Musikpsychologie. Hogrefe, Göttingen, S 767–843
Tahlier M, Miron AM, Rauscher FH (2012) Music choice as a sadness regulation strategy for resolved versus unresolved sad events. Psychol Music 41(6):729–748. https://doi.org/10.1177/0305735612446537
Tamir M (2011) The maturing field of emotion regulation. Emot Rev 3(1):3–7. https://doi.org/10.1177/1754073910388685
Tamir M (2016) Why do people regulate their emotions? A taxonomy of motives in emotion regulation. Personal Soc Psychol Rev 20(3):199–222. https://doi.org/10.1177/1088868315586325
Thoma MV, La Marca R, Brönnimann R, Finkel L, Ehlert U, Nater UM (2013) The effect of music on the human stress response. PLoS One 8(8):e70156. https://doi.org/10.1371/journal.pone.0070156
Urry HL, Gross JJ (2010) Emotion regulation in older age. Curr Dir Psychol Sci 19(6):352–357. https://doi.org/10.1177/0963721410388395
Västfjäll D (2002) Emotion induction through music. A review of the musical mood induction procedure. Music Sci Special Issue 2001–2001:173–211. https://doi.org/10.1177/10298649020050S107
Västfjäll D, Juslin PN, Hartig T (2012) Music, subjective wellbeing, and health. The role of everyday emotions. In: MacDonald RAR, Kreutz G, Mitchell L (eds) Music, health, and wellbeing. Oxford University Press, Oxford, pp 405–423
Vidas D, Larwood JL, Nelson NL, Dingle GA (2021) Music listening as a strategy for managing COVID-19 stress in first-year university students. Front Psychol 12:647065. https://doi.org/10.3389/fpsyg.2021.647065
Warth M, Keßler J, Hillecke TK, Bardenheuer HJ (2015) Music therapy in palliative care. A randomized controlled trial to evaluate effects on relaxation. Dtsch Arztebl Int 112(46):788–794. https://doi.org/10.3238/arztebl.2015.0788
Weinberg MK, Joseph D (2017) If you're happy and you know it. Music engagement and subjective wellbeing. Psychol Music 45(2):257–267. https://doi.org/10.1177/0305735616659552
Williams E, Dingle GA, Jetten J, Rowan C (2019) Identification with arts-based groups improves mental wellbeing in adults with chronic mental health conditions. J Appl Soc Psychol 49(1):15–26. https://doi.org/10.1111/jasp.12561
Wosch T (2011) Musik und Alter in Therapie und Pflege. Grundlagen, Institutionen und Praxis der Musiktherapie im Alter und bei Demenz [Music and older age in therapy and nursing. Fundamentals, institutions and practice of music therapy in older age and dementia], 1. Aufl. Kohlhammer Verlag, Stuttgart
Ziv N, Hollander-Shabtai R (2022) Music and COVID-19: changes in uses and emotional reaction to music under stay-at-home restrictions. Psychol Music 50(2):475–491. https://doi.org/10.1177/03057356211003326

Music as a Trigger for Strong Emotions

18

Eckart Altenmüller and Günther Bernatzky

18.1 Music as a Trigger for Strong Emotions

There is no doubt that music is capable of evoking particularly strong emotions. Its seductive but also destructive power has found its way into legends and has occupied writers and philosophers alike. The emotional effect of music is often cited as the most important reason for the popularity of musical activities. In Germany, for example, around seven million Germans regularly make music or sing. The music industry there achieved a turnover of almost 2 billion euros in 2021, besides still recovering from the coronavirus crisis, despite dumping prices for streaming services and pirated copies.[1] It is therefore surprising that, despite the ubiquity of music, the neurobiological and anthropological foundations of this preference have only been researched to a limited extent. However, these questions are currently the subject of intensive research, and it is becoming increasingly clear how music unfolds its effects on the emotional systems and how these effects can be used beneficially in music therapy.

In this chapter, we first want to clarify what emotions are and then turn to the strong emotions when listening to music, so-called SEM and their music-psychological prerequisites. As a particularly well-researched example of a strong emotion, we will discuss the chill effect in detail and clarify which music triggers a chill in which people under which conditions. We will then look at the brain

[1] https://miz.org/en/search?term=Music%20Industry, last updated August 17, 2024.

E. Altenmüller (✉)
Institute for Music Physiology and Musicians' Medicine, Hanover University of Music, Drama and Media, Hanover, Germany
e-mail: eckart.altenmueller@hmtm-hannover.de; altenmueller@hmthannover.de

G. Bernatzky
Department of Biosciences and Medical Biology, University of Salzburg, Salzburg, Austria

G. Kreutz, G. Bernatzky (eds.), *Music and Medicine*, Neurocultural Health and Wellbeing, https://doi.org/10.1007/978-3-662-72175-9_18

physiology behind the emotional experience of listening to music and end the chapter with the question of how emotions work and can be used in music therapy.

18.2 What Are Emotions?

We are all familiar with emotions because everyone has been happy, sad, angry, or anxious. Colloquially, the term emotion usually refers to a feeling. However, scientifically, the term feeling refers to the subjective experience within an emotion. For example, we have the feeling of "fear," but it only becomes a fully-fledged emotion when our eyes are wide open, and our heart is pounding at the same time. In other words, in humans, emotions include feelings as well as motor signs (wide-open eyes) and reactions of the autonomic nervous system (faster heartbeat). The emotions of fear, joy, sadness, anger, and disgust are distinguished not only by the feelings associated with them but also by their physical side effects. Feelings often cannot be expressed in words; they remain private.

In contrast to an emotion, a mood is a longer-term state that usually lasts for hours or days. Interestingly, our own mood sometimes remains hidden from us. For example, a depressive state of mind can cover our perceptions like mildew and make everything appear gray and dull without us even realizing it. When emotions convey strong impulses to act or even trigger spontaneous actions that we can no longer control, we speak of affects or, in legal terms, acts of affect/passion. During our emotional maturation in childhood and adolescence, in many cultures, it is important that we learn to control and, above all, suppress these impulses to act.

Of the numerous scientific emotion theories, we would like to present only the three most important ones here. As early as the nineteenth century, the psychologist Wilhelm Wundt (1905) characterized emotions according to three dimensions, which are shown in Fig. 18.1: (1) Arousal: arousal—calming (e.g., "boiling anger" versus "resigned displeasure"), (2) Valence: pleasure—displeasure (e.g., joy versus sadness) and (3) Tension—release (e.g., tense curiosity versus passive contemplation). All human emotions can be assigned to a point in this three-dimensional axial cross. The problem, however, is that the assignment is not unambiguous. For example, disgust and anger, two undoubtedly different emotions, can appear at the same point in the emotion space—both therefore receive the same value from arousal, displeasure, and tension.

An alternative to Wundt's dimensional model is the model of basic emotions or basic feelings. It is usually based on seven basic emotions which, according to Paul Ekman, are universal in all societies regardless of culture: joy, fear, anger, sadness, disgust, contempt, and surprise (Ekman 1972). However, the expression and recognition of basic emotions are partly culture-dependent. In East Asian cultures, for example, it is important not to show disgust in public. Accordingly, Japanese people are less able to recognize disgusted facial expressions in photos than Germans. In practice, everything is much more complicated because mixed emotions usually arise, such as anger at the boss mixed with fear of dismissal. It becomes even more problematic when we talk about emotions triggered by music: Music cannot usually

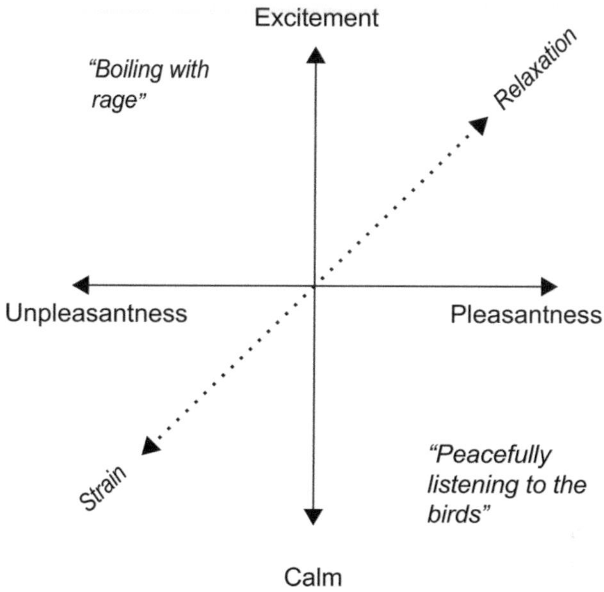

Fig. 18.1 The three-dimensional emotion model according to Wilhelm Wundt. Theoretically, all emotions at a certain point in time can be categorized in this space. The examples "Boiling with rage" and "Peacefully listening to the birds" are shown to illustrate this

evoke disgust or contempt, but it can evoke joy, sadness, and fear. The renowned emotion researcher Klaus Scherer (2005) therefore distinguishes between "aesthetic" emotions, which in his view are purposeless with respect to their adaptive value, and "utilitarian" emotions, which are useful in terms of survival. In the last decade, however, the concept of "purposeless" aesthetic emotions has been questioned by scholars, and the adaptive nature of aesthetic emotions has been emphasized. Music (and probably dance), for example, may evolutionary have played an important role in community building, group synchronization, emotional communication, and emotional self-regulation (for a review see Mehr et al. 2021).

In view of the shortcomings of the abovementioned definitions, together with zoologists Sabine Schmidt and Elke Zimmermann, we developed a third definition. It was important to us that our definition adequately accounts for emotions in non-human animals, reflecting a comparative approach: "*An emotion is a reaction to a certain stimulus based on the evaluation of the stimulus*." (Altenmüller et al. 2013a, b). The emotional reaction depends on motivation, which in turn is linked to hormones and the activity of certain neuronal networks.

To illustrate this somewhat dry and sober definition, let's imagine the following scenario: We are listening to a performance of Johann Sebastian Bach's St. Matthew Passion in a Gothic cathedral. In a touching scene shortly after the interrogation by the high priests, Jesus is brought before the crowd by Pilate, who asks: "So when they had gathered, Pilate said to them", "Whom do you want me to release for you: Barabbas, or Jesus who is called Christ?" In response, the crowd, incited by the high priests, shouts: "Barabbam!" Musically, the composer has shaped the Barabbas cry as a sudden, very loud, and harmonically unexpected dissonant chord in the choir and orchestra. Even with modern listeners, this unexpected sound often evokes a strong emotional reaction, which manifests itself in a shiver running down the spine, a feeling of goose bumps.

Let us now apply the definition and terms we have discussed to the Barabbas call. The stimulus is the acoustic signal produced by the choir and orchestra. The reaction is the involuntary raising of the body hair, a reflex triggered by the autonomic nervous system, which we become aware of as goose bumps. The stimulus evaluation is not entirely clear in this case. An innate form would be fright caused by a sudden increase in volume. The stimulus evaluation could then be described as follows: "Be careful, there is an unexpected event, I have to be careful that nothing happens to me." Neurobiologists refer to this stimulus response, which occurs very quickly and unconsciously, as an orientation response. A learned form of stimulus evaluation would be feelings of pity at the thought of an innocent person and benefactor being unjustly sentenced to death by the mob. Motivation will be high in most audiences as they are usually awake and alert and have attended the performance voluntarily. In a particularly boring, poor-quality performance, however, motivation can drop, and then it is questionable whether a goosebump effect will occur at all in a dozing or annoyed listener. An experienced listener who knows the work very well, on the other hand, may get goosebumps in anticipation of the powerful musical moment, and perhaps even the mere idea of this passage will lead to it. In this case, we would be dealing with a conditioned stimulus-response scheme.

When we try to transfer our definition of emotion to this musical example, the difficulty in describing emotions becomes apparent: Subjective feelings are not considered, even though they play a very important role in our understanding of emotions. We therefore need to expand the definition:

> In humans, an emotion is understood as a reaction pattern that becomes effective on four levels: a.) as a subjective feeling, b.) as a motor expression, e.g. as expressive behavior in facial expressions, gestures, and voice, c.) as a physiological reaction of the autonomic nervous system, e.g. as goose bumps, and d.) as a conscious evaluation.

We are often unable to talk about our subjective feelings because they defy words. This is why we often feel misunderstood when we want to communicate intense emotional experiences to others. And this is probably also why poets are unable to put deep musical impressions into words. Motor expressions, on the other hand, are often altered by cultural influences and are often even actively suppressed, as it is considered inappropriate in many cultures to show emotions through facial expressions or gestures. Tears of emotion are usually shamefully concealed, as we do not want to give too many insights into our inner life. Finally, the conscious evaluation of an emotion does not have to be congruent with the perceived, true emotion. There are even people who have great difficulty feeling their own emotions. This kind of emotional blindness is called alexithymia.

But what is the overarching meaning of the above musical scene from Bach's St. Matthew Passion? One way of looking at this is to understand music as a model of acoustic communication of emotions. Figure 18.2 shows this in a simplified way.

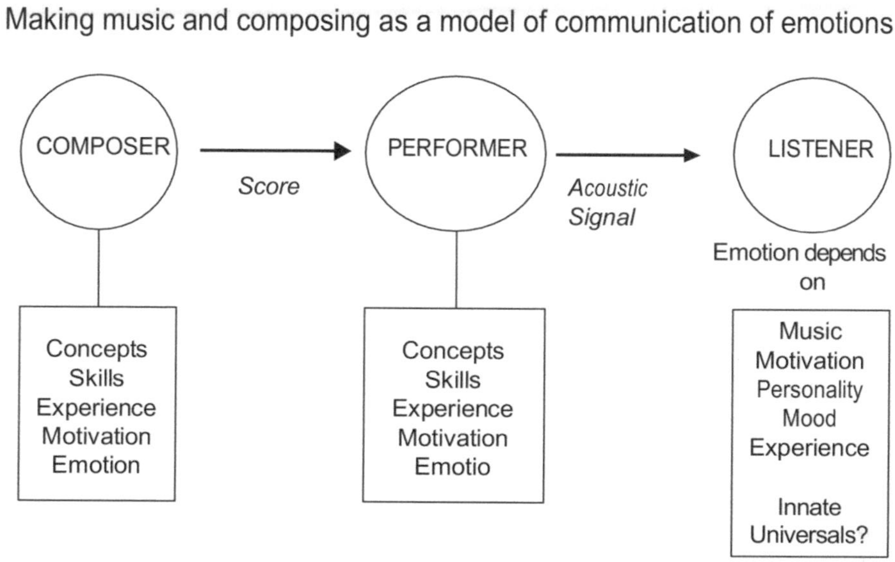

Fig. 18.2 Making music and composing as communication of emotions. Further explanations in the text

On the left-hand side of the model is the composer, who creates new representations of music and documents them in the symbol system of musical notation. The performer reads these notes and produces acoustic signals that trigger an emotion in the listener. The compositional achievement depends on the artistic concepts pursued by the composer. Compositional experience, the affective state while composing, and the composer's motivation, as well as the client's ideas and, of course, the aesthetic fashions of the time, are further factors that influence the composition. On the performer's side, the interpretation of the piece of music also depends on his artistic concepts, technical skills, experience, motivation, and emotions at the moment of interpretation. In terms of signal theory, the interpreter can therefore also be seen as a "disturbance" or "noise" factor who actively filters the composer's message on its way to the listener.

The type of emotion generated in the listener depends not only on what they hear. Important for the emotional evaluation is the momentary motivation. In addition, personality traits acquired early on, possibly innate, certainly play a significant role. Furthermore, listening experience and familiarity with the music listened to are important for the emotional experience. Finally, it can be speculated that innate emotional reaction patterns to certain acoustic signal characteristics can trigger emotions.

18.3 Strong Emotions When Listening to Music

A special feature of listening to music and making music is the particular quality of the emotions. These "aesthetic emotions" lead to measurable reactions of the autonomic nervous system. These reactions are often referred to as "strong emotions when listening to music," or SEM for short (Gabrielsson 2001). These are musical experiences that can lead to goose bumps, tears, a lump in the throat, fluttering in the stomach, or a racing heart. Such strong emotional experiences and corresponding autonomic responses when listening to music are probably a fairly common phenomenon. According to Panksepp (1995), 86% of American students experience this phenomenon regularly, Sloboda (1991) found it in 90% of adult study participants, and Goldstein (1980) in 90% of music students, but only in 53% of the hospital employees studied.

In the search for objectively measurable strong emotions when listening to music, we have looked at the chill response when listening to music, which is one of the SEMs. Such chills, thrills, or goosebumps are associated with the feeling of shivering and with shivers running down the spine. In humans, chills can be induced by auditory, visual, tactile, somatosensory, gustatory, and enteroceptive (e.g., pressure on the bladder wall) stimuli. Although most studies on the phenomenon concern the chill response to pleasant, sad-nostalgic music (Guhn et al. 2007), it should not be forgotten that unpleasant acoustic stimuli, such as the scratching sound of chalk on a blackboard or a dentist's drill, trigger such a chill response even more reliably (Grewe et al. 2010). These aversive stimuli are psychoacoustically characterized by high volume, a high frequency spectrum and often a high degree of roughness ("scratchiness"). According to new studies by Bannister (2019), three chill categories can be distinguished: "warm chills," which are associated with positive, happy emotions, "cold chills," which are coupled with aversive stimuli and finally "moving chills," which tend to be accompanied by tears in the eyes, a lump in the throat and nostalgic emotions.

The chill response also occurs in other hairy mammals in response to cold, anger, and fear. When it is cold, the raised hairs reduce heat dissipation from the skin; when angry or frightened, the animal appears larger and thus frightens its enemies. This can be observed in chimpanzees, but also in mice, rats, and frightened cats (overview in Panksepp 1996). A special case of the acoustically triggered chill response appears to occur with maternal separation calls in some monkey species. These calls cause the hair to stand up in the laid-down monkey babies. Jaak Panksepp (1995) argues that feelings of loss and social coldness can thus be alleviated by the maternal sounds. In his opinion, this could explain why chill reactions often occur in humans to sad or longing music. Critically, it should be noted that no systematic study of this chill response has yet been carried out in primates. Even though Panksepp's thesis is often quoted, it is still somewhat anecdotal (see also Panksepp and Bernatzky 2002).

Physiologically, the chill response is accompanied by an activation of the sympathetic autonomic nervous system. This results in a contraction of the tiny hair erector muscles (Musculi arrectores pilorum) in the hairy skin. Chills are also accompanied by other reactions of the sympathetic nervous system. For example, the heart rate, blood pressure, respiratory rate, and sweat production often increase. As detailed below, pleasant "warm" chills are accompanied by dopaminergic activation in the reward centers of the striatum and the accumbens nucleus. The resulting increase in arousal and motivation thus supports memory formation. In this way, events that lead to chill reactions are increasingly transferred to long-term memory. This fact is important when we later discuss the therapeutic value of the chill response.

If we consider music as a form of acoustic communication of affects, then a major advantage of the SEM is that it can be measured using psychophysiological methods. This way, the time course of the emotional reaction can also be determined. To achieve this, we designed an experimental setup with which objective psychophysiological markers of emotional experience could be registered while listening to music on the one hand, and on the other hand, the subjects could give a self-report about their changing emotional state in real time, so that we could record the temporal dynamics of the emotional effect of music. For this purpose, they moved a cursor while listening, with which they could continuously indicate their emotional "arousal." A chill experience was indicated by pressing the middle mouse button (Nagel et al. 2007).

It should be noted in advance that chill responses are rare events. Even in a selected group of amateur choral singers, only 72% experienced a chill when listening to highly emotional choral music for 30 min under laboratory conditions (Grewe et al. 2009). Such responses obviously are fleeting and not easily reproducible. For example, an experiment showed that even typical individual "chill stimuli," music that elicited strong emotions in a familiar environment, did not regularly trigger the same reactions on seven consecutive days in the laboratory. On the contrary, chill-responses became increasingly rare, i.e., the test subjects became habituated (Grewe et al. 2009–2010). In addition, chill reactions are strongly context dependent. We were able to show that listening to emotionally powerful music in a group of friends leads to fewer chill reactions than when the music was listened to by the participants alone (Sutherland et al. 2009). This points to another interesting facet of the phenomenon: at least in our culture, chill responses are perceived as very intimate and may also be associated with feelings of shame (Egermann et al. 2011). In a series of further studies, we attempted to determine musical factors that increase the likelihood of chill responses. The hypothesis was that certain harmonic progressions, timbres, human voices, or an increase in volume and high-frequency partials contribute to this phenomenon. The results were sobering: First, we did not find a simple stimulus-response relationship, i.e., even with emotionally very stimulating music, chill responses are rather rare and not easily reproducible (Nagel et al. 2008). Second, there was no combination of musical factors that reliably produced chill responses in different listeners. The only feature that was found in our experiments as a necessary but not sufficient condition for the emergence of a chill response was an unexpected break in the musical structure, i.e., a nonfulfillment of expectations (Grewe et al. 2007). The construction, fulfillment, and deception of musical expectations has been discussed as a major trigger of emotions when listening to music since Leonard Meyer (1956) and is presently in the center of research concerning the role of predictive coding in music (Vuust et al. 2022). Violations of expectations create a moment of arousal; attention is drawn to what is being heard. This seems to be another important condition of strong emotions. This also explains why listening to the human voice significantly increases the frequency of chill experiences, as voices also significantly increase arousal (Loui et al. 2013).

In his book "Sweet Anticipation" (2006), David Huron elaborated on this idea of fulfilled anticipation and emotional arousal. According to this, a certain emotional satisfaction arises when expectations are fulfilled. If musical expectations remain unfulfilled, this does not necessarily lead to negative feelings, but the result can be laughter, amazement, or even a strong reaction in the form of "goose bumps." Apparently, in an overarching sense, the positive experience of music is dependent on surprising moments. Together with colleagues (Gold et al. 2019), we believe that the process of listening to good music consists of transforming uncertainty at the beginning of the listening experience into certainty as the listening progresses. Certainty is achieved through repetitive structures, fulfilled expectations, etc. This transformation process is then often accompanied by positive emotions and occasionally also by "chills" and feelings of flow. The associated learning process leads to the activation of the dopaminergic reward system (Schoeller et al. 2024).

Numerous listener characteristics influence the frequency and strength of chills. For example, there is a "chill personality." Listeners with frequent chill reactions (chill responders) differ psychologically from those who do not experience chills. Chill responders were familiar with classical music, rated music as more important to their lives, identified more with the music they preferred, and listened to music more often in everyday life. In terms of psychological characteristics, chill responders showed a general tendency toward lower stimulus thresholds, were more sensitive, and were more dependent on other people and emotional care (Grewe et al. 2007). These findings have been replicated several times and expanded in recent years: "chill responders" are also more open to new experiences (Colver and El-Alayi 2015) and listen to music in a cognitive–empathic perceptual style (Linnemann et al. 2018).

Since familiarity with the musical genre and personal emotional memories appeared to be important factors for triggering chill responses, we wanted to examine this in more detail in a further experiment. We recruited 54 patients from three different amateur choirs that had performed Mozart's Requiem (hereafter referred to as the "Mozart group") and 41 participants from gospel and pop choirs (hereafter referred to as the "control group"). The latter were not familiar with the Mozart Requiem or with classical music. We played emotionally moving excerpts from Mozart's Requiem (Lacrimosa, Confutatis, Rex tremendae, Tuba mirum, Dies irae) to these participants, using both our own recordings from the Mozart group and an interpretation by Herbert v. Karajan. In addition, excerpts from Puccini's Requiem and from the Bach motet "Unser Leben ist ein Schatten" were played, each sung by only one of the three choirs of the Mozart group. The subjective intensity of the feelings and the perceived chill reactions were measured with the EMuJoy program. In addition, skin conductance, heart rate, and respiratory rate were recorded. Figure 18.3 shows an example of this measurement.

Only about two-thirds of the participants reported a chill response. There was a high inter-individual variability. The maximum number of chills during the experiment, which lasted about an hour, amounted to 88 "goose bumps" for one participant! On average, each participant experienced nine chill reactions. Interestingly, there was no correlation with age, gender, or preference for classical music.

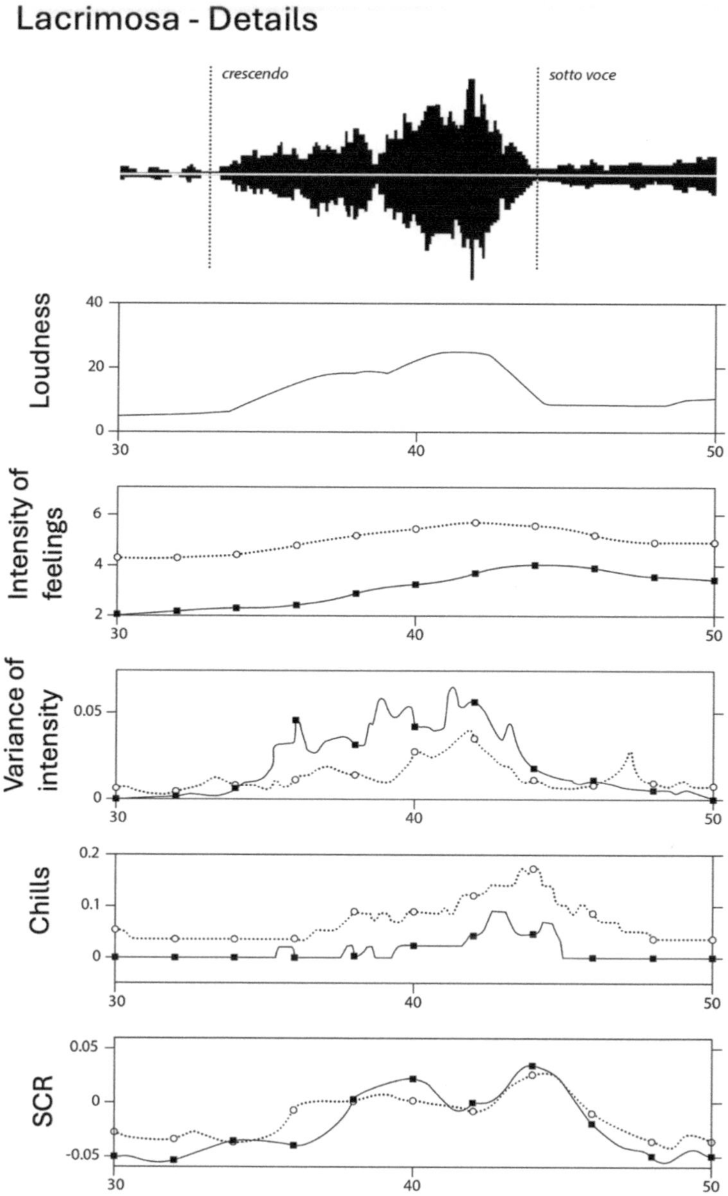

Fig. 18.3 Measurement data from the goose bumps experiments. The test subjects listen to a 20-s excerpt from the Mozart Requiem. The curves show the mean values of the two groups; the Mozart group is indicated by the dotted line. The sonogram at the top shows the volume curves of the piece. The feelings of emotional arousal indicated with the computer mouse are plotted on a scale from 2 to 6. The more "intense" the feelings, the higher the value. The goosebump experiences are shown in absolute figures; 0.2 means that one in five listeners had goosebumps at that moment. It is immediately apparent that the Mozart group experienced many more goose bumps than the control group. The course of the "sweating curve" (SCR stands for "skin conduction response") is given in microsiemens and is very similar in both groups

However, familiarity with the music influenced the frequency of chill reactions. They occurred far more frequently in the Mozart group than in the control group (72% vs. 56% of participants), and the total number of chill responses was much higher in this group than in the control group (679 vs. 173 chill responses). When listening to the Bach motet and the Puccini Requiem, chill responses were also significantly more frequent among the choristers who had sung these pieces. It seemed to be less important whether they had heard their own or someone else's interpretation (Grewe et al. 2009). Obviously, familiarity with the stimulus is an important factor in triggering chill responses. In addition, the musical biography and individual associations (for example, memories of an uplifting performance in a magnificent venue) promote the susceptibility to a chill response enormously.Overall, it became clear that strong emotional reactions occur less frequently than previously reported in the literature. This is also due to the fact that we only consider validated reactions with agreement between self-report and psychophysiological markers. In addition, it became clear that although there are inter-individual similar reaction patterns, which can be considered as universals, these in turn depend heavily on intra-individual factors.

18.4 Brain Physiological Correlates of Strong Emotions

What are the brain-physiological correlates of the emotions triggered by music?

In 2010, Stefan Koelsch published a compilation of the results of numerous functional imaging studies on music and emotion. In healthy subjects, listening to pleasant music leads, as expected, to changes in activation in the so-called limbic system, in the brain structures that program emotions. These include the regions of the nucleus accumbens, the amygdala, the hippocampus, and the cingulate cortex, shown in Fig. 18.4. Consonant-sounding and pleasantly perceived music led to activation on both sides in the basal forebrain, the hippocampus, the accumbens nucleus, and in the area of the median girdle winding, as well as in the anterior part of the right frontal brain. Dissonant music perceived as unpleasant, on the other hand, led to activation of the amygdala and activation in the right parahippocampal gyrus, a region located next to the hippocampus deep in the temporal lobe.

Chills are associated with brain activation in the reward centers of the limbic emotional system. The brain regions involved include areas of the midbrain and the accumbens nucleus, as well as the lower frontal part of the forebrain (orbitofrontal cortex) and the right upper temporal lobe (superior temporal gyrus); however, the activity of the amygdala is inhibited (Sescousse et al. 2013). This "chill network" can also be found in the brain structure. The group from the BRAMS Institute in Montreal was able to show that the nerve fiber connections between the accumbens nerve, the orbito-frontal cortex and the right upper temporal lobe were stronger in people who frequently had music-induced chills (Martinez-Molina et al. 2019). An earlier study by the same group also described the time course of the release of dopamine during intense goosebump experiences caused by music. The brain regions responsible for mediating feelings of reward and happiness in the midbrain,

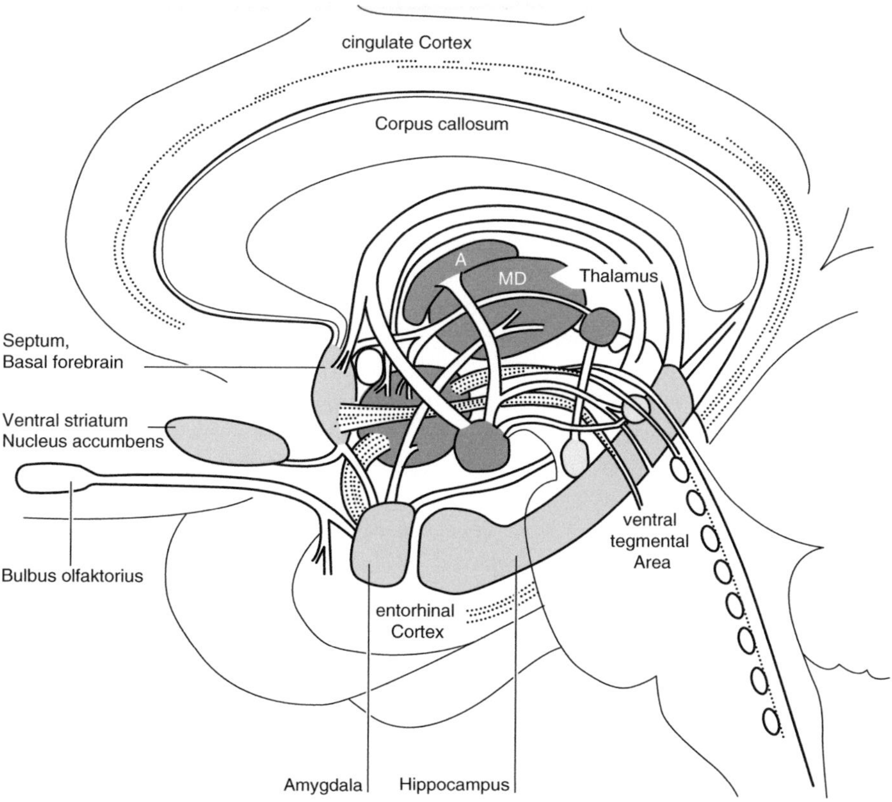

Fig. 18.4 The limbic system. The regions of the amygdala, the hippocampus, the accumbens nucleus, the basal forebrain, and the cingulate gyrus located deep inside the brain are shown schematically. This is where emotions are programmed. They are evaluated cognitively by the cerebral cortex

the accumbens nucleus, the striatum, and the orbitofrontal lobe were activated (Salimpoor et al. 2013). Interestingly, the release of the motivation and reward hormone dopamine was detectable in the striatum a few seconds before the actual feeling of pleasure during the anticipation of the forthcoming chill experience. The actual chill-response led to the release of dopamine in the accumbens nucleus (Salimpoor et al. 2011). A similar time course of neurohormonal release is also found in other strongly pleasure-inducing activities, such as eating after a long period of hunger or during sexual activity.

These results may also explain why music is accorded such high value in all human societies. The dopaminergic activation described above regulates and increases attention, supports motivation, and memory formation in episodic and procedural memory. This massively supports the recollection of musical events that are strongly emotionally evaluated. According to new studies, other regions of the cerebrum are also involved in the development of strong emotions. For example, measurements using the high-resolution EEG method during chilling experiences with music also showed increased activation in the motor areas of the right hemisphere of the brain responsible for rhythmic movements (Chabin et al. 2020). The authors assume that the anticipation of rhythmic movements and the musical "drive" are element of strong emotional arousal.

The brain structures involved are often referred to somewhat casually as the brain's "pleasure system" and are also activated in a similar way during other pleasure-based activities. Stefan Koelsch (2014) pointed out that, interestingly, the hippocampal structures that were otherwise activated during pleasant musical performances were not involved in chill activations. This means that music can appeal not only to the pleasure system, but also to other emotional dimensions. For example, the activity in the hippocampus formation generates a class of emotions that can be described as "attachment-related emotions." This refers to emotions that contain a social element, are experienced as gentle, tender, and positive, and are often described with terms such as "joy" or "happiness," or also with terms such as "being touched" or "being moved." Here, Koelsch uses a memorable image to illustrate the difference to pleasure: *"The rewarding feeling I have when I drink a glass of water when I am very thirsty is hardly described as "being moved." We are moved or touched, for example, when the hungry boy shares his last piece of bread with his little sister"* (Koelsch 2014). Creating and maintaining social bonds has probably been a central function of music in evolutionary terms, and still is: when we make music, sing or dance together, we have contact with other people, we communicate, coordinate our movements, and cooperate with each other. This naturally strengthens social cohesion.

18.5 Possible Role of SEM for Music Therapy

The information presented on the emotional effects of music has resulted in treatment approaches for adjuvant therapy for a variety of psychosomatic complaints and illnesses (Bernatzky et al. 2011; Bernatzky and Hesse 2012). However, the transferability of these research results regarding possible rehabilitation therapies for patients with neuropsychiatric disorders remains largely unexplored. Some publications describe the high potential of receptive music stimulation in everyday clinical practice (Bringman et al. 2009). Music used preoperatively to promote relaxation leads to less pain postoperatively, combined with a reduction in medication (Bernatzky et al. 2011). The mechanisms of neurological music therapy in stroke patients and patients with Parkinson's syndrome and neurodegenerative diseases have also been well elucidated in recent years. In addition to the emotional effect and the stress reduction induced by correctly applied music therapy, direct and indirect effects of music on the autonomic nervous system also play a role (Sihvonen et al. 2017; Altenmüller and Stewart 2020).

In the following, we want to relate our findings to the potential evolutionary role of the analyzed strong emotions when listening to music. We have seen that the chill response is biologically based on a phylogenetically old, reflex-like response of the sympathetic nervous system in connection with thermoregulation and threatening and intimidating gestures. It is biologically associated with an increase in arousal and facilitates memory formation. In humans, the auditory response occurs on the one hand in connection with negatively evaluated, loud, high-frequency, and harsh noises, and on the other hand in connection with pleasant musical stimuli, which are associated with activation of the dopaminergic reward system in the brain. Factors that promote these positive chill responses include: sudden structural changes in the music, the onset of something new, increasing the volume in the high register, association with positive emotional memories, and a general preference for the genre of music in question (Nagel et al. 2008; Harrison and Loui 2014; Schoeller et al. 2024).

The evolutionary adaptive value of the chill response is obvious, considering the biological concomitants mentioned above. Negative chill responses may have been the reactions to the shrieking, panicked cries of conspecifics attacked by an enemy. They can be regarded as remnants of an evolutionarily old affective communication system. Such vocalizations can be found in many social mammals when threatened. In addition, the negative emotions promote avoidance behavior, so that the distance to the sound source is increased. In this way, a safe distance is achieved, and hearing is protected. Finally, in the context of hostile confrontations, the opponent is intimidated by the raised hair, and at the same time, memory consolidation for the situation is promoted. In this way, situations are better memorized, and the associated acoustic patterns are also stored in memory. Perhaps the roots of such behavior go back some three million years, when our one-meter small ancestor, Australopithecus afarensis, roamed the tall grass of the Central African dry steppes and was panicked by the cries of the large African eagles hunting him.

The situation for the positive chill response when listening to music is more complicated. The frequently cited separation call hypothesis by Jaak Panksepp, mentioned above, has not yet been empirically proven. The lack of evidence of acoustically evoked chill reactions in infants and young children, for example, when listening to soothing lullabies, speaks against the separation call as the original source of the chill response. It is possible that such a phenomenon has been overlooked so far. However, according to our informal surveys of children and adolescents, the positive chill reactions appear to occur at the earliest shortly, before puberty is reached. Admittedly, there is still a lack of empirical research on this interesting topic.

There are two further possibilities for attributing an evolutionary adaptive value to positive chill responses. Since chill responses occur primarily in response to new, unexpected acoustic stimuli and facilitate memory formation, they increase our ability to recognize acoustic patterns and expand our repertoire of familiar acoustic shapes. In addition, the chill response is associated with the activation of neural reward networks, which positively evaluate experiences and increase our curiosity about unexpected acoustic events. This, in turn, was of evolutionary importance, as a fast and precise classification of acoustic stimuli was a prerequisite for optimal behavior. This enabled us to reliably recognize the sounds of a predator sneaking up on us at night, as well as the subtle nuances of the emotional vocalizations of our conspecifics. We therefore suspect that the driving force behind the development of our superior auditory memory was precisely the chill-mediated reward of identifying new acoustic patterns. Presumably, the first songs and chants, the first sounds of primitive musical instruments, e.g., beating hollow tree trunks with wood, also provided a safe framework for training auditory discrimination. In addition, vocal abilities were improved and thus the prerequisites for a highly differentiated acoustic communication system, namely speech, were created. The second evolutionary adaptive feature of the chill response is the generation of positive emotions. By activating the sympathetic nervous system and the reward system, music has been able to provide moments of happiness and comfort in the hard lives of early modern humans for decades.

This effect can, of course, also be used in music therapy: an increase in the availability of dopamine when experiencing chills can improve joylessness, a major symptom of depression and schizophrenia. This effect certainly also explains the great successes that Teppo Särkämo achieved with stroke patients in Helsinki (Särkämo et al. 2008; overview in Sihvonen et al. 2017). In his study, stroke patients were asked to listen to their favorite music for at least 1 h a day for a total of 2 months. A control group listened to their favorite audiobooks for one hour a day, while another "blank" control group received no additional stimulation. The results after 3 months were overwhelming: not only was the music group less depressed, but their attention, word memory, and even language skills were better than in both other groups. G. Bernatzky's working group was also able to show in a study on Parkinson's patients that fine motor skills improved significantly immediately after listening to strongly stimulating music (Bernatzky et al. 2004) (see chapter by Thaut, Chap. 11, this volume).

We suspect that these effects are due to the elevated mood and increased attention of the music group. The neurohormones associated with this are dopamine in the accumbens nucleus, discussed in detail above, and noradrenaline, which controls attention. In addition, our favorite music reduces stress, creating better conditions for new learning and neuroplasticity (for a review, see Altenmüller and Stewart 2020). Finally, music can remind us of happier days in our lives and evoke numerous associations that arise not only as sounds, but also as words, scenes, images, and emotions. The power of these strong biographical memories, which are particularly shaped by chilling experiences, presumably also plays an important role in music therapy for patients affected by dementia. Initial studies have already been carried out in this area, but research will certainly be able to contribute further significant findings in the coming years (Moreno-Morales et al. 2020).

References

Altenmüller E, Stewart L (2020) Music supported therapy in neurorehabilitation. In: Dietz V, Ward N (eds) Oxford textbook of neurorehabilitation. Oxford University Press, Oxford, pp 421–431

Altenmüller E, Kopiez R, Grewe O (2013a) Strong emotions in music: are they an evolutionary adaptation? In: Bader R (ed) Sound—perception—performance. Current research in systematic musicology, vol 1. Springer, Heidelberg. https://doi.org/10.1007/978-3-319-00107-4_5

Altenmüller E, Schmidt S, Zimmermann E (2013b) Evolution of emotional communication: an introduction. In: Altenmüller E, Schmidt S, Zimmermann E (eds) Evolution of emotional communication. From sounds in nonhuman mammals to speech and music in man. Oxford University Press, Oxford, pp IX–XIV

Bannister S (2019) Distinct varieties of aesthetic chills in response to multimedia. PLoS One 14(11):e0224974. https://doi.org/10.1371/journal.pone.0224974. PMID: 31725733; PMCID: PMC6855651
Bernatzky G, Hesse HP (2012) Music in palliative care. In: Bernatzky G, Sittl R, Likar R (eds) Pain treatment in palliative medicine, 3rd edn. Springer, Vienna/New York. ISBN 978-3-211-88876-6, 320 pages, pp 229–234
Bernatzky G, Bernatzky P, Hesse H-P, Staffen W, Ladurner G (2004) Stimulating music increases motor coordination in patients afflicted with Parkinson's disease. Neurosci Lett 361:4–8
Bernatzky G, Presch M, Anderson M, Panksepp J (2011) Emotional foundations of music as a non-pharmacological pain management tool in modern medicine. Neurosci Biobehav Rev 35(9):1889–1899
Bringman H, Giesecke K, Thörne A, Brigman S (2009) Relaxing music as pre-medication before surgery: a randomized controlled trial. Acta Anaesthesiol Scand 53:759–764
Chabin T, Gabriel D, Chansophonkul T, Michelant L, Joucla C, Haffen E, Moulin T, Comte A, Pazart L (2020) Cortical patterns of pleasurable musical chills revealed by high-density EEG. Front Neurosci 14:565815. https://doi.org/10.3389/fnins.2020.565815. PMID: 33224021; PMCID: PMC7670092
Colver MC, El Alayli A (2015) Getting aesthetic chills from music: the connection between openness to experience and frisson. Psychol Music 44:413–427. https://doi.org/10.1177/0305735615572358
Egermann H, Sutherland ME, Grewe O, Nagel F, Kopiez R, Altenmüller E (2011) The influences of a group setting on the experience of music: a physiological and psychological perspective on emotion. Music Sci 15:307–323
Ekman P (1972) Universals and cultural differences in facial expression of emotion. In: Cole JR (ed) Nebraska symposium on motivation, vol 19. University of Nebraska Press, Lincoln, pp 207–283
Gabrielson A (2001) Emotions in strong experiences with music. In: Juslin P, Sloboda J (eds) Music and emotion: theory and research. Oxford University Press, Oxford, pp 431–452
Gold BP, Pearce MT, Mas-Herrero E, Dagher A, Zatorre RJ (2019) Predictability and uncertainty in the pleasure of music: a reward for learning? J Neurosci 39(47):9397–9409. https://doi.org/10.1523/JNEUROSCI.0428-19.2019. Epub 2019 Oct 21. PMID: 31636112; PMCID: PMC6867811
Goldstein A (1980) Thrills in response to music and other stimuli. Physiol Psychol 8(1):126–129
Grewe O, Nagel F, Kopiez R, Altenmüller E (2007) Emotions over time: synchronicity and development of subjective, physiological, and facial affective reactions to music. Emotion 7(4):774–788. https://doi.org/10.1037/1528-3542.7.4.774. PMID: 18039047
Grewe O, Kopiez R, Altenmüller E (2009) The chill parameter: goose bumps and shivers as promising measures in emotion research. Music Percept 27(1):61–74
Grewe O, Altenmüller E, Nagel F, Kopiez R. (2009–2010) Individual emotional reactions towards music: evolutionary-based universals? Music Sci (Special Issue): 261–287
Grewe O, Katzur B, Kopiez R, Altenmüller E (2010) Chills in different sensory domains—frisson elicited by acoustical, visual, tactile and gustatory stimuli. Psychol Music 39(2):220–239
Guhn M, Hamm A, Zentner MR (2007) Physiological and musico-acoustic correlates of the chill response. Music Percept 24(5):473–483
Harrison L, Loui P (2014) Thrills, chills, frissons, and skin orgasms: toward an integrative model of transcendent psychophysiological experiences in music. Front Psychol 23(5):790. https://doi.org/10.3389/fpsyg.2014.00790. PMID: 25101043; PMCID: PMC4107937
Huron D (2006) Sweet anticipation: music and the psychology of expectation. A Bradford Book, Cambridge, MA
Koelsch S (2014) Brain correlates of music-evoked emotions. Nat Rev Neurosci 15(3):170–180. https://doi.org/10.1038/nrn3666. PMID: 24552785
Linnemann A, Kreutz G, Gollwitzer M, Nater UM (2018) Validation of the German version of the music-empathizing-music-systemizing (MEMS) inventory (short version). Front Behav

Neurosci 12:153. https://doi.org/10.3389/fnbeh.2018.00153. Erratum in: Front Behav Neurosci. 2018 12:228. PMID: 30135649; PMCID: PMC6092492
Loui P, Bachorik JP, Li HC, Schlaug G (2013) Effects of voice on emotional arousal. Front Psychol 4:675. https://doi.org/10.3389/fpsyg.2013.00675. PMID: 24101908; PMCID: PMC3787249
Martínez-Molina N, Mas-Herrero E, Rodríguez-Fornells A, Zatorre RJ, Marco-Pallarés J (2019) White matter microstructure reflects individual differences in music reward sensitivity. J Neurosci 39(25):5018–5027. https://doi.org/10.1523/JNEUROSCI.2020-18.2019. Epub 2019 Apr 18. PMID: 31000588; PMCID: PMC6670256
Mehr SA, Krasnow MM, Bryant GA, Hagen EH (2021) Toward a productive evolutionary understanding of music. Behav Brain Sci 44:e122. https://doi.org/10.1017/S0140525X21000030. PMID: 34588071; PMCID: PMC10625480
Meyer LB (1956) Emotions and meaning in music (Paperback edition 1961 ed.). The University of Chicago Press, Chicago/London
Moreno-Morales C, Calero R, Moreno-Morales P, Pintado C (2020) Music therapy in the treatment of dementia: a systematic review and meta-analysis. Front Med (Lausanne) 7:160. https://doi.org/10.3389/fmed.2020.00160. PMID: 32509790; PMCID: PMC7248378
Nagel F, Kopiez R, Grewe O, Altenmüller E (2007) EMuJoy: software for continuous measurement of perceived emotions in music. Behav Res Methods 39(2):283–290
Nagel F, Kopiez R, Grewe O, Altenmüller E (2008) Psychoacoustic correlates of musically induced chills. Music Sci 12(1):101–113
Panksepp J (1995) The emotional sources of "chills" induced by music. Music Percept 13(2):171–207
Panksepp J (1996) Affective neuroscience: a paradigm to study the animate circuits for human emotion. In: Kavanaugh RD, Zimmerberg B, Fein S (eds) Emotions: interdisciplinary perspectives. Lawrence Erlbaum, Mahwah, pp 29–60
Panksepp J, Bernatzky G (2002) Emotional sounds and the brain: the neuro-affective foundations of music appreciation. Behav Process 60:133–155
Salimpoor V, Benovoy M, Larcher K, Dagher A, Zatorre RJ (2011) Anatomically distinct dopamine release during anticipation and experience of peak emotion to music. Nat Neurosci 14:257–262
Salimpoor VN, van den Bosch I, Kovacevic N, McIntosh AR, Dagher A, Zatorre RJ (2013) Interactions between the nucleus accumbens and auditory cortices predict music reward value. Science 340(6129):216–219. https://doi.org/10.1126/science.1231059. PMID: 23580531
Särkämö T, Tervaniemi M, Laitinen S, Forsblom A, Soinila S, Mikkonen M, Autti T, Silvennoinen HM, Erkkilä J, Laine M, Peretz I, Hietanen M (2008) Music listening enhances cognitive recovery and mood after middle cerebral artery stroke. Brain 131:866–876
Scherer KR (2005) What are emotions? And how can they be measured? Soc Sci Inf 44(4):695–729
Schoeller F, Jain A, Pizzagalli DA, Reggente N (2024) The neurobiology of aesthetic chills: how bodily sensations shape emotional experiences. Cogn Affect Behav Neurosci 24(4):617–630. https://doi.org/10.3758/s13415-024-01168-x. Epub 2024 Feb 21. PMID: 38383913; PMCID: PMC11233292
Sescousse G, Caldú X, Segura B, Dreher JC (2013) Processing of primary and secondary rewards: a quantitative meta-analysis and review of human functional neuroimaging studies. Neurosci Biobehav Rev 37(4):681–696
Sihvonen AJ, Särkämö T, Leo V, Tervaniemi M, Altenmüller E, Soinila S (2017) Music-based interventions in neurological rehabilitation. Lancet Neurol 16(8):648–660. https://doi.org/10.1016/S1474-4422(17)30168-0. Epub 2017 Jun 26. PMID: 28663005
Sloboda J (1991) Music structure and emotional response: some empirical findings. Psychol Music 19:110–120
Sutherland ME, Grewe O, Egermann H, Nagel F, Kopiez R, Altenmüller E (2009) The influence of social situations on music listening. Ann N Y Acad Sci 1169:363–367
Vuust P, Heggli OA, Friston KJ, Kringelbach ML (2022) Music in the brain. Nat Rev Neurosci 23(5):287–305. https://doi.org/10.1038/s41583-022-00578-5. Epub 2022 Mar 29. PMID: 35352057
Wundt W (1905) Principles of physiological psychology. Engelmann, Leipzig

Health Aspects of Amateur Singing

19

Gunter Kreutz

The exploration of health-relevant effects of communal singing in everyday life is the subject of social and health science studies since the beginning of the millennium. Models that equally consider salutogenetic, cultural, and biological aspects often serve to classify the empirical literature. The diversity of singing practices and traditions does not contradict the specific emotional, cognitive, and social effects of singing on individual well-being. The promotion of well-being and quality of life and the aestheticization of everyday life through communal singing are equally important goals.

19.1 Introduction

Singing is a widespread ability that shapes the everyday life and cultural consciousness of many people. The vast majority of the population is easily able to reproduce tones and melodies and learn songs (Welch 1979; Dalla Bella and Berkowska 2009). People who intonate inaccurately without proven tone deafness do not necessarily lack practice (Berkowska and Dalla Bella 2013). Rather, at least in some cases, the implementation of perceived pitches into motor reproductions seems inadequate (Pfordresher and Mantell 2014).

Singing is a domain almost subordinate to language, yet important for its development. It is close to dance and movement, yet due to its physiological foundations,

G. Kreutz (✉)
Systematic Musicology, Carl von Ossietzky University Oldenburg, Oldenburg, Lower Saxony, Germany
e-mail: gunter.kreutz@uni-oldenburg.de

G. Kreutz, G. Bernatzky (eds.), *Music and Medicine*, Neurocultural Health and Wellbeing, https://doi.org/10.1007/978-3-662-72175-9_19

it is a model for musical instruments (Titze and Martin 1998). Natural science studies dominated its research until the 2000s (Sundberg and Rossing 1990).

Health meanings of communal singing have been increasingly in the focus of social and health science studies since the beginning of the millennium (e.g., Clift and Hancox 2001; Clift 2012; Vickhoff et al. 2013). A steadily growing number of research reports suggest that communal singing can be helpful in different ways for various groups of patients (Lewis et al. 2016; Gold et al. 2019; Irons et al. 2020). Systematic overviews of nonclinical reports show that amateur choir singers can benefit in their individual physical, mental, and emotional well-being (Clift et al. 2010b). The psychological effects are comparable to other group activities (Stewart and Lonsdale 2016; Lonsdale and Day 2021). Singing offers in health facilities are therefore particularly useful as they reach different populations, expand existing strategies, and can be considered almost side-effect free (Kreutz et al. 2014a).

The Covid-19 pandemic has revealed a number of health risks associated with communal singing (Hamner et al. 2020; Mürbe et al. 2021; Miller et al. 2021). However, a detailed discussion including effective countermeasures is beyond the scope of this overview.

19.2 How Did Humans Come to Sing?

Our current understanding and appreciation of singing as a cultural asset can be partially explained by analyzing its conditions of origin and contexts of musical behavior (Brown 2000; Cross 2001). The ability of vocal learning, thoroughly researched in its genetic and behavioral foundations in songbirds and other species (Jarvis 2019), is particularly pronounced in humans and allows prelinguistic children to participate in the surrounding singing culture (Trehub 2003).

There is no doubt that communal singing has accompanied human prehistory and early history and has spread to all known cultures (Mithen 2007). According to one of the oldest origin theories, human singing arose through the imitation of nature. Even today, natives of the Amazon rainforest communicate in song while hunting for birds or monkeys. Other theories point to the social-emotional functions of singing, such as between mother and child, or between members of communities. Rituals, celebrations, and ceremonies in secular and sacred contexts are often associated with songs and play a significant role in helping people remember and recall these occasions. Thus, singing experiences become part of the semantic memory, which often remains accessible even in late stages of dementia (Sherratt et al. 2004).

It seems sensible to distinguish clearly between songs, singing styles, practices, and repertoires as cultural techniques on the one hand, and musicality in the sense of human ability to sing as a biological phenomenon on the other. Savage et al. (2021) characterize communal singing as a human ability that can be justified both culturally and biologically for the purpose of establishing social bonds between individuals (Savage et al. 2021). Cultural aspects of singing can serve to distinguish communities from each other and create quasi-territories for the practice of specific practices. Musicality, however, refers to overarching mechanisms that enable people to perceive, produce, and enjoy music and singing, regardless of culture.

In addition to social and cognitive meanings, musical origin theories point to the regulation of emotions as a fundamental reason why communal singing has survived human development since prehistoric times. Communal singing promotes the perception of one's own voice, but on the other hand, it's merging into communal sounds shifts attention away from the individual to the group of singing people. This creates a superior sense of identity that allows one to understand oneself as part of a whole while subordinating individual differences to the sense of community. Hagen and Bryant (2003) speculate that communal singing and dancing, therefore, represent an outwardly directed signal system for group readiness to defend. Evolutionary theorists who focus on inwardly directed, psychological effects and especially the promotion of empathy through synchronization (Kirschner and Tomasello 2010) contradict this. Communicative, outwardly directed, and emotion-regulating, inwardly directed functions do not mutually exclude each other. However, since communal singing can evoke strong feelings of reward, which can also include the release of endogenous opiates (Stone et al. 2018), it seems unlikely that the protection or defense of the group is a primary motive.

Brown (2000) advocates the theory of an originally integrated, linguistic-musical vocal behavior, a "musilanguage." The overlap of cerebral networks for processing both linguistic and musical information seems to support this assumption to support. What influences ultimately led to a dichotomous processing of language and music is not clarified. What is likely crucial is that humans can only exist as a functioning community and can successfully adapt to changing environmental conditions. An important basis of singing and dancing lies in the fact that individuals physically synchronize with each other. Every individual must be able to follow an external pace setter. This ability is attributed with outstanding importance in terms of language evolution.

From a developmental psychology perspective, the maturation of the organism and especially of the brain at least partially retraces evolutionary processes. This assumption can also be applied to the hypothesis of the "Musilanguage." McMullen and Saffran (2004), for example, consider the so-called baby talk as a phenomenological equivalent of an integrated language and music module in the infant brain, from which the different domains only develop in the course of development. This assumption of fundamental musical competencies in newborns is important for various processes such as emotion regulation to social behavior. Without being able to fully address the facets revealed in the course of musical developmental research in recent years, the picture of profound influences of singing behavior in early childhood development on the maturing personality of a human being is becoming increasingly clear. On the other hand, singing and corresponding—even rudimentary—predispositions and competencies emerge as resources that represent health preventive as well as rehabilitation suitable potentials.

19.3 Salutogenesis and Context Model of Health Effects of Singing

The so-called Salutogenesis (Antonovsky 1997), which goes back to the Israeli physician Aaron Antonovsky (1923–1994), forms a counter-draft to the orientation favored in medical research on the origin of disease (Pathogenesis). The salutogenetic approach focuses on human resources and potentials that promote individual well-being as well as improve psychological, physical, and mental states (Mittelmark and Bull 2013). Behind this is the idea that self-determined human behavior toward environmental influences and genetic dispositions is the decisive factor for maintaining health (Deci and Ryan 2015).

Health-promoting actions must, from a salutogenetic perspective, be individually perceived as *comprehensible, manageable,* and *meaningful.* Although the salutogenetic terms and dimensions are subject to ongoing discussions and empirical tests, the basic idea that avoidance and overcoming of diseases is closely linked to available cognitive, emotional, and especially social resources is very compatible with general notions of health according to the WHO definition.

Regardless of the multifaceted and sometimes controversial discussions, the salutogenetic approach appears to be excellently suited from a pragmatic point of view to unlock the health potentials of artistic and cultural activities. These are especially recognizable in the broader context of prevention, healing, and the fight against secondary diseases. After all, many sick people need psychosocially effective, adjuvant therapies that help mediate between medical treatments and reintegration into everyday life. Such music-based strategies are only associated with very few contraindications, side effects, or other disease patterns negatively affecting side effects.

Figure 19.1 shows a salutogenetically inspired model of the health effects of singing. The basic idea is that the complex reality of life contributes to the construction and the influencing of self-images has a high proportion. The reality of communal singing includes a variety of factors in addition to the activity itself, which can be summed up as situation and context, and in the sum, allow a reconstruction of the self and thus indirect changes of the disease pattern. It would be speculative to suggest that the salutogenic basic understanding rather abstract concept of *coherence*, which also aims at the great health importance of social cohesion, in communal singing quasi-materializes.

The model focuses on individual and social factors that are inextricably linked with singing. In short, singing is neither necessarily novel nor unique to be individually effective. After all, singing as a human activity is based on already existing resources in the organism. Psychoactive effects of singing alone or in a group are thus repercussions of specific behaviors, which a person perceives as singing. Self-reports are therefore a primary and differentiated source of information about the effects of singing significant. In addition, the model implies potential changes in perception, consciousness, or physical indicators that need to be uncovered using suitable diagnostic procedures. A controlled methodology is required to identify factors influencing changes associated with singing activity in given experimental or empirical settings. Mechanisms of action of singing are thus basically only indirectly detectable and within the framework of temporal sequences, and in contrast with alternative interventions.

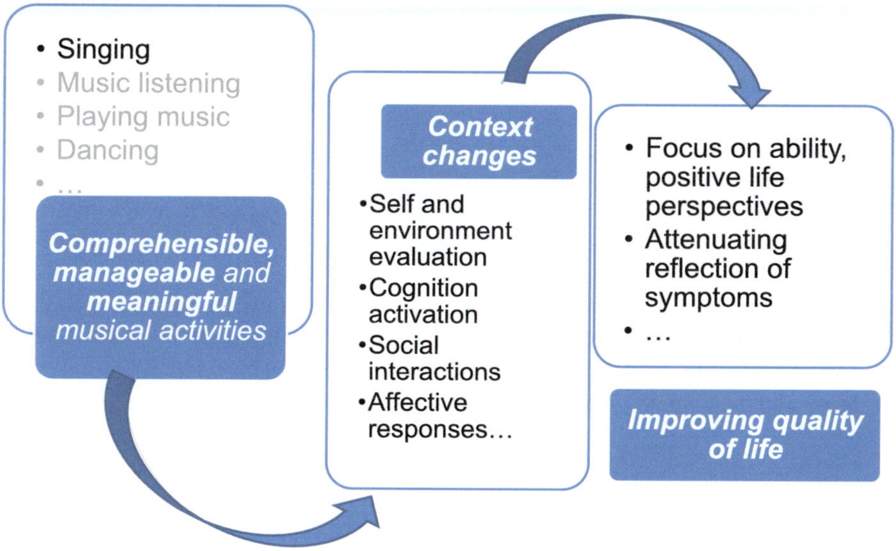

Fig. 19.1 Salutogenetically inspired simple model of hypothetical mechanisms or mediators which associate singing (preferably in groups) on the one hand, and improvements of quality of life, on the other

The form of the singing activity, the quality of the transmission, and other variables closely associated with singing are in the proposed model as significant as those that are not specifically designed for singing. In addition to the individual physical and psychological conditions, attitudes, and attributions, as well as the implicit and explicit cultural knowledge of a person, from which (positive) changes are possible. Thus, even the quality of the transmission is measured from complex variable constellations, which can indirectly and directly influence singing activity.

Potential changes attributed to communal singing thus include not only health status, but also general well-being and perceived quality of life. This fact is conceptually and methodologically significant.

Conclusion
It is important for the classification of empirical findings to view the changes associated with singing as a holistic process that can only be understood in the combination of different facets. Such a holistic view is still lacking in the current research efforts. It is to be realized through polyvalent, qualitative, and controlled quantitative methods, including strategies.

19.3.1 Psychological Effects of Singing

Singing as a group activity is subject to latent inclusion and exclusion conditions that require individuals to have musical and social competencies (Kreutz and Brünger

2012b). Singing groups can appear as legally binding organizations in the form of clubs and associations. These framework conditions are important as they regulate access and can certainly present barriers. Although the literature often describes socially inclusive aspects and individual advantages (Stewart and Lonsdale 2016), this requires, on the one hand, relatively low-threshold offers and on the other hand a correspondingly widespread affinity for singing. Thus, individual musical development in childhood and adolescence is decisive, to what extent and in what form people engage in singing in later life (Kreutz and Brünger 2012b).

Singing alone (Grape et al. 2003; Valentine and Evans 2001) and especially in groups (Clift et al. 2010a) promotes the emergence of positive emotions, at least among amateur singers (Clift 2012). Self-reports from singers point to a multitude of factors that are at least indirectly involved in this psychological process. Summarized these in a systematic overview as follows:

- "Physical relaxation and a release of physical tension
- Emotional release and reduction of stress
- A feeling of happiness, good mood, cheerfulness, joy, and elation
- A feeling of more personal, emotional, and physical well-being
- A feeling of increased stimulation and energy
- Stimulation of thinking abilities—attention, concentration, memory, and learning
- A feeling of being absorbed in an activity that demands capacities of body and mind in multiple ways
- A feeling of collective connection through coordinated activities, following the same pulse
- The potential of personal contact with others who are similarly minded, and the development of personally supportive friendships and constructive collaborative relationships
- A feeling of contributing to a whole that is greater than the sum of its parts
- A feeling of personal transcendence beyond the profane and everyday reality, making contact with a sense of beauty and with something beyond words, that moves and "is good for the soul"
- A feeling of growing self-confidence and self-esteem
- A feeling of therapeutic relief regarding long-standing psychological and social problems (e.g., depression, a biography of abuse, problems with drugs and alcohol, social disadvantage)
- A feeling of making a societal contribution through public performances
- A feeling of training physical systems, especially the lungs
- A feeling of disciplining one's own skeletal-muscular system through the adoption of good posture
- Being involved in an estimated, significant, and valuable activity that conveys a sense of purpose and motivation" (Clift et al. 2008, p. 5ff., translated by G.K.)

Within these subjective assessments, at least seven superordinate facets can be derived, which can partly be empirically supported, namely (i) improved moods and general psychological well-being; (ii) relaxation and stress reduction; (iii) mental activation; (iv) protection of mental and physical health; (v) experiences of spirituality and deeper emotional experiences; (vi) improved self-image and increased self-efficacy; and (vii) feelings of social connectedness.

It is noteworthy that an increased positive emotionality *after* singing can also be observed with a neutral to positive basic mood *before* (Beck et al. 2000); half an hour between two mood assessments proved to be sufficient. However, the intervention durations are very different between the individual studies. The lower and upper limits of time intervals within which psychological effects can be demonstrated are not clarified today.

Clift (2012) laments the heterogeneous methodological quality of empirical studies that could objectify and justify these facets. He feels a strong contrast between the undifferentiated promises of healing on the one hand, which circulate on numerous internet sites, and the only partially reliable scientific literature on the other hand. Missing details about interventions, uncertainties in the sung repertoires, the lack of control groups or comparison conditions, as well as inconsistent presentations of research results, only form part of the problem. In addition, the mechanisms which produce positive emotional well-being in the case of singing are still inadequately clarified.

19.3.2 Physiological Effects of Singing

Physiological effects of singing have been observed on different temporal levels, especially short-term neurohumoral and psychological (Beck et al. 2000) as well as long-term physiological changes of the vocal apparatus. A number of studies provided indications that communal singing seems to increase the production of immunoglobulin A in the mucous membranes of the upper respiratory tract (Beck et al. 2000; Kuhn 2002). In addition, there are indications that solo or communal singing may promote the release of the hormone oxytocin (Grape et al. 2003; Kreutz 2014a) and contribute to the synchronization of the cardiovascular system among choir singers (Olsson et al. 2013; Vickhoff et al. 2013).

Practical Tip
Singing mantras at a breathing rate of 0.1 Hertz (10 s duration for one breathing cycle) is associated with a vagal (calming) influence on heart activity, measured by the so-called heart rate variability (HRV).

Conducted an extensive longitudinal study over the period of a school year with 5th-grade students who participated in a weekly voice training of 45 min duration. The control group consisted of students from the same classes who only participated in regular music lessons, which included singing in class. Voice fields were recorded from all children at the beginning and end of the school year. Voice fields are mathematical–physical representations of the range of pitch and volume, which the children's voices are capable of producing. At the end of the school year, children in the voice training group showed highly significant improvements in vocal range and volume of their voice, while children in the control group showed almost unchanged voice fields. The author suspects that voice training, measured by the positive changes she observed in the so-called Dysphonia Severity Index derived from the voice fields, could be prophylactically significant for child voice health.

Hormonal changes through communal singing, such as with regard to local immune responses in the respiratory tract (Beck et al. 2000; Kuhn 2002; Kang et al. 2018) or altered concentrations of oxytocin in saliva (Grape et al. 2003; Kreutz 2014b; Schladt et al. 2017; Kang et al. 2018) leave many questions unanswered. In the case of the immune response, it is not certain that systemic components are involved at all. Furthermore, it is not clear to what extent psychological, physical, or contextual factors may have caused the observed changes. Similar fundamental problems arise when assessing the effects of oxytocin. Despite statistical correlations between peripheral oxytocin concentrations in saliva, blood plasma, and urine (Feldman 2012), there is no evidence of a close correlation between peripheral and central nervous system biological activities of this hormone. This interpretative limitation applies to all hormones, which are only indirectly associated on both sides of the physiological barrier between the brain and the bloodstream.

Choir singing among older people has rarely been studied for its long-term effects, although positive results have entered the professional discussion in recent years. For example, reports have been made of reduced medication intake, doctor visits, and falls among participants in a 1-year choir project (Cohen et al. 2006). The validity of such studies is rightly being critically questioned (Grebosz-Haring et al. 2022).

19.3.3 Singing Groups in Health Facilities

A growing number of singing groups in health facilities have been recorded in recent years. The international network "Singing Hospitals e.V." (www.singende-krankenhaeuser.de) is partly responsible for this development with its further education offers and certification procedures (Kreutz et al. 2014b). Since 2003, numerous singing groups with at least four and up to 70 participants have been founded in this network alone. In addition to opening up and developing further health areas for high-quality guided, communal singing, the network's goal is to document relevant research and conduct its own studies with acquired funding, with the long-term goal of establishing evidence-based singing in health facilities as therapy-related offers.

Extensive interviews with singing leaders (Kreutz et al. 2014a) revealed, for example, that many psychiatric clinics, in addition to hospitals, doctors' offices, and rehab clinics, are committed to setting up singing groups. The educational backgrounds of the individual singing leaders are often, but not exclusively, in music therapy and vocal pedagogical areas. The professionalization of singing leaders in health facilities, which is developing between music pedagogical and therapy-related offers, has not yet reached institutional training courses.

Singing offers are used by current and former patients as well as their relatives. Furthermore, singing groups also find approval among nursing staff and a circle of other people with unclear relation to the respective facility. The social structure in the singing groups already fulfills a kind of bridgehead function between therapy and everyday life. The skills acquired during the singing hours, musical procedural knowledge (exploration of the singing voice, acquisition of repertoires) form a second aspect that favors the everyday usability and sustainability of these offers.

Choir leaders use diverse strategies, which, due to the continuing education of the network, have common characteristics. This includes centrally aligning the singing offers according to the individual illnesses and singing experiences of the participants. This goes so far that the song repertoires are jointly determined, and specific rituals can unfold in the singing groups. Rarely are singing groups aimed at developing stage-ready repertoires.

Behavioral changes, such as the reduction of medication intake, showing positive effects or the increased uptake of social contacts even outside the singing group, cannot be causally linked to the singing offers. Nevertheless, anecdotal insights are also crucial for the evaluation and classification of such singing offers. After all, their benefit for health facilities in their overall effect internally and externally must be considered.

Conclusion

Singing offers in health facilities mobilize people in their vicinity and create social contacts. These aspects alone, mobility and social contact, can promote individual self-efficacy in the long run and are already of health relevance.

19.4 Meanings of Singing from the Perspective of Laypeople

A survey among a total of 725 choir singers, of whom 325 were from nonclinical lay choirs and 400 from singing groups in health facilities were recruited, revealed similar that regarding the self-reported (positive) effects of singing between the different subpopulations (lay singers, current patients, former patients). Table 19.1 shows a high degree of agreement with the individual items of an inventory used in German translation from a preliminary study (Clift and Hancox 2001). Nevertheless, the patient groups feel restricted compared to the laypeople in terms of their general quality of life (see Kreutz 2014a, b).

Table 19.1 shows that former patients overall agree most with the positive effects of singing. These differences are significant for some scales in the average comparison. However, the duration of participation in singing groups seems to be of subordinate importance.

Significant limitations of the quality of life on the part of the current and former patients compared to the nonclinical comparison group were indeed also observed, however, long-term observations are still pending in order to be able to narrow down any changes, as they appear in the self-reports of the patient groups (Kreutz et al. 2014b).

Conclusion

Singing groups in health facilities fulfill diverse functions. From the perspective of both group leaders and participants, they are cultural offerings that can have an impact both internally and externally in individual facilities. They represent holistic views in health services research, which places comprehensive human well-being, as defined by the WHO, at the center. Even in the case of serious illnesses, individual needs for cultural participation remain, which in turn enable the activation of personal resources. This can lead to a positive spiral of expression, activation, and increased well-being, resulting in improved quality of life over time.

Table 19.1 Means (and standard deviations) of singers and singers in various choirs and singing groups about effects of singing

Item	Group		
	Patients (n = 205)	Former patients (n = 93)	Laypeople (n = 325)
Singing improves my mood	4.30 (.82)	4.63 (.57)	4.31 (.69)
Singing makes me feel better afterward	4.29 (.82)	4.49 (.73)	4.05 (.76)
Singing relaxes and helps cope with stress	4.24 (.90)	4.43 (.78)	4.09 (.82)
Singing does not promote my general well-being	1.93 (1.11)	1.60 (.98)	1.86 (.91)
Singing promotes a positive attitude toward life	4.12 (.87)	4.29 (.81)	4.09 (.78)
Singing helps me become a happier person	3.91 (.99)	4.15 (.92)	4.01 (.80)
Singing does not dissolve negative feelings in my life	2.49 (1.26)	2.03 (1.21)	2.38 (.96)
Singing does not give me any feelings of elation	2.07 (1.09)	1.88 (1.17)	2.05 (.89)
Singing has no deeper meaning compared to other things	2.52 (1.18)	1.91 (0.97)	1.91 (.97)
Singing improves my general well-being	3.91 (1.01)	4.29 (.82)	3.86 (.88)
Singing causes me to have less bad mood	4.14 (.87)	4.34 (.82)	4.02 (.75)
Singing improves my quality of life	4.16 (.87)	4.45 (.75)	4.35 (.63)

Note: The averages are on a scale of 1–5 (1 = "does not apply at all"; 5 = "applies completely")

19.5 Methodological Aspects and Open Questions

Systematic studies on the effects of singing in nonclinical and clinical areas are of utmost importance for evidence-based further development and continuous review of the health implications of singing offers. Pragmatic, multicenter, randomized controlled studies provide impressive evidence of the effectiveness of communal singing even in severe and irreversible neurodegenerative diseases (Baker et al. 2022). These methodological challenges must be accepted in order to justify conclusions for practice through reliable observations. Therefore, epidemiological and intervention-led strategies are still needed to reveal the health potentials of communal singing.

The investigation of individual differences in the effects of communal singing is only just beginning. The preliminary finding that neither the extent of previous singing experience nor specific disease patterns limit potentials for creased well-being and quality of life seems significant. Furthermore, the conditions for good singing practice are scientifically little secured. The ethical quality criteria developed in the Singing Hospitals network and implemented in training courses provide initial points of reference, the transfer of which to nonclinical areas is fundamentally unopposed.

19.6 Future Perspectives

The question raised within the context of the salutogenetically inspired context model (see above) as to how musical interventions such as singing or dancing influence individual disease patterns is the subject of ongoing discussions. Methodologically high-quality studies contribute to reassessing and utilizing the therapeutic significance of communal singing. Musical and vocal activities are associated with psychophysiological and socio-emotional effects, which give them a wide range in very different disease patterns. The aim is to socialize future generations musically in order to bring the associated health potentials to fruition as much as possible.

References

Antonovsky A (1997) Salutogenese. Dgvt Verlag, Tübingen

Baker FA, Lee Y-EC, Sousa TV et al (2022) Clinical effectiveness of music interventions for dementia and depression in elderly care (MIDDEL): Australian cohort of an international pragmatic cluster-randomised controlled trial. Lancet Health Longev 3:e153–e165. https://doi.org/10.1016/S2666-7568(22)00027-7

Beck RJ, Cesario TC, Yousefi A, Enamoto H (2000) Choral singing, performance perception, and immune system changes in salivary immunoglobulin a and cortisol. Music Percept 18:87–106

Beck RJ, Gottfried TL, Hall DJ, Cisler CA, Bozeman KW (2006) Supporting the health of college solo singers: the relationship of positive emotions and stress to changes in salivary IgA and cortisol during singing. J Learn Through Arts 2(1). https://doi.org/10.21977/D92110079

Berkowska M, Dalla Bella S (2013) Uncovering phenotypes of poor-pitch singing: the Sung Performance Battery (SPB). Front Psychol 4:714. https://doi.org/10.3389/fpsyg.2013.00714

Brown S (2000) The 'Musilanguage' model of music evolution. In: Wallin N, Merker B, Brown S (eds) The origins of music. MIT Press, Boston, pp 271–300

Clift S, Hancox G (2001) The perceived benefits of singing: findings from preliminary surveys of a university college choral society. J R Soc Promot Heal 121:248–256. https://doi.org/10.1177/146642400112100409

Clift S, Hancox G, Morrison I et al (2010a) Choral singing and psychological wellbeing: quantitative and qualitative findings from English choirs in a cross-national survey. J Appl Arts Health 1:19–34. https://doi.org/10.1386/jaah.1.1.19/1

Clift S, Nicol J, Raisbeck M et al (2010b) Group singing, wellbeing and health: a systematic mapping of research evidence. UNESCO Obs 2. http://www.abp.unimelb.edu.au/unesco/ejournal/pdf/clift-paper.pdf

Clift, S. (2012) Singing, wellbeing, and health. In R. A. R. MacDonald, G. Kreutz, & L. Mitchell (Eds.), Music, health, and wellbeing (pp. 113–124). Oxford: Oxford University Press.

Cohen GD, Perlstein S, Chapline J et al (2006) The impact of professionally conducted cultural programs on the physical health, mental health, and social functioning of older adults. Gerontologist 46:726–734. https://doi.org/10.1093/geront/46.6.726

Cross I (2001) Music, cognition, culture, and evolution. Ann N Y Acad Sci 930:28–42. https://doi.org/10.1111/j.1749-6632.2001.tb05723.x

Dalla Bella S, Berkowska M (2009) Singing proficiency in the majority. Ann N Y Acad Sci 1169:99–107. https://doi.org/10.1111/j.1749-6632.2009.04558.x

Deci EL, Ryan RM (2015) Self-determination theory. In: International encyclopedia of the social & behavioral sciences. Elsevier, Amsterdam, pp 486–491

Feldman R (2012) Oxytocin and social affiliation in humans. Horm Behav 61:380–391. https://doi.org/10.1016/j.yhbeh.2012.01.008

Gold C, Eickholt J, Assmus J et al (2019) Music Interventions for Dementia and Depression in ELderly care (MIDDEL): protocol and statistical analysis plan for a multinational cluster-randomised trial. BMJ Open 9:e023436. https://doi.org/10.1136/bmjopen-2018-023436

Grape C, Sandgren M, Hansson L-O et al (2003) Does singing promote well-being?: an empirical study of professional and amateur singers during a singing lesson. Integr Physiol Behav Sci 38:65–74. https://doi.org/10.1007/BF02734261

Grebosz-Haring K, Thun-Hohenstein L, Schuchter-Wiegand AK et al (2022) The need for robust critique of arts and health research: young people, art therapy and mental health. Front Psychol 13:821093. https://doi.org/10.3389/fpsyg.2022.821093

Hagen EH, Bryant GA (2003) Music and dance as a coalition signaling system. Hum Nat 14:21–51. https://doi.org/10.1007/s12110-003-1015-z

Hamner L, Dubbel P, Capron I et al (2020) High SARS-CoV-2 attack rate following exposure at a choir practice. Morb Mortal Wkly Rep 69(19):606–610

Irons JY, Sheffield D, Ballington F, Stewart DE (2020) A systematic review on the effects of group singing on persistent pain in people with long-term health conditions. Eur J Pain (United Kingdom) 24:71–90. https://doi.org/10.1002/ejp.1485

Jarvis ED (2019) Evolution of vocal learning and spoken language. Science (80-) 366:50–54. https://doi.org/10.1126/science.aax0287

Kang J, Scholp A, Jiang JJ (2018) A review of the physiological effects and mechanisms of singing. J Voice 32:390–395. https://doi.org/10.1016/j.jvoice.2017.07.008

Kirschner S, Tomasello M (2010) Joint music making promotes prosocial behavior in 4-year-old children. Evol Hum Behav 31:354–364. https://doi.org/10.1016/j.evolhumbehav.2010.04.004

Kreutz G (2014a) Ist Singen gesund? In: Altenmüller E, Willich S (eds) Klang, Körper und Gesundheit. Wißner-Verlag, Augsburg, pp 77–84

Kreutz G (2014b) Does singing facilitate social bonding? Music Med 6:51–60

Kreutz G, Brünger P (2012a) A shade of grey: negative associations with amateur choral singing. Arts Health 4(3):230–238. https://doi.org/10.1080/17533015.2012.693111

Kreutz G, Brünger P (2012b) Musikalische und soziale Bedingungen des Singens: Eine Studie unter deutschsprachigen Chorsängern. Music Sci 16:168–184. https://doi.org/10.1177/1029864912445109

Kreutz G, Böhm K, Bossinger W, Clift S (2014a) Singen im Krankenhaus aus Sicht von Singleitern: Eine qualitative Untersuchung. Musik Umschau 35:5–15

Kreutz G, Clift S, Bossinger W (2014b) Singing in hospitals: bridging therapy and everyday life. In: Clift S, Camic P (eds) Oxford textbook of creative arts, health, and well-being: international perspectives on practice, policy and research. Oxford University Press, Oxford

Kuhn D (2002) The effects of active and passive participation in musical activity on the immune system as measured by salivary immunoglobulin A (SIgA). J Music Ther 39(1):30–39

Lewis A, Cave P, Stern M et al (2016) Singing for lung health—a systematic review of the literature and consensus statement. NPJ Prim Care Respir Med 26:1–8. https://doi.org/10.1038/npjpcrm.2016.80

Lonsdale AJ, Day ER (2021) Are the psychological benefits of choral singing unique to choirs? A comparison of six activity groups. Psychol Music 49:1179–1198. https://doi.org/10.1177/0305735620940019

Mcmullen E, Saffran JR (2004) Music and language: a developmental comparison. Music Percept 21:289–311

Miller SL, Nazaroff WW, Jimenez JL et al (2021) Transmission of SARS-CoV-2 by inhalation of respiratory aerosol in the Skagit Valley Chorale superspreading event. Indoor Air 31:314–323. https://doi.org/10.1111/ina.12751

Mithen S (2007) The singing neanderthals: the origins of music, language, mind, and body. Harvard University Press, Boston

Mittelmark MB, Bull T (2013) The salutogenic model of health in health promotion research. Glob Health Promot 20:30–38. https://doi.org/10.1177/1757975913486684

Mürbe D, Kriegel M, Lange J et al (2021) Aerosol emission of adolescents voices during speaking, singing and shouting. PLoS One 16:e0246819. https://doi.org/10.1371/journal.pone.0246819

Olsson EMG, von Scheele B, Theorell T (2013) Heart rate variability during choral singing. Music Med 5:52–59. https://doi.org/10.1177/1943862112471399

Pfordresher PQ, Mantell JT (2014) Singing with yourself: evidence for an inverse modeling account of poor-pitch singing. Cogn Psychol 70:31–57. https://doi.org/10.1016/j.cogpsych.2013.12.005

Savage PE, Loui P, Tarr B et al (2021) Music as a coevolved system for social bonding. Behav Brain Sci 44:e59. https://doi.org/10.1017/S0140525X20000333

Schladt TM, Nordmann GC, Emilius R et al (2017) Choir versus solo singing: effects on mood, and salivary oxytocin and cortisol concentrations. Front Hum Neurosci 11:1–9. https://doi.org/10.3389/fnhum.2017.00430

Sherratt K, Thornton A, Hatton C (2004) Music interventions for people with dementia: a review of the literature. Aging Ment Health 8:3–12. https://doi.org/10.1080/13607860310001613275

Stewart N, Lonsdale A (2016) It's better together: the psychological benefits of singing in a choir. Psychol Music 44:1240–1254. https://doi.org/10.1177/0305735615624976

Stone NL, Millar SA, Herrod PJJ et al (2018) An analysis of endocannabinoid concentrations and mood following singing and exercise in healthy volunteers. Front Behav Neurosci 12:269. https://doi.org/10.3389/fnbeh.2018.00269

Sundberg J, Rossing TD (1990) The science of singing voice. J Acoust Soc Am 87:462–463. https://doi.org/10.1121/1.399243

Titze IR, Martin DW (1998) Principles of voice production. J Acoust Soc Am 104:1148–1148. https://doi.org/10.1121/1.424266

Trehub SE (2003) The developmental origins of musicality. Nat Neurosci 6:669–673. https://doi.org/10.1038/nn1084

Valentine E, Evans C (2001) The effects of solo singing, choral singing and swimming on mood and physiological indices. Br J Med Psychol 74:115–120. https://doi.org/10.1348/000711201160849

Vickhoff B, Malmgren H, Åström R et al (2013) Music structure determines heart rate variability of singers. Front Psychol 4:1–16. https://doi.org/10.3389/fpsyg.2013.00599

Welch GF (1979) Poor pitch singing: a review of the literature. Psychol Music 7:50–58. https://doi.org/10.1177/030573567971006

The Potential of Singing-Based Interventions to Support Communication and Psychosocial Well-Being in People Living with Communication Challenges

20

Frank A. Russo, Arla Good, and Bridget Boyle

20.1 Introduction

Communication challenges (CCs) encompass a wide range of conditions that affect an individual's ability to effectively communicate. These challenges can manifest as primary symptoms of a disorder, such as aphasia, stuttering, or hearing loss, or as secondary symptoms associated with conditions, such as Parkinson's disease or breathing disorders. Regardless of their origin, CCs can significantly impact various aspects of psychosocial well-being:

1. Social isolation and loneliness: Impaired communication can lead to reduced social interactions and feelings of isolation (Hilari et al. 2010; Palmer et al. 2016). This isolation can be particularly pronounced in social settings where effective communication is crucial, such as family gatherings, workplace environments, and community events.
2. Disability focus: Individuals may develop the belief that they are incapable of engaging in conversations, social activities, and meaningful relationships. This self-limiting mindset can hinder personal growth and social participation, even in situations in which accommodations or support are available.
3. Stigma: People with CCs may internalize negative perceptions of their condition, affecting their social identity (Kang and Chasteen 2009; Latrofa et al. 2010). Internalized stigma can lead to decreased self-esteem.
4. Reduced participation in social activities: Due to communication difficulties, individuals with CCs may avoid social gatherings, community events, or group activities, leading to a narrowing of their social circle and decreased opportunities for social engagement.

F. A. Russo · A. Good (✉) · B. Boyle
Department of Psychology, Toronto Metropolitan University, Toronto, ON, Canada
e-mail: Arla.good@torontomu.ca

G. Kreutz, G. Bernatzky (eds.), *Music and Medicine*, Neurocultural Health and Wellbeing, https://doi.org/10.1007/978-3-662-72175-9_20

5. Negative mood: CCs are often associated with mood disorders, including depression and anxiety (Brink and Stones 2007; Goldman and Postuma 2014). The frustration and stress of struggling to communicate exacerbate underlying mental health conditions.
6. Strain on existing relationships: CCs can put strain on relationships with family members, friends, and romantic partners, as communication barriers may lead to misunderstandings, frustration, and reduced intimacy.
7. Professional challenges: In the workplace, CCs can affect an individual's ability to participate in meetings, collaborate with colleagues, or advance in their career, potentially leading to reduced job satisfaction and economic hardship.

Although singing has been an important cultural practice throughout history (Jones and Baraka 2015), the establishment of choirs specifically for individuals with CCs is a relatively recent phenomenon. This trend aligns with the growing recognition of social activities as a means to promote well-being and the increasing emphasis on inclusive and accessible community programs to mitigate disease. These initiatives are aligned with the "social cure" approach (Haslam et al. 2018), wherein individuals are referred to nonmedical activities or community-based services to improve their health and well-being (i.e., a social prescription). This approach is part of a broader movement to address social, emotional, and psychological factors that contribute to overall well-being. Instead of relying solely on medication or clinical treatments, patients may be "prescribed" activities such as exercise groups, art classes, volunteering, or group singing to support their mental and physical health. Group singing offers several important benefits to individuals living with CCs.

1. Improved breath control and vocal strength: The techniques used in singing can help individuals with certain CCs, such as those related to breathing disorders or Parkinson's disease, to improve their vocal control and projection.
2. Functional communication gains: The specific functional gains will depend on the type of CC, but may include improved voice quality, vocal fluency, or speech reception.
3. Increased communication confidence: As participants improve their singing skills and experience positive social interactions, they develop greater confidence in their ability to communicate and engage with others. A systematic review by Boster et al. (2021) found that music-based interventions (inclusive of group singing) tend to improve communication outcomes such as initiation of communication, turn-taking, and joint attention.
4. Enhanced social connections: Participation in a choir creates opportunities for social interaction and the formation of new friendships with individuals who share similar experiences. These experiences may engender trust between members (Pearce et al. 2015; Good et al. 2017).
5. Cognitive stimulation: Learning and performing songs can provide cognitive benefits, potentially improving memory.

6. Personal expression and mastery: Singing provides an alternative form of self-expression and opportunity for accomplishment that does not rely solely on spoken language.
7. Stigma: Group singing has been observed to reduce feelings of stigma (Clift et al. 2010; Irons et al. 2021). Presumably, this emerges from the experience of engaging in an activity that challenges the negative biases that underlie stigma. Over time, the group may start to challenge stereotypes, leading to a feeling of empowerment and causing the individual to reassess internalized stigma.

The *SingWell Project (singwell.org)* is an international research network studying the potential benefits of group singing for people with CCs. Our awareness of activities from members across the network provides us with a unique vantage point from which to view the positive impact of group singing for communication and psychosocial well-being. The project's findings contribute to a growing body of evidence supporting the use of music-based interventions in healthcare and community settings. As research in this area continues to expand, group singing and other creative social interventions will likely play an increasingly important role in supporting individuals with CCs. These approaches offer a holistic and engaging way to address complex social and communication needs, potentially improving the overall quality of life and fostering greater social inclusion.

20.1.1 An Inclusive and Ability-Focused Approach

Establishing singing groups for individuals with communication challenges (CCs) may present significant challenges owing to inherent concerns regarding communication and the high likelihood of pre-existing stigmas. Researchers in the SingWell project have initiated numerous group-singing intervention studies, some of which have resulted in self-sustaining programs that operate independently of the research. The standard approach involves the establishment of a new singing group for individuals with a specific CC (e.g., Parkinson's disease), followed by the recruitment of participants from the established singing group for optional participation in research. In some instances, caregivers of individuals with CCs are invited to participate in group singing. Since these groups are non-auditioned, they are open to all participants, regardless of their musical, vocal, or auditory capabilities; poor singing ability is never considered an exclusion criterion. To implement this inclusive approach, simple, familiar, and culturally appropriate songs that may encourage participation are preferred (Silvestri et al. 2018). Additionally, resources are provided for participants to enhance their singing ability outside choir sessions (e.g., sing-along videos or alternative forms of singing practice).

Another critical feature of our approach is the focus on abilities (asset model) rather than the disability focus, which tends to characterize many support groups for people with CCs (Jones 1996; Revenson et al. 1991). An ability-focused group emphasizes the strengths and potential of its members rather than focusing on their limitations, disabilities, or challenges. In the context of singing, this means celebrating whatever aspect of participation is possible. This may include being a leading voice in the choir, but it may also mean showing up and mouthing the words.

By establishing groups with a shared identity and engaging in an ability-focused activity that runs counter to conventional stigmas, we provide organic opportunities to quickly generate feelings that are conducive to the transformation of personal identity. The following is a comment about the identity transformation made by one member of a Parkinson's choir established after 6 months of participation.

> I don't feel like my Parkinson's defines me as much as it used to. Now that I've been singing with the group for a while … I feel that I'm also a singer who is part of a vibrant community. KB

Although there are effective and established interventions to support communication skills in people with CCs, such as the Lee Silverman Voice Therapy (LSVT/LOUD) for Parkinson's disease (Sapir et al. 2007) and Melodic Intonation Therapy (MIT) for Aphasia (Van der Meulen et al. 2014), group singing is an efficacious activity that may support the existing standard of care treatments. This complementarity is supported by several factors: (i) scalability because the intervention can be executed in a group format; (ii) high intrinsic motivation, contributing to adherence and promoting cumulative benefits (Livesey et al. 2012); (iii) the availability of people to lead such groups following a brief accreditation training program, which would address the critical need for support of people living with CCs in small or isolated communities (Winn et al. 2014); and (iv) the potential for caregivers to receive benefits from observing (or participating in) loved ones in a meaningful activity that is ability-focused (Forbes 2021; Tamplin et al. 2013). Thus, we believe that group singing for people living with CCs is worthy of in-depth consideration as a complementary intervention from scientific, practical, economic, and ethical perspectives.

20.1.2 Social Bonding Capacity of Group Singing

What features of group singing yield the social bonding capacity? One feature to consider is emotional alignment. Group singing may have strong abilities to align the emotional experiences among those singing together because of its ability to influence mood (Juslin and Sloboda 2001; Juslin and Västfjäll 2008). In addition, group singing often demands a high degree of cooperation and collaboration among the participating members. Furthermore, unlike most other group activities, musical rhythm provides a rich oscillatory framework that induces a coordinated internal rhythm among participants. Sharing in the rhythmic pulse fosters synchronized nervous systems and motor activity among groups of individuals of any size. The propensity to rhythmically entrain the beat (i.e., to synchronize movements with the rhythmic pulse) is a central aspect of participation in music.

Although the movements required to sing in unison may not be easily perceived visually, these forms of movement synchrony can be auditorily perceived. First, singing in unison requires synchronization of the laryngeal and orofacial muscles (e.g., lip opening) (Echternach et al. 2016). Second, the pitch interval structure of the song exerts subtle effects on the facial and head movements (Thompson and Russo 2007). Third, the phrasing of lyrics influences the synchronization of respiratory patterns (Müller and Lindenberger 2011).

Over the past 30 years, research has consistently demonstrated that moving synchrony leads to increased affiliation between individuals. More specifically, synchronized movements lead to higher ratings of preference, likeability, and rapport among those involved (Bernieri 1988; Hove and Risen 2009; Demos et al. 2012; Launay et al. 2013; Valdesolo et al. 2010; Wiltermuth and Heath 2009). The tendency toward increased affiliation following synchronized movements appears to develop as early as 12 months (Tunçgenç et al. 2015). Several sociobiological mechanisms have been proposed to account for the increased sense of affiliation following group singing, such as decreased cortisol (Kreutz et al. 2004; Good et al. 2020), increased beta-endorphin (Tarr et al. 2014), and increased oxytocin levels (Chanda and Levitin 2013; Good and Russo 2016; Kreutz 2014).

As theorists such as McNeill (1997) and Durkheim (2005) argue, moving in synchrony with others may blur the distinction between the self and the group. McNeill (1997) describes this notion as "*we-ness*" or "*boundary loss*." Through the loss of individual boundaries, a new collective identity is established. We become a type of superorganism, not unlike a flock of birds or a colony of bees, working in harmony to achieve something bigger than ourselves. The construct of self-other merging can be measured using a tool called the Inclusion of Other in Self Scale (IOS) scale, a pictorial measure of social closeness (Aron et al. 1992; see Fig. 20.1). This measure assesses social closeness by asking participants to choose between increasingly overlapping circles representing the self and the group. Decreasing the distance between circles suggests increased social closeness or self-other merging. Research using this tool empirically validates the notion that movement synchrony leads to increased self-other merging (Rabinowitz and Knafo-Noam 2015; Pearce et al. 2015).

The remainder of this chapter will focus on the five primary CCs that SingWell has been working on to date. Following a brief overview to situate considerations for each CC, communication outcomes are considered, followed by psychosocial

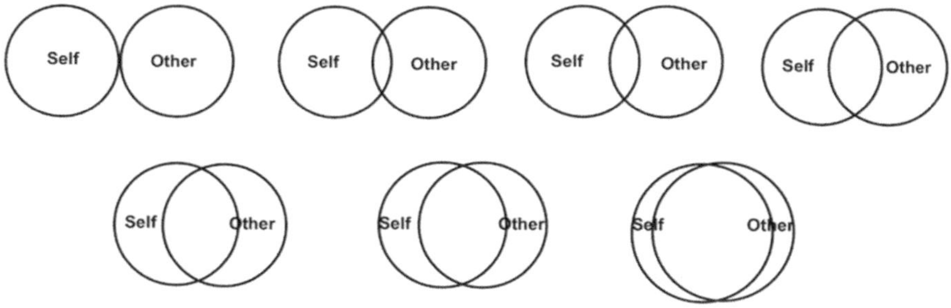

Fig. 20.1 The Inclusion of Other in Self Scale. (Reproduced with permission from Aron et al. 1992)

outcomes. In addition, where feasible, we address the mechanisms underlying these improvements.

20.2 Considerations for Specific Communication Challenges

20.2.1 Parkinson's Disease

20.2.1.1 Overview

Parkinson's disease is a neurodegenerative disorder that causes motor deficits, including rigidity and tremors. Characteristic communication deficits accompany a range of motor challenges intrinsic to the disease. These communication deficits can negatively influence social, emotional, and psychological domains, greatly reducing quality of life (Stegemoller et al. 2017). The global prevalence of Parkinson's disease in people over 60 years of age is less than 1%, but this estimate has been increasing since the 1980s and tends to be higher in more developed countries (Zhu et al. 2024).

20.2.1.2 Communication Outcomes

Extensive research has been dedicated to the therapeutic effects of movement interventions such as dance and exercise groups for adults with Parkinson's (Barnish and Barran 2020). However, comparatively few studies have considered singing interventions and how they uniquely benefit individuals with Parkinson's. The muscles of the lungs and vocal tract are compromised as a result of Parkinson's disease (Ma et al. 2020). Respiratory training has been shown to improve various measures related to speech function in individuals with Parkinson's disease that may affect speech perception (Reyes et al. 2020). These measures included subglottal pressure, maximum phonation duration, and voice intensity. Other research suggests that LSVT/LOUD, a treatment focusing on maximizing voice intensity, may have similar effects (Mahler et al. 2015).

It seems reasonable to expect that group singing, which also involves respiratory training and a focus on increasing vocal intensity, may lead to similar outcomes in speech function. Indeed, two studies that measured respiratory outcomes after choral singing reported enhancements in lung capacity, pressure, and control (Di Benedetto et al. 2009; Stegemoller et al. 2017). With respect to vocal quality measures, some studies have reported positive changes in vocal loudness, pitch, shimmer, and voice-related quality of life after 2, 3, and 12 months of a group singing intervention (Good et al. 2023; Mathews 2018; Tamplin et al. 2020).

20.2.1.3 Psychosocial Outcomes

Reductions in self-reported anxiety scores after group singing have been reported in some studies; however, psychosocial outcomes have not been explored to the same degree as physical outcomes (Irons et al. 2021; Tamplin et al. 2020). This discrepancy prompts a demand for robust research efforts to measure vocal and psychosocial outcomes following singing interventions for Parkinson's disease (Barnish et al. 2016).

20.2.2 Aphasia

20.2.2.1 Overview

Aphasia is an impairment of language function that may affect speech production and/or speech perception with associated deficits in auditory working memory (Wright and Shisler 2005). It has been estimated that 64% of people who develop aphasia and/or related speech disorders (dysarthria and apraxia of speech) do so following a stroke (Mitchell et al. 2021). The worldwide prevalence of post-stroke aphasia has been estimated to be between 7% and 77%. The broad range of this estimate reflects variability in treatment options and assessment protocols worldwide. The second most common cause of aphasia is traumatic brain injury.

20.2.2.2 Communication Outcomes

Because singing is often preserved in aphasia and rated as a highly pleasurable experience (Racette et al. 2006), many patients with aphasia are willing to participate in singing-based interventions. One such intervention, Melodic Intonation Therapy (MIT), has made its way into standard clinical practice. When administered soon after the onset of aphasia, significant improvements in communication were observed compared to a control group receiving other types of language rehabilitation (Van der Meulen et al. 2014). However, MIT is a one-on-one intervention that is relatively expensive to administer. Group singing is an attractive, complementary activity that may provide similar communication gains at a lower cost.

In a blinded randomized control pilot (Zumbansen et al. 2017), 6 months of group singing was not found to be effective in improving any objective measure of communication function. However, this study was limited in size (22 participants across the experimental and control conditions). Another pilot study involving ten participants found that 13 weeks of group singing led to increases in vocal confidence, but no improvements in objective measures of communication function (Pachete et al. under review). These mixed findings may be related to the statistical power issues. In what is likely the best powered and most intensive group singing study to date for people living with aphasia (Siponkoski et al. 2023), improvements were observed in speech production and everyday communication after the midpoint of the trial (5 months). These results were obtained in a crossover randomized control trial that involved 54 aphasia patients who participated in standard care followed by standard care and a singing intervention, or vice versa. It is important to note that the singing intervention involved multiple components: group singing, melodic intonation therapy, and singing homework.

20.2.2.3 Psychosocial Outcomes

In the aforementioned cross-over randomized control trial, participants also demonstrated an increase in social participation, and their family caregivers reported a diminished sense of caregiver burden, all of which were sustained at midpoint (5 months) and endpoint (9 months) measurements (Siponkoski et al. 2023).

20.2.3 Hearing Loss

20.2.3.1 Overview

Hearing loss due to peripheral (cochlear) and/or central (brain) losses affects over 5% of the world's population (WHO 2024). Hearing loss is particularly relevant for older adults, with as many as 60–70% of adults over the age of 70 meeting the clinical criteria for hearing loss (Yamasoba et al. 2013). For people with hearing loss, particularly older adults, one of the most common real-world difficulties is understanding speech in the presence of background noise (Pichora-Fuller et al. 2016).

20.2.3.2 Communication Outcomes

A relationship between musicianship and speech in noise ability has been established with a potential suite of neural mechanisms involving changes in cortical and subcortical auditory processing and attention (Coffey et al. 2017), suggesting that group singing may have the potential to ameliorate some of the consequences of central hearing loss. However, most of the available evidence is correlational (Alain et al. 2014) or cross-sectional (Tremblay and Perron 2023; Perron et al. 2021). To the best of our knowledge, there is only one available interventional study. Participants with age-related hearing loss experienced improvements in speech-in-noise perception after 10 weeks of group singing and singing homework (Dubinsky et al. 2019). These improvements were mediated by enhancements in the neural representation of pitch, suggesting that the extra-musical benefits to speech perception were not merely a consequence of increased motivation. However, the active singing group and do-nothing control groups in this study were not randomized; instead, the singing group was self-selected, and the controls were selected to match age and hearing loss. Consequently, some reasonable questions can be raised about whether improvements in speech perception were attributable to pre-existing differences between the two groups (McKay 2021). These significant limitations in the study design have yet to be resolved and retested, prompting the need for a controlled multisite trial of group singing for hearing loss (Lo et al. under review).

20.2.3.3 Psychosocial Outcomes

To date, there have been no direct studies of group singing benefits on psychosocial outcomes for people living with age-related hearing loss. However, given the prevalence of hearing loss in older adults and the known psychosocial benefits of group singing in an older adult population (Skingley et al. 2016), it stands to reason that these psychosocial effects would be observed if formally studied.

20.2.4 Breathing Disorders

20.2.4.1 Overview

Breathing disorders can arise from problems in the lungs, airways, muscles, and structures that support breathing. These include obstructive pulmonary disease (COPD), asthma, and other chronic respiratory difficulties. People living with breathing disorders often face challenges that affect speech production, such as reductions in inspiratory/expiratory pressure and increases in breathlessness and hoarseness. The prevalence of COPD is estimated to be 10.3% of the population worldwide, aged between 30 and 79 years (Adeloye et al. 2022). Moreover, this estimate has steadily increased since the 1960s (López-Campos et al. 2016). Although the primary cause of COPD is smoking, there are various other causes, including work-related exposure to airborne contaminants.

20.2.4.2 Communication Outcomes

Researchers studying the efficacy of singing interventions for individuals with breathing disorders and lung disease have measured several functional deficit outcomes that are intrinsic to these conditions, notably dyspnea and maximal expiratory pressure (Bonhila et al. 2009; Engen 2005; Lord et al. 2012). Noteworthy findings from group singing and singing-based therapy studies have shown improvements in maximal expiratory pressure in COPD patients (Bonhila et al. 2009), as well as maintenance and improvement of lung function in individuals living with asthma (Wade 2002). The observed improvements in expiratory pressure are thought to be caused by the intensive demands of singing on the expiratory muscles (Bonhila et al. 2009). A promising randomized controlled trial by Kaasgaard et al. (2022) found that a single lung health intervention provided COPD participants with the same lung function, dyspnea, and emotional state as traditional exercise-based pulmonary rehabilitation. The authors propose that singing may be a viable replacement for traditional rehabilitation programs for individuals with COPD, as the outcomes align with the rehabilitation outcomes (Kaasgaard et al. 2022). Replication in this field is necessary, with a focus on extended-length interventions to fortify evidence for group singing as an effective intervention for lung diseases and breathing disorders in the long term (Gick and Nicol 2016).

20.2.4.3 Psychosocial Outcomes

This growing body of research has shown consistent enhancements in psychosocial outcomes, including decreases in self-reported anxiety and increases in health-related and overall quality of life after several weeks of a group-singing intervention (Bonhila et al. 2009; Lewis et al. 2016; Lord et al. 2012). Psychosocial interventions to relieve the symptoms of dyspnea in patients with COPD have been studied and measured as moderately effective, suggesting that the psychosocial improvements obtained from group singing may lend themselves to symptom reduction (Norweg and Collins 2013).

20.2.5 Stuttering

20.2.5.1 Overview

Stuttering is a developmental speech motor disorder characterized by disruptions in speech flow. These disruptions, referred to as disfluencies, include repetition of phonemes, syllables, or whole words, elongation of phonemes, or involuntary blockages (pauses where no sound is produced). The prevalence of stuttering is 1.4% for children under 10 years of age and 0.72% across their lifespan (Craig et al. 2002).

20.2.5.2 Communication Outcomes

Singing uniquely offers respite from stuttering symptoms, granting fluency and voice control, which are otherwise absent in normal speech for those who stutter. Singing is thought to provide strengthened motor control and decrease the occurrence of stuttering, suggesting that it is an advantageous fluency-enhancing activity (Falk et al. 2020). However, beyond the promising evidence reported in pilot studies, no systematic research has been conducted to date on the effects of group singing on communication in stutterers.

A mechanistic explanation for why singing may induce fluency in stutterers is not clear; however, some researchers have hypothesized that altered vocalizations, motor timing enhancements, and the amending of auditory feedback allow for fluent speech (Glover et al. 1996; Healey et al. 1976).

20.2.5.3 Psychosocial Outcomes

Individuals who stutter also suffer from intense stigma and anxiety, occasionally resulting in social isolation or phobia (Blumgart et al. 2010; Iverach et al. 2009; Tran et al. 2011). Given the evidence for the potential of group singing to mitigate stigma in other disorders leading to communication challenges (e.g., Parkinson's disease; Irons et al. 2018; 2021), it seems that group singing could have similar benefits for adults who stutter. Dr. Simone Falk of the Université de Montreal is currently leading a multi-site trial as part of the SingWell project to assess the efficacy of group singing in adults who stutter.

20.3 Summary and Future Directions

Singing together offers an opportunity to support communication and to cultivate psychosocial well-being. Through the act of group singing, participants harness their collective strengths, overcome stigma, and freely express themselves without fear of judgment or misunderstanding. Over time, these experiences may lead to deep social connections and a strong sense of community within the group (Bullack et al. 2018). Indeed, some theorists contend that music may have evolved to develop and maintain social bonds among individuals, resulting in a more coordinated and cooperative social group (Huron 2001; Roederer 1984; Savage et al. 2021).

Although initiatives such as the SingWell project have begun to demonstrate the promise of singing-based interventions to support people living with communication challenges (CCs), much work remains to be done to fully understand the breadth and depth of both the communication and the psychosocial benefits these interventions may offer. Comprehensive research is needed to investigate how such approaches can be tailored to different types of communication challenges as well as how they may improve social connectedness, reduce isolation, and enhance the quality of life of individuals across their lifespan. According to our partners in Speech-Language and Audiology Canada, an estimated 10% of Canadians live with a communication challenge, with prevalence rates significantly higher among the elderly population (see the Speech-Language and Audiology Canada website for current reports, https://www.sac-oac.ca/). This is not only a personal and social issue but also an economic concern. In the United States, a recent study found that the cost of care and economic potential lost due to communication challenges amounted to between 154 and 186 billion USD annually, equivalent to 1% of the country's GDP (Ruben 2000). If we broaden the scope of what is meant by a communication challenge to encompass people living with cognitive decline or newcomers who are struggling to adapt to a new language and culture, the percentage of people living with communication challenges will rise sharply.

As the proportion of elderly individuals is expected to double by 2050, and the prevalence of communication challenges rises alongside this demographic shift, these annual costs are expected to increase substantially (Fougère et al. 2009). Addressing this growing burden requires not only research-based initiatives such as the SingWell Project, but also robust policy support, increased funding for social prescription of singing, and collaborative efforts across healthcare, education, and community sectors to develop sustainable, evidence-based solutions that can mitigate the personal, social, and economic impacts of communication challenges.

References

Adeloye D, Song P, Zhu Y, Campbell H, Sheikh A, Rudan I (2022) Global, regional, and national prevalence of, and risk factors for, chronic obstructive pulmonary disease (COPD) in 2019: a systematic review and modelling analysis. Lancet Respir Med 10(5):447–458

Alain C, Zendel BR, Hutka S, Bidelman GM (2014) Turning down the noise: the benefit of musical training on the aging auditory brain. Hear Res 308:162–173

Aron A, Aron EN, Smollan D (1992) Inclusion of other in the self scale and the structure of interpersonal closeness. J Pers Soc Psychol 63(4):596–612

Barnish MS, Barran SM (2020) A systematic review of active group-based dance, singing, music therapy and theatrical interventions for quality of life, functional communication, speech, motor function and cognitive status in people with Parkinson's disease. BMC Neurol 20(1):371. https://doi.org/10.1186/s12883-020-01938-3. PMID: 33038925; PMCID: PMC7547481

Barnish J, Atkinson RA, Barran SM, Barnish MS (2016) Potential benefit of singing for people with Parkinson's disease: a systematic review. J Parkinsons Dis 6(3):473–484

Bernieri FJ (1988) Coordinated movement and rapport in teacher-student interactions. J Nonverbal Behav 12:120–138. https://doi-org.ezproxy.lib.torontomu.ca/10.1007/BF00986930

Blumgart E, Tran Y, Craig A (2010) An investigation into the personal financial costs associated with stuttering. J Fluen Disord 35(3):203–215. https://doi.org/10.1016/J.JFLUDIS.2010.03.002

Bonilha AG, Onofre F, Vieira ML, Prado MYA, Martinez JAB (2009) Effects of singing classes on pulmonary function and quality of life of COPD patients. Int J Chron Obstruct Pulmon Dis 4:1

Boster JB, Spitzley AM, Castle TW, Jewell AR, Corso CL, McCarthy JW (2021) Music improves social and participation outcomes for individuals with communication disorders: a systematic review. J Music Ther 58(1):12–42

Brink P, Stones M (2007) Examination of the relationship among hearing impairment, linguistic communication, mood, and social engagement of residents in complex continuing-care facilities. The Gerontologist 47(5):633–641. https://doi.org/10.1093/geront/47.5.633

Bullack A, Gass C, Nater UM, Kreutz G (2018) Psychobiological effects of choral singing on affective state, social connectedness, and stress: influences of singing activity and time course. Front Behav Neurosci 12:223

Chanda ML, Levitin DJ (2013) The neurochemistry of music. Trends Cogn Sci 17(4):179–193. https://doi.org/10.1016/j.tics.2013.02.007

Clift S, Hancox G, Morrison I, Hess B, Kreutz G, Stewart D (2010) Choral singing and psychological wellbeing: quantitative and qualitative findings from English choirs in a cross-national survey. J Appl Art Health 1(1):19–34

Coffey EB, Mogilever NB, Zatorre RJ (2017) Speech-in-noise perception in musicians: a review. Hear Res 352:49–69

Craig A, Hancock K, Tran Y, Craig M, Peters K (2002) Epidemiology of stuttering in the community across the entire life span. J Speech Lang Hear Res 45(6):1097–1105

Demos AP, Chaffin R, Begosh KT, Daniels JR, Marsh KL (2012) Rocking to the beat: effects of music and partner's movements on spontaneous interpersonal coordination. J Exp Psychol Gen 141(1):49–53. https://doi.org/10.1037/a0023843

Di Benedetto P, Cavazzon M, Mondolo F, Rugiu G, Peratoner A, Biasutti E (2009) Voice and choral singing treatment: a new approach for speech and voice disorders in Parkinson's disease. Eur J Phys Rehabil Med 45(1):13–19

Dubinsky E, Wood EA, Nespoli G, Russo FA (2019) Short-term choir singing supports speech-in-noise perception and neural pitch strength in older adults with age-related hearing loss. Front Neurosci 13:1153

Durkheim É (2005 [1914]) The dualism of human nature and its social conditions (trans. Eulriet I, Watts Miller W). Durkh Stud/Études Durkheimiennes 11:35–45

Echternach M, Burk F, Burdumy M, Traser L, Richter B (2016) Morphometric differences of vocal tract articulators in different loudness conditions in singing. PLoS One 11(4):e0153792–e0153792. https://doi.org/10.1371/journal.pone.0153792

Engen RL (2005) The singer's breath: implications for treatment of persons with emphysema. J Music Ther 42(1):20–48

Falk S, Schreier R, Russo FA (2020) Singing and stuttering. In: Advancing interdisciplinary research in singing, volume 3: singing and wellbeing. Routledge

Forbes M (2021) "We're pushing back": group singing, social identity, and caring for a spouse with Parkinson's. Psychol Music 49(5):1199–1214

Fougère M, Harvey S, Mercenier J, Mérette M (2009) Population ageing, time allocation and human capital: a general equilibrium analysis for Canada. Econ Model 26(1):30–39

Gick ML, Nicol JJ (2016) Singing for respiratory health: theory, evidence and challenges. Health Promot Int 31(3):725–734

Glover H, Kalinowski J, Rastatter M, Stuart A (1996) Effect of instruction to sing on stuttering frequency at normal and fast rates. Percept Mot Skills 85(2):511–522. https://doi.org/10.2466/PMS.1996.83.2.511

Goldman JG, Postuma R (2014) Premotor and nonmotor features of Parkinson's disease. Curr Opin Neurol 27(4):434–441

Good A, Russo FA (2016) Singing promotes cooperation in a diverse group of children. Soc Psychol 47(6):340–344. https://doi.org/10.1027/1864-9335/a000282

Good A, Choma B, Russo FA (2017) Movement synchrony influences intergroup relations in a minimal groups paradigm. Basic Appl Soc Psychol 39(4):231–238. https://doi.org/10.1080/01973533.2017.1337015

Good A, Kreutz G, Choma B, Fiocco A, Russo F, World Health Organization (2020) The SingWell project protocol: the road to understanding the benefits of group singing in older adults. Public Health Panorama 6(1):141–146

Good A, Earle E, Vezer E, Gilmore S, Livingstone S, Russo FA (2023) Community choir improves vocal production measures in individuals living with Parkinson's disease. J Voice 39(3):848.e7–848.e20

Haslam C, Jetten J, Cruwys T (2018) The new psychology of health: unlocking the social cure. Routledge, Taylor & Francis Group

Healey EC, Mallard AR, Adams MR (1976) Factors contributing to the reduction of stuttering during singing. J Speech Hear Res 19(3):475–480

Hilari K, Northcott S, Roy PI, Marshall J, Wiggins RD, Chataway J, Ames D (2010) Psychological distress after stroke and aphasia: the first six months. Clin Rehabil 24(2):181–190. https://doi.org/10.1177/0269215509346090

Hove MJ, Risen JL (2009) It's all in the timing: interpersonal synchrony increases affiliation. Soc Cogn 27(6):949–960. https://doi.org/10.1521/soco.2009.27.6.949

Huron D (2001) Is music an evolutionary adaptation? Ann N Y Acad Sci 930:43–61. https://doi-org.ezproxy.lib.torontomu.ca/10.1111/j.1749-6632.2001.tb05724.x

Irons J, Hancox G, Stewart D (2018) Sing to Beat Parkinson's (R): a group singing intervention for people with Parkinson's and their carers. Mov Disord 33:S486–S487

Irons JY, Hancox G, Vella-Burrows T, Han EY, Chong HJ, Sheffield D, Stewart DE (2021) Group singing improves quality of life for people with Parkinson's: an international study. Aging Ment Health 25(4):650–656

Iverach L, O'Brian S, Jones M, Block S, Lincoln M, Harrison E, Hewat S, Menzies RG, Packman A, Onslow M (2009) Prevalence of anxiety disorders among adults seeking speech therapy for stuttering. J Anxiety Disord 23(7):928–934. https://doi.org/10.1016/j.janxdis.2009.06.003

Jones CJ (1996) An introduction to the nature and needs of students with mild disabilities: mild mental retardation, behavior disorders, and learning disabilities. C.C. Thomas

Jones L, Baraka A (2015) A Black Mass: for the brothers and sisters of the Black Arts. In: SOS—calling all Black people. University of Massachusetts Press, p 443

Juslin PN, Sloboda JA (2001) Music and emotion: theory and research. Oxford University Press

Juslin PN, Västfjäll D (2008) Emotional responses to music: the need to consider underlying mechanisms. Behav Brain Sci 31(5):559–575

Kaasgaard M, Rasmussen DB, Andreasson KH, Hilberg O, Løkke A, Vuust P, Bodtger U (2022) Use of singing for lung health as an alternative training modality within pulmonary rehabilitation for COPD: a randomised controlled trial. Eur Respir J 59(5):2101142

Kang SK, Chasteen AL (2009) The moderating role of age-group identification and perceived threat on stereotype threat among older adults. Int J Aging Hum Dev 69(3):201–220. https://doi.org/10.2190/AG.69.3.c

Kreutz G (2014) Does singing facilitate social bonding. Music Med 6(2):51–60

Kreutz G, Bongard S, Rohrmann S, Hodapp V, Grebe D (2004) Effects of choir singing or listening on secretory immunoglobulin A, cortisol, and emotional state. J Behav Med 27(6):623–635

Latrofa M, Vaes J, Cadinu M, Carnaghi A (2010) The cognitive representation of self-stereotyping. Personal Soc Psychol Bull 36(7):911–922. https://doi.org/10.1177/0146167210373907

Launay J, Dean RT, Bailes F (2013) Synchronization can influence trust following virtual interaction. Exp Psychol 60(1):53–63. https://doi.org/10.1027/1618-3169/a000173

Lewis A, Cave P, Stern M, Welch L, Taylor K, Russell J et al (2016) Singing for lung health—a systematic review of the literature and consensus statement. NPJ Prim Care Respir Med 26(1):1–8

Livesey L, Morrison I, Clift S, Camic P (2012) Benefits of choral singing for social and mental wellbeing: qualitative findings from a cross-national survey of choir members. J Public Ment Health 11(1):10–26. https://doi.org/10.1108/17465721211207275

Lo CY, … Russo FA (under review) Speech-in-noise, psychosocial, and heart rate variability outcomes of group singing or audiobook club interventions for older adults with unaddressed

hearing loss: a SingWell Project multisite, randomized controlled trial, registered report protocol. PLOS ONE
López-Campos JL, Tan W, Soriano JB (2016) Global burden of COPD. Respirology 21(1):14–23
Lord VM, Hume VJ, Kelly JL, Cave P, Silver J, Waldman M et al (2012) Singing classes for chronic obstructive pulmonary disease: a randomized controlled trial. BMC Pulm Med 12(1):1–7
Ma A, Lau KK, Thyagarajan D (2020) Voice changes in Parkinson's disease: what are they telling us? J Clin Neurosci 72:1–7
Mahler LA, Ramig LO, Fox C (2015) Evidence-based treatment of voice and speech disorders in Parkinson disease. Curr Opin Otolaryngol Head Neck Surg 23(3):209–215
Mathews R (2018) Acoustic, respiratory, cognitive and wellbeing comparisons of two groups of people with Parkinson's disease participating in voice and choral singing group therapy (VCST) versus music appreciation activity. Doctoral thesis
McKay CM (2021) No evidence that music training benefits speech perception in hearing-impaired listeners: a systematic review. Trend Hear 25:2331216520985678
McNeill WH (1997) Keeping together in time: dance and drill in human history. Harvard University Press, Cambridge, MA
Mitchell C, Gittins M, Tyson S, Vail A, Conroy P, Paley L, Bowen A (2021) Prevalence of aphasia and dysarthria among inpatient stroke survivors: describing the population, therapy provision and outcomes on discharge. Aphasiology 35(7):950–960. https://doi.org/10.1080/02687038.2020.1759772
Müller V, Lindenberger U (2011) Cardiac and respiratory patterns synchronize between persons during choir singing. PLoS One 6(9):e24893
Norweg A, Collins EG (2013) Evidence for cognitive–behavioral strategies improving dyspnea and related distress in COPD. Int J Chron Obstruct Pulmon Dis 8:439–451
Pachete A, Pachete C, Good A, Russo FA (under review) Understanding group singing in older adults with aphasia from a psychosocial perspective: a pilot study. Aphasiology
Palmer AD, Newsom JT, Rook KS (2016) How does difficulty communicating affect the social relationships of older adults? An exploration using data from a national survey. J Commun Disord 62:131–146. https://doi.org/10.1016/j.jcomdis.2016.06.002
Pearce E, Launay J, Dunbar RI (2015) The ice-breaker effect: singing mediates fast social bonding. R Soc Open Sci 2(10):150221
Perron M, Theaud G, Descoteaux M, Tremblay P (2021) The frontotemporal organization of the arcuate fasciculus and its relationship with speech perception in young and older amateur singers and non-singers. Hum Brain Mapp 42(10):3058–3076
Pichora-Fuller MK, Dupuis K, Smith SL (2016) Effects of vocal emotion on memory in younger and older adults. Exp Aging Res 42(1):14–30. https://doi.org/10.1080/0361073X.2016.1108734
Rabinowitch TC, Knafo-Noam A (2015) Synchronous rhythmic interaction enhances children's perceived similarity and closeness towards each other. PLoS One 10(4):e0120878
Racette A, Bard C, Peretz I (2006) Making non-fluent aphasics speak: sing along. Brain (London, England: 1878) 129(10):2571–2584. https://doi.org/10.1093/brain/awl250
Revenson TA, Schiaffino KM, Majerovitz SD, Gibofsky A (1991) Social support as a double-edged sword: the relation of positive and problematic support to depression among rheumatoid arthritis patients. Soc Sci Med 33(7):807–813
Reyes A, Castillo A, Castillo J, Cornejo I, Cruickshank T (2020) The effects of respiratory muscle training on phonatory measures in individuals with Parkinson's disease. J Voice 34(6):894–902
Roederer JG (1984) The search for a survival value of music. Music Percept 1(3):350
Ruben RJ (2000) Redefining the survival of the fittest: communication disorders in the 21st century. Laryngoscope 110(2):241–241. https://doi.org/10.1097/00005537-200002010-00010
Sapir S, Spielman JL, Ramig LO, Story BH, Fox C (2007) Effects of intensive voice treatment (the Lee Silverman Voice Treatment [LSVT]) on vowel articulation in dysarthric individuals with idiopathic Parkinson disease: acoustic and perceptual findings. J Speech Lang Hear Res 50(4):899–912. https://doi.org/10.1044/1092-4388(2007/064)
Savage PE, Loui P, Tarr B, Schachner A, Glowacki L, Mithen S, Fitch WT (2021) Music as a coevolved system for social bonding. Behav Brain Sci 44:e59

Silvestri J, Ehrenberg H, Dick L, Shim P (2018) Universal design for music: exploring the intersection of deaf education and music education. J Am Sign Lang Literat 1–11

Siponkoski ST, Pitkäniemi A, Laitinen S, Särkämö ER, Pentikäinen E, Eloranta H et al (2023) Efficacy of a multicomponent singing intervention on communication and psychosocial functioning in chronic aphasia: a randomized controlled crossover trial. Brain Commun 5(1):fcac337

Skingley A, Martin A, Clift S (2016) The contribution of community singing groups to the well-being of older people: participant perspectives from the United Kingdom. J Appl Gerontol 35(12):1302–1324

Stegemöller EL, Radig H, Hibbing P, Wingate J, Sapienza C (2017) Effects of singing on voice, respiratory control and quality of life in persons with Parkinson's disease. Disabil Rehabil 39(6):594–600

Tamplin J, Baker FA, Jones B, Way A, Lee S (2013) "Stroke a Chord": the effect of singing in a community choir on mood and social engagement for people living with aphasia following a stroke. NeuroRehabilitation (Reading, Mass) 32(4):929–941. https://doi.org/10.3233/NRE-130916

Tamplin J, Morris ME, Marigliani C, Baker FA, Noffs G, Vogel AP (2020) ParkinSong: outcomes of a 12-month controlled trial of therapeutic singing groups in Parkinson's disease. J Parkinsons Dis 10(3):1217–1230

Tarr B, Launay J, Dunbar RI (2014) Music and social bonding: "self-other" merging and neurohormonal mechanisms. Front Psychol 5:1096

Thompson WF, Russo FA (2007) Facing the music. Psychol Sci 18(9):756–757. https://doi.org/10.1111/j.1467-9280.2007.01973.x

Tran Y, Blumgart E, Craig A (2011) Subjective distress associated with chronic stuttering. J Fluen Disord 36(1):17–26. https://doi.org/10.1016/j.jfludis.2010.12.003

Tremblay P, Perron M (2023) Auditory cognitive aging in amateur singers and non-singers. Cognition 230:105311

Tunçgenç B, Cohen E, Fawcett C (2015) Rock with me: the role of movement synchrony in infants' social and nonsocial choices. Child Dev 86(3):976–984. https://doi.org/10.1111/cdev.12354

Valdesolo P, Ouyang J, DeSteno D (2010) The rhythm of joint action: synchrony promotes cooperative ability. J Exp Soc Psychol 46(4):693–695. https://doi.org/10.1016/j.jesp.2010.03.004

van der Meulen I, van de Sandt-Koenderman W, Mieke E, Heijenbrok-Kal MH, Visch-Brink EG, Ribbers GM (2014) The efficacy and timing of melodic intonation therapy in subacute aphasia. Neurorehabil Neural Repair 28(6):536–544. https://doi.org/10.1177/1545968313517753

Wade LM (2002) A comparison of the effects of vocal exercises/singing versus music-assisted relaxation on peak expiratory flow rates of children with asthma. Music Ther Perspect 20(1):31–37

Wiltermuth SS, Heath C (2009) Synchrony and cooperation. Psychol Sci 20(1):1–5

Winn CS, Chisolm BA, Hummelbrunner JA (2014) Factors affecting recruitment and retention of rehabilitation professionals in Northern Ontario, Canada: a cross-sectional study. Rural Remote Health 14(2):233–239

World Health Organization (2024, February 2) Deafness and hearing loss. Retrieved from https://www.who.int/news-room/fact-sheets/detail/deafness-and-hearing-loss#:~:text=Over 5% 25 of the world's, will have disabling hearing loss

Wright HH, Shisler RJ (2005) Working memory in aphasia: theory, measures, and clinical implications. Am J Speech Lang Pathol 14(2):107–118. https://doi.org/10.1044/1058-0360(2005/012)

Yamasoba T, Lin FR, Someya S, Kashio A, Sakamoto T, Kondo K (2013) Current concepts in age-related hearing loss: epidemiology and mechanistic pathways. Hear Res 303:30–38. https://doi.org/10.1016/j.heares.2013.01.021

Zhu J, Cui Y, Zhang J, Yan R, Su D, Zhao D et al (2024) Temporal trends in the prevalence of Parkinson's disease from 1980 to 2023: a systematic review and meta-analysis. Lancet Healthy Longev 5(7):e464–e479

Zumbansen A, Peretz I, Anglade C, Bilodeau J, Généreux S, Hubert M, Hébert S (2017) Effect of choir activity in the rehabilitation of aphasia: a blind, randomised, controlled pilot study. Aphasiology 31(8):879–900

Health Aspects of Amateur Dancing 21

Gunter Kreutz and Cynthia Quiroga Murcia

21.1 What Is Dancing?—Cultural and Biological Origins

Dancing means moving freely or through choreography to music. Often this happens in groups as a synchronous activity. Dancing is widespread in all cultures and is an important part of life for many people. The cultivation of dance as a cultural asset encompasses diverse areas between sports, amateur and high culture, and reaches people at different stages of life and socio-demographic backgrounds. Finally, dancing has health benefits that include preventive, therapeutic, and rehabilitative elements. Over the course of music history, various types of dance music have developed, which are more or less closely related to the actual performance of dances. For example, instrumental music in the Baroque era used the forms of dance to indicate a musical gesture. Nevertheless, it can be assumed that music has always played an important role in accompanying dance performances. Dance traditions are not only widespread as an art form but also as elements of everyday cultures. This raises questions about the ontogenetic and phylogenetic meanings to be attributed to dancing for individual human development.

Dancing means moving freely or through choreography to music. Often this happens in groups as a synchronous activity. Dancing is widespread in all cultures and is an important part of life for many people. The cultivation of dance as a cultural asset encompasses diverse areas between sports, amateur and high culture, and reaches people at different stages of life and socio-demographic backgrounds. Finally, dancing has health benefits that include preventive, therapeutic, and

G. Kreutz (✉)
Systematic Musicology, Carl von Ossietzky University Oldenburg, Oldenburg, Lower Saxony, Germany
e-mail: gunter.kreutz@uni-oldenburg.de

C. Q. Murcia
Registered Psychological Psychotherapist, Frankfurt, Germany

G. Kreutz, G. Bernatzky (eds.), *Music and Medicine*, Neurocultural Health and Wellbeing, https://doi.org/10.1007/978-3-662-72175-9_21

rehabilitative elements. Over the course of music history, various types of dance music have developed, which are more or less closely related to the actual performance of dances. For example, instrumental music in the Baroque era used the forms of dance to indicate a musical gesture. Nevertheless, it can be assumed that music has always played an important role in accompanying dance performances. Dance traditions are not only widespread as an art form, but also as elements of everyday cultures. This raises questions about the ontogenetic and phylogenetic meanings to be attributed to dancing for individual human development.

Rhythmic music can trigger movements in humans. The human brain is prepared from the start to receive and physically process musical impulses. In fact, infants are sensitive to musical rhythms from birth (Winkler et al. 2009). With some practice and loving attention, children learn to increasingly coordinate their own physical movement with rhythmic stimulation and to dance to music during the first years of life. Phillips-Silver and Keller (2012) refer to coordinated simultaneous and sequential movements between parents and child as a basis enabling musical learning.

The evolutionary origins of dancing are unclear. A prehistoric connection between singing, dancing, and playing percussion instruments is widely assumed. Pictorial traditions show that dance has been practiced in sacred and secular forms for thousands of years in early high cultures and is still practiced in numerous ethnic groups today. The meanings of such dances are hardly fully comprehensible, but there is a broad consensus in associating them particularly with healing rituals.

The extent to which adaptive behavior and survival value are associated with dancing is disputed, yet it is the subject of speculation. Miller (1999) assumes that dancing was an element of heterosexual advertising behavior. Dances can, for example, communicate health status, virility, aerobic fitness, and creativity, and influence partner choice as secondary characteristics of an individual's resilience and immune competence. Other researchers point to the social functions of dancing, such as promoting coordination, cooperation, and cohesion of groups, thus increasing the chances of survival (McNeill 2009). Similarly, Hagen and Bryant (2003) interpret dancing as a signaling system for communicating qualitative characteristics of group cohesion. According to this theory, dancing increased the individual's willingness to face hostile attacks in the service of the group or to join such attacks. There seems to be agreement that dancing, on the one hand, represents an original form of social communication and, on the other hand, is shaped by individual mental, physical, and psychological repercussions. These aspects also justify the question of the health potential of dancing activities.

Rhythmic properties of music, especially the temporal structure of musical structures based on regular time intervals, so-called "beats" or "beats," favor the individual coordination of music and body movement. Regardless of whether a dance is performed alone or, as is more often the rule, in smaller or larger groups, the continuous sequence of repeating and varied body movements gives the impression of a rhythmically coordinated, learned behavior.

Merker et al. (2009) point out that perceptual-motor synchronization between an external "timekeeper" and physical movements is only found in a few species in the animal kingdom. Patel et al. (2009) conducted a case study with a cockatoo living under human care. It was found that the bird is capable of synchronously executing its own body movements to rhythmic music and even partially adapting to tempo changes. Patel believes that such synchronization abilities have contributed to language development in humans (Patel 2014). Their temporal organization thus reaches the foundations of vocal-motor learning. Thus, the connections between dance elements are not random, but are subject to quasi-syntactic rules.

21.2 Neurobiological Foundations

The choreographer and dance scientist Ivar Hagendoorn (2004) puts the observation and execution of dances in a close relationship. The author suspects that watching dances, similar to listening to music, can stimulate premotor areas of the brain (Kreutz et al. 2003). Also referring to music-related studies, he suspects that strong emotions can be triggered by fulfilled or refuted expectations in the course of movement when observing dancers. Thus, the experience and practice of dances are intrinsically intertwined with aesthetic sensations of pleasure, desire, pleasantness, or rejection.

How strongly motor representations are associated with emotions and emotional evaluations of neutral stimuli is impressively demonstrated by a study by Sedlmeier et al. (2011). The authors demonstrated that the targeted manipulation of Movement gestures and facial expressions significantly influenced affective evaluations of pieces of music. The authors interpret the findings in such a way that the affects associated with physical movements and gestures color simultaneous judgments. The basis of this transfer is that these are gestures that are firmly associated with specific emotions (aversive or appetitive) due to learning and experience.

To internally carry out movements, anticipate, and estimate courses is based on the interaction of extensive cerebral networks, including so-called mirror neurons. In short, these neurons fire equally when a movement is executed by the own organism or the execution of the movement is only observed (Gallese et al. 1996). However, the significance of these neurons goes much further. Because with the representation of a movement, meanings are simultaneously encoded as movement knowledge, which includes the consequences of movements (Berrol 2006;

Hagendoorn 2004). Nevertheless, theoretical speculations have so far been followed by only a few systematic studies. Brown et al. (2006) conducted a study using positron emission tomography (PET) among amateur dancers, whose brain activity was recorded during the execution of learned dance movements. Contrast analyses of the test conditions revealed a network of structures between the midbrain, neocortex, and cerebellum, which probably underlie the sensorimotor processes. According to the authors, the following partly parallel and partly sequential working subsystems are necessary for dancing: The secondary auditory areas in the temporal lobe (melodic and harmonic analysis of the music); parallel to this, structures running from the brainstem to the cerebellum (temporal information about the basic beat of the music), which in turn control the selection and selection of well-predictable action segments via the basal ganglia and putamen; the thalamus, which is involved in the linking of somatosensory and motor parameters and reacts to novel or deviating rhythms; somatotopic areas for muscle control in the lower extremities, which encode information flows in the motor, premotor, and supplementary motor areas regarding the starting and ending points of movements (including the necessary muscle contractions). Part of these areas and possibly the cerebellum support the interhemispheric coordination of the two limbs during cyclic-repetitive movements. The right frontal operculum, the authors continue, is involved in movement sequencing, while the right cingulate motor area regulates aspects of movement intention and allocation of motor resources. Finally, activations of areas of the parietal cortex are interpreted in such a way that the kinesthetically mediated spatial guidance of the leg movements is encoded in these networks (Brown et al. 2006, p. 1161ff.). Although these functional relationships have not yet been verified, these interpretations seem quite plausible in the light of research on other movement sequences.

Karpati et al. (2015) attribute great potential to dancing in their research overview to better understand the structures and functions of the human brain, especially in connection with physical processes. The background is the observation that, as already indicated, very different perceptual-motor, cognitive, and social-affective are claimed in the course of dance performances. This results in many questions: how are these networks activated? Which organismic processes control and influence them? And how do all these processes affect individual well-being?

21.3 Dancing in Clinical Contexts

21.3.1 Dance and Movement Therapy (DMT)

The treatment forms classified under the collective term Dance and Movement Therapy (DMT; Goodill 2005) have their origins in this country in the 1920s and are associated with the Hungarian dancer Rudolf von Laban (1879–1958). Regardless of its still unsecured legal status, dance therapy has become known as an artistic psychotherapeutic method. DMT serves to activate individual physical, mental, emotional, and communicative resources. Often, the focus is on increasing well-being and quality of life, as well as changes in psychological areas such as self-efficacy, communication, and stress reduction.

Practical Tip
Music and dance can enhance physiotherapy even in irreversible neurological diseases. The inclusion of the patient and their musical preferences, as well as openness to creative therapies, is essential for this.

Scientific studies have so far only dealt with the effectiveness of dance therapeutic interventions in some areas, albeit with many positive findings. An overview of the numerous facets of this research field, which also includes socio-political aspects of contemporary dance activities in various countries, is provided by the nearly 1000-page Oxford Handbook of Dance and Wellbeing (Karkou et al. 2017). Without being able to adequately appreciate the numerous chapters here, a growing research interest is evident, also with an increase in systematic research overviews, especially about different target groups (Karkou and Meekums 2017; Mansfield et al. 2018).

The objectives of DMT seem quite comparable to other artistic therapy forms. In this respect, DMT is fundamentally suitable for comparative intervention studies. The consensus is that dance and movement-induced modifications of emotional experience are the keys to sustainable changes in the organism. Scientific studies show positive effects of DMT as a therapeutic intervention in different clinical contexts. Millman et al. (2021) conducted a systematic research overview of the effects of DMT on mental health in psychiatric clinical populations (e.g., in patients suffering from depression, schizophrenia, autism, and somatoform disorders). The authors attest to DMT's significant potential in the adjuvant treatment of a wide range of mental disorders.

DMT is subject to hardly any restrictions in its application. Especially in the case of restrictions of the musculoskeletal system, as is typical for chronic neurological diseases (e.g., multiple sclerosis, Parkinson's), DMT can effectively expand the treatment spectrum.

21.4 Parkinson's

Parkinson's disease is a slowly progressive disease of the nervous system, which includes the massive death of dopaminergic brain structures and decreased activity of the basal ganglia. The disease leads to a loss of movement control with numerous physical and psychological sequelae. For example, Parkinson's patients suffer more than three times as many falls with hip fractures (Earhart 2009). In addition, depending on their psychological adjustment to the disease, patients report a lower quality of life and suffer more frequently from depression.

From an epidemiological perspective, there seems to be a causal relationship between physical activity (leisure sports) and the occurrence of Parkinson's disease in that both too little and too much sports activity increase risks, while moderate sports reduce such risks (Thacker et al. 2008).

The medical treatment of Parkinson's disease with drugs and surgeries requires, according to widespread opinion, complementary and long-term interventions, especially physiotherapies.

Practical Tip

Rhythmic music can help improve the mobility of Parkinson's patients. The basis for this is to actively involve them in the music and also to consider preferences and aversions in musical taste (Bernatzky et al. 2004).

A Cochrane Review on the effect of physiotherapy compared to placebo or no treatment (Tomlinson et al. 2013) concludes that physiotherapies are helpful to such an extent that they can help patients to noticeable improvements in their mobility, balance, and walking behavior, and thus to a higher quality of life. However, it remains unclear which form of physiotherapy is best suited to achieve maximum improvements in symptoms.

Based on informal observations, various research groups conducted systematic investigations into the effectiveness of different dance forms on disease pattern and course in Parkinson's patients. The common basic idea is that in dancing central, otherwise isolated physiotherapeutic elements such as rhythmic movement, balance exercises, cognitive movement strategies, and strength exercises can be integrated holistically. In addition, dancing can be performed as a cultural activity in a context that promotes social interactions. The social aspect led in a number of projects and studies to an emphasis on couple dancing, with the Argentine tango proving to be particularly suitable (Westheimer et al. 2015).

Hackney and Earhart (2009a) compared three intervention groups in a randomized, controlled study. Patients were assigned to groups that either received tango lessons, waltz/foxtrot lessons, or no dance lessons. The results showed that both dance groups, unlike the controls, could benefit in terms of balance, walking range, and strength of stepping backward. However, the authors point out advantages in some aspects of movement performance changes of the tango dancers compared to the other two groups. The same research group (Duncan and Earhart 2012; Foster et al. 2013) conducted further randomized, controlled studies with the aim of investigating interactions between disease progression and tango dancing over a period of 12 months. Indeed, the results showed a significant improvement in motor skills in the tango group compared to controls without intervention. However, only participants who were not taking any medication at the time of the survey were included. The study did not provide for control of social influences and a possible Hawthorne effect.

While the studies cited so far usually choose durations of one to two dance lessons over a period of at least several weeks, comparable effects are shown in the case of an intensification of such interventions. For example, Parkinson's patients in a study by Hackney and Earhart (2009b) received daily 90-min tango lessons over a period of 2 weeks with the result that the balance of the dancers on a standardized scale could improve by three points compared to four points of improvement with a longer-lasting intervention with low weekly frequency (for an overview see Earhart 2009).

Despite the fact that physiotherapies, including dance therapies, are indicated in the early stages of Parkinson's disease, Hackney and Earhart (2010) conducted a case study on a patient in an advanced stage. In this case, too, improvements in motor skills and balance, as well as increases in quality of life, were demonstrated after 20 one-hour dance lessons, although the patient primarily relies on the wheelchair in everyday life.

Practical Tip

Studies only provide limited information about the form of effective interventions. In order for standardized procedures to develop, detailed replication studies are necessary from both a scientific and a practical point of view.

Meta-analyses of randomized controlled trials ($n = 6$) consistently suggest positive effects of dance-based movement therapies for Parkinson's patients and list improved quality of life, mobility, and balance as central outcomes (de Dreu et al. 2012; Dos Santos Delabary et al. 2018). The improvement of the basal symptoms affects the motor skills primarily of patients with mild to moderate symptoms (Carapellotti et al. 2020). Even statistically subthreshold improvements appear noteworthy and can certainly give rise to the demand for expansion of interventions in this and other patient groups (Clair et al. 2012). In fact, the long-term application of music-based movement therapies is considered safe without restriction (States et al. 2011). Heiberger et al. (2011) argue for dance-based therapies not only because of symptomatic effects, but they refer to the emotional experience and the effects on health-related quality of life of long-term interventions in the affected individuals and in the caring persons.

21.5 Multiple Sclerosis and Other Diseases

Multiple sclerosis (MS) is a chronic disease of the nervous system with various accompanying symptoms such as pain, fatigue, motor failures, spasms, incontinence, and sexual dysfunction. Unsurprisingly, the physical symptoms often come with significant psychological stress, in individual cases, up to symptoms comparable to bipolar disorders.

A single case study on a 45-year-old MS patient was conducted by Salgado and de Paula Vasconcelos (2010) with the aim of presenting changes in the patient's health assessment after a 5-month dance therapy intervention. The first phase of the study was designed to familiarize the patient at the center of this study with the intervention as part of a physiotherapeutic treatment. The entire study period covered 5 months with two weekly sessions. Accumulated, this means a therapy of over 40 sessions of approximately 66 h duration. A characteristic of the intervention is the continuous use of music to promote movement sequences, as well as the ending of each session with relaxation and stretching exercises. During the course of the measure, a choreography was also developed and recorded. Measured by standardized medical-diagnostic tests and parameters, there were overall clear improvements in the patient's health condition. This manifested itself in such a way that the patient was able to walk alone with a walking stick at the end of the measure, while at the beginning of the measure she relied on a walking stick and additional help (wall, accompanying person). Improvements were also shown in numerous specific neurological indicators, particularly regarding the functionality of the cerebellum. According to the patient's statements, an increase in joy of life and self-esteem is clearly linked to dance therapy. A systematic review suggests, despite the explicit method criticism, the reliability of such observations (Lopes and Keppers 2021).

The results achieved so far on the application of dance and movement therapies (with music) often suffer from methodological limitations. Nevertheless, the insights gained from Parkinson's and MS patients can be transferred in many respects to populations with other disease patterns, especially severe mental disorders (Barton 2011), depression (Jeong et al. 2005; Karkou et al. 2019; Pinniger et al. 2012), arthritis (Noreau et al. 1995), spastic paralysis (Joung et al. 2021), cancer (Ginsburgs and Goodill 2009; Ho 2005; Ho et al. 2007), fibromyalgia (Baptista et al. 2012; Bojner-Horwitz et al. 2003) and heart failure (Belardinelli et al. 2008). The variety and breadth of DMT in clinical applications is impressive. The studies also leave no doubt about the importance of music as a central element of effective movement therapies. Finally, the outlined clinical studies can also be considered from a prevention perspective.

Conclusion

Particularly, patients with neurological restrictions are exposed to increased dangers of falls and thus further risks that can have a correspondingly negative effect on the primary disease. Music-based movement therapies can help to break the vicious circle between neurological disorders and their almost inevitable physical and psychological sequelae and to convey positive life perspectives to patients. However, many questions about the mechanisms of possible changes remain open, despite significant advances in neurobiological basic research.

The targeted and effective use of music- and dance-based movement therapies in patient populations suffering from motor as well as cognitive and psychological restrictions or burdens seems very well justified. Patients with physical diseases and symptoms often also benefit in terms of their psychological well-being. If dance and movement promote motor coordination, body awareness, muscle tone, and other aspects of the musculoskeletal system, this is also justified by motivational factors and a stabilization of the individual psychological constitution, which only allows long-term participation in the corresponding programs. Dance and movement therapies are recommended for inclusion in prevention and rehabilitation programs due to negligible side effects and improvements in health-related quality of life in many areas (Gomes Neto et al. 2014; Koch et al. 2019).

21.6 Opportunities and Risks for Health and Well-Being in Recreational Dancing

Dancing in nonclinical areas carries both health opportunities and risks for the practicing dancers themselves. Special roles are played on the one hand by the degree of professionalization of dancing and on the other hand by the living environments and socio-economic conditions within which dance cultures form and opportunities for individual self-realization, without which one can achieve the stated goal of professionalization. There are partly controversial health implications in both areas.

Basically, a growing professionalization of dancing, similar to other musical activities, is associated with increased risks. For example, between 67% and 95% of all professional dancers in ballet and 17–24% in modern dance suffer stress fractures in the foot and ankle during their career (Kadel 2014). Are positive effects for health and well-being to be expected in the amateur sector in return?

Physical activities generally protect against physical and mental disorders (e.g., Erickson and Kramer 2008; Malm et al. 2019). Dancing in particular strengthens aerobic fitness, balance, coordination, elasticity, muscle strength, joint mobility, as well as kinesthetic awareness and body control (e.g., Zhang et al. 2008). Such observations justify intervention studies with the goal of understanding dancing in leisure time as a contribution to prevention and addressing healthy populations accordingly.

Modern urban music cultures in the sign of hip hop, rave, or techno are highly controversially discussed with regard to health aspects. Some researchers point to a number of physical and psychological risks, while others emphasize prevention aspects. Ojofeitimi et al. (2012) recognize comparatively high injury risks in hip hop dancing. The authors consider this dance to be as physically demanding as gymnastics and call for appropriate preventive measures. Popular music styles, including hip hop, are also considered robust markers for drug abuse among teenagers (Lee et al. 2011; ter Bogt et al. 2012). Finally, sociologists point to commercialization and consumer fixation within modern hip hop, where sexuality plays a significant role as a commodity (Hunter 2011). Research comes to very different conclusions, according to which the mentioned musical subcultures are central elements of prevention programs against obesity or to support cultural identity among teenagers in socially disadvantaged environments are particularly suitable (Beaulac et al. 2011; Romero 2012).

In summary, dancing in the leisure sector is not fundamentally harmless. Environmental factors such as sound pressure level, population density, and other conditions in relevant discos and dance clubs play a major role. In addition, there are personal influences and behavior of dancers, especially teenagers and young adults. The widespread consumption of legal and illegal pleasure substances at dance events raises questions. Individual and contextual factors make it difficult to estimate the chances and risks for mental and physical health of dance activities. Many of the environmental or milieu-related risk factors are absent in socially elevated milieus, from which many amateur dancers from areas of standard and couple dancing are recruited.

Changes in music taste are also closely linked with changes in dance cultures. While standard couple dances and folk dances can certainly be considered constants in a heterogeneous dance culture here and in many countries around the world, the varieties within dance-related subcultures go back to epochal changes that also indicate generational differences.

The ubiquity of the internet and the spread of mobile devices and online platforms such as TikTok and YouTube have also, in recent years, changed the way people create content through dancing. Create, consume, connect with each other, and communicate strongly influenced (Warburton 2022). Through *dance challenges,* people are encouraged to perform short dance routines of varying complexity to popular songs, which are re-enacted by other users, and to spread these. Thus, the culture of dances and dancing is also likely to undergo significant changes in the course of digitalization.

It therefore seems sensible to also ask the question of the effectiveness of dancing as a means of prevention and the enhancement of quality of life and well-being in healthy populations, differentiating between age groups, without thereby questioning the generations-connecting, integrative effect—which, by the way, has social-hygienic implications and is worthy of its own consideration.

21.7 Children and Adolescents

Lack of physical activity combined with poor nutrition is considered a major cause of mortality worldwide (Zhao et al. 2020). Based on observations about the stability of (healthy or unhealthy) lifestyles over the lifetime, children and adolescents have come into the focus of prevention programs. Although such programs have not yet led to a containment of the problem, research interest is increasingly focusing on specific forms of intervention, such as dancing in the leisure time of children and adolescents, and its health implications. For example, Flores (1995) conducted an intervention study with the declared aim of examining the long-term influence of dancing on cardiovascular indicators in children from socially disadvantaged environments in a randomized and controlled study. Indeed, the author found significant reductions in both body mass index (BMI) and resting pulse in the model group compared to a control group. Unfortunately, the study does not report on effect size, nor is there an F-statistic, which would have indicated an interaction effect between time and group. Nevertheless, central findings about positive effects of dancing in children and adolescents in comparable environments are confirmed in recent studies, for example, with regard to increased motivation for physical activities, increased self-efficacy in girls, and improved social behavior in boys (Romero 2012).

Against these backgrounds, Burkhardt and Brennan (2012) developed a systematic research overview on the question to what extent this target group can benefit in terms of health and well-being. Of the originally 1129 entries screened in scientific databases, 14 studies, including the study by Flores (1995) just outlined, proved to be methodologically reliable and—with remaining reservations—interpretable. The authors recognize positive effects of dancing on cardiovascular and bone health, as well as—albeit with mixed findings—in terms of self-image, body awareness, and the reduction of fears. It is essential to note that dancing can make a significant contribution to the prevention and reduction of overweight in children and adolescents. Since both age ranges, target group milieus, dance forms, intervention strategies (duration, control, and comparison groups), as well as dependent variables vary greatly from study to study, no concrete action guideline can be derived from this overview. Nevertheless, it can be assumed that individual motivation, music preferences, and attitudes toward music and dance styles strongly influence the chances of success and sustainability of any interventions.

Instructive for the importance of preference, taste and socioeconomic backgrounds regarding adolescent music and dance cultures and their health implications appears to be a study by Harris et al. (2012). Regardless of partial negative associations between youth music cultures and health (Miranda and Claes 2009), the authors point to rather overlooked positive aspects of dancing, especially with regard to target groups in socio-economically disadvantaged milieus. Particularly here, according to the authors, the potential seems particularly large when it comes to changing lifestyles using cultural resources. For this purpose, over a period of 12 weeks, workshops on Hip Hop and Street Dance were held once or twice a week with professional dance teachers and choreographers. Participants were two cohorts of a total of 171 adolescents between twelve and 18 years old (37 males; 134 females). At the end of the event, there were public performances and a dance competition. A qualitative interview survey among the participants included four general questions about (positive) experiences with the dance project, through which the nature and extent of perceived changes were also recorded. Initially, it was found that with a dropout rate of only 8%, the implementation of the project itself can be considered a success. Content analyses of the responses by the adolescents showed that consistent participation can be attributed to high motivations and positive experiences with the intervention. Positive life experiences, cooperation and solidarity, connection with the school, and self-expression were identified as central themes. The authors, in their interpretation, do not address methodological deficiencies such as inadequate controls and the omission of the collection of objective indicators. Nevertheless, they point to the importance of differentiated youth cultures as principal starting points for intervention studies. Interventions can only be sustainable if they are directed at the living environment of the adolescents and their cultural experiences and values themselves (Harris et al. 2012).

21.8 Adults

Health effects of dancing in nonclinical areas among adult amateur dancers have so far been little researched been. A study among young adults who participated in one of four 12-week interventions (Modern Dance, Sport, Music, and Mathematics) revealed that participants in the dance intervention reported comparatively stronger decreases in anxiety states (Lesté and Rust 1990). A quasi-experimental study by Quiroga et al. (2009) among couple dancers revealed differential effects of music and partner on psychometric and biological variables. Dancing with a partner to music had a stronger mood-enhancing and reducing effect regarding negative mood components compared to dancing alone and/or dancing without music. Accompanying music to dance also led to a stronger reduction in the cortisol concentrations measured in the participants' saliva. Less clear were the effects on the second biological marker, the hormone testosterone. Nevertheless, the patterns of observed changes suggest the importance of social interaction on the release of this hormone (in both genders) in the sense that dancing with a partner led to increased concentrations. Although the authors point to a limited validity due to the small sample size, it seems that short-term positive psychophysiological changes are associated with couple dancing, especially for combating stress and promoting mental well-being.

An exploratory study with the aim of capturing dancers' self-assessed health effects of dancing was undertaken by Quiroga Murcia et al. (2010). A total of 475 amateur dancers (304 female, 171 male; age range 18–74 years) filled out an online questionnaire, which in addition to demographic information, a number of details about the form of dance, musical backgrounds and especially psychological and health effects closely based on a questionnaire about health effects of singing (Clift and Hancox 2001) were elicited. It was found that especially folk and standard dancers participated in the study. However, three-quarters of the respondents indicated having experience with various dance forms. Interestingly, the dancers were active for an average of 17.6 h in the last month, and on average, over a period of 10.2 years. So, how do amateur dancers benefit according to the results of the study? A factor-analytical evaluation of the rating scales points to a special importance of dancing for emotional well-being. Given the high degree of explained variance for this factor (32.6%), which is only slightly explained by the further factors, this form of data reduction is nevertheless questionable. For example, physical aspects play a much larger role in the free expressions than the factor-analytical evaluations suggest. The greatest agreement with 95% was found for the statement that dancing improves balance and body awareness. Although no statement met with overwhelming rejection, the respondents were rather reserved to indifferent regarding statements about spiritual and artistic aspects. In short, health and well-being can be considered as essential motivations for amateur dancing from the perspective of the respondents. Psychological aspects such as improving moods, increased feelings of happiness, and reduction of tension play a major role. It is noteworthy, for example, that the statement "Dancing hardly helps me to improve my general emotional well-being" is rejected by 88% of the participants. The free expressions about the health effects of dancing in this study appear instructive for further studies. For example, some respondents report suffering from chronic diseases and being able to benefit from dancing in terms of their general condition. It is also not only referred to improvements in self-image, moods, or relaxation, but also to effects in partner relationships, which are often perceived as more intense and happier through dancing (Quiroga et al. 2010). The intensity of the dance activities measured here is roughly equivalent to the observed exposure in a study by Kreutz (2008) on a specific population of couple dancers. However, whether dancing has preventive effects on physical health in adult amateur dancers has not yet been demonstrated.

21.9 Older Adults

Healthy amateur dancers in higher adulthood (>60 years) have so far been less frequently chosen as target groups unless they have come into the focus of clinical studies (see above). Nevertheless, this population group is both interesting from the point of view of prevention of musculoskeletal (Guzmán-García et al. 2011) as well as neurodegenerative diseases (Verghese et al. 2003). Studies show that activities like Tai Chi Chuan, aerobic exercises, and dancing lead to improved body balance. Physical activities, including dancing, also reduce risks of falls (Keogh et al. 2009).

A pilot study with the aim of exploring the effect of a 30-min dance instruction on the body balance and posture of over 60-year-old dance inexperienced couple dancers was undertaken by Guzmán-García et al. (2011). The authors assume that dancing activates a variety of cognitive resources, which can also improve the automation of movement sequences and reflexes. On the other hand, it is not ensured that couple dancers benefit in a similar way from such advantages. The authors used physical pressure measurements as well as kinematic motion recordings in before-and-after comparisons to objectify changes of individual balance in standing. The results show immediately improved balance (less swaying) in all dependent measures after the dance instruction. Differentiations revealed regarding the leading or following roles in dance pairs, as well as a visual condition (open versus closed eyes). Leading dancers showed a stronger reduction of fluctuations. Keeping the eyes closed led to difficulties for individual dancers. Nevertheless, the significantly positive changes in a small sample suggest that a physically moderately demanding dance instruction in a very short time can contribute to a significant improvement in balance and posture in older people.

A widely noticed prospective study on the development of age-related dementia was undertaken by Verghese and colleagues (Verghese et al. 2003) with the aim of linking the onset of the disease in a population with mental and physical activities. It turned out that several different mental activities, including playing musical instruments, in the area of physical activities, however, only one, dancing, was associated with a reduced risk of dementia onset. The authors point out, however, that the development of dementia and its accompanying symptoms are still too little researched and understood to be able to establish a causal relationship between increased musical and dancing activities on the one hand and the prevention or delay of the onset of dementia on the other hand. The same applies to the classification of dance interventions for fall prevention and coping with the fear of falling in older people. The current state of research is insufficient to make recommendations beyond the hint that dancing is a safe, motivating, and positive mood-enhancing activity also, and especially for senior citizens (Hwang and Braun 2015; Veronese et al. 2017).

21.10 Future Perspective

With reference to Charles Darwin, Sheets-Johnstone justifies the therapeutic effect of dancing through its life-affirming meaning on the one hand and its non-reducibility to mere motor aspects (Sheets-Johnstone 2010). Without the complex considerations of the author, why dancing is therapeutic, to be reproduced here in detail, they are in line with theories of effect of other music and art therapeutic procedures. Movement is both a prerequisite and a result of vital processes. Physical movement is always accompanied by psychological and emotional correlates. Feelings of immobility in the case of a supposedly or actually impending danger contrasts with the expression of joy and happiness feelings, also manifested in movement. In addition, she considers the kinesthetic sense, the ability to assess the position and movement of the body, which makes movement learning possible, to be greatly underestimated and, in relation to our other sensory equipment, inadequately researched.

Conclusion

The research literature presented here is characterized by a growing number of methodologically demanding studies, including systematic reviews, which refer to health implications of dancing across clinical and nonclinical populations. The results appear to encourage further research programs, both from the perspective of prevention and adjuvant therapy, even in severe mental and physical diseases.

References

Baptista AS, Villela AL, Jones A, Natour J (2012) Effectiveness of dance in patients with fibromyalgia: a randomized, single-blind, controlled study. Clin Exp Rheumatol 30(6 Suppl 74):18–23. Retrieved from http://www.ncbi.nlm.nih.gov/pubmed/23020850

Barton EJ (2011) Movement and mindfulness: a formative evaluation of a dance/movement and yoga therapy program with participants experiencing severe mental illness. Am J Dance Ther 33(2):157–181. https://doi.org/10.1007/s10465-011-9121-7

Beaulac J, Kristjansson E, Calhoun M (2011) 'Bigger than hip-hop?' Impact of a community-based physical activity program on youth living in a disadvantaged neighborhood in Canada. J Youth Stud 14(8):961–974. https://doi.org/10.1080/13676261.2011.616488
Belardinelli R, Lacalaprice F, Ventrella C, Volpe L, Faccenda E (2008) Waltz dancing in patients with chronic heart failure: new form of exercise training. Circ Heart Fail 1(2):107–114. https://doi.org/10.1161/CIRCHEARTFAILURE.108.765727
Bernatzky G, Bernatzky P, Hesse H-P, Staffen W, Ladurner G (2004) Stimulating music increases motor coordination in patients afflicted with Morbus Parkinson. Neurosci Lett 361(1–3):4–8. https://doi.org/10.1016/j.neulet.2003.12.022
Berrol CF (2006) Neuroscience meets dance/movement therapy: mirror neurons, the therapeutic process and empathy. Arts Psychother 33(4):302–315. https://doi.org/10.1016/j.aip.2006.04.001
Bojner-Horwitz E, Theorell T, Maria Anderberg U (2003) Dance/movement therapy and changes in stress-related hormones: a study of fibromyalgia patients with video-interpretation. Arts Psychother 30(5):255–264. https://doi.org/10.1016/j.aip.2003.07.001
Brown S, Martinez MJ, Parsons LM (2006) The neural basis of human dance. Cereb Cortex 16(8):1157–1167. https://doi.org/10.1093/cercor/bhj057
Burkhardt J, Brennan C (2012) The effects of recreational dance interventions on the health and well-being of children and young people: a systematic review. Arts Health 4(2):148–161. https://doi.org/10.1080/17533015.2012.665810
Carapellotti AM, Stevenson R, Doumas M (2020) The efficacy of dance for improving motor impairments, non-motor symptoms, and quality of life in Parkinson's disease: a systematic review and meta-analysis. PLoS One 15(8):e0236820. https://doi.org/10.1371/journal.pone.0236820
Clair AA, Lyons KE, Hamburg J (2012) A feasibility study of the effects of music and movement on physical function, quality of life, depression, and anxiety in patients with Parkinson disease. Music Med 4(1):49–55. https://doi.org/10.1177/1943862111425680
Clift SM, Hancox G (2001) The perceived benefits of singing. J Royal Soc Promot Health 121(4):248–56. https://doi.org/10.1177/146642400112100409
de Dreu MJJ, van der Wilk ASDSD, Poppe E, Kwakkel G, van Wegen EEHEH (2012) Rehabilitation, exercise therapy and music in patients with Parkinson's disease: a meta-analysis of the effects of music-based movement therapy on walking ability, balance and quality of life. Parkinsonism Relat Disord 18 Suppl 1(October 2016):S114–S119. https://doi.org/10.1016/S1353-8020(11)70036-0
Dos Santos Delabary M, Komeroski IG, Monteiro EP, Costa RR, Haas AN (2018) Effects of dance practice on functional mobility, motor symptoms and quality of life in people with Parkinson's disease: a systematic review with meta-analysis. Aging Clin Exp Res 30(7):727–735. https://doi.org/10.1007/s40520-017-0836-2
Duncan RP, Earhart GM (2012) Randomized controlled trial of community-based dancing to modify disease progression in Parkinson disease. Neurorehabil Neural Repair 26(2):132–143. https://doi.org/10.1177/1545968311421614
Earhart GM (2009) Dance as therapy for individuals with Parkinson disease. Eur J Phys Rehabil Med 45(2):231–238. https://doi.org/10.1016/j.bbi.2008.05.010
Erickson KI, Kramer AF (2008) Aerobic exercise effects on cognitive and neural plasticity in older adults. Br J Sports Med. https://doi.org/10.1136/bjsm.2008.052498
Flores R (1995) Dance for health: improving fitness in African American and Hispanic adolescents. Public Health Rep (Washington, DC: 1974) 110(2):189–193. Retrieved from http://www.ncbi.nlm.nih.gov/pubmed/7630998
Foster ER, Golden L, Duncan RP, Earhart GM (2013) Community-based Argentine tango dance program is associated with increased activity participation among individuals with Parkinson's disease. Arch Phys Med Rehabil 94:240–249. https://doi.org/10.1016/j.apmr.2012.07.028
Gallese V, Fadiga L, Fogassi L, Rizzolatti G (1996) Action recognition in the premotor cortex. Brain 119(2):593–609. https://doi.org/10.1093/brain/119.2.593

Ginsburgs VH, Goodill SW (2009) A dance/movement therapy clinical model for women with gynecologic cancer undergoing high dose rate brachytherapy. Am J Dance Ther 31(2):136–158. https://doi.org/10.1007/s10465-009-9076-0

Gomes Neto M, Menezes MA, Oliveira Carvalho V (2014) Dance therapy in patients with chronic heart failure: a systematic review and a meta-analysis. Clin Rehabil 28(12):1172–1179. https://doi.org/10.1177/0269215514534089

Goodill SW (2005) An introduction to medical dance/movement therapy: health care in motion. Jessica Kingsley Publishers, London

Guzmán-García A, Johannsen L, Wing AM (2011) Dance exercise for older adults: a pilot study investigating standing balance following a single lesson of danzón. Am J Dance Ther 33:148–156. https://doi.org/10.1007/s10465-011-9114-6

Hackney ME, Earhart G (2009a) Effects of dance on movement control in Parkinson's disease: a comparison of Argentine tango and American ballroom. J Rehabil Med 41(6):475–481. https://doi.org/10.2340/16501977-0362

Hackney ME, Earhart GM (2009b) Health-related quality of life and alternative forms of exercise in Parkinson disease. Parkinsonism Relat Disord 15(9):644–648. https://doi.org/10.1016/j.parkreldis.2009.03.003

Hackney ME, Earhart GM (2010) Effects of dance on balance and gait in severe Parkinson disease: a case study. Disabil Rehabil 32(8):679–684. https://doi.org/10.3109/09638280903247905

Hagen EH, Bryant GA (2003) Music and dance as a coalition signaling system. Hum Nat 14(1):21–51. https://doi.org/10.1007/s12110-003-1015-z

Hagendoorn I (2004) Some speculative hypotheses about the nature and perception of dance and choreography. J Conscious Stud 11(3–4):79–110

Harris N, Wilks L, Stewart D (2012) HYPEd-up: youth dance culture and health. Arts Health 4(3):239–248. https://doi.org/10.1080/17533015.2012.677849

Heiberger L, Maurer C, Amtage F, Mendez-Balbuena I, Schulte-Mönting J, Hepp-Reymond M-C, Kristeva R (2011) Impact of a weekly dance class on the functional mobility and on the quality of life of individuals with Parkinson's disease. Front Aging Neurosci 3:14. https://doi.org/10.3389/fnagi.2011.00014

Ho RTH (2005) Effects of dance movement therapy on Chinese cancer patients: a pilot study in Hong Kong. Arts Psychother 32(5):337–345. https://doi.org/10.1016/j.aip.2005.04.005

Ho RTH, Ng SM, Chan CLW (2007) Effects of dance movement therapy on improving mental health in cancer patients. In: *Psycho-oncology*, vol 16, pp 1–287. https://doi.org/10.1002/pon.1266

Hunter M (2011) Shake it, baby, shake it: consumption and the new gender relation in hip-hop. Sociol Perspect 54(1):15–36. https://doi.org/10.1525/sop.2011.54.1.15

Hwang PW-N, Braun KL (2015) The effectiveness of dance interventions to improve older adults' health: a systematic literature review. Altern Ther Health Med 21(5):64–70. Retrieved from http://www.ncbi.nlm.nih.gov/pubmed/26393993

Jeong Y-J, Hong S-C, Lee MS, Park M-C, Kim Y-K, Suh C-M (2005) Dance movement therapy improves emotional responses and modulates neurohormones in adolescents with mild depression. Int J Neurosci 115(12):1711–1720. https://doi.org/10.1080/00207450590958574

Joung HJ, Yang HK, Lee Y (2021) Effect of dance on balance, mobility, and activities of daily living in adults with cerebral palsy: a pilot study. Front Neurol 12:663060. https://doi.org/10.3389/fneur.2021.663060

Kadel N (2014) Foot and ankle problems in dancers. Phys Med Rehabil Clin N Am 25(4):829–844. https://doi.org/10.1016/j.pmr.2014.06.003

Karkou V, Meekums B (2017) Dance movement therapy for dementia. Cochrane Database Syst Rev 2017(2). https://doi.org/10.1002/14651858.CD011022.pub2

Karkou V, Oliver S, Lycouris S (eds) (2017) The Oxford handbook of dance and wellbeing. Oxford University Press. https://doi.org/10.1093/oxfordhb/9780199949298.001.0001

Karkou V, Aithal S, Zubala A, Meekums B (2019) Effectiveness of dance movement therapy in the treatment of adults with depression: a systematic review with meta-analyses. Front Psychol 10:936. https://doi.org/10.3389/fpsyg.2019.00936

Karpati FJ, Giacosa C, Foster NEV, Penhune VB, Hyde KL (2015) Dance and the brain: a review. Ann N Y Acad Sci 1337(1):140–146. https://doi.org/10.1111/nyas.12632

Keogh JWL, Kilding A, Pidgeon P, Ashley L, Gillis D (2009) Physical benefits of dancing for healthy older adults: a review. J Aging Phys Act 17(4):479–500

Koch SC, Riege RFF, Tisborn K, Biondo J, Martin L, Beelmann A (2019) Effects of dance movement therapy and dance on health-related psychological outcomes. A meta-analysis update. Front Psychol 10:1806. https://doi.org/10.3389/fpsyg.2019.01806

Kreutz G (2008) Does partnered dance promote health? The case of tango Argentino. J R Soc Promot Heal 128(2):79–84. https://doi.org/10.1177/1466424007087805

Kreutz G, Russ M, Bongard S, Lanfermann H (2003) Cerebral correlates of music listening. An fMRL-study on the effects of happy and sad classical music. Nervenheilkunde 22(3):150–156

Lee JP, Battle RS, Soller B, Brandes N (2011) Thizzin'-Ecstasy use contexts and emergent social meanings. Addict Res Theory 19(6):528–541. https://doi.org/10.3109/16066359.2010.545156

Leste A, Rust J (1990) Effects of dance on anxiety, 4, 195–197. American therapy. J Dance Therapy 12(4):19–25

Lopes J, Keppers II (2021) Music-based therapy in rehabilitation of people with multiple sclerosis: a systematic review of clinical trials. Arq Neuropsiquiatr 79(6):527–535. https://doi.org/10.1590/0004-282X-ANP-2020-0374

Malm C, Jakobsson J, Isaksson A (2019) Physical activity and sports—real health benefits: a review with insight into the public health of Sweden. Sports 7(5):127. https://doi.org/10.3390/sports7050127

Mansfield L, Kay T, Meads C, Grigsby-Duffy L, Lane J, John A et al (2018) Sport and dance interventions for healthy young people (15-24 years) to promote subjective well-being: a systematic review. BMJ Open 8(7):e020959. https://doi.org/10.1136/bmjopen-2017-020959

McNeill WH (2009) Keeping together in time. Harvard University Press. https://doi.org/10.2307/j.ctvjf9wq6

Merker BH, Madison GS, Eckerdal P (2009) On the role and origin of isochrony in human rhythmic entrainment. Cortex 45(1):4–17. https://doi.org/10.1016/j.cortex.2008.06.011

Miller GF (1999) Evolution of human music through sexual selection. In: Wallin N, Merker B, Brown S (eds) The origins of music. The MIT Press, Boston, pp 329–360. https://doi.org/10.1177/004057368303900411

Millman LSM, Terhune DB, Hunter ECM, Orgs G (2021) Towards a neurocognitive approach to dance movement therapy for mental health: a systematic review. Clin Psychol Psychother 28(1):24–38. https://doi.org/10.1002/cpp.2490

Miranda D, Claes M (2009) Music listening, coping, peer affiliation and depression in adolescence. Psychol Music 37(2):215–233. https://doi.org/10.1177/0305735608097245

Noreau L, Martineau H, Roy L, Belzile M (1995) Effects of a modified dance-based exercise on cardiorespiratory fitness, psychological state and health status of persons with rheumatoid arthritis. Am J Phys Med Rehabil 74(1):19–27. https://doi.org/10.1097/00002060-199501000-00004

Ojofeitimi S, Bronner S, Woo H (2012) Injury incidence in hip hop dance. Scand J Med Sci Sports 22(3):347–355. https://doi.org/10.1111/j.1600-0838.2010.01173.x

Patel AD (2014) Can nonlinguistic musical training change the way the brain processes speech? The expanded OPERA hypothesis. Hear Res. https://doi.org/10.1016/j.heares.2013.08.011

Patel AD, Iversen JR, Bregman MR, Schulz I (2009) Studying synchronization to a musical beat in nonhuman animals. Ann N Y Acad Sci 1169:459–469. https://doi.org/10.1111/j.1749-6632.2009.04581.x

Phillips-Silver J, Keller PE (2012) Searching for roots of entrainment and joint action in early musical interactions. Front Hum Neurosci 6. https://doi.org/10.3389/fnhum.2012.00026

Pinniger R, Brown RF, Thorsteinsson EB, McKinley P (2012) Argentine tango dance compared to mindfulness meditation and a waiting-list control: a randomised trial for treating depression. Complement Ther Med. https://doi.org/10.1016/j.ctim.2012.07.003

Quiroga Murcia C, Kreutz G, Clift S, Bongard S (2010) Shall we dance? An exploration of the perceived benefits of dancing on well-being. Arts Health 2(2):149–163. https://doi.org/10.1080/17533010903488582

Quiroga C, Bongard S, Kreutz G (2009) Emotional and neurohumoral responses to dancing Tango Argentino: the effects of music and partner. Music Med 1(1):14–21. https://doi.org/10.1177/1943862109335064

Romero AJ (2012) A pilot test of the Latin active hip hop intervention to increase physical activity among low-income Mexican-American adolescents. Am J Health Promot 26(4):208–211. https://doi.org/10.4278/ajhp.090123-ARB-24

Salgado R, de Paula Vasconcelos LA (2010) The use of dance in the rehabilitation of a patient with multiple sclerosis. Am J Dance Ther 32(1):53–63. https://doi.org/10.1007/s10465-010-9087-x

Sedlmeier P, Weigelt O, Walther E (2011) Music is in the muscle: how embodied cognition may influence music preferences. Music Percept 28(3):297–306. https://doi.org/10.1525/mp.2011.28.3.297

Sheets-Johnstone M (2010) Why is movement therapeutic? Am J Dance Ther 32(1):2–15. https://doi.org/10.1007/s10465-009-9082-2

States RA, Spierer DK, Salem Y (2011) Long-term group exercise for people with Parkinson's disease: a feasibility study. J Neurol Phys Ther 35(3):122–128. https://doi.org/10.1097/NPT.0b013e31822a0026

ter Bogt TFM, Gabhainn SN, Simons-Morton BG, Ferreira M, Hublet A, Godeau E et al (2012) Dance is the new metal: adolescent music preferences and substance use across Europe. Subst Use Misuse 47(2):130–142. https://doi.org/10.3109/10826084.2012.637438

Thacker EL, Chen H, Patel AV, McCullough ML, Calle EE, Thun MJ et al (2008) Recreational physical activity and risk of Parkinson's disease. Mov Disord 23(1):69–74. https://doi.org/10.1002/mds.21772

Tomlinson CL, Patel S, Meek C, Herd CP, Clarke CE, Stowe R et al (2013) Physiotherapy versus placebo or no intervention in Parkinson's disease. Cochrane Database Syst Rev 2013(9):CD002817. https://doi.org/10.1002/14651858.CD002817.pub4

Verghese J, Lipton RB, Katz MJ, Hall CB, Derby CA, Kuslansky G et al (2003) Leisure activities and the risk of dementia in the elderly. N Engl J Med 348:2508–2516. https://doi.org/10.1056/NEJMoa022252

Veronese N, Maggi S, Schofield P, Stubbs B (2017) Dance movement therapy and falls prevention. Maturitas 102:1–5. https://doi.org/10.1016/j.maturitas.2017.05.004

Warburton EC (2022) TikTok challenge: dance education futures in the creator economy. Arts Educ Policy Rev:1–11. https://doi.org/10.1080/10632913.2022.2095068

Westheimer O, McRae C, Henchcliffe C, Fesharaki A, Glazman S, Ene H, Bodis-Wollner I (2015) Dance for PD: a preliminary investigation of effects on motor function and quality of life among persons with Parkinson's disease (PD). J Neural Transm (Vienna, Austria: 1996) 122(9):1263–1270. https://doi.org/10.1007/s00702-015-1380-x

Winkler I, Haden GP, Ladinig O, Sziller I, Honing H (2009) Newborn infants detect the beat in music. Proc Natl Acad Sci 106(7):2468–2471. https://doi.org/10.1073/pnas.0809035106

Zhang J-G, Ishikawa-Takata K, Yamazaki H, Morita T, Ohta T (2008) Postural stability and physical performance in social dancers. Gait Posture 27(4):697–701. https://doi.org/10.1016/j.gaitpost.2007.09.004

Zhao M, Veeranki SP, Magnussen CG, Xi B (2020) Recommended physical activity and all cause and cause specific mortality in US adults: prospective cohort study. BMJ:m2031. https://doi.org/10.1136/bmj.m2031

Part V

Musical Education and Well-Being

Health of the Child's Voice

22

Tadeus Nawka, Magnus Gaul, and Michael Fuchs

The voice function undergoes enormous development in childhood. Objective data for assessing the developmental status of the child's voice are rare. If children are already expected to meet higher vocal demands, certain performances are expected depending on their age, which so far have been derived mainly from the experiences of parents and educators, as well as voice trainers. Voice diagnostics in children and adolescents must be adapted to their age and developmental status. It can help to identify deviations from a harmonious, balanced, and safe development. The care of the child's voice has experienced various forms of expression in institutional settings and in leisure time, especially since the beginning of the twentieth century. Meanwhile, a singing culture can be demonstrated using a variety of successful models for solo and choir/class/ensemble singing, which promote the musical expression possibilities of children and make them aware of the richness of vocal training.

T. Nawka (✉)
Department of Audiology and Phoniatrics, Charité - Universitätsmedizin Berlin, Berlin, Germany
e-mail: Tadeus.nawka@charite.de

M. Gaul
Department of Music Education, University of Regensburg, Regensburg, Germany

M. Fuchs
Department of Phoniatrics and Audiology, University of Leipzig, Leipzig, Germany

G. Kreutz, G. Bernatzky (eds.), *Music and Medicine*, Neurocultural Health and Wellbeing, https://doi.org/10.1007/978-3-662-72175-9_22

22.1 Development of Vocal Performance and Quality

The first vocal performance is the newborn's cry. It is close to the frequency of 440 Hz, the concert pitch a', and is pure phonation, a vocal utterance that is not overlaid by the communication function of language and speech. Prerequisites are a normal breathing function for the generation of subglottic pressure and movable, vibration-capable vocal cords. Even if the voice sound when crying can be characterized by hoarseness (roughness and breathiness) as well as by a pressed voice production, the phonations can already be audibly distinguished from pathological inspiratory or expiratory breathing noises in the first few days of life. Already in the first weeks and months of life, melodic, tonal, and rhythmic elements develop, which initially express the infant's current emotions and needs and then increasingly differentiate into precursors of speech and singing (Wermke 2007).

22.1.1 Average Speaking Voice Pitch

The development of the average relaxed speaking voice pitch takes place before the voice change (mutation) in boys and girls alike. On average, the middle frequencies are between 220 Hz (a) and 262 Hz (c1) for boys and between 211 Hz (gis) and 281 Hz (cis1) for girls. There are no significant differences between the two genders, neither audibly nor statistically. As a result of the growing larynx and the associated vocal cord lengthening, the average speaking voice pitch of men moves between 104 Hz (GIS) and 147 Hz (d), women between 147 Hz (d) and 233 Hz (b) (Nawka et al. 2011).

22.1.2 Vocal Range, Dynamics, and Note Duration

Pitch range and dynamics increase with age. The extent of the increase is significantly influenced by socio-cultural and (vocal) pedagogicalfactors, which depend on regular vocal activity and voice training (Frank and Sparber 1970; Fuchs et al. 2009). Figure 22.1 shows the course of the lowest and highest tones for trained and untrained voices in boys and girls.

The measurement of dynamics and tone duration is most widespread in clinical practice. Normal value ranges for this can be found in the literature (Fuchs et al. 2008; Carding et al. 2006; Heylen et al. 1998). As a rough overview, the dynamic range can be considered to increase from about 25 dB in early childhood (4 years) to about 40 dB after the mutation. The tone duration increases from 10 s before to about 18 s after the mutation (Fuchs et al. 2008). For the pitch ranges, so-called normal voice fields (voice range profiles) exist. They are less suitable for representing age development, but are practical for diagnostics. Nevertheless, there are particular gaps in current knowledge about normal values for small children.

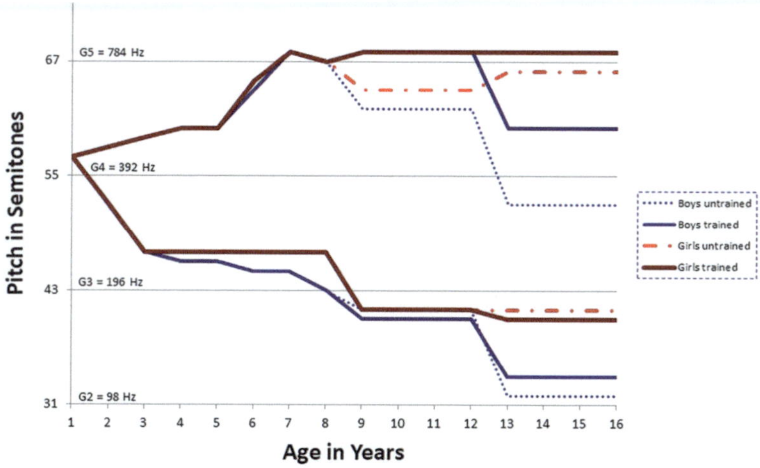

Fig. 22.1 Pitch range over the course of life in boys and girls, trained and untrained (Fuchs et al. 2007, 2008). Vocal ranges over the course of life. Starting from the reflexive newborn cry, which is around a[1] (A4 = 440 Hz), the speaking pitch gradually decreases during growth and is in the range between a (A3 = 220 Hz) and e[1] (E4 = 330 Hz) at the age of 9. Along with this, the vocal range expands to about 2 octaves. From about the 9th year of life, the voice development between girls and boys begins to differ. The ordinate shows the pitch in semitones (ST) above Subcontra C (C0 = 16 Hz, hearing threshold for the lowest perceivable frequency). The 31st ST corresponds to G (G2 = 98 Hz), followed by an octave higher the 43rd ST, g (G3 = 196 Hz), the 55th ST, g[1] (G4 = 392 Hz), and the 67th ST, g[2] (G5 = 784 Hz)

22.2 Course of Voice Development

Anatomical and histopathological knowledge is the necessary basis for clinical assessment. The vocal cord length is about 2.5–3.0 mm at the time of birth. During growth, the vocal cords become thinner and differentiate in their histological structure, forming the typical three-layer lamina propria. The development of the glottis and subglottis in the first 6 years of life has been described in detail on plastinated child larynges (Eckel et al. 2000). Since the growth of the voice apparatus does not occur at a constant speed, the individual voice development must be assessed according to the age of life. The phase of relatively slow, continuous development can be distinguished from those of rapid growth. Major organic changes in a short time occur in the first 2 years of life and during the voice change (mutation).

22.3 Normal Course of Voice Change

The voice change, the mutation, is a normal stage in the development of the child's voice. Before the voice change the voices of the boys can hardly be distinguished from those of the girls, but young men speak and sing significantly lower than women after the mutation. The differently strong growth of the larynx takes place with the general body development during puberty and is controlled by hormones. In boys, the increased production of androgens during puberty leads to a growth of the larynx. The thyroid cartilage plates protrude more and become visible as the Adam's apple. This also extends the vocal cords by about 1 cm. This increase in length and mass of the vocal cords is the cause of the deepening of the voice during puberty. In terms of progression, we distinguish between the pre-puberty phase (approx. 9–12 years of age), the actual puberty phase (approx. 12–16 years of age), and the post-puberty phase (approx. 16–18 years of age). During the actual puberty phase, the boy's voice drops by an octave. During this time, the voice can become hoarse and less efficient. A characteristic is also the disappearance of the head voice, with which boys can sing particularly intensely and powerfully just before the voice change.

The voice change usually begins around the age of 12 or 13; however, due to the general acceleration of development, but also due to ethnic characteristics, the first signs can already appear at the age of 9. While girls often do not notice their voice change, it becomes noticeable in boys through a hoarse and rough voice and through a lower resilience, which can sometimes be accompanied by an involuntary flipping of the voice from the modal register to the falsetto ("voice break"). On average, the voice change in boys lasts about 9 months and varies between 6 and 24 months. It should be completed by the age of 16 and not last longer than 2 years. During this developmental phase, the interaction between the growing structures of the larynx (muscles, mucous membrane, cartilage, control by nerves) and the other parts of the vocal apparatus (lung, resonance spaces of the throat and the head) must be constantly readjusted. Especially in boys' choirs, the children immediately before the voice change ("pre-puberty") stand out with a maximum vocal range for the child's voice and a beautiful voice. They also have a longer musical experience compared to their younger fellow singers.

At the end of puberty, the conditions stabilize, the new modal register strengthens, the falsetto register forms, and the resilience of the voice increases again. The young men must accept the new vocal range as part of their personality. In girls, the growth of the larynx is less pronounced and more continuous. The vocal cord length only increases by about 3–4 mm. The voice change sets in 1–2 years earlier, is much less noticeable, and is only rarely accompanied by a restriction of vocal performance. The average speaking voice, i.e., the pitch range in normal speech, drops by about a third. In adulthood, the vocal cords in women are between 11 and 15 mm, in men between 17 and 21 mm long (Cho et al. 2012). This is the reason why women sing in the high voice categories (soprano, mezzo-soprano, and alto) and men in the deep voice categories (tenor, baritone, and bass).

22.4 Diagnostics of the Vocal Apparatus

22.4.1 Laryngoscopy and Stroboscopy

Video laryngoscopy is mainly performed in newborns and toddlers with a flexible fiber endoscope with a diameter of 2.8–3.4 mm. When using flexible optics with a camera chip at the tip (chip-on-the-tip, Fig. 22.2), stroboscopic assessments are already possible in newborns. However, there are also good clinical experiences with rigid optics, where the tongue is not pulled out, but only slightly pressed down.

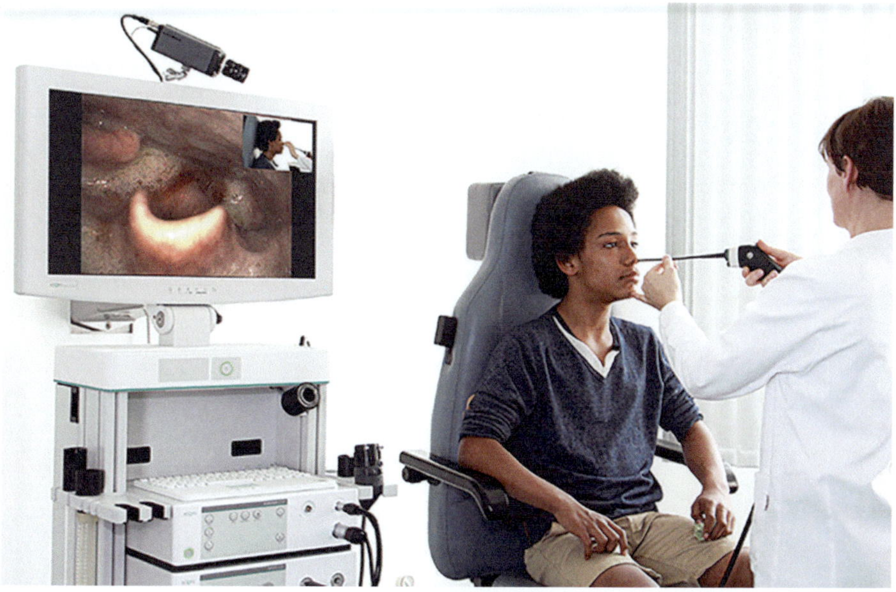

Fig. 22.2 Examination situation with a flexible videolaryngostroboscope and digital image processing

From about the 3rd year of life, the use of rigid optics predominates. In small children, the use of special pediatric optics with a shortened distance between the handle and the endoscope tip with a diameter of 7 mm has proven successful. Rigid optics with an even smaller diameter (4 mm) at not significantly larger image section than with flexible optics pose a higher risk of injury due to the narrow endoscope tip in case of defensive movements of the child. The camera systems for high-speed video recordings need optics with a heat protection attachment. These have the largest diameter (12 mm) and, according to clinical experience, due to the anatomical conditions in the oropharynx, they are tolerated from the 10th year of life at the earliest, usually from puberty.

22.4.2 Functional Diagnostics

In the diagnosis of vocal performance and quality, the auditory analysis of the voice is paramount in the first years of life. Initially, the parameters roughness, breathiness, and hoarseness, the average speaking voice pitch, and the voice production can be recorded and analyzed based on spontaneous vocal and linguistic expressions. From preschool age, additional parameters (effort, fatigue, instability) as well as the determination of the pitch range are added. Standardized, phonetically balanced texts should be used as soon as the child can read confidently. For the measurement of a speaking voice profile, the minimum voice intensity and two to three additional increase levels up to the maximum intensity are required. Experience

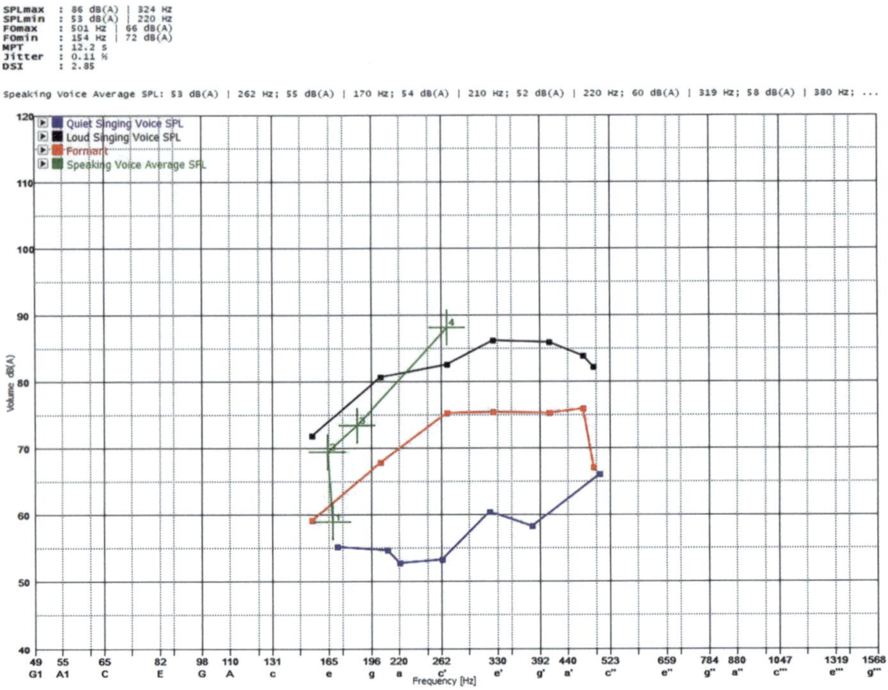

Fig. 22.3 Singing and speaking voice profile of a musically active boy at the beginning of mutation with noticeable limitations of the pitch range and dynamic range when singing, as well as a reduced ability to increase the speaking voice. The line marked with crosses shows the mean fundamental frequency of the speaking voice at different loudness levels: soft level, conversational level, raised lecture voice, calling voice. The relaxed average speaking pitch is still in the range of a boy's voice (165 Hz, E3, see the line with cross marks)

shows that children can do this from school age. For the measurement of singing voice profiles, the child must be able to sing given tones as quietly and as loudly as possible (Fig. 22.3). Singing active children can do this already in preschool age. In addition, the new generation of software for recording voice range profiles captures the fundamental frequency of sustained tones, even if they deviate from the frequency specification. The advantages of the singing voice profile and the simultaneous presentation of the findings of the speaking voice profile in the form of a diagram are that the current vocal performance can be quickly captured (Fig. 22.3). Current software also records every single tone sung during the measurement of the singing voice profile, so that acoustic analyses for explaining the respective vocal performance become possible. For the quantitative evaluation of the singing voice field, the Voice Range Profile Index for Children is also available (Heylen et al. 1998). In addition, numerous acoustic analysis methods are applicable for individual assessments of voice quality, which already work with vocal expressions of a few seconds duration (Fuchs et al. 2007). For the diagnosis of vocal performance and quality in children and adolescents, the auditory voice finding, as well as the speaking and singing voice profile, including acoustic analyses, are meaningful.

22.4.3 Supplementary Diagnostic Procedures

There is currently only limited experience with questionnaires, with which own vocal restrictions and their effects on the well-being and quality of life in children are examined. For this purpose, forms such as the pediatric Voice Handicap Index (Zur et al. 2007) are used. Standardized interviews have also proven to be effective, taking into account physical, functional, social, and emotional factors (Connor et al. 2008). Comprehensive concepts are available for psychosomatic diagnostics (Connor et al. 2008; Kollbrunner 2006). The doctor who is usually the first to confront a child's voice disorder—the specialist for speech, voice, and child hearing disorders or for ENT medicine—must know these etiological relationships and the corresponding methodology, including counseling and therapy. A cooperation with psychosomatically active. Indeed, colleagues must also be able to be on site. Diagnostic methods, in addition to anamnestic interviews, include special instruments for parental questioning, such as questionnaires on the topic of voice and family sociograms (Connor et al. 2008).

Practical Tip

In children and adolescents, as part of the clinical voice diagnostics, it should also be determined whether psychosomatic reasons or an unfavorable family dynamic situation could be responsible for the development of voice disorders. In this case, it is advisable to consult child and adolescent psychologists.

The representation of the vocal apparatus with imaging techniques (particularly CT and MRI) is only considered for organic causes of voice disorders and is then reserved for special questions regarding the narrowing of the airway and impending shortness of breath.

22.4.4 Clinical Assessment of Suitability for more Demanding Vocal Activities

Children who regularly sing in choirs, or as soloists or also take on speaking parts in the theater, have an increased vocal load. These girls and boys, especially during the voice change, require supervision by a singing teacher and voice doctor to avoid voice disorders that can arise from an overload during the growth phase of the larynx. Since the changes during the voice change do not occur abruptly and each child goes through their physical development at a different time, it is often a particular problem to recognize the beginning of the voice change in time and thus avoid singing too long "into the mutation."

If it is to be determined whether a child's vocal apparatus is suitable for an increased vocal load—for example, as a member of a children's and youth choir or for solo tasks in opera and theater—the above-mentioned diagnostic methods, taking into account the specified standard values, can provide a first assessment possible. If organic or functional limitations of the voice performance and quality are excluded, it should also be found out in a detailed anamnestic conversation whether the child brings the musical and psychosocial prerequisites for the vocal task. If the evaluator faces the problem that so far no vocal training and load have taken place, and therefore the effects of increased vocal load cannot be estimated, repeat examinations at 3- to 6-month intervals make sense. On this basis, the development of dynamics and training results can be assessed. Thus, an initially constitutionally "small voice" under a singing pedagogical training can experience a significant increase in vocal performance and quality and thus be better able to meet the increased vocal demands. On the other hand, a high vocal load without simultaneous voice training can lead to voice disorders if it chronically overtaxes the constitutional voice conditions of the child. For the assessment of vocal activity in clinical everyday life and for scientific investigations, the Leipzig working group has developed a classification that allows a reliably reproducible classification regardless of the evaluating professional group (doctors, voice trainers, choir directors, music teachers, laypeople) (Heylen et al. 1998; Table 22.1).

The previously determined normal value ranges can help to detect deviations from physiological development in time and to treat them (Fuchs et al. 2006). Voice disorders before adulthood are often left to run their course, especially when they are not pronounced and do not clearly worsen. The negative consequences of untreated voice disorders not only have an immediate impact in childhood and adolescence, but extend into adulthood. Functionally induced voice disorders deserve the same attention as organic ones. Diagnostic and therapeutic measures should definitely be age- and development-specific. With today's

Table 22.1 Classification of the singing activity of children and adolescents

Vocal strain			
A Only spontaneous, not in front of an audience	B Occasional organized singing and/or frequent singing in the family or occasional public singing	C Regular organized singing in concerts: average time of rehearsals/week + total time of concerts/year = up to 6 h	D Regular organized singing in concerts: average time of rehearsals/week + total time of concerts/year = more than 6 h
Vocal training			
	1 Not at all 2 In a large group (more than 3) 3 Individual singing lessons or in a small group (up to 3)		
Instrumental play			
Z Additional strain from playing a wind instrument with high pressure			

According to Fuchs et al. (2007)
The description is composed of the three categories voice load, voice training, and instrumental play together. A description can, for example, read: A (very low voice load), D3Z (highest voice load due to regular rehearsals and concert activity, with individual singing training and additional playing of a wind instrument with high blowing pressure, e.g., oboe, bassoon, trumpet)

endoscopes and microphones, digital recordings for precise diagnostics in early childhood are also possible on an outpatient basis. The endoscopic and acoustic findings can be precisely documented and compared. The voice only reaches its final expression after the completion of the post-mutation phase (for boys: 18th year of life; for girls: 16th year of life). Only then should professional singing training begin.

22.5 Voice Function Disorders in Childhood and Adolescence

The prevalence of voice disorders in children and adolescents is reported in the international literature to be between 6% and 24% (Zur et al. 2007). Voice disorders have an immediate relevance for young patients. They have a negative impact on their communication behavior and their self-esteem.

> Adults, as well as other children, and adolescents perceive the personality and physical factors of children with voice disorders more negatively than those of children without voice disorders.

Voice diagnostic criteria for adults cannot be directly applied to children and adolescents. The developmental stage and resulting norms must be taken into account. The wide range of variation in the frequency with which voice disorders are recorded corresponds to experiences in clinical practice: The hoarseness of a child or adolescent as a leading symptom of dysphonia is often not sufficiently perceived by parents or other caregivers, so that there is a long delay before a doctor is consulted. In a current and representative British study of 7389 8-year-olds, an atypical voice sound was diagnosed in 6%, which only 22% of the affected parents had noticed (Carding et al. 2006). Even in the context of medical examinations, hoarseness as an incidental finding is not always referred for further diagnostics by the relevant specialists for phoniatrics and paedaudiology or ENT medicine. Organic causes are possible and may require therapy. Apart from that, the voice disorder has further consequences for the affected child: Children with a pathological voice sound are judged more negatively by peers and adults than voice-healthy children. In addition, voice sound changes have emotional effects (sadness, anger, frustration) in 40–80% of children and impair social contacts (reduced vocal engagement in class and in leisure activities) (Connor et al. 2008). Medical care during voice development requires knowledge of the relationships between physical and vocal development, including the assessment of whether both are age-appropriate. Equally necessary is knowledge of socio-cultural and educational influences. Only then can the advice and support accurately assess whether it is a physiological process, whether there is suitability for increased vocal activity in the context of voice training or membership in choirs and theatre ensembles, or whether a dysphonia or dysodia in childhood and adolescence needs to be diagnosed and treated.

22.6 Typical Symptoms

Children and adolescents with voice disorders complain—like adults—typically about symptoms that can be assigned to three groups:

Changes in voice sound
Limitation of voice performance
Physical discomfort in the head/neck area

At a young age, instabilities of the fundamental frequency (involuntary change between the voice registers and diplophony) and open and closed nasalization are primarily observed as sound changes. In clinical everyday life, combined voice and speech disorders predominate, which are characterized as rhinophonolalia or palatophonolalia. Until about the age of 4, the sound changes are not perceived by the children themselves, but by the parents and other caregivers. Later, children are increasingly able to assess the sound of their own voice, its effect on other people, but also the peculiarities of the voice of other children and adults (Fuchs et al. 2009). Limitations of voice performance refer to the pitch range, the dynamic range, and the duration for which the child's voice can be used without complaints. The children can then, on the one hand, not speak or sing loudly or very loudly. This results in problems in communication situations with high noise levels in asserting their needs and their personality in the group. In the case of restrictions on the minimum intensity, on the other hand, the affected children are less able to speak and sing softly than voice-healthy children. Rapid vocal fatigue is evident in a significant deterioration in voice quality after a short voice load (loud speaking, voice-intensive leisure activities, singing) and in a prolonged recovery phase. Normally, the complaints disappear completely overnight. Due to these restrictions, the vocal and emotional expression possibilities ultimately become impoverished. In children and adolescents, discomfort, (burning) sore throats, feelings of exertion, the need to clear the throat, coughing, and the feeling of being out of breath dominate. Such voice-related complaints are reported by affected children from the age of 4 in 45–65% of cases, and in adolescents in about 25–40% of cases (Connor et al. 2008). The typical globus sensation is only complained about as the most common symptom in adulthood.

22.7 Disorders During the Voice Change

During the voice change, problems can occur for various reasons. On the one hand, the timing can be disturbed. The voice change occurs prematurely, late, or does not occur at all. On the other hand, the speaking voice pitch and the associated pitch range can decrease or drop too much compared to normal development. The result is abnormally high voices in men or unusually deep voices in women.

Mutational voice disorders occur in both girls and boys, but are much more common and noticeable in boys.

During the voice change, the entire larynx is undergoing profound remodeling and is in a performance-wise unstable state with limited resilience. Therefore, the mutation represents a critical period of voice development, especially in males. We refer to disorders in the physiological course of the mutation as mutational voice disorders (Fig. 22.4). Causes can be local, psychological, hormonal, and sensory. Local causes are primarily an incorrect muscle tone with disturbed interaction of the laryngeal muscles.

During the rapid growth of the larynx in the mutation, anomalies and asymmetries of the laryngeal framework can also develop. Psychological factors play a significant role, especially in the sensitive phase of puberty. If adolescents stubbornly cling to their child's voice, they fear—consciously or unconsciously—the transition to adulthood. This can be associated with a particularly strong attachment to the mother, rejection of the father, or emotional retardation.

The hormonal situation always needs to be clarified in the case of mutation disorders. If the physiological formation of sex hormones fails, the mutation with all morphological and functional manifestations does not occur. The larynx remains small and childlike, the voice high. The lack of testosterone can be due to illness. Since antiquity, but also in church and baroque music, there are castrato singers who kept their childlike voice through castration and the inevitable absence of mutation. The opposite is also possible, in the form of perverse mutation in girls: Their voice becomes deep due to exogenous androgen supply or pathological production of androgenic hormones in the adrenal cortex. The reasons for an incomplete mutation with only a slight drop in the speaking voice pitch with normal general sexual development and normal laryngeal growth are not always found.

Sensory factors are a co-cause in the development of mutational voice disorders. After the growth of the larynx, the new, deep voice must be audibly perceived, and the corresponding new phonation patterns must be practiced. In the absence of acoustic Feedback, e.g., in the case of hearing loss or amusia, this adjustment can make difficult. The mutation fistula voice, with which the childlike voice pitch is maintained by habitual fixation with a normally grown larynx, also belongs to this type of adjustment disorder.

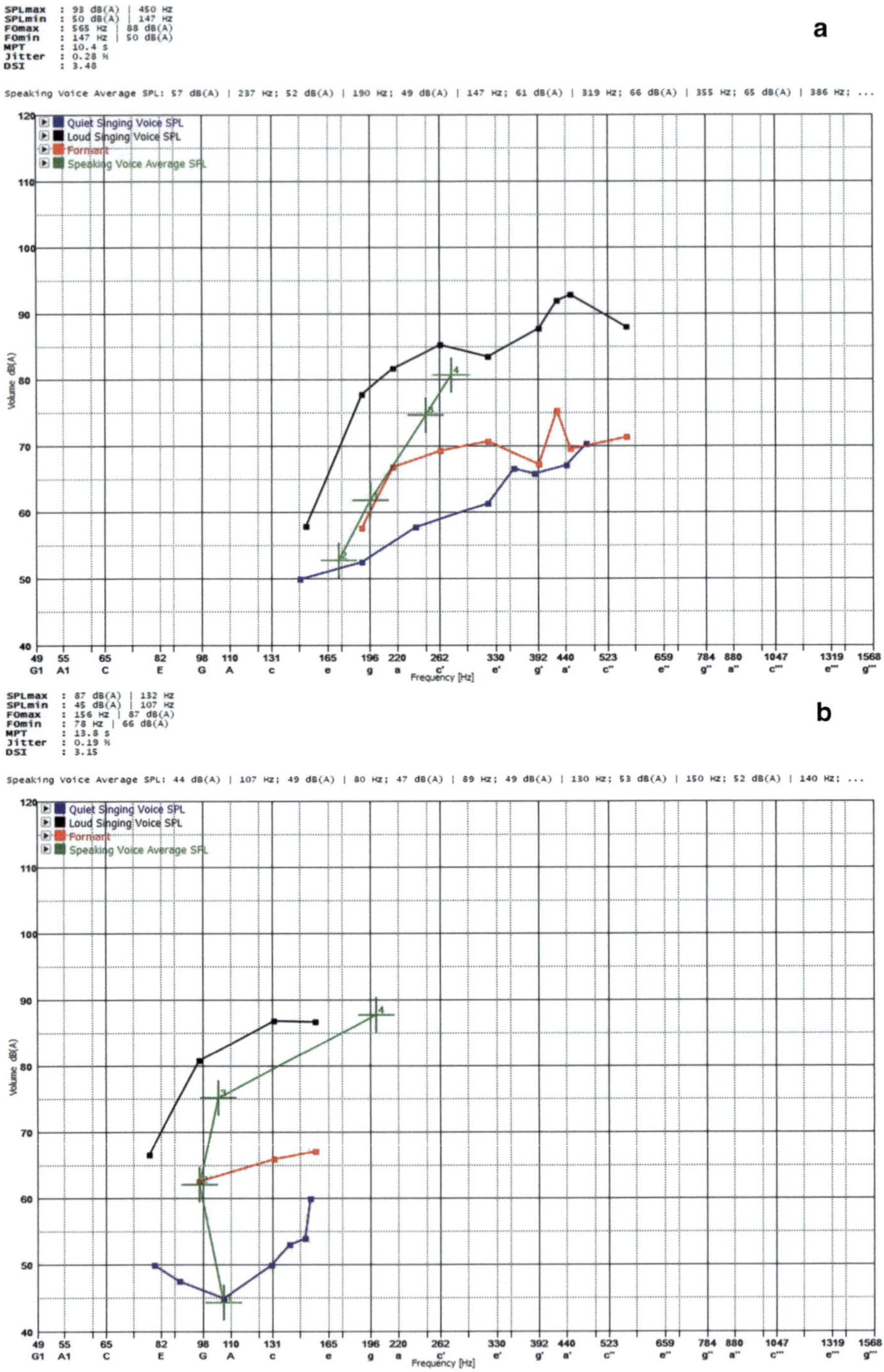

Fig. 22.4 (**a**, **b**) Mutational fistula voice in a 19-year-old; vocal range profile before (**a**) and after (**b**) Botox therapy of the cricothyroid muscle. The voice has dropped from the child's voice range to the modal range. The falsetto voice cannot yet be used

22.8 Vocal Fold Nodules

The most common question in children who use their voice musically and have voice function disorders is about vocal fold nodules. The prevalence of vocal fold nodules in school children was 16.9% in a study from Turkey, with boys being twice as likely to be affected as girls (Akif Kilic et al. 2004). Other studies show significantly lower frequencies (Dobres et al. 1990, cit. in Akif Kilic et al. 2004), namely 0.7% in a population of 18,000 children of a children's clinic, with the vocal fold nodules accounting for 17.5% of all pathological laryngeal findings. A general statement about the frequency cannot be made. However, the suspicion of vocal fold nodules can now be relatively well confirmed or ruled out by the phoniatrician or a relevantly experienced ENT doctor. A correlation between the size of the nodules and the severity of the voice function disorder was found and points to a causality (Nuss et al. 2010).

22.9 Therapy

Choir directors, voice trainers, and phoniatricians largely agree today that young singers should not actively participate in choir work (rehearsals, concerts) in the presence of vocal fold nodules and during mutation. However, individual voice training and a controlled singing effort are not excluded during the course of mutation with appropriate motivation. The duration of voice exercises should be 10–15 min and can be done two to three times a week. Primarily vocalises, i.e., sequences of tones following vowels, should be practiced, which do not reach the voice range limits and where the singer feels comfortable. Regular control by the phoniatrician is recommended. Speech therapy should also be tried for vocal cord nodules, although convincing studies on effectiveness are still lacking (Signorelli et al. 2011). The treatment of mutation voice disorders depends on the cause (e.g., disorders in hormone balance, psychological factors) and is primarily through a voice exercise therapy. If success is not achieved, there is the possibility of surgery to change the speaking voice pitch. However, such operations do not result in the voice meeting artistic requirements. In rare cases, hormone treatment is required.

> Even though malignancies are only the cause of voice disorders in exceptional cases in children and adolescents (Ohlms et al. 1994), endoscopic clarification is necessary for any hoarseness that lasts longer than 3 weeks, due to the more frequent other organic causes in this age group.

In case of lack of cooperation, and if the larynx cannot be adequately visualized videolaryngoscopically, an accurate diagnosis can only be made by examination under anesthesia. Direct laryngoscopy under anesthesia is possible from the newborn age and even in premature babies. The younger the child, the more intensive the preoperative cooperation between the surgeon and the anesthetists and pediatricians (neonatologists, pediatric intensive care physicians) must be prepared.

The surgical treatment of vocal fold nodules must be particularly carefully indicated. As a rule, until the completion of larynx growth and the differentiation of the vocal cords, surgical procedures to remove vocal fold nodules should not be performed due to the risk of permanent vocal restrictions due to scarring of the vulnerable tissue, and also ignoring the cause (Fig. 22.5).

In childhood, vocal fold nodules form due to overuse. This can be avoided by improving vocal technique or by reducing the strain. With voice rest, the nodules recede, only to reappear with renewed strain/overuse. Surgery suggests a cure that starts at the wrong end (Fig. 22.6).

On the other hand, it cannot be denied that in cases of severe hoarseness, improvement through surgery is possible (Mori 1999). However, clinical observations show that vocal fold nodules in children recur even with appropriate surgery and that

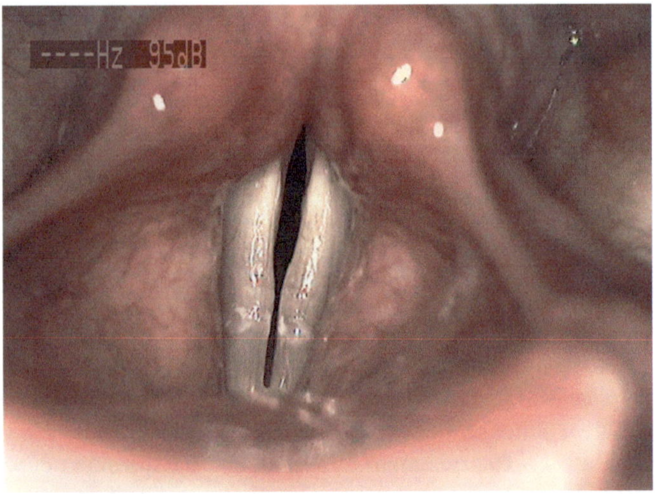

Fig. 22.5 A 13-year-old girl with flat thickening of the vocal fold margins and indications of a so-called hourglass glottis. The voice sounds breathy in the high range. Such minor findings should not be operated on

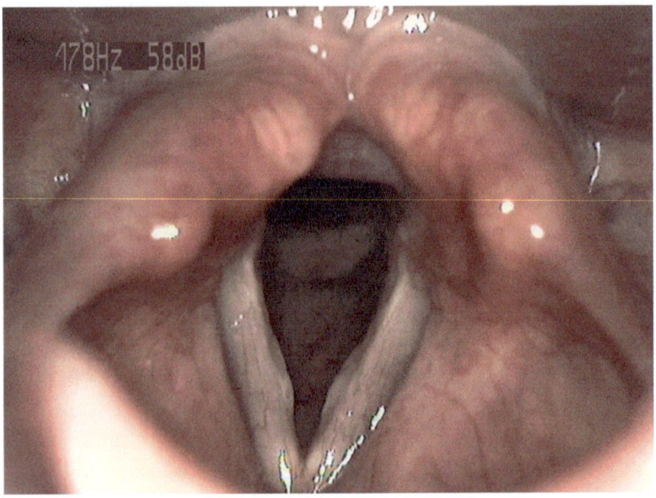

Fig. 22.6 Clear edematous thickening of the vocal fold margins, which can be considered advanced nodules. The vocal performance of the 9;2-year-old boy is limited, and the stronger the strain, the hoarser the voice becomes. Surgery is not recommended at this age

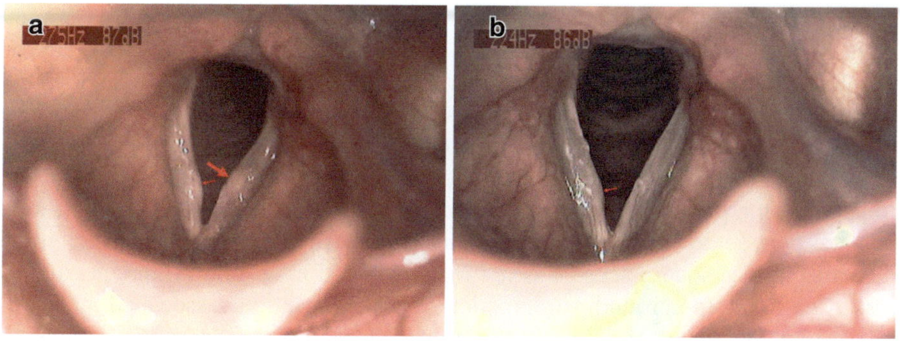

Fig. 22.7 (**a**, **b**) 12;7-year-old boy with left vocal fold cyst. (**a**) Condition before the operation. The finding is seen on the right in the picture and is marked by a thicker arrow. The thinner arrow points to a swelling of the right vocal fold, which has formed in response to the vocal fold cyst. (**b**) Condition 4 months after the operation. The cyst on the left vocal fold is no longer present. The swelling of the right vocal fold still exists. On this side, surgery should only be considered after the mutation

surgical therapy is not superior to conservative therapy in the long run. In contrast, surgical interventions on the vocal folds are indeed indicated in childhood for cysts (Fig. 22.7), juvenile larynx papillomas, or the rare tumor-suspected changes (Saha et al. 2013).

22.10 Vocal Didactics

The term "vocal didactics" in the context of the child's voice corresponds to the widely used term "instrumental didactics," which refers to the didactically guided handling of instruments in instrumental lessons (cf. also Mahlert 1997). "Vocal didactics"—used in this sense analogously as dealing with the "inherent" human instrument—goes far beyond the intentions of song didactics and includes different approaches for singing with small groups and (choir) classes, which opens up new forms of vocal music making, from vocal music to creatively developed vocussion. It deals with different introductions to vocal music making in dealing with the (child's) voice, such as the "warming-up," the initiation and implementation of voice training with child-friendly exercises, the preparation of the child's voice for more demanding literature and the implementation of a song elaboration through variative exercise forms and didactic aids.

22.11 Historical Roots

Singing is one of the most important forms of action in music education today and in the past. However, for a long time, it was neither cultivated as a personality building measure nor could one speak of a promoted vocal culture in adolescents. The cultivation of singing as a human "primal instrument" goes back far in its origins and is already attested among Indigenous peoples. The historical roots of a care for the child's voice, as well as the didactic embedding in music lessons and in the curricula of the different federal states, lie in singing lessons (sic!) in the nineteenth and twentieth centuries. This is to be terminologically distinguished from singing lessons, as the latter were given as individual soloistic training for talented child voices in parallel in a private or ecclesiastical context. The distinction can be found well into the twentieth century. However, in the history of the subject of music, vocal didactics in the modern sense was not intended for a long time. Although singing was often in the foreground, participation by students and the associated inclusion of songs were always possible. In the historical context, however, they primarily aimed to include mainly (song) texts in the lessons. This happened with both religious texts in the chorales and with political thought that was dressed in songs. Singing songs could thus be a guarantee for a "participatio actuosa" of the congregation in religious contexts or the adoption of Lutheran chorales in the design of church services.

On the other hand, singing songs with a political direction transported glorifying and obedient ideologies. In this context, many songs, at the latest during the time of National Socialism, lost their political innocence. Didactically, until well into the nineteenth century, there was no thought of a tonal-vocal competence of adolescents, and there was no sensitivity for it. Although children were only institutionalized together in primary school by a general compulsory education in the twentieth century, up to that point, the elementary school was primarily determined by the elementary methodology in the singing education theory according to Pestalozzi. The following textbooks are particularly worth mentioning:

J. M. Pfeiffer's and H. G. Nägeli's "Singing Education Theory according to Pestalozzian Principles" (1810)
J. T. Abs' "Presentation of my Application of the Pestalozzian Education Method" (1811)
B. Natorp's "Guide to Singing Instruction for Teachers in Elementary Schools" (1820)

Finally, the Stiehl's regulations (1854) are to be valued as important steps on the way to promoting (children's) voices and their training. In particular, the latter Prussian school laws were—embedded in the obligatory 9 hours of religious instruction per week—a guarantee for the cultivation of folk, fatherland, and church song singing. However, the institutional basis and the organizational framework for a structurally building care of the child's voice and proper training, which only a class formation could provide, were not yet given, because compulsory schooling was lacking.

The fact that people began to take a greater interest in the concerns of the child in the twentieth century is not least due to Ellen Key. Key advocated in her groundbreaking work published in 1902 for child-friendliness in Western industrial societies, for the prohibition of child labor, finally for compulsory schooling and thus at the same time for the realization of educational goals in an institutional structure.

The bourgeois constitution of the Weimar Republic prepared the federal legal basis for the introduction of a general compulsory primary school, which entered the new constitution in the Primary School Act of April 28, 1920. Thus, for the first time in German school history, the primary school was legally legitimized. Although this was an advantageous organizational framework for singing, at the beginning of the twentieth century, initially, the extracurricular amateur music making with the rediscovery and singing of traditional German folk songs in the youth music movement gave singing space.

Fritz Jöde (1887–1970) was one of the leading figures who attempted to create a "singing youth" and a "singing people" in his "open singing hours." Until the 1930s, the youth music movement was also characterized as a "singing movement" that included traditional instruments such as the recorder, zither, or mandolin. However, the care of the child's voice in singing lessons of those times cannot be compared with today's standards. Consequently, Leo Kestenberg also tried to improve the training of music teachers with his reform until the 1920s, as did Hermann Kretschmar (1848–1924). However, the war years prevented a continuous productive development of this type of school, also with regard to the inclusion of didactic models. Further approaches were therefore initially limited to abroad.

The lifelong learning process begins in early childhood, and singing in school institutions with homeland-related songs should be initiated early on, was adopted by the Hungarian music educator and ethnologist Zoltàn Kodály (1882–1967) as one of the first music educators in his efforts to research folk songs. Kodály compiled a remarkable collection of folk songs and researched the origins of his songs. He was the one who, based on solmization, further advanced the methodical teaching of songs and placed his understanding of tonality at the center of music education efforts.

In solmization, the pitch levels are represented and sung by syllables regardless of the key. A distinction is made between "relative" and "absolute" solmization.

Kodály's methodical suggestions, which he implemented after the Second World War together with his students in the state Hungarian school system, found widespread use, including in the USA, Canada, Asia, and Italy. The work on a song using the Ward method, which goes back to the American music educator Justine Bayard Ward (1879–1975), includes (relative) solmization and was originally developed for music lessons at Catholic elementary schools in America in cooperation with the Catholic University of America, Washington D.C., since the 1920s.

In Germany, the singing lessons of the pre-war years were continued as musical education after 1945. However, the songs collected in this process were rightly increasingly questioned (Abraham and Segler 1966). Carl Orff (1895–1982) and Gunild Keetmann (1904–1990) provided an important basis for creative interaction with the elements of music, language, and movement with their "Music for Children"

(1950–1954). In 1955, Leo Rinderer contributed valuable elements to ear and voice training in his course on "Holistic Teaching in School Singing" and also continued to use the Tonika-Do method. It was not until the end of the 1960s that the position of the primary school in the school system was consolidated and thus a secure institutional framework was provided for the carefully structured training of children's voices. Subsequently, there was a gradual interest in voice training (Nitsche 1969), and the productive work on the song continued. A new understanding of singing soon emerged that went far beyond musical promotion and led to new creative design possibilities.

22.12 Conceptual Design of Vocal Didactic Models

The primary school is the place that offers a home for targeted promotion of the child's voice, as all children, regardless of their cultural origin, social status, financial background, and musical socialization, are taught here, including music. The tradition of large children's and boys' choirs can demonstrate how children's voices can be specifically promoted and guided to remarkable successes on this path. (Brünner 1985; Schmidt-Gaden 1991). With a didactic emphasis on singing in recent teaching materials, it was vice versa taken into account that singing is no longer practiced in many parental homes. This alarming fact is a consistent development from the circumstances that bring about a new role for the family and a changed presence of reference persons in the parental home (Fölling-Albers 1989). Not insignificant is the fact that also in the educational programs of many kindergartens or daycare centers, a changed song selection can be registered, which does not in all cases take into account the promotion of the child's voice (Brünger 2003). An institutionalized promotion in the form of school offers and—above all—within the framework of private choir singing (e.g., in a school-organized all-day care, whose creative-musical possibilities are far from being exhausted) is therefore an indispensable demand on school practice, as only here can all children be reached equally. For the rehearsal of songs there are ways available that appeal to the students in different ways.

Basically, the work on a song should be clearly structured, varied and ideally contain appealing practice elements. As long as the rehearsal follows a basic pattern that always shows a same sequence in the rehearsal, this habit serves the receptiveness of the children. For the learning process transparent understandable and for the practice phases, firmly agreed signs and conventions of the guiding teacher or ensemble/choir director enrich the rehearsal and prevent misunderstandings. This includes that the instruction remains centrally related to the teacher, who can provide important aids to secure the melodies and can positively influence the course of the rehearsal with targeted measures. As long as the text lines are not overloaded with movements, a tracing of the melody with the associated kinesthetic interpretation is easily feasible for children. Creative ways of children's voice training are shown for example by Andreas Mohr (2013) and Robert Göstl (2006).

One way of song rehearsal can be the *sensory* guided learning, which is extremely effective, especially for children in pre- and primary school age. Since they are particularly responsive through seeing, hearing, touching, smelling, tasting, and movement, each musical sense section can be assigned a gesture or dramatic movement that helps the children to memorize the text and to identify with the song. For this "holistic" elaboration of songs, it is recommended to rehearse the melodies in direct contact and to follow them without song sheets, in order to have the hands free for the assigned movements. Even if the visual and auditory perception are primarily addressed within this methodical approach, the other senses are never completely excluded. Posture and possibly movements while singing can be announced and possibly corrected by the choir director in a semi-circle singing arrangement. In a song work that focuses on body movement and coordination, the vestibular sense (balance sense) is also addressed. Haptic learning is also addressed through tactile perception, where the "grasping," anticipating, and tracing of a melody can be done with the help of didactic aids, e.g., a scale rod (Gaul 2005).

Ideally, a variative work on a song addresses as many senses as possible. It shows a varied design, maintains concentration at the same time and is adequately comprehensible with the different learning types preferred already in childhood. The melody progression can finally also be fixed in writing with symbols on a board or on a sheet of paper, in order to be able to sing more extensive melodies with the corresponding texts. This understanding of working with children's voices is based on the realization that learning is easier when different senses are addressed than when cognitive addressing occurs too early (see also Fuchs 2007). Melodies can also be indicated by conducting signs, with freely invented or text-bound gestures, and finally by showing the pitch. A good aid for maintaining pauses and for timely progression of the melody can be to fill the pauses in the form of sound gestures, by using body instruments (body percussion) or simple percussion instruments.

22.13 Creative Forms of Singing in Everyday School Life

To bring the singing of children more into consciousness, since the 1990s, nationwide in music education individual singing (promotion) programs with specific emphases have been integrated, which are largely no longer school-structured, i.e., supported solely by the respective state government, but increasingly originate from public-law foundations and are transferred to school institutions. According to the federal system, these support programs are based on nationwide subsidies only in exceptional cases and, if they are successfully implemented in practice at all, are exclusively project-related. The largest proportion of the support programs remains limited to the respective local offshoots in individual federal states, but is accompanied by a flood of didactic-conceptual handouts on (choir) singing as a special form of class music-making (e.g., Kamphues 2011). For example, the development of a tonal-vocal competence in the project "Primacanta" (Frankfurt/Main), the model "Singing Classes" in Baden-Württemberg (Schnitzer 2011), the initiative "Choir Classes" (2005, Lower Saxony and Bavaria), and finally the Münster project

"JEKISS—Every Child His Voice," which sought to fundamentally link children's choir work and teacher training. In addition, "Canto elementar," the intergenerational singing project in cooperation with kindergartens in the city of Hamburg, "Choir: Class!," "Class-we sing," "SingPause" (North Rhine-Westphalia) are successful in the accentuation of the respective federal state. Creative ways to explore the voice can now also be found in open teaching formats, such as "Voice-Parcours" (von Blanckenburg and Gaul 2012).

The possibility of including new vocal voice qualities in the field of vocal percussion, rap, beatboxing, leads the children's voices already in childhood to also vocally creative register variants. The vocal facets can be extremely diverse in this area and are found in distribution already in elementary school age. Last but not least, choir singing was also discovered by the print media as a fruitful and profitable field of activity, a not-to-be-underestimated factor in music didactic work with children. In this context is also the initiative of the "Constructive Music Lessons" (Fuchs 2010; Jank et al. 2010), which recommends building steps also for song didactics in a firmly structured course. Due to sometimes missing musical-professional supervision in school practice or an unfavorable organizational framework of music education, as it was structurally given, for example, in the conception of an extended music education with extended teaching assignment (cf. also Weber et al. 1993; Gaul 2009), this variant will, however, not be fully realized in school practice—despite valuable content suggestions—but only in selected practice modules.

22.13.1 Relative Solmization

Solmization, in which the tones of a scale are designated with (singable) tone *syllables* instead of their original tone names, has a special significance in the consideration of the training of children's voices.

In its origins, solmization goes back to medieval (tone) aids in organum teaching from the eleventh century, which showed a way into early polyphony by means of a tone sign system. In consistent application, the significant music theorist Guido of Arezzo (around 991–1033), in his theoretical treatise "Micrologus de disciplina artis musicae" (1025), and with the help of his "Guidonian Hand," provided aids for the conception of tone-bound ideas in the hexachord system (ut, re, mi, fa, sol, la), which he systematically recorded for the first time. The symbols he used and the assignment of tones in the zones of a palm were initially intended as tone-bound visual aids for singing and as memory aids. Further important sources are the Milanese treatise "Ad organum faciendum" (around 1100) and the text "De musica cum tonario" by Johannes Affligemensis (after 1100).

The merit of this binding of tones to concrete symbols—especially in the explanations of Guido of Arrezzo—must be rated as invaluable from a music didactic point of view, as it already ensured early notation on lines and a tone progression according to symbols, but also a (early polyphonic) singing according to conduct. The fact that the set tone syllables referred in their pitch to the respective keynote, the term "relative solmization" was established (Fig. 22.8). If a modulation was present in the melody, a new reference tone was also determined.

Since the nineteenth century, solmization has experienced a revival and aimed at more effective teaching processes in school singing. Thus, with the music educator Sarah Anna Glover (1877–1970) and her "Norwich sol-fa," a manual that offered simplified melodic-rhythmic pointing aids for tone memorization, and with John Curwen's (1816–1880) "Tonic sol-fa," important representatives can initially be identified in the English-speaking world. They particularly developed solmization for school use and thus made it suitable for music didactic purposes. In Germany, the instruments were adopted by Agnes Hundoegger's (1858–1927) Tonic-Do-Method and by the Tone Word Method adapted by Carl Eitz (1848–1927) in 1892, which was used in schools until after the Second World War. The controversial music educator Richard Münnich (1877–1970), who played a major role in the Kesterberg reform, provided another approach with his JALE concept (1930), which sought to combine the Tonic-Do teaching and Eitz's "Tone Word" and was later used in music education in the GDR. The fact that solmization was still promoted in post-war Germany, but was increasingly abandoned in song didactics, may be a reason why those responsible were looking for a new beginning in music education and therefore neglected the increasingly complex tonal language of solmization. The current renaissance of singing in newer music didactic orientations now allows for a renewed

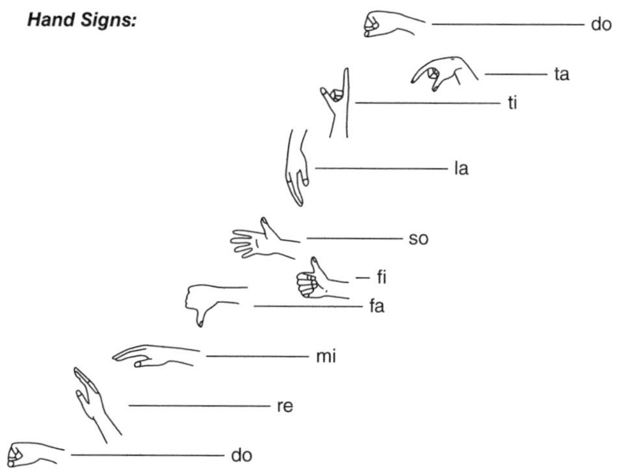

Fig. 22.8 Tonic Sol-fa method. (Kodály Concept, according to Szőnyi 1966; Losert 2011)

conceptual inclusion of solmization and a return to meaningful didactic measures in the training of the child's voice. The revived didactic representation of tones using functional syllables (do, re, mi, fa, so, la, ti, do) aims at a conscious tone conception, associated with an easier to learn "sight-singing,"recognizing tonal relationships and not least improved intonation.

Different manifestations can be registered in Europe, mainly in England and Italy. In the latter place, the Kodály student Roberto Goitre (1927–1980) achieved remarkable successes in the training of his "voci bianche," which are still noticeable to this day. He published his Cantar leggendo teaching method adapted for Italy in 1972, after extensive studies on prima-vista singing and the transfer of solmization into the ambitus of an octave (cf. also Goitre 1984). Solfège as a subfield of music theory includes, among other things, the tonal imagination with solmization syllables, in order to successively promote the note-bound sound imagination in the combination of ear training and singing. The originally United States-based *Ward Movement, which also includes relative solmization,* is today also internationally recognized in primary school and children's choir work and introduces children primarily through singing and the inclusion of their own bodies to musical experiences.

An enrichment for the didactic teaching of speech chants and songs also comes from the research-based findings of Edwin Gordon (*1927). His Music Learning Theory was developed in the 1970s. The audiation is based on the realization that hearing and the associated tonal imagination, so to speak the anticipation, are crucial as a starting point for music learning. The systematically building tonal and rhythmic pattern exercises provide a course that initiates a tonal and rhythmic competence and includes relative solmization as important support. The levels of distinguishing learning proposed by Gordon lead from hearing and responding to the verbal linkage to the symbol linkage in reading and writing of tones. To think music, Gordon sees the engagement with voice material and scores as meaningful only in the further course. On the basis of familiar content, children learn successively to unlock new melody building blocks and patterns. Anyone who plays an instrument knows how important it is to have the tonal imagination present before playing a melody. And so, according to Gordon's view, the children introduced to the principles of audiation can very effectively transfer their sound imagination—always starting from hearing and singing—to their instrument and to further musical literature.

> Neurobiological findings support the thesis that listening experiences are indispensable for understanding music.

The listening vocabulary developed by Gordon also proves to be a crucial help in introducing children to an intonation-safe interpretation of song melodies.

22.14 School-Structural Prerequisites

Currently, the media dissemination of different casting shows, which in the past were spread by television offers especially private media institutions (e.g., "Germany is looking for the superstar," since 2002; "The Voice of Germany," since 2011, etc.), or also the use of various karaoke games (e.g., "Singstar," since about 2004) in the effect on children and adolescents a noticeable motivation. The success of these entertainment formats is not least due to the fact that these are largely influenced by a mainstream orientation of popular music. However, the quality of the offers is in terms of the promotion of children's and youth voices strongly in doubt, since here stereotypical sound images are exposed and a transparent presentation of quality criteria for the training of a child's voice in terms of voice training and technique remains obscured. Nevertheless, a drive to sing caused by these media offers is still noticeable in school institutions. At its core, however, sustainable singing motivation, which is not only based on technical-media contact (cf. also Pilaj 2011), but even more strongly can be generated in direct encounter on an intrinsic path, requires fixed teaching principles and structures, such as those provided by the institution school or in the context of professional children's choir work. Examples here are not only the professional boys' choirs (Vienna Boys Choir, Leipzig Thomanerchor, Dresden Boys' Choir and Chapel Boys, Regensburg Cathedral Sparrows, Windsbach and Tölz Boys' Choir, etc.), but the structured development of a singing culture through regular singing in many primary school classes.

With the learning that builds from early childhood, the realization has matured in many educational institutions that singing, in addition to the use of the child's voice in a versatile repertoire of songs and the associated noticeable potential of school motivation, can be used in many didactic contents and contexts. This applies to learning in the subject of music per se as well as in other (interdisciplinary) areas, but also in social learning fields, in the area of German as a second language, or in learning a foreign language with the help of suitable songs (from the third grade). Although research in this area is deficient, music publishers often resort to the use of primarily English-speaking musical models. The inclusion of a media-conveyed repertoire of songs is already in vogue in kindergarten. Since many daycare centers are not yet distinguished by professionally trained staff who could prepare for guided singing in voice training and a meaningful design and singing technique, primary school time, which is uniformly provided for all school-age children as an entry level into the three-tier regular school system, offers ideal conditions for the training of the child's voice and a compensation for the missed opportunities in many parents' homes to train an expressive need in the form of singing. The fact that in most federal states, at best, two teaching hours per week are available for the subject of music often leaves little room for school vocal didactics, as all musical learning areas should be covered in the available time. A progressive course that aims at the correct singing, the professional transmission of meaningful voice physiological and didactic measures, also requires specialist teachers who have learned the tools in their university or college education that are indispensable for the training of children's voices.

The school conditions that shape the three-tier German school system in its offer and in the individual implementation at the school location quickly make it clear that the conceptual design of music lessons by the school authority will inevitably affect the possibilities of voice training in the school framework. While the concept of Extended Music Lessons, which was widespread in Bavaria since the 1970s and in Berlin among others since the 1990s, saw a diverse musical experience space, also for the child's voice, through an additional teaching assignment, elsewhere hour reductions in the subject of music at many primary schools nationwide contributed to the fact that the care of the child's voice no longer received the due attention in everyday school life. This was noticeable, for example, at schools where music lessons could not be given due to a lack of staff. Also structural changes, even if perhaps not initially intended, implicitly led to a reduction of the subject of music in the timetable, as in Baden-Württemberg since the school year 2004/05, where with the introduction of the educational standards for the subject combination "Human—Nature—Culture" (MeNuK) the aesthetic subjects were combined. MeNuK proved to be a fatal curricular experiment, as the musically used trial (time) spaces—also with regard to the care of the child's voice—in practice led to a significant subordination of musical experience spaces.

22.15 Outlook

The music didactician Georg Brünger hits the nail on the head:

> The universally noticeable post-Pisa activism offers opportunities. Even the very big ones are discovering the little ones. (Brünger 2003, p. 138)

approach to evoked. In fact, the didactic approach to children's voices, especially in recent times, has awakened particular scientific and didactic interest in singing in educational institutions and extracurricular music programs. Moreover, many teaching ideas are based on the realization that singing or music, especially in the context of special education, is often the only connection to the child (cf. also Adamek 1996). Singing thus presents itself not only as a rediscovered societal task but also as a (school) political challenge, which—due to the federal diversity—is met in the federal states with different project ideas. The current offers of initiatives for singing with children are remarkable. Many projects already start in primary school, as this is where all children are united for the first time due to compulsory schooling. However, this approach does not yet guarantee singing in the class, nor careful voice training for children or the conscientious introduction to the care of a culturally appealing song repertoire. Singing practice in schools and other educational institutions requires professionally trained teachers to avoid incorrect postures. Future vocal didactics will not be able to avoid training future educators, music teachers, and primary school educators, who—professionally trained and educated in vocal didactics—can enable music didactic and artistic work on children's voices nationwide due to their role as class teachers. The importance of singing, however, goes far beyond everyday school life and the personality-enhancing qualities of voice training for children. No less significant are the positively stimulating health aspects. As evidence for this, the fact that, according to medical findings, active singing can improve the quality of life of COPD patients (Lord et al. 2010), but also the fact that—in relation to the child's voice—the promotion of the singing voice is associated with qualities that can be clearly read from voice performance parameters (Gütay and Kreutz 2011). The call "Children need strong voices" (Kreutz and Gütay 2013) is therefore to be strongly resonated, especially in the environment of school education, as the structural conditions for the care of children's voices are particularly given here.

The models described, especially the relative solmization, can be a valuable didactic aid and initiate an introduction to the song. However, they primarily emphasize functional-technical aspects of singing. They are not a substitute for the careful didactic selection of suitable songs, the motivating and inspiring children's choir direction, a varied design of the song rehearsal, and the lasting effect of the presented models. These aspects can ideally have at least the same positive effect on voice position and intonation when working with children's voices. It is hoped that the school authorities will also take the creation of the necessary framework conditions seriously in order to give the care of the children's voice the appropriate importance. In choral and instructional work with children, this includes not only the development of an appealing song repertoire but also voice care in the form of voice training that enables children to appreciate their own body instrument and to understand it as an important medium for personal expression and personality development.

References

Abraham LU, Segler H (1966) Musik als Schulfach. Waisenhaus-Verlag, Braunschweig

Adamek K (1996) Singen als Lebenshilfe. Zu Empirie und Theorie von Alltagsbewältigung. Waxmann, Münster New York

Akif Kilic M, Okur E, Yildirim I, Guzelsoy S (2004) The prevalence of vocal fold nodules in school age children. Int J Pediatr Otorhinolaryngol 68:409–412

Brünger P (2003) Singen im Kindergarten. Eine Untersuchung unter bayerischen und niedersächsischen Kindergartenfachkräften. Wißner, Augsburg

Brünner R (1985) Gesangstechnik. Feuchtinger, Regensburg

Carding PN, Roulstone S, Northstone K, Team AS (2006) The prevalence of childhood dysphonia: a cross-sectional study. J Voice 20:623–630

Cho W, Hong J, Park H (2012) Real-time ultrasonographic assessment of true vocal fold length in professional singers. J Voice 26(819):e811–e816

Connor NP, Cohen SB, Theis SM, Thibeault SL, Heatley DG, Bless DM (2008) Attitudes of children with dysphonia. J Voice 22:197–209

Dobres R, Lee L, Stemple JC, Kummer AW, Kretschmer LW (1990) Description of laryngeal pathologies in children evaluated by otolaryngologists. J Speech Hear Disord 55:526–532

Eckel HE, Sprinzl GM, Sittel C, Koebke J, Damm M, Stennert E (2000) Zur Anatomie von Glottis und Subglottis beim kindlichen Kehlkopf. HNO 48:501–507

Fölling-Albers M (1989) Veränderte Kindheit—veränderte Grundschule. Novuprint, Hannover
Frank F, Sparber M (1970) Stimmumfänge bei Kindern aus neuer Sicht. Folia Phoniatr (Basel) 22:397–402
Fuchs M (ed) (2007) Singen und Lernen. Kinder-Jugendstimme. Logos, Berlin
Fuchs M (2010) Musik in der Grundschule neu denken—neu gestalten. Theorie und Praxis eines aufbauenden Musikunterrichts. Esslingen, Rum/Innsbruck
Fuchs M (2012) Stimmdiagnostik bei Kindern und Jugendlichen. In: Seidner W, Nawka T (Hrsg) Handreichungen zur Stimmdiagnostik. Xion, Berlin, S 201–214
Fuchs M, Heide S, Hentschel B, Gelbrich G, Makuch A, Thiel S, Taschner R, Dietz A (2006) Stimmleistungsparameter bei Kindern und Jugendlichen: Einfluss der körperlichen Entwicklung und der sängerischen Aktivität. HNO 54:971–980
Fuchs M, Froehlich M, Hentschel B, Stuermer IW, Kruse E, Knauft D (2007) Predicting mutational change in the speaking voice of boys. J Voice 21:169–178
Fuchs M, Meuret S, Geister D, Pfohl W, Thiel S, Dietz A, Gelbrich G (2008) Empirical criteria for establishing a classification of singing activity in children and adolescents. J Voice 22:649–657
Fuchs M, Meuret S, Thiel S, Taschner R, Dietz A, Gelbrich G (2009) Influence of singing activity, age, and sex on voice performance parameters, on subjects' perception and use of their voice in childhood and adolescence. J Voice 23:182–189
Gaul M (2005) Der Tonleiterstab—didaktische Hilfe oder Spielerei? In: Bäßler H (Hrsg) Aktiv hören—innovativ gestalten. Schott, Mainz, S 44–51
Gaul M (2006) Lied-Erarbeitung in der Grundschule—Lernen mit allen Sinnen. In: Grundschulmagazin. Oldenbourg, München 1:41–45
Gaul M (2009) Musikunterricht aus Schülersicht. Eine empirische Studie an Grundschulen. Schott, Mainz
Goitre R (1984) far musica è … Suvini Zerboni, Milano
Gordon E (1980) Learning sequences in music. Skill, content, and patterns. GIA-Publications, Chicago
Gordon E (1981) Wie Kinder Klänge als Musik wahrnehmen—eine Längsschnittuntersuchung zur musikalischen Begabung. Musikpädagogische Forschung, vol 2. In: Behne KE (Hrsg) Musikalische Sozialisation. Laaber-Verlag, Laaber, S 30–63
Gordon E, Bolton BM, Hicks WK, Taggart CC (1993) Experimental songs and chants without words. GIA, Chicago
Göstl R (2006) Singen mit Kindern. Modelle für eine persönlichkeitsbildende Kinderchorarbeit. ConBrio, Regensburg
Gruhn W (2003) Geschichte der Musikerziehung. Eine Kultur- und Sozialgeschichte vom Gesangunterricht der Aufklärungspädagogik zu ästhetisch-kultureller Bildung, 2. Aufl. Wolke, Hofheim
Gütay WG, Kreutz G (2011) Entwicklung der Singstimme von Kindern in Chorklassen: Eine medizinisch-physikalische Längsschnittuntersuchung von Stimmleistungsparametern. In: Schwarz B, Nenniger P, Jäger RS (Hrsg) Erziehungswissenschaftliche Forschung—nachhaltige Bildung. Verlag Empirische Pädagogik, Landau, S 461–468
Heylen L, Wuyts FL, Mertens F, De Bodt M, Pattyn J, Croux C, Van de Heyning PH (1998) Evaluation of the vocal performance of children using a voice range profile index. J Speech Lang Hear Res 41:232–238
Jank W et al (2010) Music step by step. Aufbauender Musikunterricht in der Sekundarstufe I. Helbling. Rum/Innsbruck, Esslingen
Kamphues J (2011) Mach mal: Stimmbildung. Zwiebelbook, Berlin
Key E (1902) Das Jahrhundert des Kindes. Fischer, Berlin
Kollbrunner J (2006) Funktionelle Dysphonien bei Kindern. Ein psycho- und familiendynamischer Therapieansatz. Schulz-Kirchner, Idastein
Kreutz G, Gütay W (2013) Kinder brauchen starke Stimmen. Zur Praxisrelevanz empirischer Forschung und Forschungsrelevanz gesanglicher Praxis. In: Fuchs M (Hrsg) Forschung, Wissen, Praxis. Logos, Berlin, S 131–140

Lord VM, Cave P, Hume VJ, Flude EJ, Evans A, Kelly JL, Polkey MI, Hopkinson NS (2010) Singing teaching as a therapy for chronic respiratory disease—a randomised controlled trial and qualitative evaluation. BMC Pulm Med 10:41. https://doi.org/10.1186/1471-2466-10-41

Losert M (2011) Die didaktische Konzeption der Tonika-Do-Methode. Geschichte—Erklärung—Methoden. Wißner, Augsburg

Mahlert U (ed) (1997) Spielen und Unterrichten. Grundlagen der Instrumentaldidaktik. Schott, Mainz

Mohr A (2013) Handbuch der Kinderstimmbildung. Schott, Mainz

Mori K (1999) Vocal fold nodules in children: preferable therapy. Int J Pediatr Otorhinolaryngol 49(Suppl 1):S303–S306

Nawka T, Belogradski D, Caffier P, Gross M, Martin A, Reinhardt A, Anders LC (2011) Automatische Bestimmung der mittleren Sprechstimmlage beim Vorlesen des Textes „Nordwind und Sonne". https://doi.org/10.3205/11dgpp35

Nienkerke-Springer A, McAllister A, Sundberg J (2005) Effects of family therapy on children's voices. J Voice 19:103–113

Nitsche P (1969) Die Pflege der Kinder- und Jugendstimme. Stimmbildung am Lied. Schott, Mainz

Nuss RC, Ward J, Huang L, Volk M, Woodnorth GH (2010) Correlation of vocal fold nodule size in children and perceptual assessment of voice quality. Ann Otol Rhinol Laryngol 119:651–655

Ohlms LA, McGill T, Healy GB (1994) Malignant laryngeal tumors in children: a 15-year experience with four patients. Ann Otol Rhinol Laryngol 103:686–692

Orff C, Keetmann G (1950–54) Musik für Kinder, vol 1–5. Schott, Mainz

Pilaj J (2011) Singen lernen mit dem Computer. Über Anwendungen und Nutzen neuer Feedbackmöglichkeiten in Stimmbildung und Gesang. Forum Musikpädagogik, vol 97. Wißner, Augsburg

Rinderer L (1955) Musikerziehung. Ganzheitlicher Unterricht im Schulgesang. Helbling, Innsbruck

Saha D, Sinha R, Pai RR, Kumar A, Chakraborti S (2013) Laryngeal cysts in infants and children—a pathologist's perspective (with review of literature). Int J Pediatr Otorhinolaryngol 77:1112–1117

Schmidt-Gaden G (1991) Wege der Stimmbildung für Kinder und Erwachsene. Hieber, München

Schnitzer R (2011) Singen ist klasse. Schott, Mainz

Signorelli ME, Madill CJ, McCabe P (2011) The management of vocal fold nodules in children: a national survey of speech-language pathologists. Int J Speech Lang Pathol 13:227–238

Szőnyi E (1966) Der Solfège-Unterricht in der Musikerziehung. In: Sándor F (Hrsg) Musikerziehung in Ungarn. Klett, Stuttgart, S 29–100

von Blanckenburg H, Gaul M (2012) „Stimm-Parcours"—Offene Unterrichtsformen als Beitrag zur Stimmerkundung und zum experimentell-entdeckenden Lernen. In: Gaul M, Lang S (Hrsg) Voice-Coaching. Zum richtigen Umgang mit der Stimme im Lehrberuf. Schneider, Baltmannsweiler, S 221–232

Weber EW, Spychiger M, Patry JL (1993) Musik macht Schule. Biografie und Ergebnisse eines Schulversuchs mit erweitertem Musikunterricht. Pädagogik in der Blauen Eule, vol 17. Die Blaue Eule, Essen

Wermke K (2007) Von einfachen zu komplexen Melodien: Über die frühesten Entwicklungsschritte auf dem Weg zur Sprache. In: Fuchs M (Hrsg) Singen und Lernen. Logos, Berlin, S 9–20

Zur KB, Cotton S, Kelchner L, Baker S, Weinrich B, Lee L (2007) Pediatric Voice Handicap Index (pVHI): a new tool for evaluating pediatric dysphonia. Int J Pediatr Otorhinolaryngol 71:77–82

The Singing Voice and Health

23

Bernhard Richter

23.1 Prosodic Elements

These "musical elements" of language are also described as prosody (from the Greek prosodía, "a singing in addition to or nearby") (Meyer-Kalkus 2001). They accompany us throughout our lives in speech, singing, and music, whereby science has still not conclusively been able to determine whether, in the process of evolution, it was speech or the singing voice that first developed (Fitch 2010). Prosody is significant for the division of speech through linguistic-articulatory phenomena such as accent, intonation, pauses, and the like. Every visitor to a modern railway station in Germany knows the "prosodic irritation" that arises when platform announcements are no longer directly spoken, but rather put together from unconnected preset pieces. Thus, it is not only important what someone expresses verbally or sings but also how it is said or sung.

23.2 Voice and Emotion

Through this "how," the voice has a direct link as an instrument of articulation to emotion. This connection is perhaps even more direct than that to cognition, as Darwin already articulated in the follow-up to the supposition already cited. He wrote "that when the voice is used under any strong emotion, it tends to assume, through the principle of association, a musical character" (Darwin 1872). The

B. Richter (✉)
Freiburg Institute for Musicians' Medicine, University of Music Freiburg, Medical Center and Faculty of Medicine – University of Freiburg, Freiburg Centre for Music Research and Teaching, Freiburg im Breisgau, Germany
e-mail: bernhard.richter@uniklinik-freiburg.de

G. Kreutz, G. Bernatzky (eds.), *Music and Medicine*, Neurocultural Health and Wellbeing, https://doi.org/10.1007/978-3-662-72175-9_23

ability to reach humans emotionally through the voice is comparatively universal, as is that attained by certain pieces of music. Thus, all over the world, Beethoven's setting to music of Schiller's "Ode to Joy" in the concluding chorus of the ninth Symphony is immediately understood as exhilarating, jubilant music, even if people do not know the German text or its meaning. A child's crying reaches us in a likewise direct manner, as does a whispered vow of love, emotionally, through the sound of the voice, regardless of language and cultural affiliation. The singing voice, too, can similarly be seen as a trans-cultural phenomenon: lullabies that are sung to calm children down all over the world, and the voices of famous singers from Enrico Caruso and Maria Callas to Luciano Pavarotti reach people's souls as directly as those of Frank Sinatra, Edith Piaf or Elvis Presley—this list could be added to almost infinitely.

23.3 Structure of the Voice as Instrument

The voice has three essential components: the breathing system, the larynx, and the resonating spaces in the vocal tract. Breathing provides a stream of air during voice generation. It is periodically divided into small air pulses by the opening and closing movements of the vocal folds, whose frequency per time determines the fundamental frequency of the sound. At the same time as the fundamental frequency, overtones always arise in the larynx, too. The primary larynx sound, which as a result is made up of the fundamental tone and its overtones, is then filtered acoustically in the resonance spaces above the vocal folds. In these resonance spaces, which basically include the throat and mouth, the sound of the voice and its projection are crucially shaped. The structure of the vocal apparatus in its broad outlines was already known in antiquity through descriptions of the legendary Greek doctor and researcher Galen (131–201 AD) and once again, in the Renaissance, through drawings created by the universal genius Leonardo da Vinci (1452–1519). However, it long remained unclear how notes and sounds are formed in the existing anatomical structures, i.e., how the voice is created.

23.4 Function of the Voice as Instrument

Physiological investigations in Paris in 1741 by Antoine Ferrein (1693–1769) brought about the breakthrough in our understanding of the physiology of the larynx. He described the larynx as an instrument that does not occur in music otherwise, which combines the characteristics of a string instrument with those of a wind instrument. He wrote: "I would like (…) to present a new instrument, which is equally unknown to anatomists and musicians. There are string instruments, such as the violin, the harpsichord; there are other instruments, the wind instruments, such as the flute or organ, but up to now we have not known of any instruments that are simultaneously string and wind instruments, such as the instrument that I have found inside the human body." (Ferrein 1741)

Even though Ferrein had not yet fully understood the mechanism of voice production, his perception that the voice is a unique instrument is most apt, as it is indeed incomparable in its variability with any other musical instrument with regard to the creation and formation of sound.

23.5 Capabilities of the Voice as Instrument

In its vocalizations regarding type, pitch, duration, volume, and color, the instrument that is the voice can produce a wide variety of sounds. The range of the voice is as broad as that of a modern concert grand piano (Richter et al. 2018b). The lowest notes of the oktavists of the Orthodox Church lie at A′ = 55 Hz, while the frequency of the lowest piano key corresponds to 27.5 Hz, meaning it is only one octave lower. In the pop song realm, frequencies are sung that lie in the area of the highest piano key, the C ′= 4186 Hz or above it. So, for example, the Australian singer Adam Lopez is able to reach a fundamental pitch of 4435 Hz. This corresponds to the note C sharp ′, which is thus even one semitone higher than the highest note on the piano. This circus-like ability earned him an entry in the Guinness Book of Records. The dynamic range of the voice is also remarkable: A soft pianissimo is already possible at 35 dB, while the fortissimo of dramatic opera singers reaches 115 dB. The human voice is thus capable of covering a dynamic range of some 80 dB. This wide range our voice possesses is something we use in our daily lives as a matter of course and unconsciously when we laugh, call, and bellow, when we whisper, sigh, and sob—but of course we can use it, too, for singing! In the case of sung vocalizations, one can distinguish between the singing voice, the voice of the untrained singer, and the singer's voice, the voice of a trained singer. Every person possesses a singing voice; it has been given to us as "basic equipment." Babies and infants employ their full vocal range when they scream—interestingly, they do not become hoarse in so doing, even when they let their voice be heard very loudly for hours on end. In general, singing does not damage the voice; on the contrary, it benefits it—even if one sings many hours a day.

Our voice is set up by nature to be constantly used every day—just as our musculoskeletal system is designed for daily walking and daily physical work. Yet just as training our body's muscles requires continuous use, so, too, does the human voice need to be constantly trained by means of constant use: anyone who just sits on the sofa and does not move cannot, as a rule, run the marathon; a person who never sings cannot perform at their best from this starting point. And in another analogy to sport, a sensible use of the voice without over-straining it is also advisable: if one bellows in an untrained, unwise manner, problems with the voice are inevitable.

23.6 Care and Cure of the Professional Voice

A professional singing voice has been artistically trained, which stands out from the mass of normal singing voices with regard to certain sound qualities. The training required to make a professional stage singer lasts many years as a rule. The necessity to train a voice over a long period applies not only to classical singing but also to popular music styles. For this reason, in recent years, educational institutions have arisen for nonclassical singers, too, such as the Institut für Musik, special area singing-musical/pop, at the Hochschule Osnabrück. A well-founded education is enhanced by the fact that young students are already trained in vocal physiology during their vocal studies (Richter et al. 2018a). Together with the vocal coach, one can then have a positive effect as a voice doctor on a singer's career plan, provided one has the appropriate skills and experience and is involved in the training process early enough and with trust on both sides. Professional singing is generally as unlikely to cause damage to the voice as a layperson singing. As with all activities frequently carried out, vocal problems can crop up time and again throughout a singer's career, which, as a rule, can be treated well. However, for the treatment to run positively, it is beneficial not to ignore problems and not to "sing one's way" through limitations of the voice. For this reason, it would be desirable if the voice doctor were also involved by the singer in the care of his voice, and not only in emergency cases, when the problems make singing impossible. For this reason, Bob Sataloff has proposed the term "care and cure" in connection with the professional singing voice (Sataloff 1991).

23.7 Reception and Use of the Voice

Throughout the world, singing is a central element both of social life and of medicine in the most varied cultures. This is the case for indigenous cultures that have not been completely swallowed up by mass civilization. But in highly developed countries, too, this cultural heritage has not disappeared yet. Thus, the choral tradition is vibrant in Scandinavia and in the Baltic states, as shown by the Estonian choral festival that takes place in Tallinn every 5 years, in which broad segments of the population take part with great commitment. Interestingly, the Estonian, Latvian, and Lithuanian singing and dancing festivals were recognized by UNESCO as intangible cultural heritage and accepted on the list of masterpieces of oral and intangible heritage of mankind. Here, too, great social willingness can still be found in the Nordic countries to promote singing in choirs and music schools across the board. Choral singing also has similar significance in Barcelona, where the amateur choir Orfeó Català is even today one of the key pillars of Catalan culture. For all the enthusiasm and affirmation of this vocal tradition, it should, however, be noted that in these countries, singing is often closely linked to questions of national identity and assertiveness, too. Following the atrocities of the Nazis, this national identity was called into question in Germany—and quite rightly so. Thus, the traditional, highly developed singing culture in Germany also came under scrutiny. Naturally, a critical discussion of the role of singing in the "mass hypnosis" of the Nazi period is both necessary and meaningful (Richter and Spahn 2018). As a counter-reaction to the manipulative and suggestive effect of public singing in the Nazi period, the singing tradition in German was not only discontinued, but it was even opposed. The consequence of this counter-movement to stop singing was, however, from today's perspective, a knee-jerk reaction with far-reaching, ill-considered negative side-effects. We can now say that in this case, cause and effect were confused: it was not singing that led to totalitarianism, but rather it was exploited by that system. Essentially, when nurturing the voice, the concern is with the abilities of the individual, not with the ideological indoctrination of a "mass." From a modern viewpoint, we can promote singing without conjuring up the specter of totalitarianism or fascism. We are certainly not alone at this moment in our demand for singing and music to be more tightly woven into our daily lives as part of our cultural preservation. In Switzerland, the promotion of musical education was taken up in Article 67a of the constitution in 2012 with an overwhelming majority of 72.7% of the votes cast in a referendum. Thus, music, along with sport, is the only school subject with its own article in the constitution. In Germany, too, there are numerous initiatives, such as the foundation "Singing with Children" in Baden-Württemberg or "Singing makes Sense" (»Singen macht Sinn« SMS) and "An Instrument for Every Child" (»Jedem Kind ein Instrument« JeKi) in North Rhine-Westphalia, which attempt to remedy the lack of vocal and musical training. The new appreciation for singing is shown in the way the German National Prize of 2012, under the patronage of the Federal President and honorary chairmanship of Helmut Schmidt, was awarded to the cross-generational initiative "Canto elementar." While such initiatives are sometimes laborious and require great patience, we should not be discouraged. We should remind ourselves that the human voice has long held a prominent place in the collective consciousness of our culture: assigned a preternatural quality, through it there existed a direct link to the divine world, as powerfully shown by the Orpheus myth. One possible reason for this assignation may have been to do with the singing voice being seen by primordial ancestors as a decisive factor in the formation of group identity. This power to bind possessed by the voice can be assumed to hold not only for the Stone Age, but it can be experienced close up today in any football stadium in the songs sung by fans.

23.8 The Voice in the Context of Individual and Social Health

According to the World Health Organization definition, health is "a state of complete physical, mental and social well-being and not merely the absence of disease or infirmity." In this context, a vital role in the creation of mental and social well-being can be played by a healthily functioning voice. The function of the speaking voice is crucial for carrying out a wide range of occupations in a modern, communication-based society. These jobs are described as vocally intensive. Included among such occupations are those of the teacher, the educator, the call-center employee, cashiers in post offices and banks, doctors, pastors, and in particular singers and actors. In these lines of work, there can be observed at present a considerable number of vocal restrictions and limitations. For example, a high percentage of teachers exhibit disorders of the voice. Regarding this, data can be found in the literature whereby around one half of teachers are affected (van Houtte et al. 2012; Nusseck et al. 2020). In this situation, the singing voice could help in promoting and training the abilities naturally present in every individual's voice. Fortunately, the instrument that is the voice is not irreparably damaged in terms of anatomy or physiology, but rather remains insufficiently nurtured and trained in its ability to unfold vocally by society in general. Our concern, therefore, is not with a defective instrument, rather with a form of behavioral archaeology, the cultural practice of which has in part been lost. As musicians, we can be encouraged by looking at the parallels to historically informed performance practice. After decades of practical experimentation, some musicians now play on the old instruments as well as—or presumably even better than—the "old" musicians, and some singers have re-perfected the eighteenth-century practice of ornamentation. The social changes described are hence in no way irrevocable, but can rather be rectified in the future.

23.9 Singing: Positive Health Aspects

A further positive factor in music and especially in singing is that culture in general and singing in particular carry with them demonstrable positive health aspects for the individual. Thus, it has long been known that people who frequently partake in cultural events show a higher life expectancy than those who are not active culturally (Bygren et al. 1996). Moreover, the working group around Gunter Kreutz was already able to show more than a decade ago that the power of resistance in the immune system is increased among those who partake in singing (Kreutz et al. 2004). Moreover, active singing leads directly to increased distribution of "happiness hormones," the endorphins (Biegl 2006; McDonald et al. 2012). For this reason, singing can be understood as a "staple food," as well (Richter et al. 2018b).

23.10 Conclusion

Every person is predisposed from birth on to a healthy functioning of the voice. Singing, as can be observed the world over, is one of the essential functions of communication and conveying feeling. Caring for the human voice is—similar to body care and regular physical exercise, and healthy nutrition—an important social and individual task. The general conditions for this should be improved again.

References

Biegl T (2006) Singen macht glücklich. In: Spahn C (Hrsg) Musik und Emotion. Tagungsreader der Jahrestagung von der Dt. Gesell. für Musikpsychologie. Burger, Freiburg, S 12–14

Bygren LO, Konlaan BB, Johansson SE (1996) Attendance at cultural events, reading books or periodicals, and making music or singing in a choir as determinants for survival: Swedish interview survey of living conditions. Br Med J 313(7072):1577–1580

Darwin CR (1872) The expression of the emotions in man and animals. John Murray, London

Ferrein A (1741) De la formation de la voix de l'homme. Histoire de l'academy royale des sciences de l'année 1741. p 409–432; http://gallica.bnf.fr. Archives de l'Académie des Sciences

Fitch WT (2010) The evolution of language. Cambridge University Press, Cambridge

Kreutz G, Bongard S, Rohrmann S, Hodapp V, Grebe D (2004) Effects of choir singing or listening on secretory immunoglobulin A, cortisol, and emotional state. J Behav Med 27:623–635

McDonald R, Kreutz G, Mitchell L (2012) Music, health and wellbeing. Oxford University Press, Oxford

Meyer-Kalkus R (2001) Stimme und Sprechkünste im 20. Jahrhundert. Akademieverlag, Berlin

Nusseck M, Spahn C, Echternach M, Immerz A, Richter B (2020) Vocal health, voice self-concept and quality of life in German school teachers. J Voice 34(3):488.e29–488.e39. https://doi.org/10.1016/j.jvoice.2018.11.008

Richter B, Spahn C (2018) Die Stimme in der Lebenszeitperspektive. In: Richter B (Hrsg) Die Stimme, 3. Aufl. Henschel, Leipzig, S 181–196

Richter B, Mürbe D, Schmid B, Sandel M (2018a) Stimmphysiologie in der Ausbildung von Sängern und Schauspielern. In: Richter B (Hrsg) Die Stimme, 3. Aufl. Henschel, Leipzig, S 144–160

Richter B, Schmid B, Sandel M, Weinhausen S (2018b) Stimmarten, Stimmgattungen, Stimmfächer. In: Richter B (Hrsg) Die Stimme, 2. Aufl. Henschel, Leipzig, S 91–131

Sataloff RT (1991) Professional voice: the science and art of clinical care. Plural Publishing Inc, New York

van Houtte E, Claeys S, Wuyts F, van Lierde K (2012) Voice disorders in teachers: occupational risk factors and psycho-emotional factors. Logoped Phoniatr Vocol 37(3):107–116

Making Music and Emotion Regulation in Children

24

Ingo Roden, Emily Frankenberg, Gunter Kreutz, and Stephan Bongard

Summary Even in ancient times, the Greeks believed that music had an emotionally positive and liberating effect on the human psyche. The musical processes in humans were divided into two categories: On the one hand, music was supposed to serve to imitate events in the real world in mimesis. On the other hand, it is supposed to purify the psyche through catharsis (a term later described by Sigmund Freud) based on emotional experiences while listening to music (Juslin and Sloboda 2001). Even today, It is widely believed that music can positively influence well-being, regulate emotions, and have a socially integrative effect. However, despite all the impressive examples from everyday life that prove the emotional power of music, the foundations of the emotional effects of music are rather poorly researched (Jäncke 2009). In particular, comparatively little scientific research has been conducted on the effects of playing music on instruments compared with listening to music. This limitation also applies to the emotional effects of music on children, which are better understood

I. Roden (✉)
Institute of Education, Carl von Ossietzky University of Oldenburg, Oldenburg, Germany
e-mail: ingo.roden@uol.de

E. Frankenberg
Differential Psychology & Psychological Diagnostics, Goethe University, Frankfurt am Main, Germany

Department of Neuropediatrics, Goethe University Hospital, Frankfurt am Main, Germany

G. Kreutz
Systematic Musicology, Carl von Ossietzky University Oldenburg, Oldenburg, Lower Saxony, Germany
e-mail: gunter.kreutz@uol.de

S. Bongard
Differential Psychology & Psychological Diagnostics, Goethe University, Frankfurt am Main, Germany
e-mail: bongard@psych.uni-frankfurt.de

G. Kreutz, G. Bernatzky (eds.), *Music and Medicine*, Neurocultural Health and Wellbeing, https://doi.org/10.1007/978-3-662-72175-9_24

when listening to music and less understood when creating music. Engaging with Music is one of the cultural achievements that begin to develop even before birth (Winkler et al. 2009). Furthermore, musical development in the early years of life is shaped by the musical culture of the respective environment (Gerry et al. 2012). This provides infants and toddlers with an extensive repertoire of implicit musical knowledge (Trehub 2003). This means that almost all children of primary school age can learn musical instruments. However, little is known about the effects of music on children's emotions and emotion regulation, as research in this area has been conducted almost exclusively with adults and adolescents. Accordingly, we will begin the presentation of children's musical emotions with results from studies involving adults and adolescents. First, however, we briefly outline the development of musical abilities, guided by the question of the extent to which the musical emotions of children resemble or differ from those of adults and adolescents.

24.1 Emotions and Emotion Regulation

To date, there is no agreement on what can and cannot be understood by the term "emotion" (Cole et al. 2004). According to Keltner and Shiota (2003), emotion is a universal functional reaction to a stimulus or change in stimulus. The construct of emotion must be distinguished from mood. Compared with emotions, moods can be described as more global, less intense, diffuse, and longer lasting. They often exhibit systematic fluctuations that persist throughout the day. In contrast to emotions, mood triggers are usually unconscious (Deckers 2009). On the other hand, emotions can be differentiated into five operationalizable emotion components that adapt to new conditions in the event of a change in the stimulus (Keltner and Shiota 2003). The affective emotion component is the subjective experience of the emotion itselves. It contains sensations and perceptions of feelings caused by a confrontation with a stimulus or stimulus change. These factors strongly depend on an individual's previous experiences and expectations. The expressive emotion component is the interpersonal, non-verbal communication of an emotion. This occurs through facial expressions, gestures, postures, and voice colouring. The motivational component states that emotions are characterised by typical behavioural tendencies aimed at improving or avoiding emotional states. The physiological emotion component is part of the centrally and continuously controlled physical activation processes that ensure that the individual acts in accordance with the emotion and manifests itself, for example, in changes in heart rate, blood pressure, and skin conductivity. The cognitive emotion component includes the influence of emotions on information processing. Emotions can cause slight changes (such as a distorted perception of a situation). Still, they can also cause more severe impairments in adequate information processing (e.g. selective access to memories and misjudgement of future situations) (Sokolowski 2007).

Emotional regulation describes the adaptation and control of different emotional components in a respective situation. Gratz and Roemer (2004) define emotion regulation as an adaptive reaction to emotions. Successful emotion regulation enables individuals to show an appropriate reaction to a situation and to have control over their behaviour, even under stress. An important prerequisite for the effective regulation of emotions is the ability to feel and differentiate the entire range of emotions. Gross and Muñoz (1995) distinguish between these two types of regulation mechanisms: antecedent-focused emotion regulation and response-focused emotion regulation.

24.1.1 Antecedent-Focused Emotion Regulation

Antecedent-focused emotion regulation is aimed at changing the situation and appraising the situation. It also involves emotion-avoiding actions that take place before an emotion is implemented. According to Gross and Thompson (2007) there are four different preceding emotion regulation strategies:

- Situation selection (situations in which desired emotions can arise or undesired emotions cannot)
- Situation modification (changing the situation towards the desired emotional reaction)
- Directing attention (e.g. turning the focus of attention away from the emotion-triggering object, especially if the situation is unavoidable or unchangeable)
- Cognitive change (change in the assessment of the significance or coping possibilities for the situation)

24.1.2 Reaction-Focused Emotion Regulation

Emotion regulation begins later in the process of emotion generation. It changes and controls the prevailing reactions on the various emotional levels in the desired direction. Gross and Thompson (2007) categorise reaction-focused emotion regulation as the strategy of reaction modulation. The physiological, subjective and behavioural reactions are directly reduced or suppressed by medication, sporting activity or relaxation, for example.

Coping—that is, coping with stress—is a construct related to emotion regulation; however, it serves only to regulate negative emotions (Gross and Thompson 2007). Although emotion regulation involves coping with negative emotions, it is not limited to this aspect. Although there is currently no consensus on the different types of coping strategies and their measurement (Eschenbeck et al. 2007), coping mechanisms are often used within two conceptual frameworks: They are either categorised into problem- versus emotion-focused coping (Lazarus and Folkman 1984) or assigned to the dimensions of approach- versus avoidance-oriented coping (Krohne 1993; Roth and Cohen 1986). Both approaches overlap strongly; problem-focused coping, such as approach-focused coping, involves direct strategies to actively resolve a situation. In contrast, emotion-focused coping and avoidance consist mainly of more passive, indirect coping strategies that concentrate on adapting to the stressor, for example, by avoiding it or alleviating the negative emotion (Eschenbeck et al. 2007). There is no consensus on which individual strategies are beneficial or harmful to the human psyche. In general, however, passive coping is seen as a rather unfavourable behaviour, whereas active coping is considered more beneficial to health. For example, it is widely accepted that adolescents who exhibit avoidant coping behaviours are more likely to suffer from mental health problems than adolescents with active coping behaviours (Ebata and Moos 1991; Herman-Stahl et al. 1995).

Children's coping with stress is usually made up of strategies from both approaches and includes certain recurring mechanisms (Eschenbeck et al. 2007):

- Problem-solving (active; includes both approach-focused and problem-focused coping)
- Searching for social support (active, instrumental, passive, and emotional)
- Avoidance (passive, emotional avoidance, and activity-related avoidance)
- Distraction (passive) and emotion-focused stress management (passive)

One emotion regulation strategy repeatedly used in many studies is the use of music and musical activities to control or induce emotions. The following section presents these findings in detail.

24.2 Music and Emotions

The human ability to perceive emotions in speech melodies is formed at an early stage of development. Schubert and McPherson (2006) found that even infants could interpret the emotional content of their caregivers' auditory expressions. For example, infants favour the so-called nursemaid language (Papoušek 1992) compared with normal speech, which is characterised by greater fluctuations in pitch, a slower rate of speech, and an emphasis on individual words (Trehub and Nakata 2001).

In addition, infants prefer happy to unhappy utterances (Nawrot 2003). The ability to perceive and express emotions in music develops during childhood. By the age of three, children are already able to correctly categorise musically conveyed emotions. 3-year-olds can distinguish between sad and happy music (Kastner and Crowder 1990). This ability continues to increase until the age of 6. For example, 4 to 6-year-olds can correctly identify musically presented emotions such as happiness, anger, and fear (Cunningham and Sterling 1988; Dolgin and Adelson 1990). According to Adachi and Trehub (1998), 4-year-olds can express emotions such as sadness and happiness when singing by manipulating pitch, dynamics, and tempo.

Based on these findings, it can be assumed that children have developed skills in recognising and expressing musical emotions from the time they enter primary school, similar to adults and adolescents. Therefore, it can be assumed that the findings obtained in studies with adults or adolescents are largely transferable to the musical emotions of children of primary school age. Nevertheless, the development of children's musical emotions may differ from that of adults because of the greater dynamics of cognitive and emotional developmental processes during childhood.

Consequently, research on musical-emotional developmental processes in childhood remains a significant area of study.

24.3 Regulation of Emotions Through Music

24.3.1 Children

The development of emotion regulation in children is a dynamic process that occurs within a social context, through interactions with others and in response to environmental situations. In the early stages of life, emotional regulation encompasses both regulation by and of others (extrinsic) as well as regulation by oneself (intrinsic) (Nigg, 2017; Moor, Burbach, and Hanson-Abromeit, 2025). It has been repeatedly reported in the literature that parents use music to influence their children's emotion. (Saarikallio 2009). According to Tafuri and Villa (2002), maternal singing alone can cause babies to stop crying, calm, and focus their attention on their mothers' voices. Shenfield et al. (2003) showed that maternal singing regulates cortisol balance in six-month-old infants.

Saliva samples showed a slight increase in cortisol levels for infants with below-average levels. In contrast, infants with above-average levels showed a slight decrease. Thus, maternal singing appears to have either an activating or a relaxing emotion-regulating effect on infants.

However, limited research has been conducted on how children use music to regulate their emotions. In a study conducted with parents, Saarikallio (2009) found four main functions of music perception in 3- to 8-year-old children.

Calming down ("calming down"): Parents reported that children use music to help them calm down and to relax, e.g. when going to sleep.

Concentrated interest: Children listen to music to distract themselves from restlessness and boredom. Concentration and interest in an activity.

Happy energy: Children reinforce or express happiness and positive energy by listening to music. Parents perceive their children as happy and full of energy when listening to music.

Fantasy imagery: The emotions and stories conveyed in music are experienced intensively by children; they are absorbed in the music.

Saarikallio's (2009, 2016) emotion regulation strategies found in children show some similarities to the emotion regulation strategies of adolescents and adults. Children appear to use fundamentally similar but not the same emotion regulation strategies. For example, children are more averse to listening to sad music than adolescents and adults (Saarikallio and Erkkilä 2007). However, children use music just as much as adults (DeNora 1999) and adolescents (Saarikallio and Erkkilä 2007) to calm down and relax.

Children, as well as adults and adolescents, also seem to use music to increase their ability to concentrate. According to Saarikallio and Erkkilä (2007), adolescents use music to concentrate on thinking (mental work) and specific tasks (DeNora, 1999). Both strategies share the aspect of concentration with children's focused interest, even though the concentration processes reported at different ages are qualitative and show differences. For example, young people report using music to reflect on and categorise their emotions, while adults use it primarily to focus on unpleasant activities. Moreover, children often playfully listen to music.

Similar to teenagers and adults, children reinforce or evoke happiness and positive emotions through music. Thus, all age groups appeared to use music to evoke positive emotions. However, the extent to which music is used across all age groups to reduce or express negative emotions remains unclear. Kreutz and Litta (2003) analysed a sample of 57 9–10-year-old primary school children and found that preferences for fast music were associated with high levels of aggression in some children. In contrast, children who danced regularly showed comparatively less aggressive attitudes compared to children who did not dance regularly. The authors hypothesised that movement in response to music could reduce primary school children's willingness to become aggressive.

The strong imaginative activity that children experience while listening to music is certainly age-sensitive, as is the strong self-definition of young people through music. Both phenomena are unlikely to be observed to this extent in other stages of life. Nevertheless, children's imaginative activities can be remotely compared with those reported by adolescents (Saarikallio and Erkkilä 2007). Even if a clear qualitative difference is assumed in the fantasy activities of adolescents and children, both age groups described how they used music to remove their thoughts and ideas from real situations and instead move into a purely mental world.

In addition to the perceptive effects of music on children's emotion regulation strategies, recent studies have pointed to the positive development of self-regulation skills through music-making in children. For example, experimental studies on prosocial behaviour through music-making have shown that music can convey synchronisation experiences through rhythmic games, instrumental playing, and singing, and thereby promoting different facets of prosocial behaviour such as helpfulness, cooperation, empathy, commitment, as well as a sense of community and identification with a group (Barrett and Bond 2015). Roden et al. (2016) investigated whether children who received extended instrumental music lessons responded to a provocation task with significantly fewer reactive-aggressive behaviour than children who attended extended science lessons. We also investigated whether the children differed in their psychological, cardiovascular, and neurohumoral stress reactions to provocation for aggressive behaviour. The children in both groups were tested individually at two points in time, approximately 18 months apart, with no differences in sex, educational level, school social behaviour, or social skills and children's migration background, as well as parents' income and level of education. The results showed different patterns of reactive-aggressive behaviour between the two groups over 18 months.

Children in the extended instrumental lessons did not show any significant changes in this measure after the first month. In contrast, an increase was observed among children in the extended science lessons. The authors concluded that the results showed that children in the extended instrumental lessons remained stable in their coping strategies. In contrast, children in the extended science lessons showed less ability to resist aggressive behaviour. However, no positive effects on the physiological (systolic and diastolic blood pressure, heart rate, and salivary cortisol) or psychological reactions of the children were observed.

Further studies also point to the positive development of self-regulation skills through music-making in children with an increased risk of poverty. For example, Brown et al. (2022) investigated the effects of early childhood music interventions on the development of self-regulation skills. In a quasi-experimental design, 191 children aged 3–5 years who experienced economic difficulties were observed. The results showed that children who participated in a music intervention showed greater gains in emotional self-control over the entire preschool year than children of the same age. In several studies, Williams and Berthelsen (2019) investigated a coordinated rhythm and movement program to promote the self-regulation skills of children from disadvantaged communities ("Rhythm and Movement for Self-Regulation; RAMSR"). The intervention was based on neuroscientific findings regarding beat synchronisation, rhythmic movements, music therapy, and music education. The RAMSR programme was tested (2019) on 113 preschool children aged 4–5 years from socioeconomically disadvantaged communities. Trained professionals delivered the programme daily in preschools for 8 weeks. The results were promising; the children who took part in the programme showed significant improvements in emotional regulation, cognitive, and behavioural self-regulation skills, as observed by the teachers. Similar results can also be found in a study, in which 213 children from eight preschools in disadvantaged communities participated. The intervention group received between 16 and 20 sessions of a rhythm and movement program over 8 weeks, while the control group completed the usual preschool programme. Initially, the children from both groups showed significant issues with self-regulation in comparison to the established norms. However, positive effects on emotional and behavioural regulation were only reported for children in the intervention group.

24.3.2 Young People

Adolescents appear to use music intensively as an emotion regulation strategy. Accordingly, this age group has often been investigated in previous studies (e.g. Christenson and Roberts 1998; Lacourse et al. 2001; North et al. 2000; Roe 1985; Ruud 1997; Saarikallio and Erkkilä 2007; Schwarz and Fouts 2003; Sloboda and O'Neill 2001; Wells and Hakanen 1991). For example, two studies will be described in more detail here, which investigated musical emotion regulation in adolescents using both qualitative and quantitative methodological approaches. North et al. (2000) conducted a quantitative study of 2465 9th-grade students between the ages of 13 and 14 years on the importance of music. They asked pupils about their musical activities using a self-constructed ten-stage questionnaire and differentiated between listening to and making music. Based on a factor analysis, the authors found three main reasons for young people's perceptions of music:

- External image ("creating external impression"; music as an expression of one's self, e.g. to appear cool or trendy)
- Fulfilment of emotional needs ("fulfilling emotional needs"; music as a help in difficult times and to reduce stress)
- Pleasure ("enjoyment"; enjoyment of music, distraction from boredom)

Similar factors could also be found in the reasons young people gave for making music.

The regulation of emotions could thus be extracted as an independent factor for listening to music and playing musical instruments, which clearly indicates the importance of musical emotion regulation in adolescents. However, the need to fulfil the demands of authorities such as teachers and parents also seems to play a role in music-making, which is an important point to consider in further research into musical emotions. Although listening to music and making music are similar in many respects, it can be assumed that making music has a greater emotional impact. This is particularly the case in relation to the fear of public performances, insofar as the need to fulfil expectations has been shown to represent an additional stressor for young musicians. Depending on the degree of severity, this has the potential to have a negative effect on their attitude towards music and their use of music as an emotion regulation strategy. Moreover, emotion regulation is influenced by temperament and attachment style, which have a protective or risk-prone function for the development of adaptive ER skills, especially in childhood (Moore, Burbach, and Hanson-Abromeit 2025).

Saarikallio and Erkkilä (2007) provided a model for musical mood regulation in adolescents. It was based on a qualitative study which used interviews and a music diary to ask eight Finnish adolescents about their musical activities. Even if this model represents the regulation of mood rather than emotion, it can be assumed that the correlations reported below are transferable to the emotion-regulatory area. It should be noted at the outset that even though this model speaks of a choice of regulation strategies, the adolescents chose music and musical self-regulation intuitively and needs-oriented and not, as one might wrongly assume, consciously and goal-oriented. The model, therefore, describes the intuitive dual patterns reported by young people that underlie this process. Figure 24.1 shows a model of musical mood regulation that we revised.

The current mood and the corresponding mood-regulating needs and aspirations mood-regulatory needs and goals influence the selection of a regulation strategy. The main goals of musical mood regulation identified by Saarikallio and Erkkilä (2007) are "mood control" and "feeling good". The authors were able to identify six regulatory strategies used by young people for musical self-regulation.

- Entertainment (Using music to entertain oneself, create an atmosphere, and feel positive emotions)
- Recreation (use of musical activities for relaxation)
- Strong feelings (experiencing and expressing strong emotional experiences and being absorbed by music)

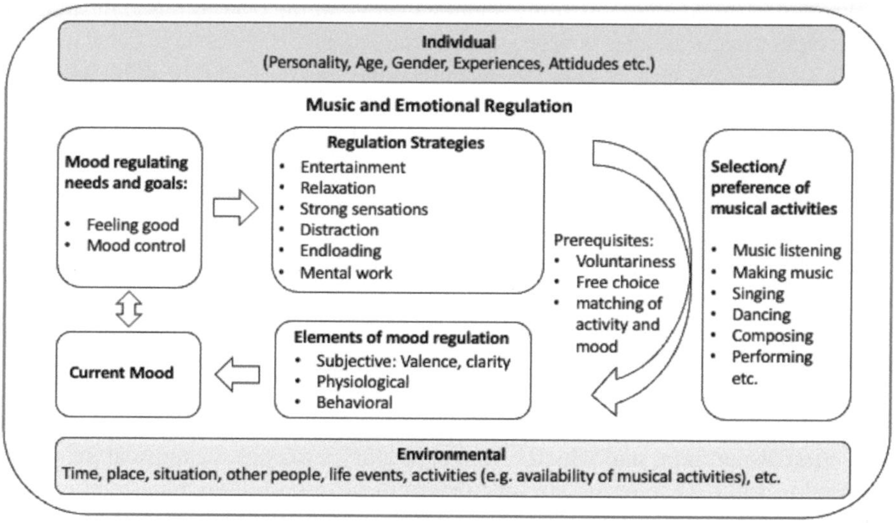

Fig. 24.1 Model of musical mood and emotion regulation

- Distraction (distract yourself from negative emotions, calm down, and lift your mood)
- Discharge (expressing negative emotions and acting them out through music, e.g. to avoid acting aggressively)
- Mental work (thinking about music, letting thoughts and images drift, thus clearing your head and working through inner conflicts)

Musical activities selected or favoured by young people for mood regulation cover a wide range of areas, such as listening to music or playing music themselves, performing, singing, writing songs, and dancing. Voluntary participation and personal choice, for example, regarding the type of music or volume, as well as the fit between music and the current mood, are prerequisites for using musical activity to regulate mood in the first place. The interplay between musical activity and regulative strategies influences three elements of subjective experience:

Valence: By reducing negative feelings and increasing positive feelings, musical activity has a strong influence on affective valence–that is, on the value young people assign to a mood or emotion.

Intensity: Music regulates the intensity of a young person's current emotional state. Music usually intensifies the perception of one's current mood.

Clarity: Musical activity also influences the clarity of emotional perception. The areas influenced by mood regulation are not limited to subjective-affective experiences. Other areas that are influenced by musical activities are subjective-physiological (such as the increase in energy levels through music and goose bumps) and behavioural (such as the expression of feelings through music). If changes in mood elements bring about a change in the overall mood desired by the regulation strategy, a new mood need can emerge. If necessary, a new regulation strategy can be activated. For example, once the desired relaxation has been achieved and a young person has recovered from a stressful school day, they switch their musical self-regulation to a musical activity that encourages them to engage in sports or meet friends. In the revision of the model, mood was assigned a position integrated into musical-emotional (whereas in the original model, it was only one of many internal variables), as we wanted to illustrate the reciprocal effects of mood and emotion regulation through music.

The regulatory process is subject to influences from both internal and external variables. In the original model, external and internal variables only influenced mood regulatory needs and processes. This model has been extended to influence the entire regulatory process. What mood is felt, which needs and goals of emotion regulation are present, and which of the regulatory strategies or musical activities are used to fulfil these needs are thus determined by both individual internal and external variables. Individual variables are, for example, the gender, age, or personality of the adolescent, as well as their attitudes and experiences towards the current situation. For example, introversion/extroversion or anxiety can be decisive for emotional needs in a situation, a chosen regulatory strategy, and musical activities. Age and sex can also influence what an individual perceives as appropriate.

In addition, environmental variables (such as the situation, the people involved, or the environment) influence the person as a whole and their mental processes and, therefore, the entire musical regulatory process. Whether a person is alone in a room, with whom they are, and the availability of musical activities such as instruments, music systems, or MP3 players can, for example, determine how they feel, which strategy, and which musical activity they use to regulate their mood.

To summarise, these two studies point to important and elementary functions of musical activities for emotion regulation in adolescents. Although these studies used different methodological approaches, they nevertheless revealed important key points for further investigation of musical emotions. For example, in studies on adults, the involvement of emotions through music and the reduction of stress were found to be the reasons for musical emotion regulation. Mood enhancement appears to be the core function of music perception and activity. Even if some regulation strategies, such as self-expression (North et al. 2000) or mental processing of situations and problems (Saarikallio and Erkkilä 2007), are less likely to be used in childhood, it is possible that other previously reported emotion regulation mechanisms, such as mood enhancement through music, are also used by children. When considering music-making as an emotion regulation mechanism, in view of the findings of North et al. (2000), it also seems important to consider the effect of other people (especially authority figures) on the development of musical emotions. Music appears to function as a reaction- and emotion-focused mechanism and is, therefore, as with adults, likelier to be classified as a passive emotion regulation strategy.

Overall, children appear to use musical emotion regulation strategies that are comparable to those used by adolescents and adults. Therefore, the consistency of these strategies across the lifespan can be assumed, even if age-typical variations in the use of music can also be decoupled. Above all, the experience, expression, and intensification of positive emotions are observed in all three age groups and, therefore, form a core element of musical emotion regulation. Therefore, it can be assumed that music has a positive emotional effect on children. Further studies investigating the emotional impact and significance of music in children's lives are desirable and will hopefully provide further insight. The emotion regulation strategies reported here are, as with adolescents, both reaction- and emotion-focused (calming down), but they also show antecedent-focused regulation mechanisms (concentrated interest). To obtain further information on the emotional effects of music, in addition to studies on musical emotion regulation, studies on the reducing and intensifying effects of music on negative emotions are presented below. Owing to the limited number of studies, the results were supplemented, as before, by studies with adult subjects.

24.4 Music and Negative Emotions

24.4.1 Reducing Stress, Anxiety, and Pain Through Music

Studies on reducing anxiety and pain through music are not directly concerned with emotion regulation. Because musical activities can reduce negative emotions and feelings, these studies can be categorised as music-related emotion regulation.

McDonald et al. (2003) showed that listening to self-selected music after surgery had an anxiety-relieving effect on patients. However, this was only observed in patients who underwent minor surgeries. This effect was not observed in patients who were about to undergo major surgery. Therefore, it is possible that above a certain level of stress (here, in the sense of pain), music no longer has any effect and is, therefore, particularly suitable for regulating low to medium levels of stress. According to Anderson et al. (1991), it can be assumed that listening to familiar music creates a sense of control over the situation. However, it has been suggested that music's ability to regulate emotions is ineffective in cases of severe stress (McDonald et al. 2003). Therefore, stress could be explained by the fact that the feeling of control and coping ability is no longer reinforced by listening to music once a situation becomes aversive enough. At the outset, the situation was assessed to be completely uncontrollable. Although this limits the effectiveness of musical stress management, it is consistent with the effectiveness of music as a stress management strategy.

Physiological correlates of the emotional effects of music have also been widely reported. Bartlett (1996) found in a review article entitled "Physiological responses to music and sound stimuli" that over half of the studies were able to demonstrate the effect of music on various parameters of the autonomic nervous system. For example, the heart rate and muscle tension increased with stimulating music, whereas these values correspondingly decreased with calming music. Kreutz et al. (2004) found an advantage of active musical activity (singing together) over listening to music without singing. In a study on amateur choir singers, active singing led to an increase in positive and negative feelings (measured by the Positive and Negative Affect Schedule, PANAS). The concentration of immune defence-promoting protein (IgA) in the saliva also increases. In this study, listening to choral ginger reduced the concentration of cortisol in saliva but also increased negative affectivity. The authors attributed this to the possible boredom experienced by the test subjects during the hour-long music performances. Thus, musical activity—in this case, singing—seems to show stronger involvement and, hence, emotion-regulatory superiority over passive listening to music. Therefore, it can be assumed that active music-making and a moderate level of activation due to situational factors can produce the best emotional-musical effects in adults. Psychological and physiological improvements have also been shown in children by listening to music and playing musical instruments. For example, Longhi and Pickett (2008) found a significant improvement in blood oxygen saturation in 21 chronically ill children and adolescents (aged 3 months to 14 years) who played music, regardless of age or sex. In a study of 101 children aged 10–12 years, Ho et al. (2011) reported significant improvements in clinical variables (e.g. depression, anxiety, and attention disorders) through daily drumming at school. However, drumming was accompanied by the uplifting of sentences or social rules, which is why these results cannot be clearly attributed to the effects of music. In contrast to the other studies reported in this paragraph, this study is based on a control group design.

Other studies investigating the effect of music therapy on children in hospitals have found a positive emotional impact on paediatric cancer patients (Barrera et al. 2002; Robb 2000). Barrera et al. (2002) studied 65 children and adolescents aged between 6 months and 17 years with a cancer diagnosis. In the music therapy programme, music was produced and listened to in an age-appropriate manner using both instruments and singing. Their parents assessed the well-being of children under the age of 3 on a rating scale, while all participants over the age of 3 assessed it themselves. The well-being of children and adolescents increased significantly before and after music therapy. The play and activity behaviours assessed by parents improved significantly during music therapy in preschool children and adolescents. However, this effect was not observed in children of primary school age, so the authors cannot provide a plausible explanation. However, qualitative analyses of the interviews with parents, children, and adolescents indicated that music therapy had a positive effect on all children and adolescents. A study by Robb (2000) reached similar conclusions and showed a positive effect of music therapy on the behaviours of ten children diagnosed with cancer. Based on video recordings of children in various situations, a significant increase in active behaviour was observed during music therapy compared to other hospital situations.

Malone (1996) concluded that music is an effective non-pharmacological method for reducing pain and stress in children. In support of this, Kenelly (2000) deduced that music attracts and influences children, distracting them from their physical problems and reducing their perception of pain and anxiety, and can, therefore, have a supportive influence. Despite the fact that music therapy is utilised in equal measure with children, adolescents, and adults in inpatient settings, the focus of treatment in outpatient music therapy is unmistakably on working with children. According to Plahl (2009), music is particularly well suited for providing therapeutic support for children whose development is hampered by disorders, illnesses, or disabilities.

Studies on stress, anxiety, and pain reduction, as well as the effects of music therapy, indicate a positive clinical effect of music as an emotion regulation mechanism in adults and children. Methodologically, however, it should be critically noted that of the studies with children, only one study (Ho et al. 2011) had a control group design. This methodological shortcoming limited the significance of our results. In the future, this aspect should be taken into account in the study design, especially as existing studies provide good indications of the effectiveness of music as an emotion regulation strategy.

Interim conclusion: Music appears to be an effective way of coping with negative emotions and physical sensations and achieving emotional balance, regardless of age.

24.4.2 Performance Anxiety

As already described, music can trigger particularly strong positive emotions in musicians and singers and reduce feelings of stress and anxiety. However, negative emotions, such as a strong fear of performing or reluctance to practice every day, are also part of a musicians emotional spectrum of experiences (Steptoe 2001). Jäncke (2009) states that professional musicians' fear of performing and failure can lead to the development of mental illnesses such as obsessive-compulsive disorder. Other studies have shown that musicians have to deal with the psychological consequences of performance anxiety. In the early 1980s, Haider and Groll-Knapp (1981) recorded the heart rate and spontaneous electrical brain activity (EEG) of 24 musicians from the Vienna Symphony Orchestra. Both parameters showed significantly higher activation in the test participants during performance than during rehearsal. This result was later replicated in various studies (e.g. Craske and Craig 1984). Fishbein et al. (1988) studied 2200 musicians from 48 U.S. orchestras. More than 20% of women and 14% of men stated that performance anxiety was a serious problem. In a study by Möller (2002), 50% of the musicians and 70% of the music students reported performance anxiety. In addition, Langendörfer et al. (2006) showed that performance anxiety plays a role not only during performance but also during rehearsals and, therefore, seems to be omnipresent for professional musicians. However, not only professional musicians but also amateur musicians are affected by performance anxiety. Hodapp et al. (2009) showed no difference in the level of performance anxiety between amateurs and professional orchestras. Therefore, musical performance appears to be associated with performance anxiety in both professional and amateur musicians, which in a certain percentage of cases has strongly impaired characteristics. Since not only performances in front of an audience but also rehearsals can cause anxiety among musicians, it seems quite possible that children also experience performance anxiety when they learn to play instruments. One implication of this is the early onset of childhood test anxiety, which, as a fear of failure in a performance situation, is comparable to emotional pressure during a performance. For example, in a meta-analysis of 562 studies across all school grades, Hembree (1988, cited in Ryan 2004) found that test anxiety was established in children around the second grade.

The first study on performance anxiety in children was conducted by Simon and Martens (1979, cited in Ryan 2005) including 749 boys aged 9–14 years. The children participated in individual and group activities, each from one of three areas (musical performance: individual addition vs. band performance; athletic performance: individual vs team sport; academic performance: individual vs. group test). Children who played the instrument alone showed the highest anxiety levels. Performing a piece of music with a band produced the highest anxiety levels among the group activities. Playing music in front of an audience appears to be emotionally stressful for children. Ryan's (2005) findings support this. Using an anxiety questionnaire, Ryan found that the state anxiety of 137 children in grades 3–7 increased significantly on the day of a school concert compared to a normal school day. In a previous study, Ryan (2004) found an increase in heart rate on stage in 26 sixth-graders who were asked to perform on a piano. Some children stated that the reason for their nervousness was fear of playing in front of many people. Others reported that they were afraid of making mistakes, and others reported that they were afraid of making mistakes in front of many people. In addition, LeBlanc et al. (1997) found that only in the condition with the highest audience (multiple scientists and classmates) did the heart rate of high school students playing an instrument increase significantly compared to two other situations (alone and alone with a scientist). Self-reported anxiety was already significantly increased when adolescents were only asked to play in front of the scientist. Thus, the inherently stressful auditioning situation seems to become more frustrating with an increase in the number of listeners.

Ryan (1998) found a negative correlation between self-confidence and performance anxiety among sixth-graders. Of the children and adolescents who indicated on an anxiety questionnaire how nervous they felt about performing in their school band, 27–42% were moderately anxious, and 5–25% were rated as highly anxious (Ryan 1999). Most of the highly anxious children were in Year 6, suggesting an effect of age or experience. Performance anxiety appears to play a role even among young musicians.

Therefore, negative affectivity associated with learning an instrument must also be considered in studies involving children and adolescents. Particularly, in view of the fact that music-making in young people can also go hand in hand with the need to please important reference persons, such as parents and teachers (North et al. 2000), the significance of performance anxiety for the use of music-making to induce and regulate emotions plays a special role. Performance anxiety and fear of failure, as well as anticipated or actual reprimands from parents or teachers, could have a long-term effect on the child's relationship with the instrument and, thus, also on its use as an emotion-regulating tool.

To round off the presentation of children's musical emotions and emotion regulation with current research data, a newly developed questionnaire for children will be presented at the end of this article, which considers the concept of musical emotion regulation and the distinction between positive and negative musical emotions.

24.5 Questionnaire on Positive and Negative Emotions During Instrument Learning (ELIS Scale)

As part of alarge, longitudinal research project called "Music Education, Child Cognition, and Affect" (Bongard et al., 2015: Roden et al., 2015), that was funded by the Federal Ministry of Education and Research Germany, a scale for positive and negative emotions in children who have just started to learn a musical instrument was developed, tested, and validated over 18 months with three time points: the "Emotions while Learning an Instrument Scale", ELIS for short (Roden et al., 2021). The ELIS scale is based on previous theoretical findings on positive and negative emotional experiences while learning a musical instrument, including social aspects such as self-esteem, self-efficacy, motivation, satisfaction with music lessons, parental support, and student-teacher relationships (e.g. Creech and Hallam 2011; Saarikallio 2008; North et al. 2000; Rife et al. 2001). Both subscales exhibited high internal reliability (Cronbach's α = .74, .86), with relatively stable retest reliabilities over 18 months (r = .11–.56). The results confirmed the structure of the measurement model. They provided evidence of the reliability and validity of the scale.

The Positive Emotions of Learning an Instrument (PELI scale) include emotional engagement and enjoyment of learning an instrument, sense of progress and musical self-esteem, satisfaction with music lessons and parental support, and general well-being from musical practice (musical emotion regulation). Negative emotions when learning an instrument (NELI scale) include the experience of stress due to musical practice and failure, a lack of fees for progress, and negative experiences in various social situations such as making music alone, playing with other children, or practising in front of parents or teachers. A complete list of all the items used in the questionnaire is presented in Table 24.1.

To validate the ELIS scale, the emotion regulation of the pupils was also measured with a shortened test inventory of the questionnaire for the survey of stress and stress management in childhood and adolescence (SSKJ 3–8; Lohaus et al. 2006) and the positive and negative affect with a shortened and child-appropriate questionnaire inventory of the "Positive and Negative Affect Schedule" (PANAS; Watson et al. 1988). Both inventories achieved adequate retest reliability (SSKJ: $r = .39–r = 71$ PANAS: $r = .74–r = .82$) and internal consistencies (SSKJ: $\alpha = .60–\alpha = .74$ PANAS: $\alpha = .84–\alpha = .90$). The results showed that positive (PELI) and negative (NELI) musical emotions were represented by one factor each, as expected. CFAs confirmed the two-factor model over 18 months, indicating a high stability of the two-factor solution (Fig. 24.2). The fit indices for testing the statistical quality of the hypothesised model also showed an acceptable fit of the two-factor model at

Table 24.1 List of items used in the ELIS questionnaire

No	Item
01	I enjoy practising my instrument
02	It makes me happy that I'm getting better and better at playing my instrument
03	I am angry when I don't get any further in playing my instrument
04	I think it is nice to learn a musical instrument
05	My parents were proud of me when I learned something new on my instrument
06	My mother or father is with me when I practice
07	It is exhausting to play on my instrument
08	I'd rather do something else and practice
09	I have enough time to practice at home
10	I like my music teacher
11	When I'm happy, I play my instrument
12	I get annoyed when others play better than me
13	I am proud when I can play something for my parents
14	I don't like playing my instrument in front of others
15	When I can't play my instrument for a long time, I start to miss it
16	It's embarrassing for me to play the wrong note on my instrument
17	When I'm sad or angry, I play my instrument to feel better
18	Music lessons at school are fun
19	I enjoy making music with other children
20	I feel good when I play my instrument
21	I hate practising
22	When I practice at home, my parents are annoyed
23	I am scared to play my instrument in front of others
24	I get mad when I have to practice, even though I'd rather do something else
25	When I make a mistake, I'm afraid my music teacher will notice
26	I'm sad when others play better than me
27	My parents get mad when I don't play well

the third measurement ($\chi 2(87) = 219.70$, $p < .001$, $\chi 2/\text{df} = 2.5$; RMSEA = .07; CFI = .90; TLI = .88; SRMR = .07).

Despite the rapid developmental changes in children, the retest reliabilities proved to be a relatively stable construct, as shown by the correlations over 6, 12, and 18 months. With internal consistencies of Cronbach's alpha $\alpha = .78$ and McDonald's $\omega = .79$ (NELI) and, $\alpha = .85$ and McDonald's $\omega = .86$ (PELI) at the third measurement time point after 18 months, the ELIS proves to be a reliable questionnaire that measures relatively stable musical emotions in children. Negative musical emotions showed a low negative correlation with positive musical emotions, with a slight increase over time. This low correlation is consistent with the results of Saarikallio (2008), which showed that musical emotions were not correlated with the expression of negative emotions through music. This suggests that negative and positive musical emotions are two relatively independent constructs. Although positive and negative affect were initially presented as two independent constructs (Watson et al. 1988), further research has shown that they are moderately interdependent (Browne and Cudeck 1992; Crawford and Henry 2004; Mineka

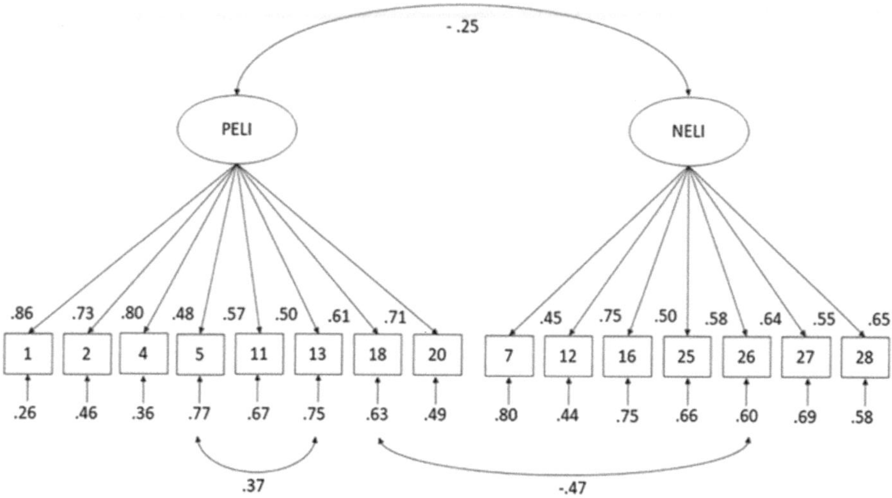

Fig. 24.2 Cross-validation of the factorial structure after 18 months with standardised estimates

et al. 1998; Schermelleh-Engel et al. 2003). Indeed, ELIS correlations between the scales appeared to increase over time, which may indicate a growing counterbalance between negative and positive emotional experiences. As previous research has suggested that positive musical emotions can counterbalance stress during performances (Beck et al. 2006), further studies are needed to determine the exact nature of the relationship between negative and positive musical emotions.

The correlation patterns between the ELIS and SSKJ scales showed the expected relationship structure, although the results for the PELI were more consistent than those for the NELI. The reduced length of the SSKJ scales in the present study may be attributable to their diminished internal consistency. Nevertheless, the overall results of divergent and convergent validities are promising. Although the gender effect was only significant for the PELI, girls scored higher on both scales. This is consistent with previous studies reporting that women experience musical emotions more intensely than men (Saarikallio 2006). Age has no significant influence on the evaluation of musical emotions. Nevertheless, the correlations were negative, which seems to contradict the results of previous studies showing that young adolescents experience musical emotions more strongly than older age groups (North et al. 2000). According to North et al. (2000), one might expect musical emotions to increase after primary school. Whether a diminishing effect is typical only for primary school children or whether it is a general phenomenon of familiarisation with a new learning experience, which could also play a role in adolescents, requires further research.

The solid factorial correlation across three measurement points and the relative stability of the measurements over 1 1/2 years demonstrate the reliability of the procedure and the stability of the characteristics. However, they also provide interesting indications of the emotional and musical development of primary school children and show that emotions are experienced relatively consistently by children when learning an instrument, whereby they relate to positive and negative experiences with the instrument, as well as with adults and other children. Similar to other studies, the experience of positive emotions was shown to be a core element of musical experiences. In this study, this was the most frequently experienced and stable emotional component of the music. In addition, children appear to use music-making as an emotion regulation mechanism over a long period. With its items on negative and positive experiences with parents and teachers, the scale provides evidence that the importance of parents and teachers for music-making in adolescents, as found by North et al. (2000), also applies in childhood.

Using the ELIS scale, it is now possible, for the first time, to measure the basic dimensions of positive and negative emotions in children who are learning to play an instrument. As the high dropout rates in Evans et al.'s (2013) study have shown, it is crucial to understand the negative emotional processes during instrumental learning and their effects. The present scale for measuring emotions during instrument learning not only covers a variety of constructs that are also included in other published scales but could also contribute to the further investigation of children's emotional experiences, as its validated and published form allows positive and negative emotions to be captured reliably and efficiently. The internal consistency and the first assessment of validity yielded acceptable to good results, indicating that the ELIS can serve as a valuable instrument for the assessment of musical emotions in primary school children.

24.6 Summary

Although emotions and their regulation through instrumental learning have been little studied to date, the studies cited were able to show that they fulfil basic functions such as the experience of positive emotions and the reduction of negative emotions. Children, adults, and adolescents use musical emotion regulation.Listening to music, instrumental playing, and other musical activities appear to function as emotion regulation mechanisms at all age levels. McDonald et al. (2003) provide evidence that listening to music is particularly suitable for coping with moderate stress. It is possible that emotional reactions to strong stressors cannot be regulated by music because of the perceived uncontrollability of the situation. Further studies on music-making would be interesting to better determine the range of effects of musical emotion regulation. There is a need for further differentiation in the study of musical emotions. Even though music listening and music-making showed similar emotion regulation mechanisms, they still exhibited a crucial difference (North et al., 2000). In contrast to music perception, music-making also included the desire to please authority figures such as parents and teachers. This may result in further stress for the musicians. Studies on performance anxiety have shown that even children experience stressful performance anxiety. The emotional impact of making music should, therefore, be analysed in a more differentiated way according to its positive and negative effects. The newly constructed ELIS questionnaire, with its scales for recording positive and negative emotions during instrument learning and its scale for emotion regulation during instrument learning, provides a measuring instrument for reliable and standardised psychometric recording and investigation of emotional processes in children of primary school age.

24.7 Conclusion

Learning about a musical instrument and its associated emotional processes is difficult to compare with simply listening to music. There is not only a need for further research into musical processes in young musicians but also for suitable instrumental pedagogy that knows how to promote the motivating potential of instrumental playing and, at the same time, does not burden the learning process with negative experiences and reservations.

To our knowledge, the Emotions of Learning an Instrument Scale (ELIS) presented here is the first scale used to measure positive and negative emotions in children learning to play instruments. With its deep variety of constructs, it contributes to further research into children's emotional experiences by enabling researchers to capture positive and negative emotions in a reliable, efficient, and time-saving way. Internal consistency and validity assessments yielded acceptable to good results, suggesting that ELIS can serve as a valuable tool for assessing musical emotions in elementary school children.

References

Adachi M, Trehub SE (1998) Children's expression of emotion in song. Psychol Music 26:133–153

Anderson RA, Baron RS, Logan H (1991) Distraction, control, and dental stress. J Appl Soc Psychol 21:156–171

Barrera ME, Rykov MH, Doyle SL (2002) The effects of interactive music therapy on hospitalised children with cancer: a pilot study. Psycho-Oncology 11:379–388

Bartlett DL (1996) Physiological responses to music and sound stimuli. In: Hodges DA (ed) Handbook of music psychology. IMR, San Antonio, pp 343–385

Barrett MS, Bond N (2015) Connecting through music: The contribution of a music programme to fostering positive youth development. Research studies in music education 37(1):37–54.

Beck RJ, Gottfried TL, Hall DJ, Cisler CA, Bozeman KW (2006) Supporting the health of college solo singers: The relationship of positive emotions and stress to changes in salivary IgA and cortisol during singing. J Learn Through Arts 2(1).

Bongard S, Frankenberg E, Friedrich EK, Roden I, Kreutz GG (2015) Auswirkungen von JeKi-Instrumentalunterricht auf Stresserleben und Stressbewältigung von Grundschulkindern, in: U. Kranefeld (Hrsg.). Instrumentalunterricht in der grundschule: prozess-und wirkungsanalysen zum programm jedem kind ein instrument 170–179.

Browne MW, Cudeck R (1992) Alternative ways of assessing model fit. Sociol Methods Res 21(2):230–258

Brown ED, Blumenthal MA, Allen AA (2022) The sound of self-regulation: Music program relates to an advantage for children at risk. Early childhood research quarterly 60:126–136.

Christenson PG, Roberts DF (1998) It's not only rock & roll: popular music in the lives of adolescents. J Commun 49(4):212–229

Cole PM, Martin SE, Dennis TA (2004) Emotion regulation as a scientific construct: methodological challenges and directions for child development research. Child Dev 75:317–333

Craske MG, Craig KD (1984) Musical performance anxiety: the three-systems model and self-efficacy theory. Behav Res Ther 22:267–280

Crawford JR, Henry JD (2004) The Positive and Negative Affect Schedule (PANAS): construct validity, measurement properties and normative data in a large non-clinical sample. Br J Clin Psychol 43(3):245–265

Creech A, Hallam S (2011) Learning a musical instrument: the influence of interpersonal interaction on outcomes for school-aged pupils. Psychol Music 39(1):102–122

Cunningham JG, Sterling RS (1988) Developmental change in the understanding of affective meaning in music. Motiv Emot 12:399–413

Deckers L (2009) Motivation: biological, psychological, and environmental. Allyn and Bacon, Boston

DeNora T (1999) Music as a technology of the self. Poetics 26:1–26

Dolgin KG, Adelson EH (1990) Age changes in the ability to interpret affect in sung and instrumentally presented melodies. Psychol Music 18:87–98

Ebata AT, Moos RH (1991) Coping and adjustment in distressed and healthy adolescents. J Appl Dev Psychol 12:33–54

Eschenbeck H, Kohlmann CW, Lohaus A (2007) Gender differences in coping strategies in children and adolescents. J Individ Differ 28:18–26

Evans P, McPherson GE, Davidson JW (2013) The role of psychological needs in ceasing music and music learning activities. Psychol Music 41(5):600–619

Fishbein M, Middlestadt SE, Ottati V, Straus S, Ellis A (1988) Medical problems among ICSOM musicians: overview of a national survey. Med Probl Perform Art 3(1):1–8

Gerry D, Unrau A, Trainor LJ (2012) Active music classes in infancy enhance musical, communicative and social development. Dev Sci 15:398–407

Gratz KL, Roemer L (2004) Multidimensional assessment of emotion regulation and dysregulation: development, factor structure, and initial validation of the difficulties in emotion regulation scale. J Psychopathol Behav Assess 26:41–54

Gross JJ, Muñoz RF (1995) Emotion regulation and mental health. Clin Psychol Sci Pract 2:151–164

Gross JJ, Thompson RA (2007) Emotion regulation: conceptual foundations. In: Gross JJ (ed) Handbook of emotion regulation. Guilford Press, New York, pp 3–24

Haider M, Groll-Knapp E (1981) Psychophysiological investigation into the stress experienced by musicians in a symphony orchestra. In: Piperek M (ed) Stress and music: medical, psychological, sociological, and legalstrain factors in a symphony orchestra musician's profession. Wilhelm Braumüller, Wien, pp 15–34

Hembree R (1988) Correlates, causes, effects, and treatment of test anxiety. Rev Educ Res 58:47–77

Herman-Stahl MA, Stemmler M, Petersen AC (1995) Approach and avoidant coping: implications for adolescent mental health. J Youth Adolesc 24:649–665

Ho P, Tsao JCI, Bloch L, Zeltzer LK (2011) The impact of drumming on social-emotional behavior in low-income children. Evid Based Complement Alternat Med 2011:1–14

Hodapp V, Langendorfer F, Bongard S, Kreutz G (2009) Arbeitsbedingungen, gesundheitliche Beschwerden und Aufführungsängste bei professionellen Orchestermusikern. Musikphysiologie und Musikermedizin 16:99–113

Jäncke L (2009) Macht Musik schlau?—Neue Erkenntnisse aus den Neurowissenschaften und der kognitiven Psychologie. Huber, Bern

Juslin PN, Sloboda JA (2001) Music and emotion. Oxford University Press, New York

Kastner MP, Crowder RG (1990) Perception of the major/minor distinction: IV. Emotional connotations in young children. Music Percept 8:189–202

Keltner D, Shiota MN (2003) New displays and new emotions: a commentary on Rozin and Cohen (2003). Emotion 3:86–91

Kenelly J (2000) The specialist role of the music therapist in developmental programs for hospitalised children. J Pediatr Health Care 14:56–59

Kreutz G, Litta G (2003) Musikpräferenzen und aggressive Einstellungen in der vierten Grundschulklasse. Musikpsychologie 17:72–88

Kreutz G, Bongard S, Rohrmann S, Hodapp V, Grebe D (2004) Effects of choir singing or listening on secretory immunoglobulin A, cortisol, and emotional state. J Behav Med 27:623–635
Krohne HW (1993) Vigilance and cognitive avoidance as concepts in coping research. In: Krohne HW (ed) Attention and avoidance: strategies in coping with aversiveness. Hogrefe und Huber, Seattle, pp 19–50
Lacourse E, Claes M, Villeneuve M (2001) Heavy metal music and adolescent suicidal risk. J Youth Adolesc 30:321–332
Langendörfer F, Hodapp V, Kreutz G, Bongard S (2006) Personality and performance anxiety among professional orchestra musicians. J Individ Differ 27:162–171
Lazarus RS, Folkman S (1984) Stress, appraisal, and coping. Springer, New York
LeBlanc A, Jin YC, Obert M, Siivola C (1997) Effect of audience on music performance anxiety. J Res Music Educ 45:480–496
Lohaus A, Eschenbeck H, Kohlmann CW, Klein-Heßling J (2006) Fragebogen zur Erhebung von Stress und Stressbewältigung im Kindes-und Jugendalter (SSKJ 3–8)
Longhi E, Pickett N (2008) Music and well-being in long-term hospitalized children. Psychol Music 36:247–256
Malone AB (1996) The effects of live music on the distress of paediatric patients receiving intravenous starts, venipunctures, injections and heel sticks. J Music Ther 33:19–33
Nigg JT (2017) Annual research review: on the relations among self-regulation, self-control, executive functioning, effortful control, cognitive control, impulsivity, risk-taking, and inhibition for developmental psychopathology. J Child Psychol Psych. 58(4):361–83.
McDonald RAR, Mitchell LA, Dillon T, Serpell MG, Davies JB, Ashley EA (2003) An empirical investigation of the anxiolytic and pain reducing effects of music. Psychol Music 31:187–203
Mineka S, Watson D, Clark LA (1998) Comorbidity of anxiety and unipolar mood disorders. Annu Rev Psychol 49(1):377–412
Möller H (2002) Lampenfieber und Aufführungsängste sind nicht dasselbe! In: Hofmann G, Trubsbach C (Hrsg) Mensch und Musik. Wißner, Augsburg, S 59–68
Nawrot ES (2003) The perception of emotional expression in music: evidence from infants, children and adults. Psychol Music 31:75–92
North AC, Hargreaves DJ, O'Neill SA (2000) The importance of music to adolescents. Br J Educ Psychol 70:255–272
Papoušek M (1992) Early ontogeny of vocal communication in parent-infant interactions. In: Papoušek H, Jürgens U, Papoušek M (eds) Nonverbal vocal communication: comparative and developmental approaches. Cambridge University Press, Cambridge, pp 230–261
Plahl C (2009) Musiktherapie: Praxisfelder und Vorgehensweisen. In: Bruhn H, Kopiez R, Lehmann AC (Hrsg) Handbuch der Musikpsychologie. Rowohlt Taschenbuchverlag, Reinbek, S 630–652
Rhythm and Movement Delivered by Teachers Supports Self-Regulation Skills of Preschool-Aged Children in Disadvantaged Communities: A clustered RCT
Rife NA, Shnek ZM, Lauby JL, Lapidus LB (2001) Children's satisfaction with private music lessons. J Res Music Educ 49(1):21–32
Robb SL (2000) The effect of therapeutic music interventions on the behaviour of hospitalized children in isolation: developing a contextual support model of music therapy. J Music Ther 37:118–146
Roden I, Kreutz G, Friedrich EK, Frankenberg E, Bongard S (2015) auswirkungen von jeki-instrumentalunterricht auf aufmerksamkeits-und gedächtnisleistungen bei grundschulkindern, in: u. Kranefeld (hrsg.). Instrumentalunterricht in der grundschule: prozess-und wirkungsanalysen zum programm jedem kind ein instrumentinstrumentalunterricht in der grundschule. Prozess-und wirkungsanalysen zum programm "jedem kind ein instrument 182–194
Roden I, Zepf FD, Kreutz G, Grube D, Bongard S (2016) Effects of music and natural science training on aggressive behavior. Learning and instruction 45:85–92.

Roden I, Friedrich EK, Etzler S, Frankenberg E, Kreutz G, Bongard S (2021) Development and preliminary validation of the Emotions while Learning an Instrument Scale (ELIS). Plos one 16(8):e0255019. https://doi.org/10.1371/journal.pone.0255019
Roe K (1985) Swedish youth and music: listening patterns and motivation. Commun Res 12:353–362
Roth S, Cohen LJ (1986) Approach, avoidance, and coping with stress. Am Psychol 41:813–819
Ruud E (1997) Music and the quality of life. Nord J Music Ther 6:86–97
Ryan CA (1998) Exploring musical performance anxiety in children. Med Probl Perform Art 9:83–88
Ryan CA (1999) Musical performance anxiety: are junior high band students affected? Opus 41:8–9
Ryan C (2004) Gender differences in children's experience of musical performance anxiety. Psychol Music 32:89–103
Ryan C (2005) Experience of musical performance anxiety in elementary school children. Int J Stress Manag 12:331–342
Saarikallio S (2006) Regulation and gratification: the emotional meanings of music in adolescence. ECDPM 2005:297
Saarikallio SH (2008) Music in mood regulation: initial scale development. Music Sci 12(2):291–309
Saarikallio S (2016). Music as emotion regulation. Musicae Scientiae 20(1):10–10.
Saarikallio S (2009) Emotional self-regulation through music in 3–8-year-old children. In: Proceedings of the 7th Triennal Conference of European Society for the Cognitive Sciences of Music (ESCOM 2009) Jyväskylä, Finland, pp 459–462
Saarikallio S, Erkkilä J (2007) The role of music in adolescents' mood regulation. Psychol Music 35:88–109
Schermelleh-Engel K, Moosbrugger H, Müller H (2003) Evaluating the fit of structural equation models: tests of significance and descriptive goodness-of-fit measures. Methods Psychol Res Online 8(2):23–74
Schubert E, McPherson GE (2006) The perception of emotion in music. In: McPherson GE (ed) The child as musician: a handbook of musical development. Oxford University Press, New York, pp 193–212
Schwarz KD, Fouts GT (2003) Music preferences, personality style, and developmental issues of adolescents. J Youth Adolesc 32:205–213
Sena Moore K, Burbach K, Hanson-Abromeit D (2025) A theory of intervention model to define the essential characteristics of music to support emotion regulation development in early childhood. Front Neurosci 19:1568789.
Shenfield T, Trehub SE, Nakata T (2003) Maternal singing modulates infant arousal. Psychol Music 31:365–375
Simon JA, Martens R (1979) Children's anxiety in sport and nonsport evaluative activities. J Sport Psychol 1:160–169
Sloboda JA, O'Neill SA (2001) Emotions in everyday listening to music. In: Juslin PN, Sloboda JA (eds) Music and emotion: theory and research. Oxford University Press, New York, pp 415–429
Sokolowski K (2007) Emotion. In: Müsseler J (ed) Allgemeine Psychologie. Spektrum Akademischer Verlag, Heidelberg, S 295–333
Steptoe A (2001) Negative emotions in music making: the problem of performance anxiety. In: Juslin PN, Sloboda JA (eds) Music and emotion: theory and research. Oxford University Press, New York, pp 292–307
Tafuri V, Villa D (2002) Musical elements in vocalizations of infants aged 2-8 months. Br J Music Educ 19:73–88
Trehub SE (2003) The developmental origins of musicality. Nat Neurosci 6:669673
Trehub SE, Nakata T (2001) Emotion and music in infancy. Musicae Scientiae Special Issue:37–61
Watson D, Clark LA, Tellegen A (1988) Development and validation of brief measures of positive and negative affect: the PANAS scales. J Pers Soc Psychol 54(6):1063

Wells A, Hakanen EA (1991) The emotional use of popular music by adolescents. Journal Q 68:445–454

Winkler I, Haden GP, Ladinig O, Sziller I, Honing H (2009) Newborn infants detect the beat in music. Proc Natl Acad Sci USA 106(7):2468–2471

Williams KE, Berthelsen D (2019) Implementation of a rhythm and movement intervention to support self-regulation skills of preschool-aged children in disadvantaged communities. Psychol Music 47(6):800–20.

Williams KE, Bentley LA, Savage S, Eager R, Nielson, C (2023) Rhythm and movement delivered by teachers supports self-regulation skills of preschool-aged children in disadvantaged communities: a clustered RCT. Early Child Res Q 65, 115–128. https://doi.org/10.1016/j.ecresq.2023.05.008

Music and Cognitive Development 25

Franziska Degé, Ulrike Frischen, and Gudrun Schwarzer

25.1 Introduction

For a number of years, extra-musical effects of music lessons have been of interest to researchers, policymakers, the media, and the public. The strong research interest in the effects of music lessons on child development can be largely attributed to the so-called Mozart effect (Rauscher et al. 1993). In this study, students were found to improve visuospatial performance after listening for 10 min to the Sonata for Two Pianos in D Major, K448, by Wolfgang Amadeus Mozart. After very heterogeneous replication experiments, Glenn Schellenberg and his colleagues postulated what they called the arousal and mood hypothesis. According to this hypothesis, a positive stimulus (in this case, a Mozart sonata) increases both mood and arousal, and this state causes an increase in performance in cognitive tasks. The researchers were able to show that the Mozart effect is a short-term improvement in a circumscribed cognitive or creative performance that can be triggered by listening to a positively valenced piece of music but also by any other nonmusical positively valenced stimulus (Nantais and Schellenberg 1999; Schellenberg et al. 2007; Thompson et al. 2001). Although passive music listening is unlikely to have the same effect that years of music lessons might have (Schellenberg 2004), the Mozart effect also sparked scientific interest in the positive transfer effects of music or instrumental lessons. In this chapter, we aim to present the state of research on the positive

F. Degé (✉)
Max Planck Institute for Empirical Aesthetics, Frankfurt a.M., Germany
e-mail: franziska.dege@ae.mpg.de

U. Frischen
University of Bremen, Bremen, Germany

G. Schwarzer
Justus Liebig University Giessen, Giessen, Germany

G. Kreutz, G. Bernatzky (eds.), *Music and Medicine*, Neurocultural Health and Wellbeing, https://doi.org/10.1007/978-3-662-72175-9_25

transfer effects of music lessons on various cognitive skills and academic achievement. In doing so, we specifically address relationships that we find to have the greatest practical significance and that are supported by studies with methodologically high-quality designs. Furthermore, we try to clarify how these effects might come about and whether they are specific to active music making or music lessons.

25.2 Transfer

Researchers have been discussing transfer effects for many years. Even today, this topic is still of high relevance (Klauer 2010). Questions arise, such as: When does transfer take place at all? Are transfer effects the rule in learning, or are they rather the exception? What exactly is transfer anyway? Learning transfer occurs as an effect of learning. Knowledge or skills learned in one requirement area can be used to master a new requirement from an independent requirement area (Mähler and Stern 2006). Not only can the positive transfer effects just outlined occur, but negative transfer can also occur: knowledge in one domain can also inhibit the acquisition of new knowledge in another domain Klauer 2001. Negative transfer, however, is less commonly reported. Within positive transfer, different effects can arise in learning and practice processes, with domain-specific effects relating to the domain practiced or learned (so-called trivial learning effects), whereas cross-domain effects can affect domains that were neither practiced nor learned (nontrivial learning effects) (Klauer 2011). For example, when learning a musical instrument over time, one would expect a child to become increasingly proficient on his or her instrument (trivial learning effect). However, if at the same time the child improves his or her working memory skills by practicing on the musical instrument, then there is a nontrivial learning effect (Roden et al. 2014).

Besides the distinction between trivial and nontrivial learning effects, there are several other ways of classifying transfer effects. These classifications are all based on the idea that the degree of dissimilarity between the learning situation and the transfer situation determines the quality of the transfer. Overall, the transfer distance is smaller for literal (skill is transferred to learning task of the same type), horizontal, and specific (certain narrowly defined skill is transferred) transfer than for vertical, figural (analogy enables transfer to a new problem), and general or nonspecific (principles of one domain are transferred to another) transfer. The greater the distance or range of the transfer, the greater its qualitative assessment and the less frequently it takes place. This aspect is summarized under the term *generalization gradient* (Osgood 1962). Consequently, since trivial learning transfers result in lower transfer distances than nontrivial learning transfers, their quality is rated lower. The transfer effects of active music making on cognitive abilities are predominantly nontrivial positive transfers, because the transfer distance between music making and cognition is large.

25.3 Methodological Considerations

25.3.1 Music Lessons

In the following sections, music lessons do not refer to regular lessons at school. We use it to refer to music lessons in the sense of instrumental or singing lessons, such as those offered at a music school, and to additional practical music programs in schools (extended school music lessons) and kindergartens.

25.3.2 Study Designs

When we look at the various studies on the effect of music lessons on cognitive abilities, we should always keep in mind some quality standards regarding the study quality and be clear about which information can be drawn from which study designs. In simple terms, this means that the higher the quality of a study design, the more far-reaching and robust the findings that can be drawn from such a study.

25.3.2.1 Correlational Design

In correlational studies, two characteristics are related to each other at a particular point in time of investigation. For example, one examines the relationship between music lessons and verbal memory performance (Degé and Schwarzer 2017). If one finds a positive correlation here, then one knows that music lessons and verbal memory performance are related, and it might be worthwhile to further research transfer effects here. However, it is not known whether participation in music lessons improves verbal memory or whether a person with better verbal memory is more likely to take music lessons.

25.3.2.2 Longitudinal Design

Longitudinal studies in which the same subjects are studied over a longer period of time are more informative than studies in which groups of subjects are compared at only one point in time (correlational or cross-sectional studies). By tracking trends over time, one gets clues about which trait influences another. For example, extended school music lessons over 2 years may improve auditory/verbal memory performance in students who participated in extended school music lessons compared to those who did not participate (Degé et al. 2011b). Critical to such study designs is the choice of control group (trained vs. untrained) and the existence of possible selection effects. Usually, one compares the development of a group with intervention (music lessons) with the development of a control group (without intervention or with a control intervention). The methodologically better way is to compare a group with control intervention, because here one can exclude the possibility that the intervention group has simply become better due to more schooling. If I compare school groups with each other, as in the example just given, then students and parents have jointly decided whether the respective student will participate in extended school music lessons. This carries a risk of selection bias: Participating students might differ systematically from nonparticipating students. To minimize the influence of such selection effects, certain characteristics (e.g., parents' educational attainment, children's personality) of the group can be recorded and statistically controlled.

25.3.2.3 Intervention Design

This is implemented in intervention or training studies. Children are randomly assigned to a music intervention group and a control group with comparable non-music intervention and trained over a certain period of time. This can be used to show, for example, that a particular precursor of learning to read and write can be improved by music training and language training but not by sports training (Degé and Schwarzer 2011). This methodological approach provides evidence for a direction of causation (causality). This study design allows for high-quality and far-reaching conclusions but is very time-consuming and costly. Therefore, such designs are implemented much less frequently than correlational or cross-sectional studies or longitudinal studies without randomization.

Overall, many different studies have addressed the question of whether certain cognitive skills are related to music lessons. Many of these studies use a correlational or cross-sectional design and are, therefore, limited to statements about associations. From this multitude of studies, a variety of cognitive abilities related to music lessons have emerged (see Fig. 25.1).

25.3.3 Influencing Characteristics of Different Subject Groups

In general, when studying children who take music lessons, one must be aware that this population has certain *characteristics* that distinguish it from other populations. Specific demographic variables associated with receiving music lessons have been shown to predict better cognitive performance. For example, children who take music lessons are more likely to have parents who earn more money and have a higher scholastic record (Orsmond and Miller 1999; Sergeant and Thatcher 1974) than children who do not take music lessons. In addition, children who take music lessons also appear to differ in personality from children who do not take music lessons (Corrigall et al. 2013). Children who choose to take music lessons score higher on the Openness to New Experiences scale of a personality test. Since parental education, parental income, and the expression of the Openness personality trait have been found to be positively related to cognitive abilities, including IQ in particular (Ceci and Williams 1997), it is much more difficult to attribute the relationship between music lessons and cognitive ability to music lessons (Schellenberg 2006a). Thus, one should always keep in mind that the comparison of children with and without music lessons is also a comparison of children with different sociodemographic backgrounds. Therefore, a positive effect of music lessons on children's cognitive abilities can only be confirmed if statistical or methodological precautions have been taken to control for sociodemographic differences. Such

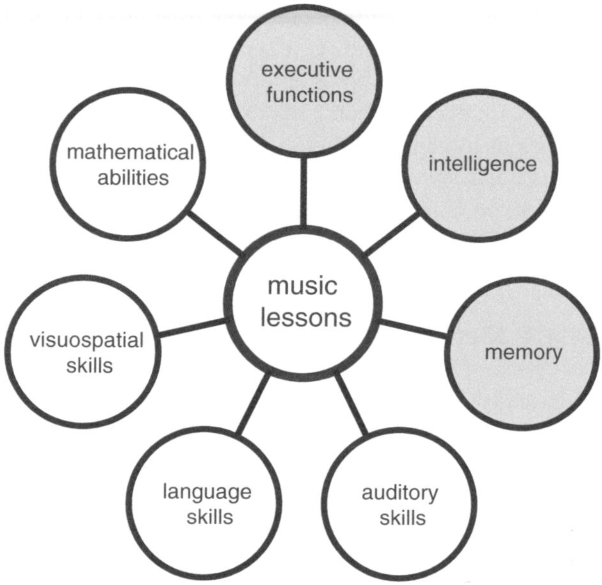

Fig. 25.1 Schematic representation of the relationships between music education and the different cognitive abilities

precautions may include deliberate recruitment of children with the same sociodemographic background, statistical control of these data, or random assignment of children with different sociodemographic backgrounds to an experimental and control group (e.g., music lessons vs. other lessons).

25.4 Music Lessons and Cognitive Skills

As Fig. 25.1 makes clear, many different cognitive abilities are associated with music lessons in childhood. Regular participation in music lessons during childhood shows correlations with better performance on intelligence tests (Schellenberg 2006b) and is associated with improved problem-solving skills (executive functions) (Degé et al. 2011a). In addition, children who take music lessons show good auditory perceptual skills for musical material (Corrigall and Trainor 2009; Orsmond and Miller 1999), and musically trained children have also enhanced auditory perceptual skills for linguistic material (Magne et al. 2006; Thompson et al. 2004). Furthermore, they show better performance in visual memory (Bilhartz et al. 1999) and in verbal memory (Ho et al. 2003) Beyond that, music lessons are associated with language skills such as phonological awareness (Anvari et al. 2002; Lamb and Gregory 1993), reading ability (Gardiner et al. 1996; Moreno et al. 2009), or vocabulary (Forgeard et al. 2008). Lastly, music lessons are related to both visuospatial skills (Rauscher et al. 1997; Rauscher and Zupan 2000) as well as with mathematical abilities (Bahr and Christensen 2000; Cheek and Smith 1999). These various associations can be systematized in terms of connections with general (shaded in gray in Fig. 25.1) and specific cognitive abilities (shaded in white in Fig. 25.1). General cognitive abilities are those that are important for solving tasks from many different domains, such as intelligence or executive functions. Specific cognitive abilities, on the other hand, relate to a specific cognitive domain (e.g., mathematical abilities or linguistic abilities).

It is clear that the topic of transfer effects of music lessons has stimulated much research, so that there are already enough studies for so-called meta-analyses (see Vaughn 2000; Hetland 2000; Butzlaff 2000; Sala and Gobet 2017, 2020).

25.4.1 Meta-analyses

Meta-analysis is essentially about summarizing evaluating the results of various quantitative primary studies on a specific question in order to be able to make more general statements. Based on the effect size estimation, statements can be made about the existence of an effect and its size. In meta-analyses on individual cognitive abilities, Butzlaff (2000) was able to prove a correlation between music lessons and reading ability in correlational studies, but not in experimental studies. However, a later meta-analysis with a larger number of included studies demonstrated a relationship between music lessons and reading ability (Standley 2008). A more recent meta-analysis suggests that the findings on music lessons and reading ability are not quite as consistent: across all measures of reading ability, no effect of music lessons on diverse measures of reading ability was found. When content areas were grouped more homogeneously, however, the relationship between music lessons and phonological awareness (an important precursor to reading ability) appears to be reliably demonstrable (Gordon et al. 2015) but not relationships with other measures of reading ability. Further work on individual cognitive skills has demonstrated small effects of music lessons on math skills (Vaughn 2000) and on visuospatial skills (Hetland 2000). In many recent papers, rather than examining individual cognitive abilities for their relationship to music lessons, different cognitive abilities are examined together. In a review paper by Benz and colleagues (2015), the authors concluded that small effects of music lessons on various cognitive abilities exist. However, in two recent meta-analyses by Sala and Gobet (2017, 2020), the authors reached a different conclusion. They examined the effects of music making on cognitive abilities in children and adolescents and concluded that there was no effect of music lessons on cognitive abilities. Overall, the results of the first meta-analysis (Sala and Gobet 2017) from 38 studies showed a rather small effect size across all content areas. When the effects of music training on individual cognitive domains such as intelligence and memory were considered, the effect sizes increased. This illustrates how misleading it is to report studies across different content areas in a meta-analysis, in this case. The resulting heterogeneity casts strong doubt on whether valid results can be found. In addition to the heterogeneity in the respective content areas, however, the heterogeneity of the interventions implemented in the studies must also be taken into account. Music lessons in the studies included in the meta-analyses ranged from computer-based lessons (e.g., Janus et al. 2016) to small group instrumental lessons (e.g., Roden et al. 2012). Therefore, other researchers decided to conduct a meta-analysis examining the effect of instrumental lessons only (Román-Caballero et al. 2022). The results of this meta-analysis showed a still small but robust effect of instrumental lessons on cognitive and academic content areas. In addition, the researchers found that the effect size appears to be dependent on the different content areas. However, further studies with a high-quality design are needed to examine this aspect more reliably. Overall, the findings of this study suggest that the heterogeneity of the studies influences the results of the reported meta-analyses. The relatively small reported effect sizes in all meta-analyses are not surprising, given that the effects of music training on the cognitive abilities studied are nontrivial or general transfer effects. In light of this, Sala and Gobet's (2017, 2020) conclusion that music training cannot reliably improve children's and adolescents' cognitive skills seems to be too pessimistic. However, the main criticism of the meta-analyses conducted by these authors is that the studies conducted in research on transfer effects of music training were predominantly not of high enough methodological quality. If this is the case, then reliable results of a meta-analysis cannot be expected to emerge from it, and the conclusion of Sala and Gobet (2017, 2020) seems hasty. Rather, the call here should be to conduct even better studies in the future to increase the set of suitable studies for a meaningful meta-analysis.

25.4.2 Music Lessons and Selected Cognitive Skills

As the meta-analyses just reported show, it is useful not to consider all cognitive abilities and their influence by music lessons together. Rather, a detailed examination of different cognitive abilities is more promising. Music lessons do not seem to affect all cognitive abilities in the same way. Moreover, as a way of improving cognitive skills, it is also not equally useful in all areas. The following sections present in more detail those cognitive abilities that have been well researched and thereby show promising relationships to music lessons or music training (e.g., executive functions, intelligence, memory, language). On the one hand, this involves promising studies in terms of methodologically high-quality designs and the resulting more robust results. On the other hand, such cognitive areas are presented in which a promotion through music lessons could have practical significance. The systematization into music lessons and domain-general cognitive abilities and music lessons and specific cognitive abilities is maintained, and preference is given to studies with a longitudinal approach, i.e., those that allow conclusions about causality.

25.4.2.1 Music Lessons and Executive Functions

Executive functions are cognitive control processes that humans use for conscious and goal-directed thought and action (Zelazo et al. 2008). Executive functions include a variety of processes such as inhibition (inhibiting automated impulses to act), selective attention (focusing attention on a target stimulus), cognitive flexibility (e.g., switching attention or switching tasks), working memory (short-term storage and manipulation of information), and planning (e.g., anticipatory action) (Diamond 2013).

Numerous cross-sectional studies confirm the suggestion that long-term music making is associated with different domains of executive functions in adults (Bialystok and DePape 2009; Okada and Slevc 2018) as well as in children (Degé et al. 2011a; Schellenberg 2011; Zuk et al. 2014). However, the results of these studies leave open the extent to which music lessons are associated only with individual (Okada and Slevc 2018; Schellenberg 2011) or with different domains of executive functions. (Degé et al. 2011a, b; Zuk et al. 2014). Furthermore, these cross-sectional studies do not answer the question of causality, i.e., to what extent music lessons may lead to an improvement in executive functions or whether individuals with very good executive functions are more likely to take music lessons. Experimental intervention studies in childhood suggest that music lessons can indeed lead to an improvement in executive functions (e.g. Bugos and DeMarie 2017; Degé et al. 2020; Frischen et al. 2019, 2021; Holochwost et al. 2017; Jaschke et al. 2018). Here, studies with preschool-aged children show that different music-based interventions can have an impact on children's inhibitory skills in particular (Bugos and DeMarie 2017; Degé et al. 2020; Frischen et al. 2019). Moreover, experimental research with school-aged children indicates that the ability to influence executive functions is not limited to early childhood (Frischen et al. 2021; Jaschke et al. 2018). For example, Frischen et al.'s (2021) study showed that eight and a half months of instrumental lessons resulted in improvements in inhibition, selective attention, and visual working memory in 6- to 7-year-old children compared with painting lessons or no additional lessons. Jaschke et al. (2018) did a similar study with elementary school-aged children in which they implemented music and painting lessons into the school curriculum and examined how the classroom-based offerings affected the executive functions of elementary school students. The results of the study showed that the children in the music group performed better on the inhibition and planning tasks than the children in the painting or control groups after 18 months and after 24 months. However, after 24 months, the children in the painting group showed greater improvement in visual working memory compared to the music and control groups.

In summary, there is a positive association between music lessons and executive functions. However, due to the use of different research methods, it is still unclear whether music lessons are associated with only some or with many different executive functions. Experimental intervention studies in childhood indicate that music lessons can lead to improvements in various executive functions in childhood. Again, more research is needed to determine exactly which executive functions benefit from music lessons, how music lessons must be structured to address executive functions, and whether there are age ranges within which music lessons can have a particular impact on executive function development.

Explanations of the Influence of Music Lessons on Executive Functions

The possible influence of music lessons on executive functions probably lies in the continuous demand on executive functions during music making. For example, cognitive flexibility is needed for successful consideration of accidentals, as are inhibitory processes. Selective attention and inhibition are also very important when playing with multiple musicians, as one must closely follow the course of one's own part, find one's cue, and inhibit the impulse to match another part in sound and rhythmic pattern (Herrero and Carriedo 2022; Jäncke 2009). Moreover, the characteristics of music lessons fit excellently with the parameters of successful executive function training named by Diamond and Lee (2011). Such training should be in the children's field of interest, should be able to involve them emotionally, and should give them the feeling of being part of a social structure. Furthermore, it should also be continuous and increase in difficulty so that challenges can be mastered. All of these are points that are naturally combined in music training.

25.4.2.2 Music Lessons and Intelligence

Intelligence describes the ability to learn from experience, solve problems, and adapt to new situations (Myers 2006).

One of the first major studies of music lessons and intelligence in Germany was a 5-year longitudinal study of elementary schools in Berlin (Bastian 2000). This longitudinal study examined the relationship between participation in extended music lessons and intelligence development. Extended music lessons consisted of additional music lessons at school and learning to play an instrument. In addition to intelligence development, Bastian also recorded the development of other skills, such as concentration and social behavior. The effect of music lessons on intelligence was mapped by means of two different test procedures: the Culture Fair Test (CFT; Weiß and Osterland 1977; captures fluid intelligence) and the Adaptive Intelligence Diagnostic (AID; Kubinger and Wurst 1991; captures fluid and crystalline intelligence). The findings regarding the CFT showed that in the first 3 years, the intelligence development of the children with and without extended music lessons was relatively parallel. Only after 4 years of music lessons did the groups differ significantly. The children with extended music lessons did better on the CFT. In contrast, no significant difference was found between children with and without extended music lessons over the entire period, considering the AID. On the one hand, this contradictory result could be explained by differences in the intelligence tests used (recording of fluid vs. recording of fluid and crystalline intelligence). On the other hand, methodological problems (e.g., inappropriate control groups without extended music lessons) could have caused the result. Therefore, based on this study, no clear conclusions can be drawn about the relationship between music lessons and intelligence (Jäncke 2008). More definite results about this relationship are provided by two international studies.

In a study of 6- to 11-year-old children and adults (college students) who had varying degrees of musical training, Schellenberg (2006b) examined the relationship between music lessons and intelligence in more detail. He recorded overall IQ with an age-appropriate intelligence test (recording fluid and crystalline intelligence) and also the academic performance of the children and adults. For both the children and the adults, there was a positive correlation between music lessons and overall IQ. However, this decreased with age: the longer the music lessons took place in the past, the smaller the increases in IQ points were. Furthermore, this study showed that the correlations between music lessons and IQ could not be explained by socioeconomic status or schooling effects. Accordingly, the duration of nonmusical leisure activities, which was also assessed in this study, did not correlate with IQ.

Since this was a cross-sectional study, the general question of causality remains unclear, i.e., whether music lessons can actually promote general intelligence. This question has been addressed by Schellenberg (2004) in a longitudinal study. He randomly assigned 144 6-year-olds to two music groups (singing or keyboarding) and to two control groups (drama or waiting control). Each group received free lessons for 1 year; only the waiting control group did not receive lessons. These children did not receive keyboard lessons until the following year. All children completed an intelligence test at the beginning of the study and again after 1 year (Wechsler Intelligence Scale for Children; WISC-III; Wechsler 1991, which measures fluid and crystalline intelligence). All four groups showed significant improvements in their intelligence after 1 year. This was entirely to be expected, since IQ usually increases after school enrollment (Neisser et al. 1996). However, it is noteworthy that the IQ of the children in both music groups had increased significantly compared to the control groups, although the difference was not very large. Here, the children in the singing group did not differ in the amount of IQ increase from those in the keyboard group. Overall, music lessons produced a small but significant increase in intelligence. In addition to the effects on IQ, this study also measured changes in social competence. No advantage was found in social skills for the children in the music groups. However, the children who had received drama lessons showed significantly better social skills after 1 year of lessons. The socially adaptive behaviors (e.g., executive behavior, adaptability) of these children improved. Based on these results, Schellenberg suggested (2006a) that extracurricular activities generally have positive effects on child development. However, different activities (e.g., music lessons or drama classes) affect different domains (e.g., IQ or social skills).

Overall, it can be stated that there is a relationship between music lessons and IQ. This is long-lasting (into adulthood) and cannot be explained exclusively by the most likely alternative explanations (socioeconomic status or schooling effects). In addition, there is experimental evidence suggesting that music lessons can increase IQ. However, this is only a small improvement.

Explanations of the Influence of Music Lessons on Intelligence

Why do music lessons influence IQ? Which mechanisms of action explain this connection? One conceivable explanation could be differences in IQ even before music lessons begin. It is possible that more intelligent children are more likely to receive music lessons than less intelligent ones. However, empirical results on this assumption are controversial. On the one hand, this assumption is supported by the substantial magnitude of IQ differences between children with and without music lessons of ten IQ points found in some cross-sectional studies (Schellenberg 2011). Indeed, such a high difference cannot be explained only by learning experiences due to music lessons without taking genetic differences into account. On the other hand, no empirical evidence could be found to support the assumption that more intelligent children are more likely to take music lessons. For example, Norton et al. (2005) found no differences in intelligence between children with and without the intention to take music lessons. In principle, according to Schellenberg (2009), if pre-existing differences in intelligence exist, they could be exacerbated by music lessons.

Another explanation refers to the fact that the connection between music lessons and intelligence is a so-called distal transfer. The large transfer distance makes the effect of one or more previously unrecorded mediating variables possible. However, the most likely mediating variable, socioeconomic status, can be ruled out based on the results of Schellenberg (2006a, b). Nevertheless, there could be other variables mediating the relationship between music lessons and intelligence that are responsible for cognitive transfer effects between music lessons and intelligence, such as the influence of executive functions.

The Role of Executive Functions

Few studies to date have examined the role of executive functions as a mediating variable of the relationship between music lessons and IQ (Degé et al. 2011a; Schellenberg 2011). Both studies tested whether there is a positive relationship between music lessons and executive functions in 9- to 12-year-old children and whether they mediate the better performance on an IQ test. In the Schellenberg study, executive functions did not mediate the relationship between music lessons and IQ. In contrast, in the study by Degé and colleagues, executive functions such as selective attention and inhibition (the ability to inhibit automated impulses to act) were found to mediate the relationship between music lessons and IQ. However, the studies used different IQ tests and measured different executive functions, so these different results can likely be attributed to differences in study design and are suggestive of further research.

25.4.2.3 Music Lessons and Memory

Memory describes the ability to permanently retain what has been learned. This is made possible through storage and retrieval (Myers 2006). The three-stage model of memory by Atkinson and Shiffrin (1968) divides memory into a very short-term storing sensory memory, a consciously processing part, the short-term memory, and a long-term storing part, the long-term memory. Today's memory researchers prefer the term working memory to short-term memory because it focuses on the active processing (Myers 2006).

Previous studies explored the relationship between participation in music lessons and memory abilities mainly by comparing memory abilities between adult musicians and nonmusicians. These studies have examined working memory skills and rarely long-term memory performance. In the area of working memory, there is overlap with studies of executive functions, as working memory is also counted among the components of executive functions. Studies show that musicians generally perform better than nonmusicians in visual, auditory, and verbal (working) memory tasks (Aleman et al. 2000; Brandler and Rammsayer 2003; Brochard et al. 2004; Chan et al. 1998; Franklin et al. 2008; Jakobson et al. 2003, 2008; Kilgour et al. 2000) However, for childhood, there are few studies that have examined the impact of music lessons on visual, auditory, and verbal memory (Degé et al. 2011b; Ho et al. 2003; Roden et al. 2012). Ho et al. (2003) showed in a study with children aged 7–11 years that music lessons increased verbal memory performance. The study was designed to examine different groups of children: one group began music lessons (beginners), another had already had music lessons and continued (continuers), and another group had dropped out of music lessons (dropouts). All children were assessed in verbal and visual memory at the beginning of the study and after 1 year, and some control variables (age, parents' income) were recorded. After 1 year, the beginners had improved by about 20% and the continuers by about 10% in their verbal memory performance. The dropouts actually performed about 10% worse in their verbal memory skills. Visual memory improved at about the same rate in all three groups over the study period. Accordingly, this study indicates a positive effect of music lessons on children's verbal, but not visual, memory.

Another longitudinal study explored the impact of 2 years of extended music lessons on visual and auditory memory in 9- to 10-year-old children (Degé et al. 2011b). Variables such as socioeconomic status, motivation, schooling, musical aptitude, and IQ of the children were controlled. Consistent with the findings of Ho and colleagues, this study demonstrates a positive impact of music lessons on auditory memory. However, in contrast to Ho and colleagues, a positive effect on visual memory was also found. The different findings on visual memory might reflect a culture effect. Namely, in the Chinese study, simple graphic designs (BVMT-R, Benedict 1997) were used to assess visual memory. Instead, the German study used color sequences (BASIC-MLT, Lepach and Petermann 2008). Since in Asian cultures written language is based on visual designs, the ability to remember graphic designs could possibly be excellently trained and music lessons could not provide any additional improvement. However, it also cannot be ruled out that the children in the German study silently spoke the color sequences and that this may have tested verbal rather than visual memory. The results of another longitudinal study with 7- to 8-year-old children also support the assumption that music lessons only improve verbal or auditory memory, but not visual memory (Roden et al. 2014). Furthermore, the results of a longitudinal study with 2 control groups (one with no additional lessons and one with additional science lessons) show that the children with additional music lessons had the greatest improvements in verbal memory (Roden et al. 2012). These studies are consistent in their reported impact of music lessons on verbal memory. However, such improvement was not found in all studies (Hallberg et al. 2017). For example, a short-term intervention of 5 weeks did not produce a measurable difference between kindergarteners who received music lessons and kindergarteners who did not receive additional lessons. Therefore, in order to prove an effect of music lessons on memory, an intervention duration of several months seems to be necessary.

Overall, similar to the adult studies, there appear to be positive effects of music lessons on verbal and auditory memory in childhood. The results regarding visual memory turn out to be rather inconsistent and require further clarification.

25.4.2.4 Music Lessons and Language

Music lessons appear to be associated with several skills relevant to language acquisition. In childhood, correlations exist between music lessons and vocabulary. In 9- to 11-year-old children, a comparison of children who had already received 4 years of music lessons with children who had not received music lessons showed a larger vocabulary in children with music lessons (Schlaug et al. 2005). An intervention study with preschool children yielded similar results: A computer-based musical intervention increased preschoolers' vocabulary (Moreno et al. 2011). Similarly, evidence of a relationship between music lessons and reading ability was found (Douglas and Willatts 1994; Hurwitz et al. 1975; Moreno et al. 2009) The results of two longitudinal studies (Hurwitz et al. 1975; Moreno et al. 2011) suggest an improvement in reading ability due to music lessons. Both studies examined the relationship at the elementary school age and showed improvement after participation in music lessons. While a Hawthorne effect cannot yet be ruled out as a possible explanation in the study by Hurwitz et al. (1975) due to an untrained control group, the evidence from the Moreno study can be interpreted quite clearly as a music-specific improvement in reading ability. One relationship between music lessons and language that may be particularly important in preschool-age is that between music lessons and phonological awareness. Phonological awareness is an essential precursor to literacy acquisition and is therefore very significant for school entry.

25.4.2.5 Music Lessons and Phonological Awareness

Phonological awareness is the insight into the sound structure of our language. It refers to the child's knowledge that phonemes are the building blocks of our language and it includes the ability to analyze and synthesize sounds (Jansen 1992). Phonological awareness is a precursor skill to written language acquisition (Bruck 1992; Pratt and Brady 1988) and, as such, is consistently the target of remedial programs to help children learn written language (reading and writing). Studies have demonstrated both short- and long-term effects of such phonological awareness support programs (Schneider et al. 1997, 1998). In addition to these specific programs to promote phonological awareness, there are also nonspecific approaches that seek to achieve improvement in phonological awareness by promoting other skills. One such approach is to promote phonological awareness through music lessons. Some studies showed a positive relationship between music lessons or musical perception skills and phonological awareness (Anvari et al. 2002; Lamb and Gregory 1993). In addition, Gromko (2005) demonstrated in a longitudinal study that kindergarten children who received music training for 4 months improved significantly in phonological awareness compared to children in a control group. However, there was no random assignment to control and experimental groups in this study. As mentioned above, such an approach could have led to systematic differences between the groups. In this case, it appears that there were indeed differences between the control and experimental groups with respect to socioeconomic status (Gromko 2005), which is why the results cannot be interpreted unambiguously. To prevent such systematic biases, Degé and Schwarzer (2011) assigned preschoolers randomly to three different groups in a longitudinal study: an experimental group that received music training, a control group that received a special phonological awareness program, and a control group that participated in a sports training program. Preschoolers in the three groups performed similarly in phonological awareness at baseline and were also comparable in the control variables (age, intelligence, and socioeconomic status). After 20 weeks of training, the music group and the phonological awareness group showed similar improvements in phonological awareness. In contrast, the sports group did not improve. Overall, based on these results, it can be concluded that phonological awareness can be promoted through music lessons. In a further study, it was shown that children with a migration background, who may have been at increased risk of developing reading and spelling difficulties, also benefited from music lessons to promote phonological awareness (Patscheke et al. 2016). In this study, the authors implemented a slightly modified form of Degé and Schwarzer's (2011) music program with children from immigrant backgrounds. Participating preschoolers were randomly assigned to a music group, a phonological awareness group, and a sports group. Also in this study, the children in the music group and the phonological awareness group improved in phonological awareness over the training period. In contrast, the children in the sports group showed no change in their phonological awareness.

Overall, the findings on the relationship between music lessons and language suggest that music lessons do indeed positively influence language and thus offer some developmental potential. Music lessons are intended as a supplement to established programs and should not replace them. The impact of music lessons does not appear to be limited to specific language skills and age levels. In general, it creates a positive learning environment in which children have positive learning experiences. Without the use of language support materials, children can virtually incidentally support their language development.

Explanations for the Relationship Between Music Lessons and Phonological Awareness

Two possible explanations for the nonspecific training effects of music lessons on phonological awareness assume neural mediation. Patel (2008) postulated the shared sound category learning mechanism hypothesis (SSCLMH), whereas Besson and colleagues postulate more sensitive processing of acoustic features (Besson et al. 2011). Patel (2008) hypothesizes that both music and speech are based on the mental representation of learned sound categories. Since there are two sound systems consisting of different categories (speech and music), a well-functioning mechanism for learning sound categories in general is very important. Therefore, he postulates that music and language use a common neural mechanism or process for learning sound categories. Another approach explains the connections between music and language at an even more fundamental level. Here, the connection between the two domains is made through sensitivity to acoustic parameters. It is hypothesized that music lessons increase sensitivity to acoustic parameters such as intonation in a sentence or even pitch perception. In this approach, it is brought together that the same brain structures and processes are involved in the different processing steps of music and speech and that musicians are more sensitive to acoustic parameters involved in both music and speech compared to nonmusicians (Besson et al. 2011; Bidelman et al. 2014). This enhanced perception of acoustic features leads musicians to form a more elaborate perceptual impression of speech than nonmusicians. This, in turn, facilitates the processing of speech.

25.5 Conclusion

Overall, many associations between music lessons and cognitive abilities are reported in the literature. Music lessons seem to be associated with both general abilities, such as intelligence, and specific cognitive abilities, such as mathematical abilities. Some cognitive abilities show a particularly promising association with music lessons. The methodological quality of the studies is such that it can be assumed that music lessons have an influence on the respective cognition and that this influence has practical significance. For example, music lessons seem to be able to promote important skills for successful school entry (executive functions, phonological awareness). Besides music lessons, other leisure activities can also have positive effects on child development. Drama lessons could not increase cognitive skills, but they could increase social skills. The effects of music lessons on child cognitive development are mostly small; however, they gain importance due to their sustainability (but see Costa-Giomi 1999 for controversial results). However, the influence of music lessons is not a miracle cure. Not all children should take music lessons as a precaution. On the one hand, the effects are not large enough for this to happen, and on the other hand, music lessons are something that also needs appropriate intrinsic motivation to be successfully implemented. This intrinsic motivation refers to the joy of making music as a cultural activity. Music lessons are, therefore, first and foremost a fulfilling leisure activity and can also be a valuable support opportunity.

References

Aleman A, Nieuwenstein MR, Böcker KBE, de Haan EHF (2000) Music training and mental imagery ability. Neuropsychologia 38(12):1664-1668. https://doi.org/10.1016/s0028-3932(00)00079-8

Anvari SH, Trainor LJ, Woodside J, Levy BA (2002) Relations among musical skills, phonological processing, and early reading ability in preschool children. J Exp Child Psychol 83(2):111–130. https://doi.org/10.1016/s0022-0965(02)00124-8

Atkinson RC, Shiffrin RM (1968) Human memory :A proposed system and its control processes. In: Spence KW (ed) The psychology of learning and motivation: advances in research and theory. Academic Press, Vol. 2, pp 89–195

Bahr N, Christensen CA (2000) Inter-domain transfer between mathematical skills and musicianship. J Struct Learn Intell Syst 14(3):187–197
Bastian HG (2000) Musik(erziehung) und ihre Wirkung (3. Auflage 2002 ed.). Schott Musik International
Benedict RHB (1997) Brief visuospatial memory test—revised. Psychological Assessment Resources
Benz S, Sellaro R, Hommel B, Colzato LS (2015) Music makes the world go round: the impact of musical training on non-musical cognitive functions—a review. Front Psychol 6
Besson M, Chobert J, Marie C (2011) Transfer of training between music and speech: common processing, attention, and memory. Front Psychol 2(94):1–12
Bialystok E, DePape AM (2009) Musical expertise, bilingualism, and executive functioning. J Exp Psychol Hum Percept Perform 35(2):565–74. https://doi.org/10.1037/a0012735
Bidelman GM, Weiss MW, Moreno S, Alain C (2014) Coordinated plasticity in brainstem and auditory cortex contributes to enhanced categorical speech perception in musicians. Eur J Neurosci 40:2662–2673
Bilhartz TD, Bruhn RA, Olson JE (1999) The effect of early music training on child cognitive development. J Appl Dev Psychol 20(4):615–636. https://doi.org/10.1016/S0193-3973(99)00033-7
Brandler S, Rammsayer TH (2003) Differences in mental abilities between musicians and non-musicians. Psychol Music 31(2):123–138
Brochard R, Dufour A, Despres O (2004) Effect of musical expertise on visuospatial abilities: evidence from reaction times and mental imagery. Brain Cogn 54(2):103–109. https://doi.org/10.1016/s0278-2626(03)00264-1
Bruck M. (1992) Persistence of dyslexics' phonological awareness deficits. Dev Psychol 28:874–886
Bugos JA, DeMarie D (2017) The effects of a short-term music program on preschool children`s executive functions. Psychology of Music 45(6):855–867
Butzlaff R (2000) Can music be used to teach reading? Journal of Aesthetic Education, 34(3-4):167–178. Go to ISI://000174688000008
Ceci SJ, Williams WM (1997) Schooling, intelligence, and income. Am Psychol 52(10):1051–1058. https://doi.org/10.1037/0003-066x.52.10.1051
Chan AS, Ho YC, Cheung MC (1998) Music training improves verbal memory. Nature 396(6707):128–128. https://doi.org/10.1038/24075
Cheek JM, Smith LR (1999) Music training and mathematics achievement. Adolescence 34(136):759–761
Corrigall KA, Schellenberg EG, Misura NM (2013) Music training, cognition, and personality. Front Psychol 4:222
Corrigall KA, Trainor LJ (2009) Effects of musical training on key and harmony perception. Ann N Y Acad Sci 1169:164–168. https://doi.org/10.1111/j.1749-6632.2009.04769.x
Costa-Giomi E (1999) The effects of three years of piano instruction on children's cognitive development. J Res Music Educ 47(3):198–212. Go to ISI://000083884900002
Degé F, Schwarzer G (2011) The effect of a music program on phonological awareness in preschoolers. Front Psychol 2:Article 124
Degé F, Schwarzer G (2017) Music lessons and verbal memor in 10- to 12-year-old children: investigating articulatory rehearsal as mechanism underlying this association. Psychomusicol Music Mind Brain 27(4):256–266
Degé F, Kubicek C, Schwarzer G (2011a) Music lessons and intelligence: a relation mediated by executive functions. Music Percept 29(2):195–201
Degé F, Müllensiefen D, Schwarzer G (2020) Musical abilities and phonological skills in 9- to 12-year-old children: Can singing abilities predict phonological awareness? Jahrbuch Musikpsychologie Vol. 29, Artikel e66. https://doi.org/10.5964/jbdgm
Degé F, Wehrum S, Stark R, Schwarzer G (2011b) The influence of two years of school music training in secondary school on visual and auditory memory. Eur J Dev Psychol 8(5):608–623. https://doi.org/10.1080/17405629.2011.590668
Diamond A (2013) Executive functions. Annu Rev Psychol 64:135–168
Diamond A, Lee K (2011) Interventions shown to aid executive function development in children 4 to 12 years old. Science 333:959–964

Douglas S, Willatts P (1994) The relationship between musical ability and literacy skills. J Res Read 17(2):99–107. http://ovidsp.ovid.com/ovidweb.cgi?T=JS&CSC=Y&NEWS=N&PAGE=fulltext&D=psyc3&AN=1995-11443-001; http://translate.google.com/#en|de|The+relationship+between+musical+ability+and+literacy+skills.Explored+a+possible+link+between+musical+ability+and+literacy+skills+in+78+children+%28aged+7.5-8.9+yrs%29.+Ss+were+tested+on+picture+vocabulary%2C+aural+awareness%2C+reading%2C+and+spelling.+Rhythm+was+significantly+related+to+reading+ability+and%2C+to+a+lesser+degree%2C+spelling+ability.+Pitch+was+significantly+related+to+reading+and+spelling%2C+except+when+vocabulary+was+partialled+out.+In+a+further+pilot+study+of+Ss+aged+8.1+to+10.8+yrs%2C+6+Ss+were+assigned+to+a+musical+program+intervention+group%2C+and+6+Ss+were+assigned+to+a+control+group.+Both+groups+were+matched+for+reading+ability+on+an+initial+test+and+were+administered+the+same+test+after+the+intervention.+Reading+scores+for+the+intervention+group+increased+from+initial+to+final+testing%2C+but+scores+for+the+controls+did+not+change.+Results+indicate+that+musical+skills+training+is+a+valuable+strategy+for+assisting+children+with+reading+difficulties.+%28French+abstract%29+%28PsycINFO+Database+Record+%28c%29+2010+APA%2C+all+rights+reserved%29

Forgeard M, Winner E, Norton A, Schlaug G (2008) Practicing a musical instrument in childhood is associated with enhanced verbal ability and nonverbal reasoning. PLoS One 3(10). https://doi.org/10.1371/journal.pone.0003566

Franklin MS, Moore KS, Yip CY, Jonides J, Rattray K, Moher J (2008) The effects of musical training on verbal memory. Psychol Music 36(3):353–365. https://doi.org/10.1177/0305735607086044

Frischen U, Schwarzer G, Degé F (2019) Comparing the effects of rhythm-based music training and pitch-based music training on executive functions in preschoolers. Front Integr Neurosci 13:41. https://doi.org/10.3389/fnint.2019.00041

Frischen U, Schwarzer G, Degé F (2021) Music lessons enhance executive functions in 6- to 7-year-old children. Learning and Instruction 74

Gardiner MF, Fox A, Knowles F, Jeffrey D (1996) Learning improved by arts training. Nature 381(6580):284–284. https://doi.org/10.1038/381284a0

Gordon RL, Fehd HM, McCandliss BD (2015) Does music training enhance literacy skills? A meta-analysis. Front Psychol https://doi.org/10.3389/fpsyg.2015.01777

Gromko JE (2005) The effect of music instruction on phonemic awareness in beginning readers. J Res Music Educ 53(3):199–209. https://doi.org/10.2307/3598679

Hallberg KA, Martin WE, McClure JR (2017) Teh Impact of Muisc Instruction on Attention in Kindergarten Children. Psychomusicology: Music, Mind, and Brain 27(2):113–121

Herrero L, Carriedo N (2022) The role of cognitive flexibility and inhibition in complex dynamic tasks: the case of sight reading music https://rdcu.be/b52wV. Current psychology (New Brunswick, N.J.) 1–13. https://doi.org/10.1007/s12144-020-00983-y

Hetland L (2000) Listening to music enhances spatial-temporal reasoning: Evidence for the Mozart Effect. Journal of aesthetic education 34(3-4):105–148. Go to ISI://000174688000006

Holochwost SJ, Propper Cb, Wolf DP, Willoughby MT, Fisher KR, Kolaczs J, Volpe V, Jaffee SR (2017) Music education, academic achievement, and executive functions. Psychology of Aesthetics, Creativity, and the Arts 11(2):147–166. https://doi.org/10.1037/aca0000112

Ho YC, Cheung MC, Chan AS (2003) Music training improves verbal but not visual memory: cross-sectional and longitudinal explorations in children. Neuropsychology 17(3):439–450. https://doi.org/10.1037/0894-4105.17.3.439

Hurwitz I, Wolff PH, Bortnick BD, Kokas K (1975) Nonmusical effects of the Kodaly music curriculum in primary grade children. J Learn Disabil 8(3):167–174

Jakobson LS, Cuddy LL, Kilgour AR (2003) Time tagging: a key to musicians' superior memory. Music Percept 20(3):307–313. https://doi.org/10.1525/mp.2003.20.3.307

Jakobson LS, Lewycky ST, Kilgour AR, Stoesz BM (2008) Memory for verbal and visual material in highly trained musicians. Music Percept 26(1):41–55. https://doi.org/10.1525/mp.2008.26.1.41

Jäncke L (2008) Macht Musik schlau? Neue Erkenntnisse aus den Neurowissenschaften und der kognitiven Psychologie. Huber

Jäncke L (2009) Planung, Handlung und Selbstkontrolle. Der Frontalkortex und die Musik [Planning, action, and self-control. The frontal cortex and music.]. In: BMBF (ed) Pauken mit Trompeten (pp 88-97). Bundesministerium für Bildung und Forschung

Jansen H (1992) Untersuchung zur entwicklung lautsynthetischer verarbeitungsprozesse im vorschul- und frühen grundschulalter. Hänsel-Hohenhausen

Janus M, Lee Y, Moreno S, Bialystok E (2016) Effects of Short Term Music and Second Language Training on Executive Control. J Exp Child Psychol 144:84–97. https://doi.org/10.1016/j.jecp.2015.11.009

Jaschke AC, Honing H, Scherder EJA (2018) Longitudinal analysis of music education on executive functions in primary school children [original research]. Front Neurosci 12. https://doi.org/10.3389/fnins.2018.00103

AR, Jakobson LS, Cuddy LL (2000) Music training and rate of presentation as mediators of text and song recall. Mem Cogn 28(5):700–710. https://doi.org/10.3758/bf03198404

Klauer KJ (2001) Handbuch kognitives Training (2 ed.). Hongrefe Verlag für Psychologie

Klauer KJ (2010) Transfer des Lernens: Warum wir oft mehr lernen als gelehrt wird. Kohlhammer

Klauer KJ (2011) Transfer des Lernens: Warum wir oft mehr lernen als gelehrt wird. Kohlhammer

Kubinger KD, Wurst E (1991) Adaptives Intelligenz Diagnostikum, 3. ergänzte Auflage ed. Beltz

Lamb SJ, Gregory AH (1993) The relationship between music and reading in beginning readers. Educ Psychol 13(1):19–27

Lepach AC, Petermann F (2008) Battery for Assessment in Children—Merk- und Lernfähigkeitstest für 6- bis 16-Jährige. Hans Huber

Magne C, Schön D, Besson M (2006) Musician children detect pitch violations in both music and language better than nonmusician children: behavioral and electrophysiological approaches. J Cogn Neurosci 18(2):199–211. https://doi.org/10.1162/089892906775783660

Mähler C, Stern E (2006) Transfer. In Rost DH (ed) Handwörterbuch Pädagogische Psychologie (3. überarb. u. erweit. Aufl. ed.). PVU

Moreno S, Bialystok E, Barac R, Schellenberg EG, Cepeda NJ, Chau T (2011) Short-term music training enhances verbal intelligence and executive function. Psychol Sci 22(11):1425–1433

Moreno S, Marques C, Santos A, Santos M, Castro SL, Besson M (2009) Musical training influences linguistic abilities in 8-year-old children: more evidence for brain plasticity. Cereb Cortex 19(3):712–723. https://doi.org/10.1093/cercor/bhn120

Myers GD (2006) Psychology. Worth Publishers, Inc

Nantais KM, Schellenberg EG (1999) The Mozart effect: an artifact of preference. Psychol Sci 10(4):370–373. https://doi.org/10.1111/1467-9280.00170

Neisser U, Boodoo G, Bouchard TJ, Boykin AW, Brody N, Ceci SJ, Halpern DF, Loehlin JC, Perloff R, Sternberg RJ, Urbina S (1996) Intelligence: knowns and unknowns. Am Psychol 51(2):77–101. https://doi.org/10.1037/0003-066x.51.2.77

Norton A, Winner E, Cronin K, Overy K, Lee DJ, Schlaug G (2005) Are there pre-existing neural, cognitive, or motoric markers for musical ability? Brain Cogn 59(2):124–134. https://doi.org/10.1016/j.bandc.2005.05.009

Okada BM, Slevc LR (2018) Individual differences in musical training and executive functions: A latent variabel approach. Mem Cognit 46(7):1076–1092

Orsmond GI, Miller LK (1999) Cognitive, musical and environmental correlates of early music instruction. Psychol Music 27:18–37

Osgood C (1962) Method and theory in experimental psychology. Oxford University Press.

Patel AD (2008) Music, language, and the brain. University Press

Patscheke H, Degé F, Schwarzer G (2016) The influence of a music programme on phonological awareness in preschoolers with migration background. Front Psychol 7(1647). https://doi.org/10.3389/fpsyg.2016.01647

Pratt AC, Brady S (1988) Relation of phonological awareness to reading disability in children and adults. J Educ Psychol 80:319–323

Rauscher FH, Zupan MA (2000) Classroom keyboard instruction improves kindergarten children's spatial-temporal performance: a field experiment. Early Child Res Q 15(2):215–228. https://doi.org/10.1016/s0885-2006(00)00050-8

Rauscher FH, Shaw GL, Ky KN (1993) Music and spatial task performance. Nature 365(6447):611. https://doi.org/10.1038/365611a0. http://www.nature.com/nature/journal/v365/n6447/pdf/365611a0.pdf
Rauscher FH, Shaw GL, Levine LJ, Wright EL, Dennis WR, Newcomb RL (1997) Music training causes long-term enhancement of preschool children's spatial-temporal reasoning. Neurol Res 19(1):2–8. https://doi.org/10.1080/01616412.1997.11740765
Roden I, Bongard S, Kreutz G (2012) Effects of a class-room based music program on verbal memory of primary school children within a longitudinal design. In: ICMPS-ESCOM 2012 joint conference, Thessaloniki/Greece
Roden I, Grube D, Bongard S, Kreutz G (2014) Does music training enhance working memory performance? Findings from a quasi-experimental longitudinal study. Psychology of Music 42(2):284–298
Român-Caballero R, Vadillo MA, Trainor LJ, Lupianez J (2022) Please don't stop the music: A meta-analysis of the cognitive and academic benefits of instrumental musical training in childhood and adolescence. Educational Research Review 35. https://doi.org/10.1016/j.edurev.2022.100436
Sala G, Gobet F (2017) Does far transfer exist? Negative evidence from chess, music, and working memory training. Curr Dir Psychol Sci 26:515–520. https://doi.org/10.1177/0963721417712760
Sala G. Gobet F (2020) Working memory training in typically developing children: A multilevel meta-analysis. Psychon Bull Rev 27, 423–434. https://doi.org/10.3758/s13423-019-01681-y
Schellenberg EG (2004) Music lessons enhance IQ. Psychol Sci 15(8):511–514. https://doi.org/10.1111/j.0956-7976.2004.00711.x.
Schellenberg EG (2006a) Exposure to music: the truth about the consequences. In: McPherson GE (ed) The child as musician: a handbook of musical development. Oxford University Press, pp 111–134
Schellenberg EG (2006b) Long-term positive associations between music lessons and IQ. J Educ Psychol 98(2):457–468. https://doi.org/10.1037/0022-0663.98.2.457
Schellenberg EG (2009) Music training and nonmusical abilities: Commentary on Stoesz, Jakobson, Kilgour, and Lewycky (2007) and Jakobson, Lewycky, Kilgour, and Stoesz (2008) [Editorial Material]. Music Perception 27(2):139–143. https://doi.org/10.1525/mp.2009.27.2.139
Schellenberg EG (2011) Examining the association between music lessons and intelligence. Br J Psychol 102:283–302. https://doi.org/10.1111/j.2044-8295.2010.02000.x
Schellenberg EG, Nakata T, Hunter PG, Tamoto S (2007) Exposure to music and cognitive performance: tests of children and adults. Psychol Music 35(1):5–19. https://doi.org/10.1177/0305735607068885
Schlaug G, Norton A, Overy K, Winner E (2005) Effects of music training on the child's brain and cognitive development. In: Avanzini G, Koelsch S, Lopez L, Majno M (eds) Neurosciences and music ii: from perception to performance. New York Acad Sciences Vol. 1060, pp 219–230. https://doi.org/10.1196/annals.1360.015
Schneider W, Kuspert P, Roth E, Vise M, Marx H (1997) Short-and long-term effects of training phonological awareness in kindergarten: Evidence from two German studies [Proceedings Paper]. J Exp Child Psychol 66(3):311–340. Go to ISI://A1997XW15700002
Schneider W, Roth E, Küspert P, Ennemoser M (1998) Kurz- und langfristige Effekte eines Trainings der sprachlichen (phonologischen) Bewusstheit bei unterschiedlichen Leistungsgruppen: Befunde einer Sekundäranalyse. Zeitschrift für Entwicklungspsychologie und Padagogische Psychologie 30(1):26–39
Sergeant D, Thatcher G (1974) Intelligence, social status and musical abilities. Psychol Music 2(2):32–57. https://doi.org/10.1177/030573567422005
Standley JM (2008) Does music instruction help children to learn to read? Evidence of a meta-analysis. Update Applied Research in Music Education 27:17–32.
Thompson WF, Schellenberg EG, Husain G (2001) Arousal, mood, and the Mozart effect. Psychol Sci 12(3):248–251. https://doi.org/10.1111/1467-9280.00345. http://pss.sagepub.com/content/12/3/248.full.pdf

Thompson WF, Schellenberg EG, Husain G (2004) Decoding speech prosody: do music lessons help? Emotion 4(1):46–64. https://doi.org/10.1037/1528-3542.4.1.46

Vaughn K (2000) Music and mathematics: modest support for the oft-claimed relationship. Journal of Aesthetic Education 34(3-4):149–166. https://doi.org/10.2307/3333641

Wechsler D (1991) Wechsler intelligence scale for children, 3rd edn. Psychological Corporation

Weiß R, Osterland J (1977) Grundintelligenztest CFT 1. Westermann

Zelazo PD, Carlson SM, Kesek A (2008) The development of executive function in childhood. In: Nelson CA, Luciana M (eds) Handbook of developmental cognitive neuroscience. MIT Press, 2 ed, pp 553–574

Zuk J, Benjamin C, Kenyon A, Gaab N (2014) Behavioral and neural correlates of executive functioning in musicians and non-musicians. PlosS One 9(6)

Positive Effects of Music Making on Perception and Cognition from a Neuroscientific Perspective

26

Annemarie Seither-Preisler and Peter Schneider

Since the end of the nineteenth century, scientists have been investigating why individuals differ in their cognitive and artistic abilities. Empirical psychology, and particularly intelligence research, has had a strong influence on the later development of creativity research. From the outset, the question of the interplay between these two domains was posed. Are intelligent individuals also particularly creative? Do activities such as painting, dancing, or making music have positive effects on the ability to solve problems or articulate well verbally? Can such effects also be demonstrated in the brain?

26.1 Measurement of Cognitive and Musical Abilities

First, a brief outline will be provided on how cognitive and musical abilities are measured to systematically investigate and relate them to each other.

Intelligence research has a history of approximately 100 years. Cattell (1941) introduced an early model of human intelligence that remains relevant today. This model distinguishes between two types of intelligence: genetically determined fluid intelligence, which is reflected in processing speed and general abilities of reasoning and problem-solving, and acquired crystallized intelligence, which manifests in vocabulary, knowledge, and specific solution strategies. Empirical studies have shown that fluid intelligence peaks around the age of 20 and then declines slightly but continuously, whereas crystallized intelligence can continue to increase into old age (Cavanaugh and Blanchard-Fields 2011).

A. Seither-Preisler (✉) · P. Schneider (✉)
Department of Psychology, Music Psychology and Brain Research Section, Karl-Franzens-University, Graz, Austria
e-mail: annemarie.seither-preisler@uni-graz.at; peter.schneider@uni-graz.at

G. Kreutz, G. Bernatzky (eds.), *Music and Medicine*, Neurocultural Health and Wellbeing, https://doi.org/10.1007/978-3-662-72175-9_26

From the early days, there was a controversial debate about whether intelligence is a unified phenomenon or consists of multiple, independent "intelligences." This question is relevant because the likelihood of transfer effects from the musical to the cognitive domain is higher if there are overarching factors that connect both domains. Moreover, it is essential to consider to what extent cognitive and musical abilities represent stable aptitudes or are viewed as plastic and learning-dependent. While Cattell supported the idea of a general intelligence factor, Thurstone (1938) proposed a series of largely independent factors covering verbal, numerical, visuo-spatial domains, as well as memory and processing speed. Later, dimensional models were developed that assumed several hierarchical factors with a general factor, the "g-factor," at the top. The first proponent of this approach was Joy Paul Guilford (1967), who presented the Structure-of-Intellect model. This model inspired many scientists to further develop the approach, and until today it is widely accepted in its basic form (Neubauer and Stern 2007; Stern and Neubauer 2013).

John B. Carroll (1993) proposed a dimensional model that includes a general factor, seven secondary abilities, and a number of additional subordinate tertiary factors. The secondary factors encompass not only the classical cognitive domains but also visual and auditory perception, thus establishing some connection to artistic and musical domains. Additionally, there have been approaches aimed at incorporating social skills and creativity into the concept of intelligence. Notably, Howard Gardner's (1983) theory of multiple intelligences is one such approach, which includes, alongside linguistic, logical-mathematical, and intra- and interpersonal intelligences (related to emotional and social abilities), aesthetic domains such as bodily kinesthetic, spatial-visual, and musical-rhythmic intelligences. Gardner identifies characteristics of musical intelligence as pitch, timbre, and rhythm perception, as well as the ability to experience the emotional effects of music. He posits that each intelligence domain is represented in the brain by its own processing system, as brain damage can lead to the loss of specific functions. This is evident, for instance, when musical abilities are impaired without significant impact on cognitive abilities. Additionally, within these domains, specific high or low talents may occur.

In addition to intelligence models that have attempted to integrate musical aspects, standalone models for assessing musicality have also been developed. Methodologically, these are closely related to intelligence research. Wing (1939/1961) advocated a general factor model of musicality, including specific areas such as rhythmic, melodic, and harmonic abilities. In contrast, Seashore (1919) in his early research proposed that these abilities are independent subdomains.

As a middle ground, Edwin Gordon (1965, 1986) proposed an eclectic model, which is favored by many researchers in musicality. While historical tests by Wing and Seashore considered musicality more as a performance characteristic ("musical achievement") assessable through auditory discrimination thresholds, Gordon focused on stable predispositions ("musical aptitude") and more complex information processing. He distinguished between melodic and rhythmic pitch representations and musical sensitivity to phrasing, suggesting that individuals have specific aptitude profiles in these dimensions. Moreover, similar to the structural models of intelligence, Gordon proposed that these subdomains are interconnected and can be viewed as aspects of the overarching trait of musicality.

According to Gordon's musical learning theory, musical aptitude is expressed in the ability of "audiation." The term was coined by Gordon himself and describes the extent of mental sound imagery.

> Audiation is the ability to hear and understand music that is not physically present but is imaginatively conceived. For music, audiation is akin to what thinking is for language.

Just as one thinks while listening to language or engages in inner speech when thinking, audiation occurs when listening to and imagining music. Thus, Gordon situates the concept of musicality close to linguistic abilities, which also play a significant role in intelligence models. From this perspective, transfer effects between the two domains seem plausible. According to existing empirical findings, the potential for sound imagery is believed to be in a sensitive developmental phase until about the age of 9 (Gordon 1986), influencing both the individual musical maturation process and the associated neural networking of specific auditory and general cognitive/emotional brain functions (Koelsch et al. 2005; Zatorre 2003). After this period, audiation appears to enter a stable phase, during which performance continues to improve, but the extent of change is largely predictable based on the inherent potential.

26.2 Musical Transfer Effects

The Göttingen professor of education, Christian Rittelmeyer, dedicated a book to the topic of aesthetic education and its transfer effects on cognitive abilities. In this work, he extensively discusses the positive side effects of arts education, music education, as well as engagement with theater and dance. Based on the available research material, he argues "in a time when artistic school subjects are increasingly marginalized in favor of mathematical, scientific, and language-related competencies" (Rittelmeyer 2012, back cover) for a revaluation of aesthetic education. At the same time, he emphasizes that the formative impact of aesthetic activities is not limited to transfer effects and should not be the primary goal of educational promotion. Similarly, the German musical aptitude researcher Wilfried Gruhn qualifies the significance of potential transfer effects (Gruhn 2003, p. 100):

> The ongoing debate regarding the cognitive effects of musical education should not obscure the primary objective, which is to introduce children to music as a fundamental means of expression. Its rhythmic and melodic foundations originate from vital human needs, rather than instrumentalizing music solely for its uncertain side effects.

Although this position should find broad support, it is a fact that transfer effects are often cited in educational policy discussions as justification for artistic and musical education. Therefore, in the following, we will examine the empirical evidence for such effects in more detail.

In the field of transfer research, various types of effects are distinguished. Positive transfer refers to an improvement, while negative transfer denotes a deterioration in performance related to the original training area. Concepts such as "near transfer" or "lateral transfer" describe the application of learned competencies to situations of comparable complexity, whereas "far transfer" or "vertical transfer" involve applying these competencies to dissimilar situations or tasks of higher complexity (Neubauer and Stern 2007; Neubauer et al. 2005). An example of near transfer is the effect of active music-making on auditory perception, including speech recognition. An example of far transfer is the effect on cognitive abilities such as problem-solving, mathematical, or literacy skills.

Research into the relationship between intelligence and creativity, as well as intelligence and musicality, typically reveals moderate but consistently positive correlations. For instance, Feist and Barron (2003) reported that highly creative individuals such as artists, scientists, and writers generally exhibit high general intelligence. Anecdotally, exceptional composers like Mozart, Bach, or Beethoven are believed to have had exceptionally high intelligence, although this assumption cannot be empirically verified post hoc. Empirical studies indicate that musically gifted individuals generally have at least above-average IQ (Kormann 1989). The correlations found between intelligence and musicality in various studies range between 0.2 and 0.45, explaining between 4% and 20% of the variance. Comparisons between adult musicians and nonmusicians have shown that the former perform significantly better in terms of perceptual speed and flexibility of perceptual organization (Helmbold et al. 2006, 2007). The authors speculate that musicians' enhanced perceptual abilities may either be inherent to musical talent or developed as a result of frequent musical training.

Gruhn (2003) explored whether there is a relationship between musical abilities and cognitive processing speed in young children aged 3–7 years. A comparison of children with and without music lessons revealed that the former performed significantly better. Furthermore, a clear positive correlation was observed between cognitive processing speed and the duration of musical training. In a study by Lynn et al. (1989) involving elementary school children, the relationship between general intelligence and the ability to discriminate rhythms and pitches was also examined, with positive correlations found between intelligence and musicality test results.

In recent years, several studies have examined the effects of active music-making on auditory abilities and whether these, in turn, affect linguistic and language-related functions. Schön et al. (2004) investigated whether adult musicians differ from nonmusicians in their ability to detect pitch deviations in musical sequences and spoken sentences. Musicians not only performed better in the musical domain, as expected, but also demonstrated superior skills in recognizing speech intonation. Additionally, brain responses measured through auditory evoked potentials and fields showed that musicians were more sensitive to pitch deviations. A subsequent study found similar differences between children at an age of about 8 years who were either playing or not playing a musical instrument (Magne et al. 2006).

A meaningful longitudinal study on cognitive near and far transfer in children and adolescents comes from a Chinese research group (Ho et al. 2003), which examined the linguistic and spatial-visual memory performance of 6- to 15-year-olds. One group had received musical training before the study began, which continued over the 1-year investigation period. Another group started receiving music lessons at the beginning of the study. At the outset, children with prior musical training performed better in linguistic memory tasks, despite similar socioeconomic background, but not in spatial-visual memory tasks. Over the study period, the linguistic memory of these children continued to improve. Even children who had not received music lessons before the study showed significantly improved linguistic memory after 1 year of musical training, but no improvement in spatial-visual memory. Conversely, children who had discontinued music lessons prematurely showed no increase in linguistic memory performance. Overall, these results indicate that music education led to positive near transfer effects in linguistic memory but not in spatial-visual memory.

Another frequently cited longitudinal study by Schellenberg (2004) involved 144 children randomly assigned to one of the four groups. One group received piano lessons, another singing lessons, a third group acting lessons, while the fourth group received no additional instruction. After 1 year, all groups showed a moderate increase in intelligence quotient (IQ), with the two music groups showing significantly greater gains. Acting training, however, led to significant improvements in social competence. The finding of a modest increase in intellectual abilities, although relatively small, was replicated in follow-up studies by the research group (Schellenberg 2006, 2011; Thompson et al. 2004). Glenn Schellenberg points out that both the mechanisms underlying the postulated transfer effects and their specificity (enhancement of linguistic and spatial abilities or general intelligence) require further research. The studies cited used the Wechsler Intelligence Scale for Children (WISC-III), which places particular emphasis on verbal abilities.

Interesting is also a large-scale study conducted in Switzerland with 1200 students (Weber et al. 1993). In the study, 17 classes with additional music lessons were compared with an equal number of control classes matched in terms of socioeconomic status regarding academic performance in the subjects of Mathematics, German, and French. In the music classes, instruction in core subjects was reduced by 1 h each. Nonetheless, in the lower grades, regular classes and music classes performed equally well in achievement tests. However, in the middle grades, there was a certain decline in performance in Mathematics and German in the music classes, likely due to the reduction in regular hours. Interestingly, the results reversed in the upper grades, where Mathematics and German performance was even better than in the control group. No effects were found for French or general intelligence development across all classes, suggesting that direct teaching practices had a strong influence on the results achieved in each class.

In another study conducted in Switzerland, Wetter et al. (2009) examined with a statistical regression model which factors influenced the academic performance of 134 children. Factors considered included school grade level, gender, parental income, instrumental lessons, and arts and crafts education (drawing, painting, working with wood and textiles). Academic performance was measured by grade point average. Both school grade level and parental income, as well as instrumental lessons, independently showed a significant influence on academic performance. Musically trained children performed significantly better in the subjects of German, French, Mathematics, History, Art, and Music—after adjusting for socioeconomic differences—but not in Sports, compared to non-musically trained children.

A longitudinal study that became widely known in the German-speaking public was conducted by Bastian (2000) over several years in elementary schools in Berlin. The sample included 170 children, with 47 receiving regular school education and the remaining 123 receiving additional music lessons. The study measured social competence and cognitive abilities, including basic intelligence, everyday knowledge, verbal-logical reasoning, spatial-visual imagination, speed of symbolic information processing in manual-visual tasks, mathematical ability, and attention performance. However, the study results should be interpreted cautiously, since the initial sample sizes were uneven, more than a quarter of the children dropped out of the study prematurely, not all tests were applied to all children, and the results were not published in peer-reviewed journals. Therefore, the results of the study published in book form are not explicitly discussed here. Short summaries in German can be found in the BMBF volume "Does Mozart Make You Smarter?" (Schumacher et al. 2006) and in Jäncke (2008).

Moreno et al. (2009) conducted a longitudinal study examining the effects of active music-making on child development. Participants were musically inexperienced children who received either music or painting lessons for 6 months as part of the study. Only children assigned to the music group showed significant improvements in the recognition of speech melody and, notably, also in a reading test at the end of the study. Additionally, in the music group's auditory brain areas, there was evidence of sensitization to language stimuli. Therefore, the study concluded on a positive near transfer from music to language and a far transfer to reading and writing skills, which were effective even in children.

The authors of the present article conducted a 12 year longitudinal study in Germany (AMseL)[1] with 220 participants as part of the JeKi accompanying research program.[2] At the beginning of the study, the tested individuals were in the primary school age, while at the end, they were young adults. Results revealed that musical training not only induced significant neuroplastic changes in auditory cortex, indicating an increase in neural efficiency, but also improved auditory skills, attention, and literacy competencies (Seither-Preisler et al. 2014; Schneider and Seither-Preisler 2015; Serrallach et al. 2016; Schneider et al. 2022, 2023).

> Children and adolescents who regularly made music showed not only better discrimination skills for pitches, timbres, tone lengths, and rhythms but also a lower tendency to ADHD,

[1] The study "Audio- and Neuroplasticity of Musical Learning" (AMseL) conducted by the authors of this chapter was funded by the Federal Ministry of Education and Research (BMBF) as part of the accompanying research for the educational program "Jedem Kind ein Instrument" (JeKi) as a joint project 01KJ0809/01KJ0810.

[2] https://www.musik.tu-dortmund.de/fileadmin/user_upload/Musikpaedagogische_Forschungsstelle/Sammelband.pdf

higher auditory and visual sustained attention, and better impulse control. Furthermore, there were clear music-related advantages with regard to reading and spelling skills.

Musically active children demonstrated superiority in reading speed, phonetic spelling (alphabetic strategy), the segmentation of words into meaningful units (morphometric strategy), the application of spelling rules (orthographic strategy), and the correct spelling of difficult word parts (grapheme hits). These effects persisted even after controlling for the influences of parental educational background, parental attention given to their children, financial resources, and children's leisure activities. This supports the notion that making music has an independent positive impact on literacy acquisition beyond social influences. However, the study did not find music-related advantages for mathematical skills and drawing creativity. This is not surprising from our perspective, as these activities activate brain regions with little relation to auditory processing.

Slevc and Miyake (2006) explored whether there is a relationship between musical ability and the ability to learn a second language after childhood. The study found a significant positive correlation between musical skills and the ability to recognize speech sounds, but not grammatical structures. In a neuroscientific study by Jentschke et al. (2005), the relationship between the processing of musical and linguistic syntax structures was investigated. Two groups of children were tested: one group consisted of boys from the Leipzig Thomaner Choir with singing training, and the other group consisted of children without musical training. The non-singing group was further divided into subgroups, one with typical development and another with deficits in language development. The study examined how the presentation of syntactically incorrect sentences and unharmonious sequences of musical chords affected cortical activation. The Thomaner choirboys exhibited stronger activation in specific brain regions in response to both syntactically incorrect sentences and unharmonious chord sequences compared to children without singing training. The authors interpreted these results as evidence of a positive near transfer from the musical to the linguistic domain, attributing it to the overlap between music and language processing regions in the brain (Jentschke et al. 2005, 2008; Patel et al. 1998; Schuppert et al. 2000). The comparison between the typically developing and language-impaired non-singing children also revealed interesting differences. While the typically developing children showed characteristic brain responses to unharmonious musical sequences, these responses were absent in children with language development deficits. Apparently, these children were unable to process the musical syntax of what they heard.

26.3 The Relationship Between Music and Literacy Skills

The ability to disengage from the semantic content of language and understand that sentences are composed of words, words of syllables, and syllables of sounds is a crucial prerequisite for acquiring literacy (Wagner and Torgesen 1987). Children suffering from dyslexia often exhibit reduced phonological awareness, which makes it difficult for them to recognize speech sounds and assign meanings to them. Various studies have shown that phonological awareness is linked to the ability to distinguish fundamental acoustic features (Anvari et al. 2002; Lamb and Gregory 1993). It is estimated that about 40% of children with dyslexia also have deficits in auditory information processing (Hämäläinen et al. 2013). Although dyslexic children frequently exhibit deficits in central auditory processing (Serrallach et al. 2016), they are also often characterized by other problems, such as attention and learning deficits (Landerl and Willburger 2010).

In cases of mild central auditory impairment, poor discrimination of fundamental acoustic features is believed to lead to a blurred perception of language, which initially hinders the development of differentiated phonological representations (Bishop et al. 1999) and later impedes literacy acquisition (Castles and Coltheart 2004; Goswami 2011; Huss et al. 2011). Issues with rapid temporal processing, such as distinguishing between plosive sounds (e.g., "b" vs. "p," "d" vs. "t," "g" vs. "k") or rhythmic patterns, seem to play a particularly significant role (Tallal and Gaab 2006).

Neuroscientific studies provide critical insights into the neural mechanisms underlying such deficits. It has been shown that at the brainstem level, where acoustic information is automatically preprocessed, speech stimuli are encoded more precisely in children with good reading skills compared to those with poor reading skills (Hornickel et al. 2009). In the auditory cortex, the left hemisphere is specialized for detecting rapid temporal changes at a rate of about 40 Hz, while the right hemisphere predominantly detects slow changes at a rate of about 4 Hz. The left-sided, rapid analysis enables fine auditory discrimination of plosive sounds, which are often confused by individuals with dyslexia during writing. Conversely, right-sided processing is crucial for the rhythmic structuring of heard syllables and words, which is essential for understanding linguistic meaning. It is likely that a disturbance in fine temporal analysis leads to a disruption in coarse rhythmic structuring, causing both issues to typically occur together (Seither-Preisler et al. 2014). This likely has negative implications for the ability to transfer acoustic elements (e.g., syllables or meaning-bearing word segments) into the phonological storage and retrieve them automatically when needed to alleviate the working memory load. As a result, the auditory working memory in individuals with dyslexia becomes overwhelmed more quickly than usual, leading to overload and stress in complex listening situations. Consistent with these assumptions, Meyer et al. (2012) demonstrated that temporal processing is impaired in both the left and right hemispheres in individuals with dyslexia. The neuroscientific longitudinal study AMseL, conducted by the authors of this chapter, further suggests that in children with dyslexia, the two auditory cortices work less synchronously compared to their non-dyslexic peers (Serrallach et al. 2016; Seither-Preisler & Schneider, in preparation). Additionally, it has been shown that the automation deficits often observed in individuals with dyslexia are associated with reduced temporal precision in auditory signal processing (Chandrasekaran et al. 2009; Strait et al. 2011).

Against this background, the question arises as to whether such abnormalities are congenital or due to learning deficits and whether they can be compensated for by special support measures. An enlightening study by Skoe et al. (2013) showed that poverty and low parental education levels are associated with reduced temporal precision in auditory signal processing at the brainstem level. Another study by Hornickel et al. (2012) demonstrated that children with reading and writing difficulties who used a special hearing aid for a year at school showed significant improvements in literacy skills. This improvement was not observed in children who did not have access to such a device. Both findings strikingly illustrate the impact of environmental factors on auditory processing. Particularly interesting is the finding that playing music can enhance the temporal precision of neural coding, with positive effects increasing with years of musical experience (Kraus and Chandrasekaran 2010; Strait and Kraus 2014). Moreover, a study by Skoe and Kraus (2012) demonstrated that individuals who played an instrument as children continued to show more precise neural response patterns as adults. These advantages were observed for both musical sounds and speech (Musacchia et al. 2007; Wong et al. 2007). For instance, musicians were better able to distinguish sounds like /ba/ and /ga/, which was evident in more precise timing of the elicited neural impulses (Parbery-Clark et al. 2012). This could explain the aforementioned near transfer from the musical to the linguistic domain and suggests that making music could also help mitigate issues in the literacy domain.

The research group led by British music psychologist Katie Overy studied children with and without reading and writing difficulties, focusing on their linguistic and musical abilities (Overy 2003; Overy et al. 2003). The results showed that children with dyslexia performed worse in both areas on tests of temporal stimulus perception. Consequently, the authors hypothesized that active music-making, particularly rhythmic training, would have a beneficial effect on dyslexia. This hypothesis was confirmed in later studies. Katie Overy developed a musical training program for children with reading and writing difficulties, primarily utilizing rhythm games. The program was implemented in a longitudinal study over a period of 15 weeks, conducted three times a week for 20–30 min each session. Compared to an untrained group, the training group showed significantly improved rhythmic, phonological, and literacy skills after this period.

26.4 Neural Correlates of Intelligence, Creativity, and Musicality

A currently prominent branch of psychological research examines how cognitive and musico-creative abilities of humans manifest in the structure and function of the brain. Although intelligence is a complex trait arising from the interplay of various brain functions, neuroanatomical investigations reveal discernible patterns. Positive correlations have been observed between intelligence and the volume of gray matter (neurons), white matter (nerve fibers), and overall brain size (Posthuma et al. 2002). Particularly, gray matter volume in the frontal cortex (frontal lobe) appears crucial for intelligence (Thompson et al. 2001). Twin studies suggest that these neurological characteristics are largely heritable (Neubauer and Stern 2007). Furthermore, the continuous increase in intelligence during childhood and adolescence correlates with a maturation-related increase in cortical thickness (Shaw et al. 2006).

Apart from these structural characteristics, individual differences and maturation-related changes in functional brain activation are evident. When repeatedly exposing individuals to visual or auditory stimuli, such as light flashes or tones, and measuring their characteristic brain responses (evoked potentials), it becomes evident that response patterns vary to some extent among individuals. During childhood development, these responses accelerate due to natural maturation of the central nervous system (Eggermont and Ponton 2002; Seither-Preisler et al. 2014; Schneider et al. 2023; Sharma et al. 1997, 2005). This acceleration is attributed to the increasing myelination of nerve fibers with age, enhancing the speed and efficiency of signal transmission in both the peripheral nervous system and the brain. In the auditory cortex, the maturation process comes to a halt in adolescence in primary regions, which are responsible for elementary sound processing. Conversely, in secondary regions, which enable complex auditory pattern recognition, this development continues into adulthood (Schneider et al. 2023). Similarly, higher human brain functions in the frontal cortex have been found to extend beyond puberty into young adulthood. Around the ages of 65–70, the myelin sheath begins to slowly decline, coinciding with corresponding declines in performance in behavioral tests, particularly in terms of reaction speed.

Interestingly, cortical response patterns in adults are influenced, among other factors, by their intelligence, with more intelligent individuals generally exhibiting slightly faster neural reactions (Bazana and Stelmack 2002; Ertl and Schafer 1969). A study conducted by the authors of this chapter (Seither-Preisler et al. 2014; Schneider et al. 2023) found a similar pattern concerning musical activities. Specifically, neuronal responses in the auditory cortex of musically trained children were faster and more synchronized compared to non-musically trained children.

> It is likely that high musical creativity is associated with a state akin to flow, which is mediated through the frontal cortex. This state enables individuals to largely ignore external stimuli and focus fully on the current musical performance.

While focused activation of specific brain regions with simultaneous inhibition of all other functions characterizes intelligent problem-solving, in the realm of creativity and the arts, the opposite applies to some extent. Here, cortical networks and activations are extensive and integrative (Bhattacharya et al. 2001; Bhattacharya and Petsche 2005), with the frontal cortex appearing to ensure undisturbed access to the diverse contents stored in memory.

However, creative achievements are not only characterized by openness to novelty (divergent phase). After the flood of ideas, there is also a need to organize and evaluate them, separating the wheat from the chaff. This requires concentration, which involves narrowing the focus once again (convergent phase). Thus, artistic and creative accomplishments represent a dynamic balance between openness and focus, which in the brain manifests as an interplay between widespread integration and restrictive neural efficiency. The creative personality would therefore be characterized by the ability to flexibly operate in either divergent or convergent modes depending on the demand and phase, and to harmonize both optimally.

26.5 Individual Differences in Auditory Perception and Neuronal Information Processing

Next, we explore the extent to which individual differences in sound perception, auditory ability, and auditory impairments can be explained from a neuroscientific point of view. How does music induce neuroplastic changes in the brain? To what extent are there structural and functional peculiarities that—possibly also predisposed—can explain the different effects of music?

As a pioneer in neural auditory research, Lawrence Parsons from Texas used positron emission tomography (PET) to investigate the neural activity during the memorized performance of virtuoso piano music in the brain. Professional pianists were placed in the scanner with a nonmetallic keyboard imitation and were asked to play the third movement of Johann Sebastian Bach's Italian Concerto. In a control condition, they were asked to play simple scales. The results showed that during memorized performance, there was a focused activation of essential centers, whereas scale playing activated additional irrelevant areas (Parsons et al. 2005).

Canadian researcher Robert Zatorre further investigated the differential processing of spectral and temporal aspects of sound perception (Zatorre and Belin 2001). He found that tone duration and rhythm predominantly mapped to the left hemisphere, while spectral components such as timbre and melody contour were predominantly processed in the right hemisphere. A more detailed analysis revealed that the focus of auditory processing was in the Heschl's gyrus, named after Viennese anatomist Richard Ladislaus Heschl and located bilaterally in the center of the auditory cortex.

Neuroanatomical studies have shown that musicians typically have significantly enlarged auditory cortices (Gaser and Schlaug 2003; Schlaug et al. 1995; Schneider et al. 2002, 2023; Seither-Preisler et al. 2014). Moreover, they exhibit larger brain waves when listening to musical stimuli (Shahin et al. 2003; Schneider et al. 2023). Already passive listening to music led to significantly stronger brain activation in musicians, especially in the primary and secondary auditory core areas (Schneider et al. 2005). Active music-making was reflected in additional connectivity with non-auditory functions, such as involvement of the audio-motor loop (Altenmüller 2008), spatial imagination (Sluming et al. 2007), and synchronization of multisensory networks (Wengenroth et al. 2013). In the following, some neuroanatomical characteristics of the auditory cortex are highlighted, which are most likely already present in early childhood and are associated with specific talents or deficits.

26.5.1 Absolute Pitch

Absolute pitch is the ability to identify or produce a specific tone immediately and effortlessly without external aids. Neuroanatomically, absolute pitch skills were found to correlate with an enlargement or medial duplication of the right Heschl's gyrus. Neurofunctionally, a processing center has been identified in that area, which is interconnected with a right-hemispheric network of motor, sensory, and visual brain regions (Wengenroth et al. 2013).

26.5.2 Tinnitus

A second specific phenomenon is tinnitus, the perception of ringing, buzzing, or hissing sounds in the ear. The occurrence of tinnitus correlates with a volume reduction (approximately 60%) in the sound-processing areas of the primary auditory cortex on the affected side. Interestingly, compared to nonmusicians, musicians show a significantly lower risk of developing tinnitus, and in cases where it does occur, they experience less emotional distress and shorter duration, suggesting a protective effect of musical training (Schneider et al. 2009).

26.5.3 Williams-Beuren Syndrome (WBS)

A third auditory specificity is the Williams-Beuren syndrome (WBS), a genetically determined condition associated with a unique auditory perception and affinity for music and everyday sounds. Patients with WBS exhibit a distinct neurocognitive profile due to a mutation on chromosome 7, characterized by significant weaknesses in the logical-spatial domain juxtaposed with strengths in the musical-linguistic domain. From early childhood, individuals with WBS show enthusiasm for rhythmically emphasized music genres such as pop, folk, country, and rock, and they exhibit a noticeable leftward asymmetry in neuronal measurements. Their Heschl's gyri display a characteristic rooted gyrification pattern similar to that seen in musicians. Due to psychomotor deficits, WBS subjects are unable to participate in conventional music education programs, making the neurological findings a genetic model of musicality and providing valuable insights into a genetic, training-independent component of musical ability (Wengenroth et al. 2010).

To further elucidate predisposed and environmentally influenced factors, longitudinal studies are necessary, which have been rare in neurological research thus far. The research group led by the German music researcher Gottfried Schlaug demonstrated in a comprehensive longitudinal study that musically trained children aged 5–7 years show a trend toward transfer effects of early musical education in the linguistic, spatial-visual, and mathematical domains, accompanied by neuroplastic changes in auditory association areas in the temporal lobe and temporal-parietal connections (Forgeard et al. 2008; Hyde et al. 2009; Schlaug et al. 2005).

The results of the longitudinal AMseL study conducted on 220 elementary school children reveal that musically trained children exhibit an enlarged Heschl's gyrus, particularly in the right hemisphere (Seither-Preisler et al. 2014; Schneider et al. 2023). Comparable findings had previously been observed in a cross-sectional study involving adult musicians and nonmusicians (Schneider et al. 2002). However, at the time of that investigation, it was unclear whether the observed differences in gray matter volume were primarily a result of long-term intensive instrumental practice or should be regarded as stable indicators of musical ability. The recent AMseL study on children now demonstrates that such morphological peculiarities are already present at a very early stage when children are still at the beginning of their musical training. Practically no changes in the shape and volume of Heschl's gyrus were observed between the first and second measurement points, 1 year apart (Seither-Preisler et al. 2014; Schneider et al. 2023). This suggests that these features are established prior to elementary school and the onset of formal music education.

Thus far, it remains unclear whether the significant individual differences in the morphological structure of the auditory cortex are genetically determined, influenced by prenatal hormonal factors, or explained by early auditory learning experiences. Particularly noteworthy from the present findings is that even after controlling for prior musical experience, the individual morphology of the right Heschl's gyrus allowed predictions regarding how much time children would invest in practicing their instruments in the future. Greater size of the right Heschl's gyrus correlated with higher practice intensities. Therefore, it is likely that individual differences in the size and shape of this structure are not merely a consequence of musical training but are already present in elementary school-aged children, indicating their musical interest or potential.

These findings also have (musical) educational implications, briefly discussed as follows. We assume that specific neuroanatomical dispositions in the auditory cortex provide insights into a person's musical aptitude. A favorable disposition apparently increases intrinsic motivation to engage in instrumental play. High practice intensity, in turn, leads to further learning effects and influences the development of perceptual abilities, cognitive skills, and brain functions positively. This results in transfer effects, improving general auditory perception, attention, language comprehension, and literacy skills.

Pedagogy plays a crucial role in fostering or, under unfavorable circumstances, inhibiting this developmental process. Therefore, it is important to identify latent talents as early as possible and support them. Sensitively observing what children engage in independently, willingly, and persistently can provide valuable insights. Furthermore, it is essential for educators to guide and support specific practice behaviors, aiming to facilitate and accelerate neuroplastic learning processes. The goal is to fully exploit the latent potentials already present in the individual's profile of talents, ultimately developing them into mature competence profiles. Given that learning success and the extent of neuroplasticity likely correlate directly with the individual's inherent potential, it seems effective to focus pedagogically on the strongest areas of talent and expect that even deficit areas will benefit from such support.

26.6 Conclusions

A comparative overview of research on musicality, intelligence, and creativity reveals commonalities, demonstrating that basic auditory perceptual abilities can influence higher cognitive functions. This is supported by findings on transfer effects from musical to cognitive domains. Musically active children not only exhibit enhanced abilities in discriminating pitch, timbre, duration, and rhythm but also show reduced tendencies toward ADHD, improved auditory and visual sustained attention, and better impulse control. Furthermore, significant musically induced advantages in reading and writing skills are evident.

Recent neuroscientific findings attribute these effects to an accelerated maturation of auditory areas induced by musical engagement, which are closely associated with brain regions involved in attentional control, working memory, and language processing. Studies have also indicated that children with ADHD and dyslexia, who often experience auditory perceptual and processing deficits, exhibit inadequate cooperation between the right and left auditory cortices. Since making music counteracts this problem, it is advisable to develop playful training programs for such children that start at the level of elementary hearing.

References

Altenmüller E (2008) Neurology of musical performance. Clin Med 8:410–413

Anvari SH, Trainor LJ, Woodside J, Levy BA (2002) Relations among musical skills, phonological processing, and early reading ability in preschool children. J Exp Child Psychol 83(2):111–130

Bastian HG (2000) Musik(erziehung) und ihre Wirkung. Eine Langzeitstudie an Berliner Grundschulen. Schott Musik International

Bazana PG, Stelmack RM (2002) Intelligence and information processing during an auditory discrimination task with backward masking: an event-related potential analysis. J Pers Soc Psychol 83(4):998–1008

Bhattacharya J, Petsche H (2005) Drawing on mind's canvas: differences in cortical integration patterns between artists and non-artists. Hum Brain Mapp 26(1):1–14

Bhattacharya J, Petsche H, Pereda E (2001) Long-range synchrony in the gamma band: role in music perception. J Neurosci 21(16):6329–6337

Bishop DVM, Carlyon RP, Deeks JM, Bishop SJ (1999) Auditory temporal processing impairment: neither necessary nor sufficient for causing language impairment in children. J Speech Lang Hear Res 42:1295–1310

Carroll JB (ed) (1993) Human cognitive abilities: a survey of factor-analytic studies. Cambridge University Press

Castles A, Coltheart M (2004) Is there a causal link from phonological awareness to success in learning to read? Cognition 91(1):77–111

Cattell RB (1941) Some theoretical issues in adult intelligence testing. Psychol Bull 38:592

Cavanaugh JC, Blanchard-Fields F (2011) Adult development and aging. Wadsworth/Cengage Learning

Chandrasekaran B, Hornickelm J, Skoe E, Nicol T, Kraus N (2009) Context-dependent encoding in the human auditory brainstem relates to hearing speech in noise: implications for developmental dyslexia. Neuron 64(3):311–319

Eggermont JJ, Ponton CW (2002) The neurophysiology of auditory perception: from single units to evoked potentials. Audiol Neurotol 7:71–99

Ertl JP, Schafer EWP (1969) Neural efficiency and human intelligence. Nature 223:421–423
Feist GJ, Barron FX (2003) Predicting creativity from early to late adulthood: intellect, potential, and personality. J Res Pers 37(2):62–68
Forgeard M, Winner E, Norton A, Schlaug G (2008) Practicing a musical instrument in childhood is associated with enhanced verbal ability and nonverbal reasoning. PLoS One 3(10):e3566
Gardner H (ed) (1983) Frames of mind: the theory of multiple intelligences. Basic Books
Gaser C, Schlaug G (2003) Gray matter differences between musicians and nonmusicians. Ann N Y Acad Sci 999:514–517
Gordon EE (ed) (1965) Musical aptitude profile. Houghton Mifflin
Gordon EE (Hrsg) (1986) Musikalische Begabung. Beschaffenheit, Beschreibung, Messung und Bewertung. Schott
Goswami U (2011) A temporal sampling framework for developmental dyslexia. Trends Cogn Sci 15(1):3–10
Gruhn W (2003) Kinder brauchen Musik: Musikalität bei kleinen Kindern entfalten und fördern. Beltz
Guilford JP (ed) (1967) The nature of human intelligence. McGraw-Hill
Hämäläinen JA, Salminen HK, Leppänen PHT (2013) Basic auditory processing deficits in dyslexia: systematic review of the behavioral and event-related potential/field evidence. J Learn Disabil 46(5):413–427
Helmbold N, Troche S, Rammsayer T (2006) Temporal information processing and pitch discrimination as predictors of general intelligence. Can J Exp Psychol 60(4):294–306
Helmbold N, Troche S, Rammsayer T (2007) Processing of temporal and nontemporal information as predictors of psychometric intelligence: a structural-equation-modeling approach. J Pers 75(5):985–1006
Ho YC, Cheung MC, Chan AS (2003) Music training improves verbal but not visual memory: cross-sectional and longitudinal explorations in children. Neuropsychology 17(3):439–450
Hornickel J, Skoe E, Nicol T, Zecker S, Kraus N (2009) Subcortical differentiation of stop consonants relates to reading and speech-in-noise perception. Proc Natl Acad Sci USA 106(31):13022–13027
Hornickel J, Zecker SG, Bradlow AR, Kraus N (2012) Assistive listening devices drive neuroplasticity in children with dyslexia. Proc Natl Acad Sci USA 109(41):16731–16736
Huss M, Verney JP, Fosker T, Mead N, Goswami U (2011) Music, rhythm, rise time perception and developmental dyslexia: perception of musical meter predicts reading and phonology. Cortex 47(6):674–689
Hyde KL, Lerch J, Norton A, Forgeard M, Winner E, Evans AC, Schlaug G (2009) The effects of musical training on structural brain development: a longitudinal study. Ann N Y Acad Sci 1169:182–186
Jäncke L (2008) Macht Musik schlau? Neue Erkenntnisse aus den Neurowissenschaften und der kognitiven Psychologie. Huber
Jentschke S, Koelsch S, Friederici AD (2005) Investigating the relationship of music and language in children: influences of musical training and language impairment. Ann N Y Acad Sci 1060:231–242
Jentschke S, Koelsch S, Sallat S, Friederici AD (2008) Children with specific language impairment also show impairment of music-syntactic processing. J Cogn Neurosci 20(11):1940–1951
Koelsch S, Fritz T, Schulze K, Alsop D, Schlaug G (2005) Adults and children processing music: an fMRI study. NeuroImage 25(4):1068–1076
Kormann A (1989) Der Zusammenhang zwischen Intelligenz und Musikalität. Internationale Zeitschrift Für Musik-, Tanz- Und Kunsttherapie 2–3:153–159
Kraus N, Chandrasekaran B (2010) Music training for the development of auditory skills. Nat Rev Neurosci 11(8):599–605
Lamb SJ, Gregory AH (1993) The relationship between music and reading in beginning readers. Educ Psychol 13(1):19–27
Landerl K, Willburger E (2010) Temporal processing, attention, and learning disorders. Learn Individ Differ 20(5):393–401

Lynn R, Wilson RG, Gault A (1989) Simple musical tests as measures of Spearman's g. Personal Individ Differ 10:25–28
Magne C, Schön D, Besson M (2006) Musician children detect pitch violations in both music and language better than nonmusician children: behavioral and electrophysiological approaches. J Cogn Neurosci 18(2):199–211
Meyer M, Elmer S, Jäncke L (2012) Musical expertise induces neuroplasticity of the planum temporale. Ann N Y Acad Sci 1252:116–123
Moreno S, Marques C, Santos A, Santos M, Castro SL, Besson M (2009) Musical training influences linguistic abilities in 8-year-old children: more evidence for brain plasticity. Cereb Cortex 19(3):712–723
Musacchia G, Sams M, Skoe E, Kraus N (2007) Musicians have enhanced subcortical auditory and audiovisual processing of speech and music. Proc Natl Acad Sci USA 104(40):15894–15898
Neubauer A, Stern E (Hrsg) (2007) Lernen macht intelligent. Deutsche Verlags-Anstalt
Neubauer A, Grabner R, Fink A, Neuper C (2005) Intelligence and neural efficiency: further evidence of the influence of task content and sex on the brain-IQ relationship. Cogn Brain Res 25(1):217–225
Overy K (2003) Dyslexia and music: from timing deficits to musical intervention. Ann N Y Acad Sci 999(1):497–505
Overy K, Nicolson RI, Fawcett AJ, Clarke EF (2003) Dyslexia and music: measuring musical timing skills. Dyslexia 9(1):18–36
Parbery-Clark A, Tierney A, Strait DL, Kraus N (2012) Musicians have fine-tuned neural distinction of speech syllables. Neuroscience 219:111–119
Parsons LM, Sergent J, Hodges DA, Fox PT (2005) The brain basis of piano performance. Neuropsychologia 43:199–215
Patel AD, Gibson E, Ratner J, Besson M, Holcomb PJ (1998) Processing syntactic relations in language and music: an event-related potential study. J Cogn Neurosci 10(6):717–733
Posthuma D, De Geus EJ, Baaré WF, Hulshoff Pol HE, Kahn RS, Boomsma D (2002) The association between brain volume and intelligence is of genetic origin. Nat Neurosci 5:83–84
Rittelmeyer C (2012) Warum und wozu ästhetische Bildung? Über Transferwirkungen künstlerischer Tätigkeiten. Ein Forschungsüberblick (2. Aufl). Athena
Schellenberg EG (2004) Music lessons enhance IQ. Psychol Sci 15:511–514
Schellenberg EG (2006) Long-term positive associations between music lessons and IQ. J Educ Psychol 98:457–468
Schellenberg EG (2011) Music lessons, emotional intelligence, and IQ. Music Percept 29:185–194
Schlaug G, Jäncke L, Huang Y, Staiger JF, Steinmetz H (1995) Increased corpus callosum size in musicians. Neuropsychologia 33(8):1047–1055
Schlaug G, Norton A, Overy K, Winner E (2005) Effects of music training on the child's brain and cognitive development. Ann N Y Acad Sci 1060:219–230
Schneider P, Seither-Preisler A (2015) Neurokognitive Korrelate von JeKi-bezogenen und außerschulischem Musizieren. In: Ulrike Kranefeld, Bundesministerium für Bildung und Forschung (Hrsg) Instrumentalunterreicht in der Grundschule: Prozess- und Wirkungsanalyse zum Programm Jedem Kind ein Instrument. Berlin. Bildungsforschung Band 41, S 19–39
Schneider P, Scherg M, Dosch HG, Specht HJ, Gutschalk A, Rupp A (2002) Morphology of Heschl's gyrus reflects enhanced activation in the auditory cortex of musicians. Nat Neurosci 5(7):688–694
Schneider P, Sluming V, Roberts N, Scherg M, Goebel R, Specht HJ, Dosch HG, Bleeck S, Stippich C, Rupp A (2005) Structural and functional asymmetry of lateral Heschl's gyrus reflects pitch perception preference. Nat Neurosci 8(9):1241–1247
Schneider P, Andermann M, Wengenroth M, Goebel R, Flor H, Rupp A, Diesch E (2009) Reduced volume of Heschl's gyrus in tinnitus. NeuroImage 45(3):927–939
Schneider P, Groß C, Bernhofs V, Christiner M, Benner J, Turker S, Zeidler B, Seither-Preisler A (2022) Short-term plasticity of neuro-auditory processing induced by musical active listening training. Ann N Y Acad Sci 1517(1):176–190. https://doi.org/10.1111/nyas.14899

Schneider P, Engelmann D, Groß C, Bernhofs V, Hofmann E, Christiner M, Benner J, Bücher S, Ludwig A, Serrallach BL, Zeidler BM (2023) Neuroanatomical disposition, natural development, and training-induced plasticity of the human auditory system from childhood to adulthood: a 12-year study in musicians and nonmusicians. J Neurosci 43(37):6430–6446. https://doi.org/10.1523/JNEUROSCI.0274-23.2023

Schön D, Magne C, Besson M (2004) The music of speech: electrophysiological study of pitch perception in language and music. Psychophysiology 41:341–349

Schumacher R, Altenmüller E, Deutsch W, Jäncke L, Neubauer A, Schwarzer G et al (2006) In: Bundesministerium für Bildung und Forschung (BMBF) (Hrsg) Macht Mozart schlau? Die Förderung kognitiver Kompetenzen durch Musik, Bd 18, S 46–48, 68–70

Schuppert M, Munte TF, Wieringa BM, Altenmüller E (2000) Receptive amusia: evidence for cross-hemispheric neural networks underlying music processing strategies. Brain J Neurol 123(Pt 3):546–559

Seashore CE (1919) Seashore measurement of musical talent. New York, revidierte Fassungen 1939, 1956, 1960; dt. Ausg. hrsg. v. H. Fischer & C. Butch, Bern 1966

Seither-Preisler A, Parncutt R, Schneider P (2014) Bilateral synchronization of auditory cortex promotes musical and attentional skills in children. J Neurosci 34(33):10937–10949

Serrallach B, Groß C, Bernhofs V, Benner J, Schneider P, Seither-Preisler A (2016) Neural biomarkers for dyslexia, ADHD, and ADD in the auditory cortex of children. Front Neurosci 10(204784). https://doi.org/10.3389/fnins.2016.00324

Shahin A, Bosnyak DJ, Trainor LJ, Roberts LE (2003) Enhancement of neuroplastic P2 and N1c auditory evoked potentials in musicians. J Neurosci 23(13):5545–5552

Sharma A, Kraus N, McGee TJ, Nicol TG (1997) Developmental changes in P1 and N1 central auditory responses elicited by consonant-vowel syllables. Electroencephalogr Clin Neurophysiol 104(6):540–545

Sharma A, Martin K, Roland P, Bauer P, Sweeney MH, Gilley P, Dorman M (2005) P1 latency as a biomarker for central auditory development in children with hearing impairment. J Am Acad Audiol 16(8):564–573

Shaw P, Greenstein D, Lerch J, Clasen L, Lenroot R, Gogtay N, Evans A, Rapoport J, Giedd J (2006) Intellectual ability and cortical development in children and adolescents. Nature 440:676–679

Skoe E, Kraus N (2012) A little goes a long way: how the adult brain is shaped by musical training in childhood. J Neurosci 32(34):11507–11510

Skoe E, Krizman J, Kraus N (2013) The impoverished brain: disparities in maternal education affect the neural response to sound. J Neurosci 33(44):17221–17231

Slevc LR, Miyake A (2006) Individual differences in second-language proficiency: does musical ability matter? Psychol Sci 17(8):675–681

Sluming V, Brooks J, Howard M, Downes JJ, Roberts N (2007) Broca's area supports enhanced visuospatial cognition in orchestral musicians. J Neurosci 27(14):3799–3806

Stern E, Neubauer A (2013) Intelligenz—Große Unterschiede und ihre Folgen. Deutsche Verlags-Anstalt

Strait DL, Kraus N (2014) Biological impact of auditory expertise across the life span: musicians as a model of auditory learning. Hear Res 308:109–121

Strait DL, Hornickel J, Kraus N (2011) Subcortical processing of speech regularities underlies reading and music aptitude in children. Behav Brain Funct 7:44

Tallal P, Gaab N (2006) Dynamic auditory processing, musical experience and language development. Trends Neurosci 29(7):382–390

Thompson P, Cannon T, Narr K, van Erp T, Poutanen V, Huttunen M, Lönnqvist J, Standertskjöld-Nordenstam CJ, Kaprio J, Khaledy M, Dail R, Zoumalan CI, Toga AW (2001) Genetic influences on brain structure. Nat Neurosci 4(12):1253–1258

Thompson W, Schellenberg E, Husain G (2004) Decoding speech prosody: do music lessons help? Emotion 4(1):46–64

Thurstone LL (ed) (1938) Primary mental abilities. The University of Chicago Press

Wagner R, Torgesen J (1987) The nature of phonological processing and its causal role in the acquisition of reading skills. Psychol Bull 101:192–212

Weber EW, Spychiger M, Patry J (1993) Musik macht Schule. Biografie und Ergebnisse eines Schulversuchs mit erweitertem Musikunterricht. Die Blaue Eule

Wengenroth M, Blatow M, Bendszus M, Schneider P (2010) Leftward lateralization of auditory cortex underlies holistic sound perception in Williams syndrome. PLoS One 5(8):e12326

Wengenroth M, Blatow M, Heinecke A, Reinhardt J, Stippich C, Hofmann E, Schneider P (2013) Increased volume and function of right auditory cortex as a marker for absolute pitch. Cereb Cortex 24(5):1127–1137

Wetter OE, Koerner F, Schwaninger A (2009) Does musical training improve school performance? Instr Sci 37(4):365–374

Wing HD (1939/1961) Standardised tests of musical intelligence. National Foundation for Educational Research

Wong PC, Skoe E, Russo NM, Dees T, Kraus N (2007) Musical experience shapes human brainstem encoding of linguistic pitch patterns. Nat Neurosci 10(4):420–422

Zatorre RJ (2003) Absolute pitch: a model for understanding the influence of genes and development on neural and cognitive function. Nat Neurosci 6(7):692–695

Zatorre R, Belin P (2001) Spectral and temporal processing in human auditory cortex. Cereb Cortex 11:946–953

Performance and Stage Fright: Acquiring Competence Through Musical Education in Childhood and Adolescence

27

Claudia Spahn

Given that stage fright – referred to as music performance anxiety (MPA) in scientific discourse – naturally arises in presentational situations, musically active people gain particularly extensive experience of performance situations while making music–and thus of MPA. In publications to date, attention has been on supportive measures to deal with MPA and in the prevention of performing anxiety arising. The fact that dealing with MPA in a positive manner can also be seen as a resource for children's and teenagers' development, in particular, has been little discussed up to now. If positive performing experiences as part of vocal and instrumental coaching are imparted early on, then significant resources may lie herein for further personality development in terms of self-confidence and skills in making presentations.

27.1 Introduction

Performing in front of an audience is tightly bound up with the making of music. Anyone who plays an instrument or sings encounters the act of performing in front of others as a matter of course. If one considers making music with this aspect in mind, an essential part of musical education consists of acquiring skills in presentational situations. In this, positive handling of the reactions received plays a central role, which go hand-in-hand with a performance and which we describe as stage fright or MPA. As part of their musical training, children and youths are introduced to making performances and learn how they can positively cope with MPA. This nurtures both their musical career and their self-confidence in situations where they perform that are unrelated to music. Musical training during childhood and

C. Spahn (✉)
Freiburg Institute for Musicians' Medicine (FIM), University of Music Freiburg, Medical Faculty University Freiburg, University Clinic Freiburg, Freiburg, Germany
e-mail: claudia.spahn@uniklinik-freiburg.de

G. Kreutz, G. Bernatzky (eds.), *Music and Medicine*, Neurocultural Health and Wellbeing, https://doi.org/10.1007/978-3-662-72175-9_27

adolescence thus constitutes the chance to acquire skills for performative situations, which play an important role over and above making music, in school and the workplace.

In the professional field, performing is part of the reality of the job of a concert-giving musician. Throughout their career, artists acquire numerous experiences of situations that contain a performance (Spahn 2011d, 2015a). A high degree of expertise in dealing with MPA thus represents an important prerequisite for a successful and healthy professional life as a musician. In the specialized field of music physiology and musicians' medicine, appropriate training to cope with performance situations and MPA already takes place in music studies today (Spahn 2006a, 2011a; Spahn et al. 2016; Spahn 2022).

Among amateur musicians, too, the subject of stage fright plays an important role, for making music is then experienced as something especially positive and can best unfold its health-promoting effect when performances are enjoyed and are not burdened by debilitating MPA. It is, therefore, important that skills in giving performances are actively taught in amateur music, as well (Spahn 2006b, 2015a).

In the following, the fundamentals of MPA are first set out, and based on this, approaches to MPA in music education for children and youths are presented from the perspective of a general educational model.

27.2 Basics

27.2.1 Definition of Terms

In the past, authors from the Anglo-American language area have repeatedly pointed out that the acquisition of scientific knowledge is limited by the prevailing diversity of terms and have therefore proposed standardized definitions (Brodsky 1996). In English, the term "music performance anxiety" (MPA) has become established in scientific terminology (Kenny 2011; Osborne and Kirsner 2022). In colloquial language and everyday literature, the term "stage fright" continues to be used. The term 'stage fright' was used in the headline to appeal to the everyday language of the readers. Terms for music performance anxiety in other European languages also express the phenomenon of excitement and fear that occurs under the spotlights on stage: in German, people speak of "Lampenfieber" and "Auftrittsangst," in Spanish of "miedo escénico," and in Italian of "paura del palcoscenico." There are comparable expressions in all languages.

Consistent terminology seems important, both for reasons of scientific methodology and for educational usage. In particular, a distinction should be made between normal psychological phenomena and psychopathological symptoms, even though these are located on a continuum and exhibit fluid borders (Möller 1999; Spahn 2012). In English, the term MPA is used for the entire spectrum from normal to severe symptoms on stage. MPA, therefore, does not automatically refer to a psychological diagnosis but is differentiated according to its severity (Osborne and Kirsner 2022). In this article, we refer to the nonpathological form of MPA.

In general, we define MPA as a specific psychophysical state that basically occurs when we expose ourselves to others and are the focus of attention. Typically, our body tension is then increased, concentration and attention are enhanced, and our capacity to experience emotions is more intense (Spahn 2012). It is assumed that everyone can experience MPA. It, thus, belongs to the repertoire of experiences common to humanity and is not to be assessed as pathological per se.

MPA can vary in the form it takes, both within a person and between individuals, and depending on the situation. If its effect is beneficial to the performance, we talk of "performance-enhancing MPA," while if it reduces our ability to perform on stage, we talk of "performance-impairing MPA" (Spahn 2012). The third form that is found takes on pathological dimensions and is characterized by the performance being greatly impaired in the actual moment or being rendered impossible. Symptoms of anxiety and depression arise, and the feelings of being overwhelmed are so great before the performance that this is often avoided altogether. This form is described as "performance-impeding MPA." As a mental disorder, MPA is coded as a performance-only subtype of social anxiety disorder in the Diagnostic and Statistical Manual for Psychiatric Disorders (Falkai et al. 2015).

27.2.2 Psychophysiology of Music Performance Anxiety

MPA arises from an ancient pattern rooted in evolutionary biology; originally, its function was to configure humans in life-threatening situations in an optimal way for "fight" or "flight." Triggered by the fright signal, a cascade of reactions is launched in the brain—emanating from the thalamus—that leads to the adrenaline and noradrenaline hormones being released. These cause:

- Activation of the cardiovascular system (Spahn et al. 2010; Spahn 2015b) with centralization of the blood supply to muscles close to the trunk
- An increase in breathing
- Enhancement of muscle tone
- Intensification of other bodily functions that can be categorized under the sympathetic part of the autonomic nervous system

These responses, which are advantageous for flight/fight situations, can be a hindrance for more fine motor demands, such as those presented by music making. Thus, trembling hands, for instance–caused by the increased muscle tonus—disturb the bowing when playing the violin, while cold and sweaty hands—caused by vasoconstriction in the periphery—affect the finger dexterity of the pianist, and rapid, superficial breathing—in order to gain more oxygen—impairs the wind instrumentalist's ability to create the sound. Concentration and memory function can be improved by an optimal form of MPA, as can emotional expressiveness yet can also be impaired by excessive MPA. In the case of pronounced MPA, memory lapses can occur, even blackouts. The fear of existential physical threat in earlier days has now given way to a fear of social humiliation. Thus, prior to a performance, fears are often to be found of not being able to hold one's own in the eyes of others, of embarrassing oneself, of not being able to fulfill one's expectations of oneself, or others' expectations, or not pass muster in competition with others.

27.2.3 Influences on Music Performance Anxiety

The form MPA takes is influenced by a range of factors. These can be divided into three areas: into factors that lie within the person performing, into those arising from the context of the performance, and from those to do with the type and difficulty of the task involved in the performance.

27.2.3.1 Personal Influences

The individual performance experiences in the performer's biography play a decisive role. Anxiety as an innate personality trait also favors the development of performance-impairing MPA (Ryan 2005; Kenny 2011).

From a time-of-life perspective, adolescence in particular represents a sensitive phase, in which the way MPA is handled, and the experience of performing assumes a special significance for further development (Kenny 2011). Thus, among those musician patients with a diagnosis-relevant MPA whom we treat in our psychotherapeutic consultation hours of the musician's medical outpatient clinic, we frequently encounter experiences of performing in adolescence that were experienced as a burden and were inadequately worked through.

The net result remaining from such negative key experiences ranges from insecurity and fears right through to avoidance of performance that span several years and get worse. However, our extensive work with musicians' life stories—in education, training, and treatment at the Freiburg Institute for Musicians' Medicine—has mainly yielded examples proving that successful experiences of performing during adolescence can promote performance self-confidence and self-efficacy in the long term.

27.2.3.2 Contextual Influences

The context, i.e., the framework in which a performance takes place, influences the extent of MPA. In an investigation at a high school, the MPA experienced by 27 girls and boys who played in a band increased in line with the increasing size of the auditorium and the importance of the performance as subjectively perceived by the performers (Le Blanc et al. 1997). The MPA is affected not only by the numbers present in the audience, but who is sitting there, too. Thus, experts in the audience trigger greater MPA responses when compared with laypersons (Eckhardt and Lüdemann 1974). However, our observation is that the reactions to the type and size of the audience are individual and can greatly depend upon the relations to individuals within the audience (Spahn et al. 2021b).

27.2.3.3 Task-Specific Influences

The type and quality of the task on the stage are as important for the form that the MPA takes as the fact of how well a person is prepared for such demands. If, for example, we think of the level of difficulty of a piece of music to be performed, this alone is not decisive but rather in combination with the level of playing and preparation on the part of the player. Excessive MPA impairs the performance on stage more in the case of highly differentiated movements requiring fine motor skills than with simple challenges (Kenny 2011). The demands placed on the performer on stage by the musical task influence the potential to enter the positive state of flow. A medium level of challenge increases the likelihood of flow and simultaneously reduces MPA (Spahn et al. 2021a).

27.2.4 Goals in Dealing with Music Performance Anxiety

In sports psychology, there exists the model of "zone of optimal functioning," in which a relationship is assumed between a certain level of arousal and the maximum performance (Robazza et al. 2004). This approach implicitly contains the assumption that a particular level of arousal should be present in order to achieve a good performance. Yerkes and Dodson, too, had presented as early as 1908 the relationship between "performance" and "arousal" as an expressive form of fear in a reverse U-curve (Yerkes and Dodson 1908). This states that the best performance can be achieved with medium arousal—neither too low nor too high. According to today's level of scientific knowledge, this relationship needs to be differentiated in consideration of other components such as the level of difficulty of the task in hand, the scope of preparation, or the basic degree of anxiety present in the person concerned (Kenny 2011). Nonetheless, it is still agreed that a minimum level of arousal remains a prerequisite for a good performance. Positive acceptance of the phenomenon of MPA should, therefore, take first priority in educational and therapeutic ways of dealing with MPA. This frequently means a shift in thinking, as it is not infrequently the case that people assume that the experience of MPA must be tackled and entirely eliminated. In the case of artistic performance, such as in singing and music-making, the target parameters are complex, encompassing several areas such as cognition, emotions, memory, and motor skills. In practice, therefore, a combination of several approaches has proven successful in dealing with MPA. A series of measures, such as mental, imaginative, and relaxational techniques in themselves already, represent an integration of different areas (Spahn 2012, 2015a, b).

27.3 Dealing with Music Performance Anxiety in Music Education with Children and Youths

27.3.1 Music Performance Anxiety Among Children and Youths

Up until the onset of adolescence, girls and boys mostly deal with performance situations in a spontaneous and natural manner. Nonetheless, small children can certainly experience MPA, too. This was the result of a study by Ryan (2005), which questioned 173 children aged 3–7 before a concert in their school. The situational fear was also correlated in the study with anxiety as a personality trait (Ryan 2005), i.e., anxious children had more MPA than less anxious children. In a further investigation by Ryan (1998), 26 piano students aged 12 were found to have a significant increase in heart rate between being calm and the performance situation, allowing the assumption of physical MPA symptoms, comparable with those of adults. Here, it was also shown that greater MPA goes hand-in-hand with lower self-esteem (Ryan 1998). The greatest sample to date of MPA among children was examined by Wang (2001), who found 23% of 1.033 music students suffered MPA so great that this impaired their musical performance. A study of 66 children aged 3–4 showed that both the number of performances and the context of the performance already has an effect on the psychophysiological characteristics of the MPA (Ryan and Boucher 2011). MPA in the children was measured during class and at two consecutive concerts, based on the fear experienced and cortisone levels in the saliva. Both measuring components increased between class and the first concert, and fell significantly before the second concert. The children reacted to an audition-type situation, perceived as unfriendly, with an increase in MPA.

During adolescence, the degree of MPA usually increases. In terms of psychological development, drastic physical and psychological changes take place here, which are only gradually integrated into the person's self-concept and only over time lead to a stable identity. In this phase of discovering one's self, the very act of presentation in front of others releases feelings of shame and insecurity. To this can be added heightened sensitivity and a critical view of oneself. Osborne and Kenny (2005) investigated 381 music students aged 11–19 and classified the extent of the MPA in three age groups (<11, 11–13, 14–19 years of age). The most pronounced MPA was found in the age group between 14 and 19. In total, anxiety, the female sex, and negative thoughts were predictors of higher MPA. In other studies, girls admitted more MPA than boys (Ryan 1998, 2003, 2004, 2005; Le Blanc et al. 1997). At the same time, girls showed a higher correlation between the physiological and psychological components of MPA than was the case with boys (Le Blanc et al. 1997; Osborne and Kenny 2005; Rae and McCambridge 2004). Nusseck et al. (2015) investigated 239 music students aged between 7 and 20 years old, of which 126 received training in classical music and 113 received training in popular music, with regard to MPA. Comparably high levels of MPA were found in both groups, which showed a different progression depending on age, however.

27.3.2 Approaches to Dealing with Music Performance Anxiety in Music Education

As already set out, experiences of performing as a child or youth—especially in adolescence—play a key role in terms of performance skills from a lifetime perspective. Teachers and parents have a special responsibility here. This is all the greater as instrumental and vocal lessons offer the opportunity to promote the students' personal development in a particularly positive and comprehensive way as part of their musical education. Musical performances represent the greatest challenges when set against sporting and academic situations. In a study of 749 boys aged from 9 to 14, the levels of fear were the highest for a musical performance and with a band performance in comparison with a school exam and sports competition (Simon and Martens 1979). From this can be inferred that, conversely, the training of musical performances may well be particularly effective.

27.3.2.1 Approaches for the Music Pedagogue in Instrumental Teaching

There are different ways for the music pedagogue to introduce the student to performance situations in a positive way. Like with the conveying of musical content, the pedagogical approach should be deliberate and well-considered.

The educational approaches are related to the three areas mentioned above of performance context, musical task, and the student's personality (Table 27.1). They thus concern aspects of the performance context, the musical performance, and measures that directly address the person of the student. The appropriate method should be selected and corresponding measures variously combined, depending on the student's and teacher's individual situation.

General recommendations for the music pedagogue in dealing with music performance anxiety:

- Observe the MPA in the student.
- Maintain an open, appropriate manner of dealing with MPA.
- Deal with MPA in an age-appropriate manner.
- Enable frequent, positive performance experiences for the student.
- Set realistic musical goals for the performance.
- Give differentiated feedback several days after the performance.
- Record positive aspects of the performance and express them to the student.
- Give the student tools for self-assessment of performance (e.g., as an app).

Table 27.1 Possible starting points for the music pedagogue to design the performance positively for the student

Performance context	Musical task	Person of the student
Supportive design of concert setting	Appropriate level of difficulty	Resource-based approach
Creating positive relationship with audience	Sufficient preparation	Individually selecting measures for dealing with MPA
Making music in an ensemble	Varying playing/singing: playing from music/off by heart/improvised	Guiding students to mutual support
Designing external conditions (room, acoustics, etc.) in most positive way possible	Varying the music genre (classical and popular music)	Promoting solidarity among musicians on stage

It is the task of the music pedagogue to observe the way the student handles MPA in the preparation phases, as well as shortly before the performance, during, and after it. The teacher creates the opportunity to communicate with the student on this topic in an open and appropriate manner. Every student, regardless of the specific performance, should be informed that everyone is familiar with MPA, as well as how it manifests itself, and what inner processes lead to the appearance of the phenomena of MPA. This includes the realization that performing represents a separate learning experience in itself, both in terms of content and process, which demands—like learning to play the instrument or singing—motivation, practice, patience, and decisiveness. If the pedagogue succeeds in making the context and the task of the performance favorable for the student, then specific person-focused measures such as relaxation exercises and specific mental techniques are not always necessary in every case. On the contrary, for students with natural self-confidence in performing, dealing with the subject of MPA should not needlessly take up too much attention. On the other hand, MPA should not be a taboo subject.

Practice Tip
As the number of positive performance experiences has a lasting effect on self-confidence in playing before others, students should regularly be given opportunities to perform that they experience as motivating.

However, performance opportunities are only conducive to the student's development if there are realistic goals for the performance that can be achieved by the student.

Performances should take place frequently enough that the individual performance is not given too much importance, but that the student can also go through a learning process when performing with corrective experiences.

Practice Tip
After a performance, it has proven to be important for subsequent performances that differentiated feedback is given by the teacher after a few days, which also explicitly mentions the positive aspects of the performance (Spahn 2011c, 2012).

Digital options are now also available for the self-assessment of a musical performance. Spahn and Nusseck (2019) developed the Stage: Cool app at the Freiburg Institute for Musicians' Medicine, which can be completed on a mobile phone after a performance. Stage: Cool is based on the validated performance questionnaire for musicians (FZAM, Spahn et al. 2021b). The questionnaire contains the three scales: MPA symptoms, functional coping with MPA, and self-efficacy with regard to performance. The questions relate to the times shortly before the performance, during the performance, and directly after the performance. In addition, each individual performance can be evaluated in the app according to musical criteria, and notes on the respective performance situation can be recorded. The Stage: Cool performance app also offers the option of creating a list of performances and viewing them afterward individually, as average values, or in a graphical overview. The Stage: Cool app can be downloaded and used free of charge for iOS and Android smartphones (https://fim.mh-freiburg.de/stagecool-app).

Practice Tip
The Stage: Cool app enables a personal self-assessment of the student's own performance skills over a longer period of time, which can also be used as a common basis for discussion for the teacher's feedback.

27.3.2.2 Performance Context

The design of the performance context offers numerous opportunities to make playing in front of an audience easier for the student and to adjust MPA in a positive way. Particularly for youths in adolescence who in this phase of life are greatly oriented toward their peer groups, making music together with others of the same age in a duo or ensemble offers a good opportunity to reduce the sense of shame during a performance (Nusseck et al. 2015). Vocal formations such as choirs or ensembles offer ideal possibilities in this age group for development in a positive direction of musical stage experience. Likewise, integrating pieces to be performed into a staged setting, relaxing the concert setting by means of conversational elements, or communal singing with the audience, as well as deliberate interaction with the specific characteristics of the performance space (acoustics, architecture, building style) can all shape the performance situation for the student in a positive way and link MPA with the joy of performing. In this, youths can actively introduce their own ideas and identify with their performance in a special way (Spahn 2011c, 2012). The relationship with the audience can be used as a resource in educational work with the children and youth. The fear of being judged by others (Eckhardt and Lüdemann 1974) can be mitigated by incorporating the musical performance into a reciprocal communication concept.

27.3.2.3 Musical Task

The music performance represents the heart of work in music education. The selection of music content is closely connected to the performance setting. Alongside the actual music performance using the voice or an instrument, other tasks on stage can be added, such as speaking, singing, or choreographed movement. Basically, it should be the case both for the choice of music and for the overall design of the performance that the tasks are easily mastered by the student on the one hand, and sufficiently demanding on the other. With regard to MPA, these conditions provide the best prerequisite for optimally fine-tuning the MPA for the performance (Kenny 2011; Osborne and Kirsner 2022). The students' own performance consists, in any case, of appropriate preparation. A performance marked by major risks from the outset, due to the piece to be performed being insufficiently practiced and rehearsed, and having only a low chance of going well, should be regarded as a threat and is not recommended from an educational point of view. With each individual case, the advantages and disadvantages of a performance need to be weighed up. Clarification of technical aspects of playing should also always be prepared and gone through in lessons with the stage situation in mind, especially as the transfer to the performance situation with MPA represents a challenge of its own for the student. A switch in music styles (e.g., incorporating improvisational elements) can help the student gain new, positive experience of performing, which can be transferred positively to other areas in the individual's work.

27.3.2.4 Person of the Student

Generally, it is recommended to start with the student's strengths and to use them positively for the performance. In the same sense, negative feelings following a performance should not lead the student to avoid further performance situations. It is important here to find positive aspects of the performance and to encourage the student firmly to take on the next performance. A selection of practical performance tips for youths can be found in the following overview.

Performance Tips for Youths (Based on Spahn et al. 2010)

- Set yourself realistic goals for your performance.
- No one, including you, has to be perfect.
- Even if you don't achieve your goal at the first try, nothing has been lost in the trying.
- Talk to your parents and teachers if you believe that your parents are expecting too much from you.
- Do not take refuge in illnesses such as a headache or stomach pains to avoid having to perform. Be brave!
- Undertake something that you find fun and that will bolster your self-confidence.
- Before the performance, practice for an emergency as realistically as you can: rehearse in front of people you know to begin with.
- Recall positive thoughts before you go on stage: imagine something pleasant and enter a state of optimal concentration for the performance.
- Afterward, think about everything that went well.

In the students' group, social aspects such as mutual support among those making music before the performance and on stage can be rehearsed. Musical training in particular opens up many opportunities for conveying these key social skills, as "listening to one another" is already an integral component of playing music together. Direct support for the student in performing and dealing with MPA covers a wide range of possibilities (Spahn 2011c, 2012). It ranges from relaxational, breathing, and specific body exercises (Spahn 2017), to mental training for performing, all the way to one-on-one discussions with individual students concerning the background to and fears regarding the performance. Essentially, the range of measures is spread over physical sensation, feelings, thoughts, and the student's behavior in the preparation stage, during the performance, and afterward. A detailed description of the individual measures can be found in Spahn (2012).

If a teenage student complains of severe MPA and cannot overcome this within the teaching context, then a referral to a musicians' medicine consultant may be helpful. Performance problems can usually be quickly addressed and treated in collaboration with an experienced musicians' medicine specialist. In our view, a multimodal therapeutic approach is always productive in this case (Spahn 2011b).

Practice Tip
Physicians must urgently warn against exclusively medical therapy, e.g., with beta-receptor blockers or tranquillizers, as this treats the actual problem inadequately and replaces it with a psychological or physical dependency.

In cooperation with an experienced musician's medicine doctor, performance problems can usually be addressed and treated quickly. In our view, a multimodal therapeutic approach is always the most effective (Spahn 2011b).

27.3.2.5 The Role of Parents

In the case of children and youths, the family setting plays a key role. MPA in particular is greatly influenced by the demands one makes on oneself in terms of achievement, as well as the expectations of others—parents, teachers, and friends. For this reason, it is important that a relationship of trust and cooperation exists between the music pedagogue and the students' parents. On account of their interest and the emotional support they offer their child during the performance, parents contribute vitally to the development over the years of assured performance skills. If, on the other hand, conflicts within the family and excessive expectations or a lack of support on the part of parents lead to performance issues for the student, this issue should be discussed by the teachers and parents. In case of serious problems, it is also advisable to recommend psychotherapeutic help to the student and his or her family (Spahn 2011b).

27.4 Music Performance Anxiety and Health

The health-promoting aspects of musical training in the area of skills acquisition for performance and presentation situations have received too little attention hitherto, as already briefly alluded to at the beginning. The results and experiences garnered from Music Physiology and Musicians' Medicine with regard to dealing with MPA are being integrated—gradually to begin with, yet increasingly so—into music pedagogy. However, it seems to us that the great potential of music training on the development of children's and youths' personalities remains insufficiently recognized. If we concentrate on the aspect of musical performance ability, then this has a value of its own for the music-making itself. Furthermore, experiences gained in musical performance offer other opportunities for the development of personality. Based on empirical observations made in practicing music pedagogy and music physiology, these are as follows:

- The experience of "flow" as a feeling of happiness (Csíkszentmihályi 2000; Spahn et al. 2021a)
- The experience of self-efficacy
- Nurturing of a positive self-concept
- Stabilization of one's feeling of self-esteem (Araújo and Spahn 2022)

The same applies to the importance of musical performance experience in childhood and adolescence as a resource for dealing with presentation situations throughout life. This aspect appears to be particularly significant, as performance skills are one of the central requirements in the modern communication society. Not least of all, MPA itself harbors potential, as it can intensify the joy of making music, promote health in its effects, and thus enable the positive health aspects of making music to develop even more powerfully.

27.5 Conclusion

Musical training as a child and teenager includes the experience of performing as an important component. Children who make music have the chance to gather extensive experience and to learn skills in dealing with music performance anxiety. The confidence in performing thereby gained can be utilized in other situations beyond making music, too. Music pedagogues should be aware of this opportunity and should teach their students basic skills in how to cope with performative situations and music performance anxiety.

References

Araújo LS, Spahn C (2022) Promoting health-related lifestyle. In: McPherson GE (Hrsg.) The Oxford handbook of music performance, vol 2. Oxford University Press, 279–306

Brodsky W (1996) Music performance anxiety reconceptualized: a critique of current research practices and findings. Med Probl Perform Art 11(3):88–98

Csíkszentmihályi M (2000) Das Flow-Erlebnis. Jenseits von Angst und Langeweile im Tun aufgehen. Klett Verlag, Stuttgart

Eckhardt I, Lüdemann L (1974) Kennen Sie Lampenfieber? Das Orchester 1:10–15

Falkai P, Wittchen HU, Döpfner M (2015) Diagnostic and statistical manual of mental disorders. Hogrefe, Göttingen, Bern, Wien

Kenny DT (2011) The psychology of music performance anxiety. Oxford University Press, Oxford/New York

Le Blanc A, Jin YC, Obert M, Siivola C (1997) Effect of audience on music performance anxiety. J Res Music Educ 45:480–496

Möller H (1999) Lampenfieber und Aufführungs.ngste sind nicht dasselbe! Üben & Musizieren 5:13–19
Nusseck M, Zander M, Spahn C (2015) Music performance anxiety in young musicians—comparison of playing classical or popular music. Med Probl Perform Art 30:30–37
Osborne MS, Kenny DT (2005) Assessment of music performance anxiety in late childhood: a validation study of the music performance anxiety inventory for adolescents (MPAI-A). Int J Stress Manag 12(4):312–330
Osborne MS, Kirsner J (2022) Music performance anxiety. In: McPherson GE (ed) The Oxford handbook of music performance, vol 2. Oxford University Press, pp 204–231
Rae G, McCambridge K (2004) Correlates of performance anxiety in practical music exams. Psychol Music 32(4):432–439
Robazza C, Pellizzari M, Hanin Y (2004) Emotion self-regulation and athletic performance: an application of the IZOF model. Psychol Sport Exerc 5:379–404
Ryan C (1998) Exploring musical performance anxiety in children. Med Probl Perform Art 13:83–88
Ryan C (2003) A study of the differential responses of male and female children to musical performance anxiety. Diss Abstr Int 63(7–A):2487
Ryan C (2004) Gender differences in children's experience of musical performance anxiety. Psychol Music 32(1):89–103
Ryan C (2005) Experience of musical performance anxiety in elementary school children. Special edition: performance anxiety in human endeavour. Int J Stress Manag 12(4):331–342
Ryan C, Boucher H (2011) Performance stress and the very young musician. J Res Music Educ 57(2):108–126
Simon JA, Martens R (1979) Children's anxiety in sport and nonsport evaluative activities. J Sport Psychol 1:160–169
Spahn C (2006a) Gesundheit für Musiker—Entwicklung des Freiburger Präventionsmodells. Schriftenreihe des Freiburger Instituts für Musikermedizin (Spahn C, Hrsg) Freiburger Beiträge zur Musikermedizin, Bd 1. Projektverlag, Freiburg, Bochum
Spahn C (2006b) Lampenfieber und Aufführungsangst bei Musikern—Grundlagen und Therapie. Med Welt 57:559–563
Spahn C (2011a) Prävention und Gesundheitsförderung. In: Spahn C, Richter B, Altenmüller E (Hrsg) MusikerMedizin. Diagnostik, Therapie und Prävention von musikerspezifischen Erkrankungen. Schattauer, Stuttgart, S 50–79
Spahn C (2011b) Psychosomatische Medizin und Psychotherapie. In: Spahn C, Richter B, Altenmüller E (Hrsg) MusikerMedizin. Diagnostik, Therapie und Prävention von musikerspezifischen Erkrankungen. Schattauer, Stuttgart, S 135–186
Spahn C (2011c) Lampenfieber bei Musizierenden im Kindes- und Jugendalter. In: Schriftenreihe Kinder- und Jugendstimme (Fuchs M, Hrsg) Stimme—Persönlichkeit—Psyche. Logos, Berlin, S 155–163
Spahn C (2011d) Das Problem kannte schon Caruso—Angst macht den Auftritt zur Tortur. MMW-Fortschr Med 153(43):46–48
Spahn C (2012) Lampenfieber: Handbuch für den erfolgreichen Auftritt. Grundlagen, Analyse, Maßnahmen. Henschel Verlag, Leipzig
Spahn C (2015a) Musikergesundheit in der Praxis: Grundlagen, Prävention, Übungen. Henschel-Verlag, Leipzig
Spahn C (2015b) Treatment and prevention of music performance anxiety. In: Altenmüller E, Finger S, Boller F (eds) Progress in brain research, vol 217. Elsevier, Amsterdam, pp 129–140
Spahn C (2017) Körperorientierte Ansätze für Musiker. Hogrefe-Verlag
Spahn C (2022) Diseases and health risks in instrumentalists. In: McPherson GE (ed) The Oxford handbook of music performance, vol 2. Oxford University Press, pp 232–259
Spahn C, Nusseck M (2019) Stage:Cool—die Auftritts-App für Musizierende. https://fim.mhfreiburg.de/transfergesund-mitmusik/praxistipps-fuer-profis-und-amateure/stagecool-app/
Spahn C, Echternach M, Zander MF, Voltmer E, Richter B (2010) Music performance anxiety in opera singers. Logoped Phoniatr Vocol 35:175–182

Spahn C, Krampe F, Nusseck M (2021a) Live music performance: the relationship between flow and music performance anxiety. Front Psychol 12:725569. https://doi.org/10.3389/fpsyg.2021.725569

Spahn C, Krampe F, Nusseck M (2021b) Classifying different types of music performance anxiety. Front Psychol 4. https://doi.org/10.3389/fpsyg.2021.538535

Spahn C, Walther J-C, Nusseck M (2016) The effectiveness of a multimodal concept of audition training for music students in coping with music performance anxiety. Psychology of Music 44:893–909.

Wang JC (2001) A study of performance anxiety in talented music students. Bull Res Element Educ 7:1–67

Yerkes RM, Dodson JD (1908) The relation of strength of stimulus to rapidity of habit-formation. J Comp Neurol Psychol 18:459–482

28 Healthy Music-Making: Prevention in Instrumental Lessons for Children and Young Musicians

Claudia Spahn

Making music can unlock great potential in terms of health-promoting effects, especially when we consider the whole lifespan. The best conditions for developing this potential are present when musical education is rooted in the early years and playing an instrument is already learned during childhood and adolescence. However, key here is that instrumental students are taught a healthy way of making music from the beginning, which extends to the body, mind and spirit. According to scientific studies, up to three quarters of children and adolescents who make music suffer from health problems related to the playing of the instrument (Ranelli et al. 2008; Gembris and Ebinger 2017; Gembris et al. 2020). This points to the great significance of prevention in early instrumental teaching. The integration of music physiology content into teaching practice nurtures musical development and achievement on the instrument, as well as obviating health problems and creating the conditions for music-making and musical education to blossom to its full potential in terms of promoting health.

As part of the establishment of the specialized area of music physiology and musicians' medicine, future music pedagogues are now trained at German universities of music in health-related aspects of music-making; likewise, working music teachers, in whose studies at the time health aspects were not yet taught, also receive further education in this field. As the positive groundwork for music-making in later life—whether as an amateur or professional musician—should already be laid during childhood and adolescence, the education of children and adolescents plays an especially important role in the teaching of instruments.

Making music carries great potential in terms of promoting health and development (Roden et al. 2014) provided the physical, psychological and cognitive

C. Spahn (✉)
Freiburg Institute for Musicians' Medicine (FIM), University of Music Freiburg, Medical Faculty University Freiburg, University Clinic Freiburg, Freiburg, Germany
e-mail: claudia.spahn@uniklinik-freiburg.de

G. Kreutz, G. Bernatzky (eds.), *Music and Medicine*, Neurocultural Health and Wellbeing, https://doi.org/10.1007/978-3-662-72175-9_28

conditions for playing an instrument are kept in mind and positively utilized (Nawrocka et al. 2014). As such, one should pay attention to these conditions from the outset (Spahn 2018, 2022).

28.1 Playing-Related Complaints Among Instrumental Students in Childhood and Adolescence

Since the 1980s, studies can be found of adolescents concerning the frequency and type of complaints occurring in relation to playing an instrument.

Lockwood (1988) investigated 120 instrumental students in a youth symphony orchestra in the USA aged between 14 and 17 and found that in around half of those questioned, slight pain occasionally arose during playing, while 17% indicated considerable pain. Complaints among string players were more frequent when playing the cello and double bass than the violin and viola. Four-fifths of adolescent musicians accepted pain while playing without further ado, considering it a part and parcel of successful music-making. Fry et al. (1988) similarly studied music students at the same age in Australian music schools. Of the participants in the study, 98 in all, 56% had already experienced pain while playing their instrument, while one-third complained that they were at that time having pain while playing. Fry and Rowley (1989) carried out a further study among 169 students of two British music schools. The students had a mean age of 14.4 and practiced 3.3 h per day on average. Half of the music students indicated pain in the area of the upper extremities at the time of the study. In these studies, girls uniformly suffered complaints more frequently than boys (Lockwood 1988; Fry et al. 1988; Fry and Rowley 1989). Brown (1997) questioned 36 members of a youth symphony orchestra in the north west of the USA, whose ages ranged from 11 to 18. Two-thirds indicated that they were having pain at that time in the musculoskeletal system while playing. In a study by Shoup (1995) of 425 music students in Arizona with an average age of 12.9, who had been playing their instrument for a mean of 3.4 years and belonged to various orchestral and band formations, around 20% of the music students complained of pains at that time while playing, specifically of the musculoskeletal system.

Britsch (2005) examined 255 music students from four youth orchestras in the Midwest of the USA concerning the frequency of playing-related pain syndromes; moreover, she inquired in a more differentiated way than in previous investigations about dealing with pain when playing an instrument. Those questioned were between 9 and 15 years of age and had received a classical instrumental education on one of the orchestral instruments, namely the flute, oboe, clarinet, horn, trumpet, trombone, percussion, violin, viola, cello or double bass. The severity of the pain was recorded on a scale of 0–5, enabling differentiation between whether the pain arose while the instrument was being played or subsequently, how long the pain endured and whether it occurred during the normal run of the day outside of music-making. About 8% of the students questioned indicated a complete absence of pain. Around half reported they had already suffered pain once while playing their instrument. Three-quarters of the students experienced the pain only when playing or shortly thereafter. Most frequent parts of the body affected were the neck, shoulders, wrists, fingers, thumbs and lower back. At least three-quarters of respondents indicated likewise that they were "really nervous" during the performance.

About 58% of the 255 music students reported that they take breaks during practice; among the younger students this was the case with less than half. Playing scales was stated by the majority of students to be the most frequent warm-up exercise, with only around one-tenth of them carrying out warm-up exercises without an instrument (Britsch 2005).

To the question "Do you think it is alright to play while feeling pain?" 55% answered with "no", 6% with "sometimes" and 35% with "yes" (Britsch 2005). In previous studies of music students of comparable age, 79% (Lockwood 1988) and 44% (Shoup 1995) had answered with "yes".

The most frequent reaction to pain while playing was named in Britsch's (2005) study as "take a break and play again later on". About 13% of respondents indicated "no change in behaviour". Most of the students had never spoken about their complaints with their instrumental teachers and had not been trained by the latter in the prevention of health risks while practicing. In those cases where a recommendation was made to the students by the instrumental teacher on how to handle complaints, these consisted of taking a break and/or changing playing technique.

Shields and Dockrell (2000) carried out a study of 182 piano students from seven Irish music schools with the goal of recording the specific areas of pain while playing the piano. A questionnaire on complaints in the hand and forearm areas was used for this. The wrist was the most common location of injury (36.6%).

Samsel et al. (2005) carried out a survey of 705 young musicians—mainly music students from eight German and nine international young symphony orchestras—by means of standardized questionnaires. Three-quarters of the sample participants were aged between 16 and 22. The participants were questioned with regard to their current mental and physical stress, their health behaviour, as well as their attitude toward preventive measures and their application (ibid). The investigators compared the musicians' data with 807 youths and young adults from the Federal Health Survey (BGS) of 1998 (Contributions to the Federal Health Report 2002). In this, general mental stress resulted in 77% of the participants with completed musical training, whereby the younger the musicians, the less the mental strain. In contrast with the group of non-musicians, around twice as many respondents from the musicians' sample complained of pain. At the same time, the scores for the musicians' group in self-assessing their health were significantly better than in the comparative group: 46% of musicians and 24% of non-musicians, who reported a high or very high degree of pain, assessed their state of health as excellent, nonetheless. The authors conclude from this finding that pain is rather accepted as inherent to the activity among musicians (Spahn 2011a).

Ranelli et al. (2008) investigated 731 instrumental students aged between 7 and 17 in Australia regarding symptoms and disorder patterns of the musculoskeletal system. About 30% suffered from a diagnosable disorder of the musculoskeletal system that impaired them during play. Around half of the respondents had noticed complaints while playing in the previous month. 67% of children and adolescents in the sample had experienced complaints in connection with playing the instrument. The frequency of the complaints linked to the age showed that the youngest in the sample already suffered complaints with similar frequency to the older ones and so were hindered in their playing, too.

Cygańska et al. (2017) examined the body posture of 101 children, aged between 7 and 12 years. Among the participants were 49 child violinists and a control group of 52 children who did not play any musical instrument. Compared to the control group, changes in body posture in children who played the violin appeared early in their training, leading to spinal curvatures.

Gembris et al. (2022) performed an investigation as part of a large-scale study (*N = 1143*) with participants at the age of 9–24 years at the national level of the "Jugend musiziert" contest. About three-quarters (76%) of the surveyed participants stated that they had experienced pain during or after playing their instrument. Female musicians were significantly more frequently affected (79%) than male musicians (71%). With increasing age, the prevalence of playing-related pain (PRP) rises from 71% (9–13 years) to 85% (18–24 years). Regarding localization of pain, results are in line with many other studies, with musculoskeletal problems the most common. Furthermore, data show a clear relationship between the duration of practice and the prevalence of PRP.

The survey of the literature shows that playing-related complaints among children and adolescents are a frequent and relevant subject. Children as young as 4–7 can develop symptoms of strain. In almost all the studies, around half of the instrumental students were negatively affected by complaints relating to playing to a greater or lesser extent. Two-third of the children and adolescents who learn an instrument have already experienced pain once while playing.

Especially, attitudes to complaints while playing are of great interest.

While 79% of adolescent instrumental players perceived pain while playing as "normal" (Lockwood 1988), the share of youths with this attitude fell to 44% (Shoup 1995) and further to 35% in 2005 (Britsch 2005).

It can be assumed that in the course of establishing and institutionalizing the subject of music physiology and musicians' medicine, complaints during the playing of an instrument are meantime assessed as problematic and needing therapy and that a process of greater awareness towards the perception of pain relating to playing an instrument is taking place. In the study by Britsch (2005), it became clear that both on the part of the students and the instrumental teachers, a limited repertoire lacking in nuance existed in dealing with playing-related complaints. This is hardly surprising, as it is only in recent years that instrumental teachers have been trained in the field of prevention and health promotion.

Prevention with regard to lifelong, healthy music-making is important, especially for young musicians who have chosen professional training. In her study of music students, Spahn (2006) established that at the beginning of their studies at the music university, a quarter of students already suffered at that time from adverse effects related to playing. Compared with other subjects of study such as medicine and sports science, music students thus begin their studies with physical complaints occurring at a significantly greater frequency (Spahn et al. 2004). This situation seems not to have changed, as current data confirm (Spahn et al. 2017).

There are also data from a musicians' medicine perspective on the nature of the complaints in adolescent musicians among corresponding patient collectives.

Warrington et al. (2002) investigated 140 musician patients who had attended a music-medical hand surgery department in London. In the group of the under 25-year-olds, non-specific pain syndromes predominated. Burkholder and Brandfonbrener (2004) analysed the distribution of the diagnosis in a patient sample, which consisted of 314 music-making youths under the age of 19 at a clinic in the USA specialized in musicians' medicine. Mostly frequently found were pain syndromes of the upper extremities and muscle tension. The symptoms were accompanied by a lack of physical fitness and with non-physiological playing technique (Burkholder and Brandfonbrener 2004; Shoup 1995; Warrington et al. 2002; Lockwood 1988). Hypermobility of the joints as a risk factor for the development of strain syndromes were found more commonly among girls than boys. Girls suffered more frequently from hand muscle weakness and scoliosis, while boys more often presented the diagnoses of carpal tunnel syndrome and tenosynovitis.

Besides primarily physical complaints, harmful forms of stage fright, so-called performance fears, represent a problem for around half of adolescent instrumentalists (Shoup 1995). In a study by Nusseck et al. (2015) high levels of MPA for classical musicians between 7 and 16 yrs were found and for popular musicians, low MPA was seen in the younger (7-11 yrs) and high MPA in the older (16+ yrs) musicians (Nusseck et al. 2015)

28.2 Preventive Approaches in Instrumental Teaching

In contrast to the prevention programmes in music university education, which were evaluated with regard to their effectiveness in intervention studies (Spahn et al. 2001, 2016, 2017, 2020; Zander 2006; Barton and Feinberg 2008; Zander et al. 2010; Ginsborg et al. 2012), the prevention approaches in instrumental teaching for children and adolescents are conceptualized but not yet so clearly evaluated. Hildebrandt (2000) reports on the music physiology consultation at a music school that he founded in 1993. This was an inter-class 2-h instructional programme with the aim of preventing playing-related health problems, which was held weekly and in which both music students and instrumental teachers at the music school took part. Topics taught were playing posture and movement, ergonomics and stage presence as well as healthy and effective learning and practicing strategies. Included in the concept is the musical and individual adaptation of certain body techniques. One-to-one consultation in music physiology also took place over and above the group lessons. The preventative approach happened on several levels, by means of the work on individual and musical expression, as well as the work undertaken with and without the instrument. As decisive factors in the prevention of playing and health problems, Hildebrandt names the training and coordination of posture, breathing and fine motor skills, the development of appropriate musical playing performance and playing motor skills, as well as individual adaptation of ergonomic aids (Hildebrandt 2000).

Nawrocka et al. (2014) assessed correlations between the level of physical activity and the occurrence of musculoskeletal pain among young instrumentalists. A total of 225 Polish music school students were investigated. The pain localized in neck, shoulders, upper and lower back was reported significantly more often by the participants who did not meet standard criteria for the recommended or minimal physical activity level. The results suggest that performing the recommended health-oriented physical activity may reduce the prevalence of musculoskeletal pain in young musicians.

Brennscheidt (2000) reports on her experiences with a comparable consultation and teaching concept at Düsseldorf Music School. In this case, individual appointments were likewise carried out for consultation of students in topics of music physiology, parents and instrumental teachers with recommended further measures, as well as teaching in small groups with students. The class covered teaching music physiological basics, playing and movement analysis as well as body-related exercises. Drawing on the experiences with the children and adolescents, the author formulates four predisposing factors which in her view are frequent and key for the development of playing disorders and complaints.

Predisposing factors for the development of playing disorders and complaints (based on Brennscheidt 2000).

- *Ergonomic questions, i.e. adapting the instrument to the player*
  For children, the risk here exists of instruments that are too large relative to their body size. This can result in an evasive posture that persists until adolescence is reached.
- *Immobility, i.e. the lack of permeability of movement and expression in the whole body while playing the instrument*
  For children, the risk exists of focusing on fine motor skills, which can become locked during puberty due to feelings of embarrassment.
- *Lopsided weight distribution*
  Especially, with asymmetrical instruments, static compensation may occur with the weight being distributed to one side of the body, which then becomes established as a lopsided pattern (Nusseck and Spahn 2020).
- *Hyperlordosis, i.e. the stretching in the lower back into the so-called hollow back*
  In the case of children, this posture can arise due to the need to hold on to the instrument. Adolescents often wrongly associate hyperlordosis with "upright posture".

Most authors emphasize as key for effective prevention the networking between instrumental teachers, music physiologists, physicians specialized in musicians' medicine (e.g. paediatricians and physicians for psychosomatic medicine), parents and others significantly involved in the education of the child and adolescent (music teachers and other specialist teachers of general schools) (Brennscheidt 2000; Ackermann and Driscoll 2013; Birkedahl 1989; Dawson 2006; Sklaire 1997).

In a 1989 article in the magazine "Medical Problems of Performing Artists", the violin teacher Nonie Birkedahl describes the tasks of the instrumental teacher in recognizing, preventing and healing the health problems of students in instrumental teaching. Based on five case studies of young violin students, who began playing the violin aged between 4 and 6, she convincingly describes how from the first violin lesson she attentively observes the posture, patterns and range of movement of her students, integrating them into the pedagogical approach as they learn to play. In this, she proceeds systematically according to a playing-based research plan developed over the years. Besides the physical prerequisites, she is equally interested in her students' activities, she regularly keeps in touch with the parents and documents each student's psychosocial situation in the family and school. In some cases, she cooperates with physicians experienced in musicians' medicine in order to be better able to categorize diagnostically the significance of certain observations made during teaching. Sklaire (1997), too, points out, from the perspective of the supervising paediatrician, that in collaboration with the music pedagogue, thorough and regular examination by the paediatrician can provide an important basis for the adolescent instrumental student's health to develop positively. Ackermann and Driscoll (2013) are concerned in a pilot study with the parents' role in health promotion in early instrumental teaching. The parents of 24 adolescent music students aged from 12 to 17 were questioned on music, physiological and health aspects of their children's music-making. Half of the adolescents in the sample were educated at a High school without music as a special subject, and the other half with. Nearly all the parents agreed that the physical health of their children represents an important precondition for them to play their instrument well, that dealing with music performance anxiety in a positive way is likewise a key contribution to this, which it is important for playing one's instrument well to understand one's body and the way it functions when one is playing and practicing. Regarding the question of whether pain is normal when one plays an instrument, half of the parents whose children attended the school with music as a special focus answered "yes". No parent in the other school found pain during playing to be something normal. Ackermann and Driscoll concluded from their results that the subject of health in instrumental teaching is considered important by parents and supported by them. The attitude of some of the parents, whereby they accept pain during music-making, should be the subject of further study (Ackermann and Driscoll 2013). The importance of the parents' role generally in terms of prevention for children is supported by broadly conceived meta-analyses (Kendrick et al. 2008). Manchester (1997) points out that the development of children and adolescents should follow criteria from developmental psychology in the first phase of learning an instrument up until studies begin or job training, i.e. up to the age of 21 depending on the educational system concerned, and thus can be divided up into three phases. These are explained by the bio-psychosocial developmental steps of each age group concerned. Manchester suggests an early phase of adolescence from 10 to 13 years of age, a middle phase of 14–17, and a late phase of adolescence from 18 to 21. From this differentiation, there arise different requirements with regard to music physiological themes (Manchester 1997).

28.3 Qualification of Music Pedagogues in the Area of Prevention and Health Promotion

28.3.1 Prevention in Instrumental Teaching in the Higher Education of Music Pedagogues

A prerequisite for conveying healthy music-making in instrumental teaching is the training of music educators in the subjects of music physiology and prevention. Graduates of music pedagogy have only been trained in this area since the integration of this material in the last 10 years due to the establishment of music physiology and musicians' medicine as a subject at universities of music.

The subject of music physiology is taught at music universities in Germany and is integrated as a compulsory subject in the education of instrumental teachers at some music universities. In practice-oriented seminars, music pedagogues learn the physiological and psychological basics of music-making and how they can convey these contents to their students in terms of prevention and health promotion. In instrumental and vocal lessons, this content should be presented in such a way that the students acquire the relevant skills. Table 28.1 summarizes the topics and learning goals for instrumental lessons as part of the subject music physiology and musicians' medicine at a glance.

28.3.2 Music Physiology for Instrumental and Vocal Teachers in Further Education

For instrumental teachers who have been working in this field for a long time, comprehensive further training is required. Hildebrandt and Nübling (2004) investigated

Table 28.1 Skills that should be taught to young students in instrumental lessons by their instrumental teachers (Spahn 2018)

Subject areas	Learning goals The student should learn
Motion Body awareness Mindfulness	To perceive his movements while playing as precisely as possible To make his playing movements as economical as possible That the whole body is involved in all activities while playing an instrument or singing To adapt the instrument ergonomically To do a warm-up and cool-down
Healthy practice Effective learning	To have a concept of practice that includes rest and balance exercises To correctly assess the mental and physical demands of playing in order to prevent overuse To respect their own limits That practice changes over the lifetime
Performance skills Development promotion	How to cope with music performance anxiety and which techniques to use What mental and psychological concepts are relevant to performance To develop a realistic and positive musical self-concept

the effects of a music physiology advanced training course on the pedagogical instruction style of the music pedagogues participating. At the same time, they were interested in whether, from the students' viewpoint, changes in instrumental teaching could be perceived that were attributable to the course. About 26 instrumental educators and 66 related music students took part in the study. One half of the educators formed the intervention group and received group teaching for two weekly semester hours over one semester. The other half of the music teachers received no further education and formed the control group. The music students were allocated to the Intervention or control group, respectively. The central elements of the course material were reflection and the optimization of playing instructions during teaching (solution-centred approach versus problem-centred approach), as well as the teaching of movement (understanding of movement chains in playing movements). In the evaluation by means of questionnaires, a significant difference was shown in the intervention group compared to the control group in that both the music teachers themselves, who had taken part in the course, and their students perceived more responsibility and clarity in the issuing of playing instructions in class.

28.3.3 Curriculum for Instrumental and Vocal Teachers in Further Education

Certified programmes are offered by music universities in Germany, Austria and Switzerland for further training in music physiology.

Spahn et al. (2009; Spahn 2018) developed a concept for instrumental and vocal teachers, which trains music teachers in the subjects of music physiology and prevention. The main subject areas and contents are shown in Table 28.2.

The curriculum consists of five modules in all (Table 28.2). From 2009 to 2013, 28 music teachers (19 women and 9 men) took part in this further education programme, made up of four small groups of seven persons, respectively. The participation enabled them as mentors to be the contact person for musicians' health at their music school. The mentor training for music teachers was part of the "healthy music school" concept, which was initiated by the Internationale Musikakademie Schloss Kapfenburg. As part of this concept, music schools can be certified as an institution with the descriptor "healthy music school", if at least one music educator on the teaching staff has successfully passed the curriculum and the music school has carried out regular activities in the area of musicians' health.

A formative evaluation of the curriculum was carried out by means of standardized questions, in which the participants could answer the questions in an open-ended way and impart their experiences. The questions focused on the personal experiences and learning gains, as well as the opportunities and experiences of applying them in the classroom with students. The participants each had the chance in between the training units to try out in practice what they had learned. Some of those who completed the course produced reports, in which the transfer of the curricular learning material into practice was presented and reflected upon.

Table 28.2 Curriculum for further education for instrumental and singing teachers for prevention at music schools (Spahn et al. 2009; Spahn 2018)

Subject area curricular modules	Content
Body awareness and somagogy	Recognizing and scrutinizing one's own movement sequences Body-oriented methods, breathing and voice
Physiological basics of making music	Breathing and uprightness Learning about movement elements for teaching music Resources-oriented approach
Psychological basics of making music	Coping with MPA and performance preparation Relaxation and preparation techniques Teacher—Student relationship Promotion of personality development
Student-oriented application of the learning content in the teaching practice	Instrument-specific movement sequences Recognizing non-physiological positions and playing movements Selection of suitable exercises in the teaching practice, ergonomic aids Reflecting on communication processes
Prevention at music schools	Mentor's task in the teaching staff of music schools Organizing further training and information events at the music school Networking—contact partner in the area of musicians' medicine

The evaluation results showed that all the participants had gained new learning experiences through the training course, which they rated as relevant and helpful for their own teaching. Indeed, a great need apparent among the majority of educators to be better able to cope with the diverse issues of music physiology and prevention that they encounter in their teaching practice. Therefore, many music teachers had already undergone further training in individual body methods, such as the Feldenkrais Method or Alexander Technique (Spahn 2011b). From the participants' perspective, the contents learned in the training could, for the most part, be implemented successfully into the teaching practice; difficulties occasionally arose concerning time management within the lessons. Communicating the topic of "making healthy music" within the teaching staff of each respective music school proceeded differently, depending on the degree of openness previously found. In some cases, a committed attitude to health issues within the team of colleagues could be achieved through the activities of the trained teacher in the medium term. This is reflected in the fact that almost all music schools where participants of the mentor training are active have attained the "healthy music school" certificate. Table 28.3 illustrates the results of the evaluation by means of examples of original quotes from participants.

Table 28.3 Formative evaluation of the continuing education programme on prevention at music schools (Spahn et al. 2009) involving 28 instrumental and vocal instructors—exemplary responses as original quotes

Subject areas curricular modules	Learning experiences of participants
Body awareness	"The whole body is involved in all activities more extensively than previously assumed" "The willingness to perceive more precisely leads to enhanced mindfulness"
Body methods	"Improvement of mobility, pain relief and resultant well-being, due to Feldenkrais lessons" "Playing-based approach to different postures while playing"
Physiological basics of making music	"The ability to sense, feel and understand sequences of movements promotes the capacity for insight into the systemic connections in the body"
Psychological basics of music-making	"One important recommendation is to consider students in the broad context of their lives (e.g. tension with parents)" "Guiding principles: Respect yourself and others—continue to work and develop your skills (while having fun and with joy, too, of course)—accept yourself and your level of achievement" "Accept stage fright and try to convert it into positive energy"
Student-oriented application of the learning content in the teaching practice	Break down movement sequences and practise without an instrument if necessary "How breathing works anatomically and physiologically" "Talk about stage fright—prepare the performance mentally—play in front of others more often (step-by-step: in front of fellow students, in front of one's parents, in a protected space, performance)"
Prevention at music schools	"Warm-up exercises, instrument-specific risks and ergonomic aids" "Enthusing my colleagues for my experiences of healthy music-making in an information/discussion session" "Collegial intervision and stress management"

28.4 Conclusion

The great potential of instrumental music-making and singing for physical and mental health, as well as for the development of the personality (Spahn 2007; Spahn and Richter 2006, 2007), can only unfold when healthy forms of music-making are conveyed in instrumental teaching from the beginning. The frequency of playing-related complaints among musicians in childhood and adolescence indicates that music educators have hitherto devoted insufficient attention to the subject of such complaints. Likewise, therapeutic support from physicians specializing in musicians' medicine (Dawson 2006) was apparently not sufficiently used by music teachers to reduce the complaints of young students.

That music's physiological and health aspects were not represented or underrepresented in the training of music educators at universities for a long time, and that competence in this area was lacking, have certainly been issues here. The integration of prevention content into the curricula of the Bachelor's and Master's Programmes for Music Education, which is now taking place in most Music Universities in European countries as well as in the United States and Australia, will lead to better training for musicians in the medium term. The improved training is complemented by further training programmes in music physiology.

This goes along with a new self-conception on the part of instrumental and singing teachers, whose knowledge and activities must move within an interdisciplinary canon of subjects. Decision-makers in the field of music schools have the important task of recognizing qualifications in the field of music physiology among graduates of music universities as an important recruitment argument and supporting further training for working music school teachers.

References

Ackermann B, Driscoll T (2013) Attitudes and practices of parents of teenage musicians to health issues related to playing an instrument: a pilot study. Med Probl Perform Art 28(1):24–27

Barton R, Feinberg JR (2008) Effectiveness of an educational program in health promotion and injury prevention for freshman music majors. Med Probl Perform Art 23:47–53

Beiträge zur Gesundheitsberichterstattung des Bundes (2002) Der Bundes-Gesundheitssurvey—Baustein der Gesundheitssurveillance in Deutschland. Robert Koch-Institut, Berlin

Birkedahl N (1989) Identification, prevention, and remediation of medical problems in very young violin students. Med Probl Perform Art 4:176–178

Brennscheidt R (2000) Frühe Instrumentalförderung erfordert frühe medizinische Prävention—Konsequenzen aus der musikmedizinischen Beratung auf Musikschulebene. Musikphysiologie und Musikermedizin 1:22–26

Britsch L (2005) Investigating performance-related problems of young musicians. Med Probl Perform Art 20(1):40–47

Brown AN (1997) Musculoskeletal misuse among youth symphony string players. Med Probl Perform Art 12(1):15–18

Burkholder KR, Brandfonbrener AG (2004) Performance-related injuries among student musicians at a specialty clinic. Med Probl Perform Art 19:116–122

Cygańska A, Truszczyńska-Baszak A, Drzał-Grabiec J, Tarnowski A (2017) Analysis of antero-posterior spinal curvatures in child violinists from music schools. Med Probl Perform Art 32(3):176–179(4). https://doi.org/10.21091/mppa.2017.3029

Dawson WJ (2006) Playing without pain: strategies for the developing instrumentalist. Music Educ J 93(2):36–41. https://doi.org/10.1177/002743210609300218

Fry HJH, Rowley GL (1989) Music related upper limb pain in school children. Ann Rheum Dis 48:998–1002

Fry HJH, Ross P, Rutherford M (1988) Music-related overuse in secondary schools. Med Probl Perform Art 3(4):133–134

Gembris H, Ebinger F (2017) Musizierbedingte körperliche Beschwerden bei Kindern und Jugendlichen. In: Gembris H (ed) Musik studieren und Abitur machen. Doppelbelastung im gesundheitlich-gesellschaftlichen Kontext. Lit, Münster, pp 129–158

Gembris H, Menze J, Heye A, Bullerjahn C (2020) High-performing young musicians' playing-related pain. Results of a large-scale study. Front Psychol. https://doi.org/10.3389/fpsyg.2020.564736

Gembris H, Menze J, Heye A, Bullerjahn C (2022) High-Performing Young Musicians' Playing-Related Pain. Results of a Large-Scale Study. Front Psychol. 16;11:564736. https://doi.org/10.3389/fpsyg.2020.564736.

Ginsborg J, Spahn C, Williamon A (2012) Health promotion in higher music education. In: MacDonald RAR, Kreutz G, Mitchell L (eds) Music, health, and wellbeing. Oxford University Press, Oxford, pp 356–366

Hildebrandt H (2000) Prävention von Spiel- und Gesundheitsproblemen bei Musikern von Anfang an. In: Klein-Vogelbach S, Lahme A, Spirgi-Gantert I (Hrsg) Musikinstrument und Körperhaltung. Springer, Berlin, S 108–140

Hildebrandt H, Nübling M (2004) Providing further training in musico-physiology to instrumental teachers: do their professional and pre-professional students derive any benefit? Med Probl Perform Art 19:62–69

Kendrick D, Barlow J, Hampshire A et al (2008) Parenting interventions and the prevention of unintentional injuries in childhood: systematic review and meta-analysis. Child Care Health Dev 34:682–695

Lockwood AH (1988) Medical problems in secondary school-aged musicians. Med Probl Perform Art 3(4):129–132

Manchester RA (1997) Musculoskeletal problems of adolescent instrumentalists. Med Probl Perform Art 12:72–74

Nawrocka A, Mynarski W, Powerska A et al (2014) Health-oriented physical activity in prevention of musculoskeletal disorders among young Polish musicians. IJOMEH 27:28–37. https://doi.org/10.2478/s13382-014-0224-5

Nusseck M, Spahn C (2020) Comparison of postural stability and balance between musicians and non-musicians. Front Psychol. https://doi.org/10.3389/fpsyg.2020.01253

Nusseck M, Zander M, Spahn C (2015) Music performance anxiety in young musicians: comparison of playing classical or popular music. Med Probl Perform Art 30(1):30–7. https://doi.org/10.21091/mppa.2015.1005

Ranelli S, Straker L, Smith A (2008) Prevalence of playing-related musculoskeletal symptoms and disorders in children learning instrumental music. Med Probl Perform Art 23:178–185

Roden I, Grube D, Bongard S, Kreutz G (2014) Does music training enhance working memory performance? Findings from a quasi-experimental longitudinal study. Psychol Music 42(2):284–229

Samsel W, Marstedt G, Möller H, Müller R (2005) Musikergesundheit: Ergebnisse einer Befragung junger Musiker über Berufsperspektiven, Belastungen und Gesundheit. Asgard-Verlag, St. Augustin

Shields N, Dockrell S (2000) The prevalence of injuries among pianists in music schools in Ireland. Med Probl Perform Art 15:155–160

Shoup D (1995) Survey of performance-related problems among high school and junior high school musicians. Med Probl Perform Art 10(3):100–105

Sklaire MW (1997) Performing arts medicine: pediatric and adolescent medical aspects. Med Probl Perform Art 12:75–78

Spahn C (2006) Gesundheit für Musiker—Entwicklung des Freiburger Präventionsmodells. Schriftenreihe des Freiburger Instituts für Musikermedizin (Spahn C, Hrsg) Freiburger Beiträge zur Musikermedizin, Bd 1. Projektverlag, Freiburg/Bochum

Spahn C (2007) Singen und musizieren für die Gesundheit: Das Freiburger Institut für Musikermedizin. Tonkünstlerforum 66:2–6

Spahn C (2011a) Prävention und Gesundheitsförderung. In: Spahn C, Richter B, Altenmüller E (Hrsg) MusikerMedizin. Diagnostik, Therapie und Prävention von musikerspezifischen Erkrankungen. Schattauer, Stuttgart, S 50–79

Spahn C (2011b) Spielende Bewegungen—Über die Integration körperorientierter Methoden in die Instrumentalpädagogik. Üben und Musizieren 2:16–20

Spahn C (2018) Musikergesundheit in der Praxis: Grundlagen, Prävention, Übungen. Henschel-Verlag Leipzig

Spahn C (2022) Diseases and health risks in instrumentalists. In: McPherson GE (ed) The Oxford handbook of music performance, vol 2. Oxford University Press, pp 232–259

Spahn C, Richter B (2006) The development of the singing voice across the lifespan. In: Gembris H (ed) Musical development from a lifespan perspective. Peter Lang, Frankfurt, pp 119–130

Spahn C, Richter B (2007) Gesundheitliche Aspekte des Singens und Musizierens. In: Gauger JD, Wilske H (Hrsg) Bildungsoffensive Musikunterricht. Rombach, Freiburg, S 133–141
Spahn C, Hildebrandt H, Seidenglanz K (2001) Effectiveness of a prophylactic course to prevent playing-related health problems of student musicians. Med Probl Perform Art 16:24–31
Spahn C, Strukely S, Lehmann A (2004) Health conditions, attitudes towards study, and health at the beginning of university study: student musicians in comparison with other student populations. Med Probl Perform Art 19:26–33
Spahn C, Gädeke D, Hausen D, Noé B, Türk A, Zander M (2009) Fortbildungscurriculum für Instrumental- und Gesangspädagogen zum Thema Gesundheit im Instrumental-unterricht (unveröff)
Spahn C, Walther J-C, Nusseck M (2016) The effectiveness of a multimodal concept of audition training for music students in coping with music performance anxiety. Psychol Music 44:893–909
Spahn C, Voltmer E, Mornell A, Nusseck M (2017) Health status and preventive health behavior of music students during university education: merging prior results with new insights from a German multicenter study. Music Sci 21:213–229
Spahn C, Immerz A, Nusseck M (2020) „Die Lücke schließen zwischen Unterricht und Musizierpraxis"—eine qualitative Studie zur Evaluation spezifischer pädagogischer Elemente im Bereich körperorientierter Gesundheitsförderung und Prävention bei Musikstudierenden. In: T. Fischinger und C. Louven: Jahrbuch Musikpsychologie—Musik im audiovisuellen Kontext, Band 29:e45
Warrington J, Winspur I, Steinwede D (2002) Upper-extremity problems in musicians related to age. Med Probl Perform Art 17:131–134
Zander MF (2006) Musiker zwischen Gesundheit und Krankheit—Evaluation des Freiburger Präventionsmodells Schriftenreihe des Freiburger Instituts für Musikermedizin (Spahn C, Hrsg) Freiburger Beiträge zur Musikermedizin, Bd 2, Projektverlag, Freiburg/Bochum
Zander MF, Voltmer E, Spahn C (2010) Health promotion and prevention in higher music education—results of a longitudinal study. Med Probl Perform Art 25(2):54–65

Part VI

Health Risks Due to Music

The Role of Emotion Modulation in Defiant Adolescence Music

29

Julia Herr and Richard von Georgi

29.1 Music and Mental Health in Adolescence

Music does not only affect the physical health of its recipients but has impact on psychological parameters as well (Juslin and Sloboda 2001). This notion of a psychoactive effect of music listening is supported by studies dealing with music-related psychobiological changes (e.g., Bartlett et al. 1993; McCraty et al. 1996; Nilsson 2009; Altenmüller and Schlaug 2012) as well as modulations of psychosomatic conditions such as depression (e.g., Chan et al. 2011), pain perception (Beck 1991; Good 1996; McDonald et al. 2003; Phumdoung and Good 2003; Nilsson 2008; Gebhardt and von Georgi 2010), or the influence of musical activities on subjective quality of life (Biley 2000; Bradt et al. 2011).

It remains unclear, however, to what extent the associations between music and an individual's mental state can be construed as causal effects. Although some animal studies do point to specific biological effects of music (e.g., Panksepp and Bernatzky 2002; Núñez et al. 2002; Angelucci et al. 2007; Xu et al. 2007; Akiyama and Sutoo 2011), there is still controversy about a causal theoretical explanation of these effects as applied to humans.

Moreover, some professional circles take general issues with the notion of a predominantly *positive* impact of music on the physical and mental health of recipients. Frequently, impact studies on different music genres arise from the fields of adolescent pediatrics and music psychology, allegedly indicating negative effects of specific musical styles.

J. Herr
SRH School of Arts, Information and Media, Berlin, Germany

R. von Georgi (✉)
SRH School of Arts, Information and Media, Berlin Institute of Biomusicology and Empirical Research (BIBER), Berlin, Germany
e-mail: Richard.vonGeorgi@srh-hochschulen.de

G. Kreutz, G. Bernatzky (eds.), *Music and Medicine*, Neurocultural Health and Wellbeing, https://doi.org/10.1007/978-3-662-72175-9_29

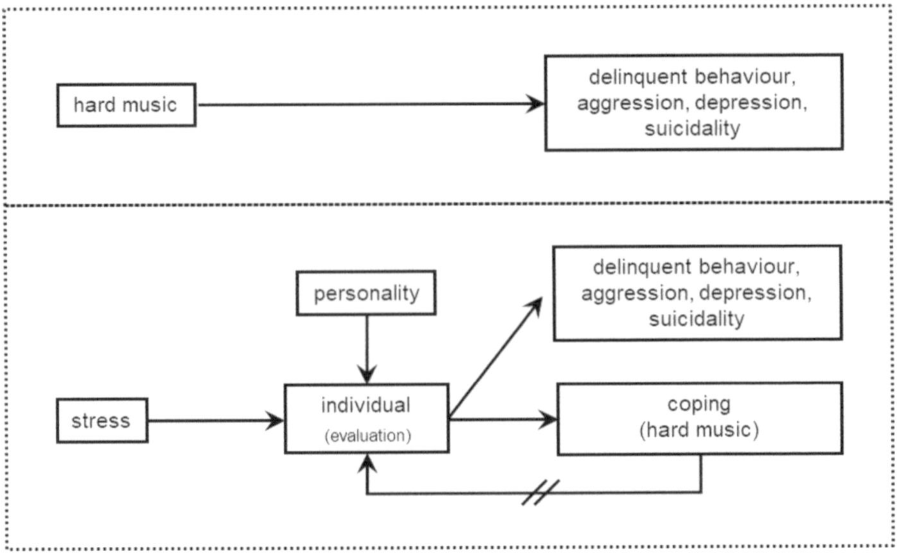

Fig. 29.1 Two models of the effect of hard music. Top: causal model (e.g., Miehling 2006); bottom: stress interaction model (e.g., Arnett 1991a, b)

Since the 1980s, so-called hard music (e.g., rock, heavy metal, alternative) in particular has repeatedly been assumed to cause certain behavioral, health-related, and/or developmental disorders (see below) in its mostly adolescent recipients. Figure 29.1 (above) represents such a hypothesis, which in professional discourses, apart from exemplary individual cases and scientifically questionable publications (e.g., Miehling 2006; for a critical discussion, see von Georgi 2011), is seemingly supported also by empirically legitimate studies.

At first sight, these studies seem to confirm that frequent reception of hard music and its associated lyrics and music videos can have the following (negative) effects:

(a) It leads to both delinquency and substance abuse and evokes aggression and violence (Pfaus et al. 1986; King 1988; McCraty et al. 1998; Weidinger and Demi 1991; Arnett 1991a, b; Martin et al. 1993; Lacourse et al. 2001; Schwartz and Fouts 2003; Mulder et al. 2007).
(b) It is related to personality traits such as sensation seeking, psychoticism, and other similar constructs (e.g., Litle and Zuckerman 1986; Wells and Hakanen 1991; Arnett 1991a; Robinson et al. 1996; Rawlings et al. 1995, 1998, 2000; Dillmann Carpentier et al. 2003; Schwartz and Fouts 2003).
(c) It induces depression, hopelessness, and suicidality (e.g., Martin et al. 1993; Stack et al. 1994; Lester and Whipple 1996; Steinhausen and Winkler Metzger 2001; Lacourse et al. 2001).

29.2 Cogency of Existing Findings

Even though abovementioned studies prompt the idea that certain music genres do indeed have harmful effects on people's health and behavior, a closer look at the findings suggests that there are a number of problematic aspects to such an interpretation. First of all, it should be noted that the methods used in many studies, i.e., correlation statistics and simple univariate mean comparisons, cannot be considered as adequate methodological tools to support the assumption of a causal relationship like the one stated. That is because these methods of analysis do not take into account the numerous superordinate variables, such as gender effects (Steinhausen and Winkler Metzger 2001; Mulder et al. 2006) or age effects (Klein et al. 1993; Took and Weiss 1994; Lacourse et al. 2001), which play a mediating role and may thus be at the actual root of the postulated relationship. This idea of indirect relationships, therefore, remains disregarded. As a consequence, when it comes to the association of certain music genres with (psychological) abnormalities of their recipients, studies tend to convey the impression of a supposedly monocausal chain of effects, which, however, most likely simplifies the systems of reference actually present in reality. The assumption of an indirect effect via mediating variables, admittedly, has yet to be sufficiently substantiated empirically, likewise. Comparison of studies, for instance, that do consider relevant mediators (e.g., Leming 1987; Wanamaker and Reznikoff 1989; Wass et al. 1991; Martin et al. 1993; Took and Weiss 1994; Rustad et al. 2003; Mulder et al. 2006; Chen et al. 2006; Baker and Bor 2008; von Georgi et al. 2009; Miranda et al. 2012), often shows heterogeneous results.

In this respect, Baker and Bor (2008) have previously urged researchers to establish a consistent research strategy for the identification of such mediators first, before exploring different music genres and their positive or negative effects on mental health (Baker and Bor 2008, p. 287). To date, however, their call has hardly been acted upon, although, e.g., Miranda et al. (2012) explicitly discuss respective mediation models in their theorization of potential models of effects. With the exception of the work of von Georgi et al. (2006, 2009), also quantitative, empirical mediation models have been left out of consideration so far.

In view of the contradictory and ambiguous results of the abovementioned studies, there is reason to suspect that the findings on the illness-promoting effect of certain types of music are more likely to be based on an empirical artifact. A similar conclusion is reached by Chen et al. (2006), who statistically controlled for a number of mediating variables in their study, such as age, gender, sensation seeking, and ethnicity. The authors discuss substance abuse, aggression, and music preference to be independent constructs, suggesting that only by means of one or more superordinate construct(s), an ostensible correlation emerges.

29.2.1 Mediating Variables

To what extent, then, is the hypothesis of harmful effects of hard music genres tenable at all? Does certain music make people ill, or are such observations rather attributable to mediating superordinate constructs and/or preexisting abnormalities on the part of the respective recipients? Three factors that seem to be crucial concerning this question can be derived from research literature: the acquired strategies of emotion modulation through music, age effects, and the resulting cohort and generational effects.

29.2.1.1 Use of Music in Everyday Life for Emotion Modulation

Regarding the assumption of a negative effect of hard music (metal, alternative, rock) on health and/or psychological condition, von Georgi et al. (2011) found that very dedicated listeners of "hard" music do not exhibit significant abnormalities neither in health (chronic mental or somatic illnesses) nor in corresponding personality variables. However, this group of people revealed to make frequent use of their preferred music to influence emotions. Adolescence, in particular, is a period when learning to regulate emotions is considered pivotal and has been widely linked to the development of mental health disorders and illnesses (e.g., Ochsner and Gross 2005; John and Gross 2004; Moore et al. 2008; Gullone and Taffe 2012; Teixeira et al. 2015; Preece et al. 2019; Martín-Albo et al. 2020). It becomes apparent by this point that a direct causal relationship between the different parameters of health and disease and certain music preferences seems unlikely. In fact, it may be the mediator variable "use of music for emotion modulation" that establishes the statistical relationship.

Yet, it remains unclear: What are the underlying structures and processes of the emotion-modulating effect of music, and in which ways does the use of music in everyday life affect the organic health and subjective well-being of its recipients?

In this respect, it has been argued by some authors that hard genre listeners use music specifically to reduce negative affective states. Listening to music may serve as a kind of coping strategy (stress management behavior) for this group, aimed at helping them deal with existing family and/or personal problems (Arnett 1995; Laiho 2004; Saarikallio and Erkkilä 2007; Miranda et al. 2012). Against this background, the correlations between listening to hard music and the aforementioned abnormalities might not be interpreted as an indication for harmful effects of music but more so as signs for failed coping behavior (e.g., Arnett 1991a, 1995) (see Fig. 29.1, below). At their core, these explanatory approaches can be traced back to R.S. Lazarus' stress model (e.g., Lazarus and Folkman 1984). However, similar models of a situation-adaptive use of music to reduce negative affective states also exist in media effects research (e.g., Zillmann 1988a, b; Knobloch and Zillmann 2002; Schramm 2005). The applicability of such media theoretical approaches to music listening and its associated psychological and somatic effects is not uncontested, though (for critical discussion on this issue, see von Georgi 2013). And those approaches that describe music reception as a coping strategy are as yet lacking sufficient support from studies that would have explicitly assessed coping behavior in this context. Beyond that, these types of scientific explanations harbor two major shortcomings: For one thing, they characterize the use of music in everyday life as being reactive in nature, invariably tied to an external stimulus (situation). Second, they confine themselves to negative stimuli. Any form of active, primarily positive emotional stimulation and modulation through music is therefore disregarded.

Incorporating the criticism briefly outlined above, the so-called AAM model (Activation and Arousal Modulation model) provides a conceptualization of the use of music in everyday life as a mediator variable, thus allowing for a theoretical integration of findings from studies on the role and use of music (e.g., North and Hargreaves 1996; Hargreaves and North 1999; Sloboda et al. 2001; Sloboda and O'Neill 2001; Pickles 2003; North et al. 2004; Juslin and Laukka 2004; Hays and Minichiello 2005; Bellstorf 2009; Schäfer and Sedelmeier 2009; Dunn et al. 2012). The AAM model construes the active use or application of music in everyday life as acquired strategies of modulating positive and negative affect and cognition. In contrast to a simple compensation model (cf. Miranda et al. 2012), however, it emphasizes the role of personality and potential action-related variables. The use and effects of music in everyday life thus take place against the backdrop of the interaction of both the individual and their specific (life) situation. Figure 29.2 depicts the AAM macromodel. It is rooted in the basic premise that listening to music involves learned, volitional processes that unfold against the backdrop of an individual's personality, current affective state, and their sociopsychological environment in order to intentionally modify emotions and states (von Georgi et al. 2006; von Georgi 2007, 2013; Gebhardt et al. 2015, 2018; Gebhardt and von Georgi 2019; Kreutz and von Georgi 2017). Since these processes are not regarded as simple upregulation and downregulation of existing basic emotions or arousal states, as in Zillmann's model (1988b), but rather imply a qualitative change in existing emotions, the term emotion *modulation* is deliberately used instead of the term *regulation*. On a micro level, the AAM model connects the use of music with the neurophysiological model of Gray and McNaughton (2000) (cf. also Corr 2008), which, at this point, will not be discussed further, though (cf. von Georgi 2013). Using the AAM model as a theoretical framework, it can now be empirically shown that the use of music for modulating negative emotions counteracts and/or compensates for potential adverse health effects that may arise from general emotional lability. This process is illustrated in Fig. 29.3 (cf. von Georgi et al. 2009).

29.2.1.2 Age and Cohort Effects

With regard to aforementioned age effects, yet largely neglected in research, Kurdek (1987) has previously argued that the empirical findings on the illness-promoting effects of youth-specific music genres may simply reflect a more general phenomenon, which he refers to as "youth rebelliousness": that is, being the result of the specific behavior, experiences, and feelings common during adolescent development, combined with the concurrently growing importance of music and its use for emotion regulation in this stage. It is known, for example, that sensation seeking, impulsivity, and general emotional responsiveness, as well as somatic symptoms and stress, surge considerably during adolescence due to developmental factors (Roth and Hammelstein 2003; Roth et al. 2007; Lohaus and Klein-Heßling 2008). During this period, adolescents then increasingly turn to music in an attempt to counteract the negative shifts in feelings and experiences on an emotional level.

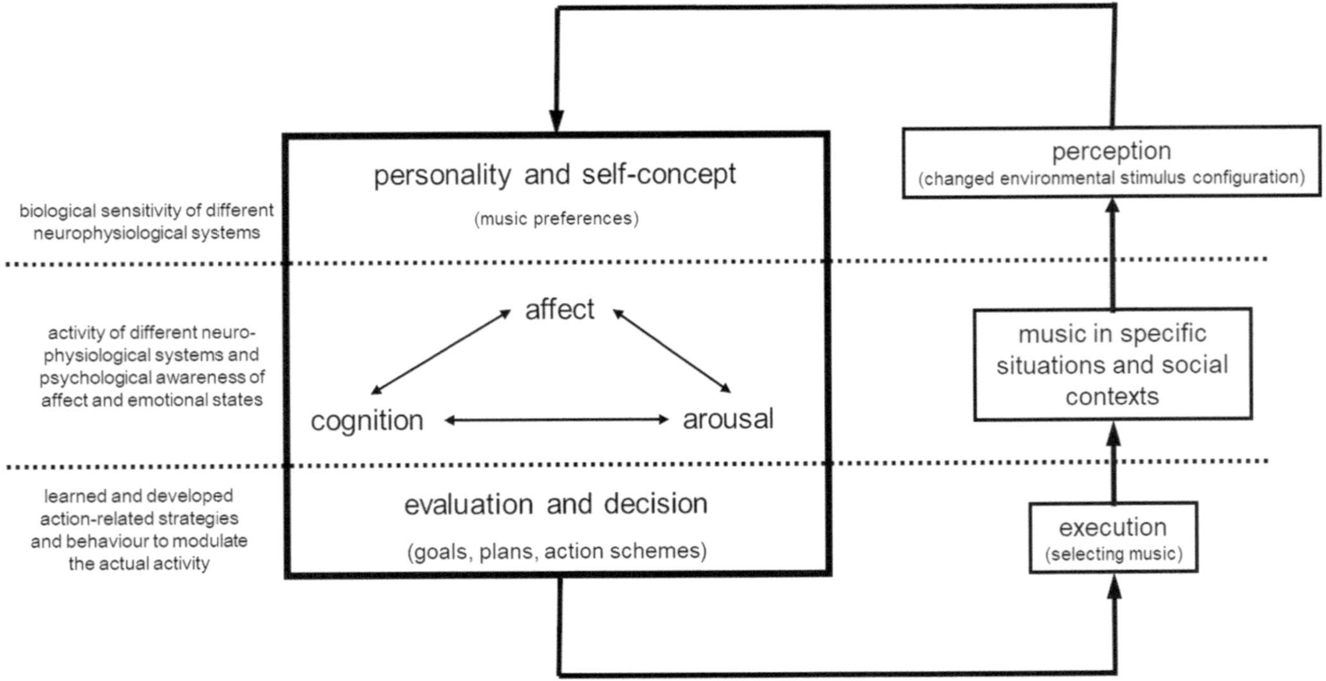

Fig. 29.2 The AAM macro model, which illustrates the use of music in everyday life based on personality, internal affective state, action planning and execution, as well as the current situation. (According to von Georgi et al. 2006; von Georgi 2013)

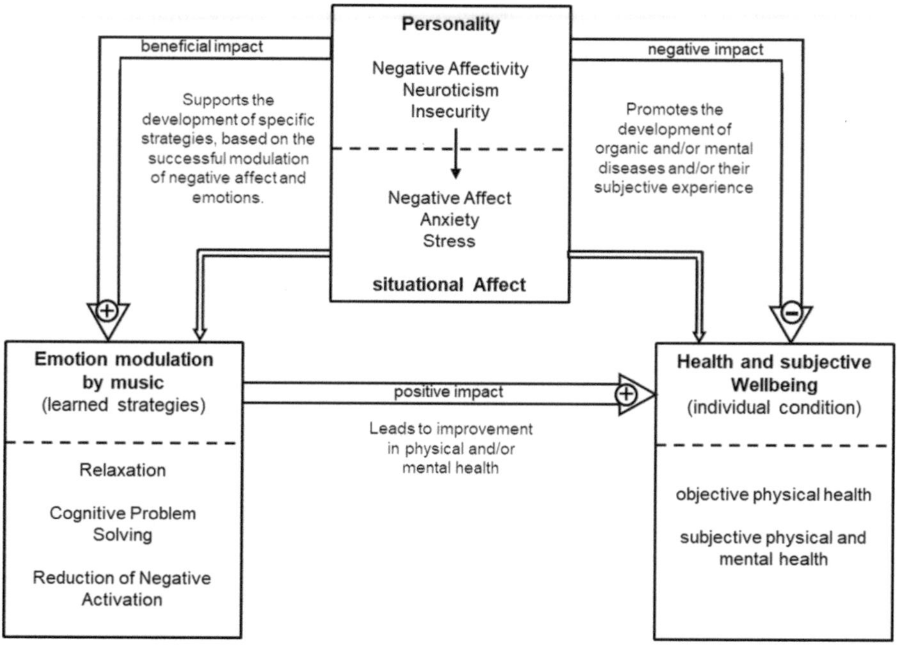

Fig. 29.3 Health and the Effects of Using Music in Everyday Life

Statistically, what becomes manifest in consequence is a spurious correlation between variables of impaired mental and/or physical health and a preference for music genres that are particularly popular among adolescents.

Adolescents' use of music in everyday life is further shown not to be limited to modulating emotions only but rather extends to establishing social connections and affecting attention and concentration, as demonstrated by the works of de Nora (1999, 2000, 2001) and other authors (e.g., Heargreaves and North 1999; Pickles 2003; North et al. 2004; Hays and Minichiello 2005) as well as contributions of music sociology on the role of music in adolescence (e.g., Baacke 1968, 1993, 1998; Pape 1998, 2001; Müller et al. 2002, 2007; Connell and Gibson 2002; Dollase 2005; Kleinen 2008). As part of the developing efforts to control and influence (modulate) emotions, music-related strategies are thus explored and applied to a greater extent in this period of life. It, therefore, seems reasonable that the degree to which different forms of music are used in adolescence is significantly higher than in older groups of people (von Georgi et al. 2008). The correlation between the reception of certain genres and existing personality or health problems in adolescents may therefore be the result of a failure to take into account the developing strategies for emotion modulation through music.

The fact that hard music in particular is deemed harmful, for that matter, appears to be nothing more than a zeitgeisty phenomenon. Indeed, from 2000 onward, outcomes in support of the assumption of harmful effects decrease in relation to hard music, while there is a substantial increase in findings related to rap and hip-hop

(Miranda and Claes 2004; van Havere et al. 2011)—those genres that have risen to prominence as youth music in the last 10 years. Given how closely the results of research on the effects of particular music genres are tied to particular generations, there is little doubt that the apparent effect ultimately reflects a purely associative relationship between mental health problems among adolescents and certain forms of music consumed primarily by adolescents. It is worth noting here that even rock 'n' roll was once reputed to have a corrupting influence on the youth. As long as age-related cohort effects like these are not taken into account, the current youth music, differing from generation to generation, will always appear to be connected to mental health problems.

29.3 Empirical Examples to Differentiate Underlying Interdependencies

It, thus, stands to reason that listening to those music genres that are tied to a youth movement's respective trends will always go hand in hand with a variety of youth-specific variables, while not necessarily being directly or even causally related to them. Nonetheless, scientific discourses continue in their efforts to single out any potential differences in music preference on this matter, without taking into account or even discussing methodological or content-related flaws. In this chapter, we will, therefore, use studies from within the ranks of our own research to demonstrate how the presumed relationship between mental and somatic health and specific music genres—whether it be causal or not—is first based on a methodological artifact that continues to influence existing results, even in more recent studies. Second, it will be shown that the results in question may be boiled down to a factor of "youth rebelliousness" which, dependent on the generation, gives rise to new or may strengthen spurious correlations between certain music genres and variables related to personality, behavior, and health.

29.3.1 Hard Music and *Sensation Seeking*

Our first study focuses on the construct *sensation seeking* (cf. Zuckerman 1994), whose sub-construct *disinhibition* (DIS: alcohol-induced social disinhibition and sexual disinhibition) has been found to be associated with a wide range of different forms of delinquent behaviors in recent years (cf. Roth and Hammelstein 2003). As a starting point for the research presented below, reference is made to the findings by von Georgi et al. (2011; see above) who conducted a study on dedicated listeners of hard music. Their results showed that dedicated listeners of hard music did not exhibit any remarkable characteristics regarding the health and personality variables assessed. How is the situation with an average student sample, though, i.e., that kinds of subjects that have been examined in so many studies of the past and present? Whether or not in their case the trait sensation seeking can be linked to a targeted use of music will be investigated in the course of this study. In addition, the study seeks to provide a direct comparison between music preference for hard music and a preference for the younger urban music genres (e.g., rap, hip-hop, house, techno). In line with the exposition outlined above, our analysis is thereby based on the following assumption: If the reception of hard music leads to deviant behavior, a preference for these music genres will correlate significantly with *sensation seeking* (SS), particularly with the subconstruct *disinhibition*. In case there is validity of the "youth rebelliousness" hypothesis (Kurdek 1987), corresponding correlations should nowadays (data collection took place in 2007) be hardly observable anymore, since younger urban music genres have replaced older hard music genres as youth music for quite some time now (von Georgi et al. 2007).

To investigate the matter, 151 first-year medical students were presented with a German translation of the SS-V scale (Zuckermann 1994 1996), along with a questionnaire categorically assessing music preference as defined by Rentfrow and Gosling (2003) (Reflexive & Complex (R&K): Jazz, Classical, Blues; Intense & Rebellious (I&R): Heavy Metal, Alternative, Grunge; Upbeat & Conventional (U&K): Pop, Top40, Country, Folk, Religious, and Film Music; Energetic & Rhythmic (E&R): Rap, Hip-Hop, Techno, Dance, Soul, Funk, Latin, Reggae). According to this classification, the genres described as "hard" in scientific literature correspond to the group Intense & Rebellious (I&R). The average age of participants (57 men, 93 women) was 21 years (SD = 2.7; min = 18; max = 34). The significance level was set at 0.05.

Table 29.1 displays the intercorrelations between the SS scales and the different preference categories. With the exception of the *Boredom Susceptibility* scale (BS: fear of boredom), SS scales do not show any correlations with the preference category that encompasses hard music. Clear and even negative correlations do emerge, however, with the preference category Upbeat & Conventional. This category of music preference comprises those individuals who in the scientific literature are often defined as so-called listeners of non-hard music—constituting the group of people that is regularly used as reference group within comparisons, being therein referred to as "normal."

Table 29.1 Intercorrelations between the preference categories according to Rentfrow and Gosling (2003) and the SS-V scales

	Reflective & Complex	Intense & Rebellious	Upbeat & Conventional	Energetic & Rhythmic
Sensation seeking (total scale)	−0.058	0.093	−0.203**	0.164*
Thrill and adventure seeking	0.019	0.087	−0.054	−0.067
Disinhibition	−0.066	0.010	−0.223**	0.301***
Experience seeking	−0.012	0.089	−0.154*	0.072
Boredom susceptibility	−0.103	0.121(*)	−0.211**	0.180*

(*)$p < 0.09$, *$p \leq 0.05$, **$p \leq 0.01$, ***$p \leq 0.001$

A subsequent multivariate analysis of variance of the SS scales correspondingly indicates a significant difference between music preferences (p[Wilks Lambda = 0.67; F = 1.83; df = 27/334] = 0.008; $\eta 2$ = 0.093). Figure 29.4 illustrates those differences on SS scales between the music preferences that are significant ($p < 0.05$) after subsequent single-testing using one-factorial analysis of variance. What can be seen clearly is that the group with "normal" music preference (Upbeat & Conventional) has noticeably low mean values on three of the five SS scales. In other words, it is not that listeners of hard music are characterized by heightened SS values, but rather that listeners of "normal" music are characterized by comparatively low SS values.

If it is only these two groups that are directly contrasted, it will appear as if listeners of hard music have higher mean values or a corresponding correlation will be found, while in fact, hard music listeners' mean values do not considerably differ from listeners of classical and jazz music (Reflexive & Complex) or urban music forms (Energetic & Rhythmic). This means that if in the present sample the group of listeners of hard music is compared solely with people who have a preference for "normal" music, it will result not only in a significant positive correlation but also in a considerable increase in effect size of mean differences as indicated by the correlations (t-test): *Sensation Seeking*-total scale (SS): r=,305 (p = 0,003) and p[df = 92; t = 3068] = 0,003; *Thrill and Adventure Seeking* (TAS): r = ,108 (p = 0,295) and p = [df = 94; t = 1054] = 0,295; *Disinhibition* (DIS): r = ,260 (p = 0,010) and p[df = 95; t = 2627] = 0,01; *Experience Seeking* (ES): r = ,222 (p = ,027) and p[df = 98; t = 2252] = 0,027; *Boredom Suspectibility* (BS): r = ,273 (p = 0,006) and p[df = 97; t = 2792] = 0,006.

Table 29.1 further shows a distinct positive correlation between the *disinhibition* scale and a preference for urban music forms (Energetic & Rhythmic)—a pattern

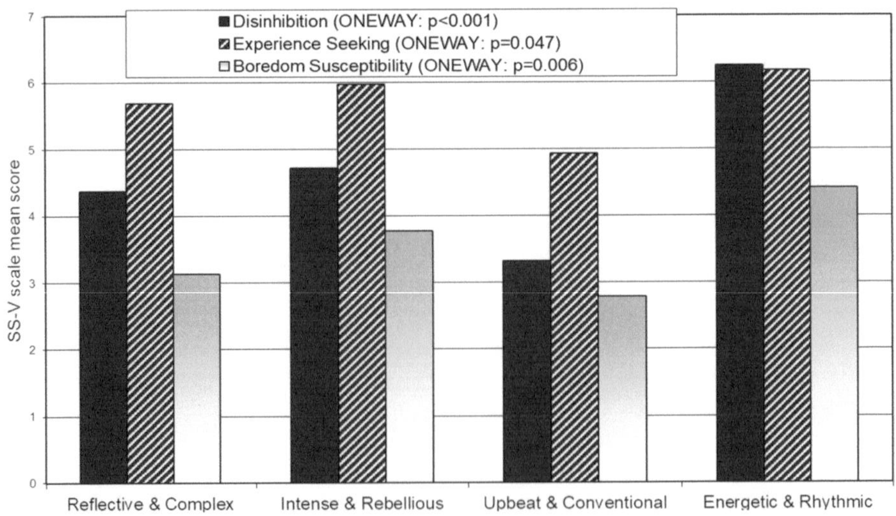

Fig. 29.4 Scale Means of the Significant SS-V Scales for the Different Preference Categories

that, in previous studies, used to be more commonly associated with listening to hard music. Again, as anticipated, the correlations and mean differences increase considerably when it is only the group of people who prefer "normal" music that is used for comparison (SS: $r = ,423$ ($p < 0,0001$) and $p[df = 62; t = 3677] = 0,0004$); TAS: $r = -,026$ $p = 0,841$) and $p[df = 62; t = 0,202] = 0,081$; DIS: $r = ,518$ ($p < 0,0001$) and $p[df = 63; t = 4810] = 0,00009$; ES: $r = ,255$ ($p = 0,041$) and $p[df = 63; t = 2089] = 0,041$; BS: $r = ,421$ ($p < 0,0001$) und $p[df = 63; t = 3682] = 0,0004$.

The results presented here provide clear empirical evidence of correlations and differences existing between various music genres and *sensation seeking*. While no conclusive evidence is found for the association between hard music and sensation seeking discussed above, there is support for the hypothesis of "youth rebelliousness" (Kurdek 1987), which refers to a shift in this relationship toward urban forms of music. What further shows is how specific characteristics of the reference group generally classified as "normal" distort the interpretation of results or may lead to them being substantially overestimated. One can clearly observe in this context, that in comparison, the group of listeners of hard music does not have a very high level of sensation seeking, but that listeners of "normal" music exhibit too low a level of this characteristic instead. Overall, there are no significant differences between any of the three remaining preference groups, as long as they are not contrasted with the group of listeners of "normal" music. Analyses conducted on a smaller sample (cf. by von Georgi et al. 2015) likewise revealed such emergence of effects in case of comparison with listeners of "normal" music and further showed that this contrasting effect is even amplified by data manipulation in terms of using only two samples. It is worth noting here that the comparison between "normal" and "hard" music or "norm deviating" music such as techno, rap, or hip-hop is often implemented in the very planning stage of many studies. Putting it exaggeratedly, however, at this point one could be tempted to wonder: Just how "normal" are the listeners of so-called normal music?

The results presented here cast considerable doubt on a normative nature of this sample: The behavior and personality of individuals with a preference for pop music (pop, Top40, country, folk, religious, film music, etc.) are strikingly less accentuated than those of other student preference groups. In other words, listeners of hard and urban music are not characterized by behavioral conspicuity; it is listeners of pop music referred to as "normal music" who are remarkably *inconspicuous* in their behavior. What further becomes noticeable concerning this group is its characteristic listening habits. As shown in other studies, listeners of "normal" music rapidly change their preferred music, often dependent on situational conditions (cf. von Georgi 2013). These observations suggest that listeners of "normal" music are not at all or only slightly attached to a specific genre of music but rather select music in accordance with their current state of mind and perception; non-music-related aspects (reference to life, fashion and style of the artists, etc.) likely being of primary importance in the process. Yet, since research is entirely based on music preferences per se, such forms of interrelatedness have not been part of the discourse on the impact and use of music to date.

29.3.2 Music Preference, Health, and Use of Music in Everyday Life Among Adolescents

Thus, it emerges that the correlations found in old studies, linking hard music to the psychological variables mentioned in the introduction, seem to disappear and—although not discussed so far—reappear when it comes to music preferences for more recent urban music forms (Miranda and Claes 2004; Escobar-Chaves et al. 2005; Mulder et al. 2007; van Havere et al. 2011). This presumed transition can be observed quite clearly in a study by North and Hargreaves (2007), involving $n = 2062$ subjects. Increased substance abuse and delinquency could not be detected in the group of subjects with a preference for rock music, it has been found, though, among participants with a preference for the emerging youth-oriented music genres (techno, rap, etc.). Results like these may indicate that there has been a shift in adolescents' music preferences—as suggested by the analyses presented above as well as other studies (e.g., North and Hargreaves 2007; von Georgi et al. 2008). In this vein, it can be seen in Fig. 29.5 that so-called hard music is no longer a music preference of a few young listeners but is indeed consumed by a large number of both young and older people. By contrast, there is a strong tendency for the broad spectrum of listeners to gravitate toward the younger urban forms of music (Energetic & Rhythmic), which seem to have replaced the hard genres in their status as youth music. In 2008, they already represented the most common preference group among young people aged 12–15. An increased popularity of Energetic & Rhythmic music

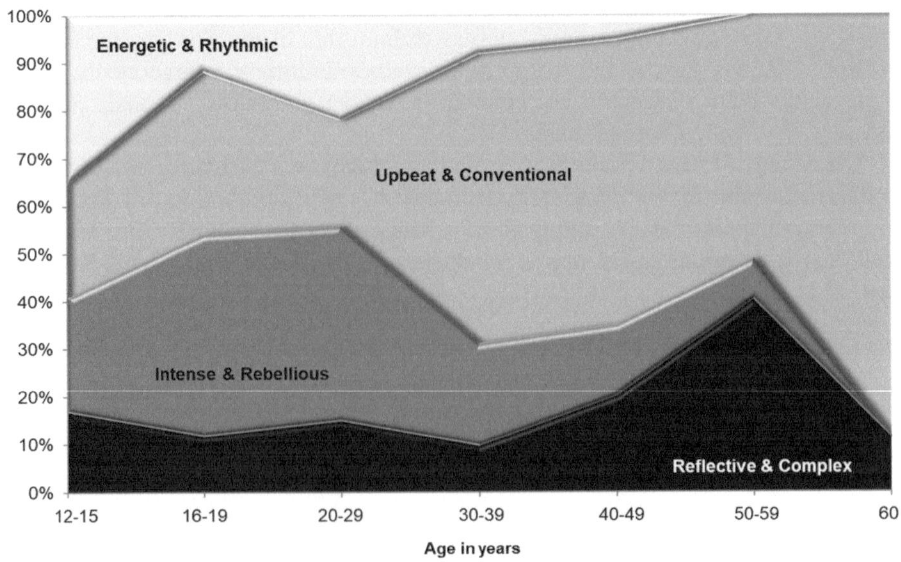

Fig. 29.5 Frequency distribution by percentage ($n = 430$) per age group for preference groups according to Rentfrow and Gosling (2003) in a cross-sectional sample. (From von Georgi et al. 2008)

can also be observed among 20- to 29-year-olds, though this may be attributable to the boom in techno music between 1990 and 2000.

So, if the notion of apparently harmful effects of certain music genres is indeed rooted in age-related effects across generations of young people—underpinning the "youth rebelliousness" hypothesis discussed above—this should reflect in empirical data. With regard to school students between 12 and 18 years of age, somatic or mental health problems should nowadays no longer be significantly detectable in those who preferably listen to hard music but be associated with a primary consumption of more recent urban forms of music.

To test these assumptions, 66 female and 30 male students aged 12–16 (grades 7–10) were interviewed in another study at a school in central Hesse (Dillenburg). The students were asked to complete a series of questionnaires (see below) during a school lesson under the supervision of the respective teacher and the examiner.

The following instruments were used for assessment: the Inventory for the Assessment of Emotion and Arousal Modulation by Means of Music in Everyday Life (IAAM: von Georgi et al. 2006; von Georgi 2013), the trait form of the Positive and Negative Affect Schedule (PANAS: Watson and Clark 1992; Watson 2000; German version: Krohne et al. 1996), and a questionnaire on health and physical discomfort, as well as questions concerning music preference and sociodemographic variables (age, gender, parents' occupation, etc.). For music preferences, again, interval-scaled mean variables were formed in accordance with the categories of Rentfrow and Gosling (2003). In order to compare mean values, the subjects were then assigned to that category in which they had scored highest. Within the categories, it emerged that in Intense & Rebellious, most people tended toward rock and metal ($n = 23$), in Upbeat & Conventional toward pop, top40 and film music ($n = 28$), and in the category Energetic & Rhythmic ($n = 35$), rap and techno almost exclusively resulted as primary music preference. Besides five responses missing, the Reflective & Complex category accounted for only $n = 5$ individuals. Due to the insufficient sample size of this group, it was excluded from the music preference comparisons ($n = 86$).

As a first step, factor analysis was performed on the 22 items composing the Health and Physical Discomfort Questionnaire. The solution that made the most sense, both statistically and content-wise, was to be applied. After examining the plot of eigenvalues, analyzing the maximum number of items with unambiguous loadings on one factor while minimizing the overlap of loadings, and interpreting the factors in terms of content and quality, it was found that a three-factor solution best described the interrelationships of the individual items with respect to both content and statistics (cf. von Georgi et al. 2015). The three factors were interpreted and labeled, respectively, as follows: F1: somatic impairment and discomfort, F2: psychological stress and mental exhaustion, F3: substance abuse. Based on this solution, factor scores per subject were calculated using regression analysis. For all subsequent statistical analyses, the significance level was set at 0.05.

Table 29.2 displays the correlations between the variables and health parameters assessed for the sample as a whole. Overall, it can first be observed that adolescents of higher age and grade show increased substance abuse. Noteworthy is, however,

Table 29.2 Intercorrelations between the health parameters and the scales of IAAM and PANAS

Measures	Scale (variable)	Somatic impairment	Mental exhaustion	Substance abuse
IAAM	Age	.001	−.030	.523***
	Gender	−.011	−.149	.107
	Grade (grades 7–10)	−.029	.093	.271**
	Relaxation	.008	.204	.123
PANAS	Cognitive problem solving	.001	.220*	.204(*)
	Reduction of negative activation	.112	.115	.190(*)
	Positive stimulation	−.097	.160	.232*
	Arousal modulation	−.045	.232*	.175
	Negative affectivity	.146	.203(*)	.176
	Positive affectivity	.063	−.102	.209*

IAAM Inventory for the Assessment of Emotion and Arousal Modulation by Means of Music, *PANAS* Positive and Negative Affect Schedule; (*)$p < 0.072$, *$p \leq 0.05$, **$p \leq 0.01$, ***$p \leq 0.001$; $n_{min} = 90$; $n_{max} = 93$ (missing: casewise)

that substance abuse is not associated with variables indicating negative emotionality but rather with positive affectivity (PA) and with the strategy of stimulating oneself positively by means of music in everyday life. The two strategies theoretically associated with negative affect (cognitive problem solving and reduction of negative activation, cf. von Georgi 2013) fail to reach statistical significance but do show slight correlations with the *substance abuse* dimension as well. The dimension of *mental exhaustion*, on the other hand, is correlated only with cognitive problem solving and, by tendency, with the modulation of arousal and concentration by means of music (cf. Table 29.2).

Looking at these findings on the dimension *substance abuse*, one still has to wonder: Does substance abuse indicate increased emotion modulation, regardless of the type of music preferred, or do increased emotion modulation and substance abuse result from a preference for hard music in the first place?

Table 29.3, to this end, provides the intercorrelations separated by preference category. Strikingly, the group of hard music listeners (Intense & Rebellious) does not show any peculiarities regarding the variables measured other than an increased positive stimulation by means of music in everyday life. It is different though, for adolescents who mostly prefer rap and techno. In their case, there are clear correlations of music preference with a use of music for emotion modulation, substance abuse, and high negative affectivity (NA). Indeed, among the listeners of "normal" music (U&C), a close relationship with the use of music in everyday life for emotion modulation is also observed; in absence, however, of associations with either health-related variables or personality (PANAS). In addition, more females (girls) seem to prefer this type of music, which may indicate an effect of gender.

Even though a one-factor analysis of variance does not reveal any differences in mean values between the preference groups, a one-to-one comparison (t-test)—the type of analysis frequently employed in other studies—shows that the group

Table 29.3 Intercorrelations between the preference categories according to Rentfrow and Gosling (2003), the scales for the use of music in everyday life (IAAM) and general affect (PANAS)

Measures	Scale (variable)	Intense & Rebellious	Upbeat & Conventional	Energetic & Rhythmic
Health	Age	.010	.066	.072
	Gender	.096	−.255*	−.148
	Grade (grades 7–10)	.127	.098	.062
	Somatic impairment (SI)	−.080	−.144	.041
	Mental exhaustion (ME)	−.011	.071	.078
	Substance abuse (SA)	−.091	.053	.258*
IAAM	Relaxation	.097	.365***	.396***
	Cognitive problem solving	.131	.380***	.444***
	Reduction of negative activation	.170	.290**	.427***
	Positive stimulation	.230*	.347***	.456***
	Arousal modulation	.128	.157	.310**
PANAS	Negative affectivity	.014	.176	.294**
	Positive affectivity	.011	.159	.223*

IAAM Inventory for the Assessment of Emotion and Arousal Modulation by Means of Music, *PANAS* Positive and Negative Affect Schedule; gender: 0 = female. 1 = male; (*)$p < 0.09$, *$p \leq 0.05$, **$p \leq 0.01$, ***$p \leq 0.001$, $n_{min} = 91$; $n_{max} = 95$ (missing: casewise)

preferring urban music forms (Energetic & Rhythmic) scores higher in positive affectivity (PA) and on the dimension of *substance abuse* (p[DF56; 2.652] = 0.01) than the group preferring hard music (p[DF = 55; t = 1.967] = 0.054). Listeners of urban music forms further exhibit significantly higher levels of negative affectivity (NA) than the latter group (p[DF = 55; t = 2.154] = 0.036) (cf. Fig. 29.6).

If potential statistical differences are calculated individually between the listeners of hard music (I&K) on the one side and the pooled group (U&K + E&R) or just the listeners of "normal" music (U&K) on the other side, no significant results are to be found. It thus becomes evident, that people with a preference for hard music (I&R), which in older studies seemed to be associated with variables of negative emotionality, now appear quite ordinary when viewed relative to those with a "normal" music preference (U&K), whereas the preference group of new urban music such as rap, techno, and hip-hop (E&C) displays conspicuous features. Once again, this serves to illustrate how the choice of a specific reference group within the context of a given method of analysis has a crucial impact on the overall statistical results.

Further differentiating the results depicted in Tables 29.3 and 29.4 shows the correlations between the three health dimensions, the use of music for emotion modulation (IAAM), and personality (PANAS), sorted by preferred type of music. The most striking finding is that substance abuse increases with age, regardless of a person's music preference. Among adolescent listeners of "normal" music (U&K),

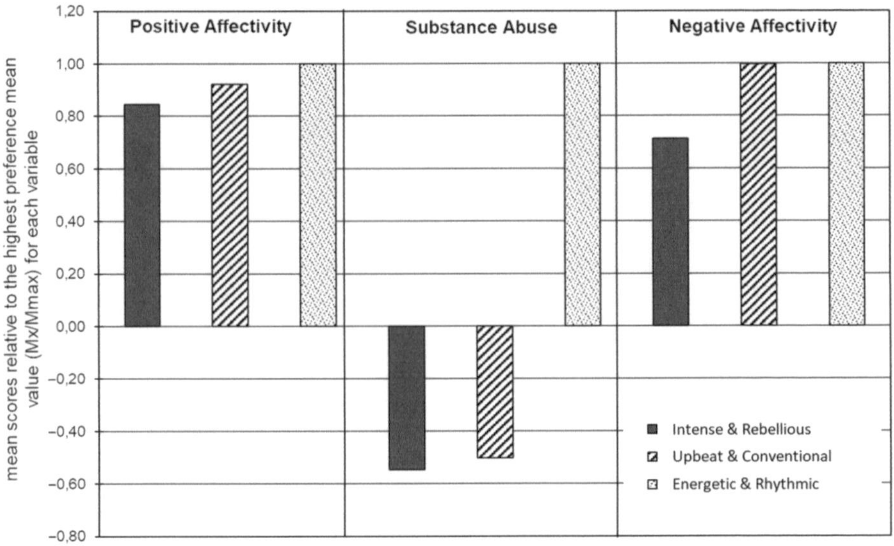

Fig. 29.6 Representation of mean differences between the preference groups in the variables "Positive Affectivity" (PANAS), "Substance Abuse," and "Negative Affectivity" (PANAS). For consistency in presentation, the means (Mx) were normalized relative to the maximum group mean (Mmax) (Mx/Mmax). **Positive Affectivity (PANAS):** *Intense & Rebellious* (M = 18.73; SD = 6.95) *Upbeat & Conventional* (M = 20.41; SD = 7.06) *Energetic & Rhythmic* (M = 22.14; SD = 6.01). **Substance Abuse:** *Intense & Rebellious* (M = -0.25; SD = 1.02) *Upbeat & Conventional* (M = -0.23; SD = 0.85) *Energetic & Rhythmic* (M = 0.45; SD = 1.02) **Negative Affectivity (PANAS):** *Intense & Rebellious* (M = 8.10; SD = 4.61) *Upbeat & Conventional* (M = 11.32; SD = 7.73) *Energetic & Rhythmic* (M = 11.34; SD = 5.74)

however, increased substance abuse is primarily tied to positive affectivity (extraversion) and to a use of music for positive stimulation and reflection about the self and social relationships (cognitive problem solving). Among adolescent listeners of younger urban music forms (E&R), substance abuse is not linked to any of the variables assessed. In this group, the increased use of music for emotion modulation—especially for the purpose of relaxation, problem solving, and reduction of activation—rather seems to be associated with a general mental exhaustion. Negative affectivity (emotional lability) in their case is accompanied by somatic stress, with music hardly being used in everyday life. In contrast, nothing in terms of emotion modulation, health parameters, or personality stands out in the group of hard music listeners.

In summary, it can thus be stated that when it comes to substance abuse, a connection to the consumption of their preferred music can be made primarily for the group of those who listen to "normal" music, especially for those who seek to activate themselves positively by means of music and who have a generally positive affect. Adolescents who favor the new urban forms of music (rap, hip-hop, techno), for their part, are more likely to experience psychological stress, which in turn is associated with greater use of music to modulate negative affect. A pronounced

Table 29.4 Intercorrelations between health parameters and scales of the IAAM and PANAS separated by music preference category

	Intense & Rebellious			Upbeat & Conventional			Energetic & Rhythmic		
	SI	ME	SA	SI	ME	SA	SI	ME	SA
Age	−.058	.173	.575**	−.315	−.060	.521**	.226	−.101	.578***
Gender	−.193	−.037	.415*	.064	−.081	.169	−.074	−.179	−.030
Grade (7–10)	−.090	.304	.339	−.249	.037	.201	.187	.079	.207
Relaxation	−.090	−.086	.102	−.289	.187	.115	.298(*)	.451**	.162
Cognitive problem solving	−.028	.114	.249	−.247	.283	.413*	.241	.334*	.042
Reduction of negative activation	.032	−.166	.305	−.082	.027	.343(*)	.356*	.424*	.011
Positive stimulation	.044	−.091	.227	−.317	.192	.546**	.161	.294(*)	−.070
Arousal modulation	−.068	.171	.215	−.421*	.081	.485*	.191	.393*	−.038
PA	−.246	−.346	.212	−.058	−.055	.462*	.159	.030	.092
NA	.228	−.087	.002	−.036	.253	.387(*)	.446**	.303(*)	.053

SI somatic impairment, *ME* mental exhaustion, *SA* substance abuse; Intense & Rebellious: $n = 22$; Upbeat & Conventional: $n = 26$; Energetic & Rhythmic: $n = 35$; (*)$p < 0.09$, *$p \leq 0.05$, **$p \leq 0.01$, ***$p \leq 0.001$

negative affectivity in terms of a personality trait, however, is coupled with somatic strain in this group. The use of music in everyday life—with the exception of reducing states of tension—hardly seems to be related hereto, though.

While it may seem surprising at first that substance abuse is most common among young listeners with a music preference for pop, top40, etc. (U&K), the explanation for that might be quite simple: As observed earlier by Rentfrow and Gosling (2003), there is a strong correlation between this "normal" pop music preference and a preference for the urban forms (rap, hip-hop, techno). Even then, this close relationship between the two pointed toward the gradual transition that rap and hip-hop would undergo from being distinct musical forms to their eventual integration into popular music. Consequently, by the time of the data analyzed here, in 2008, rap and hip-hop could more and more be considered part of pop music (a development that is almost complete today, in 2020, as was the case with metal from the 1980s and techno from the 1990s). Furthermore, it should be taken into account that the recipients of "normal" music (U&K) for most parts are not dedicated consumers of these genres but use and listen to music more as a function of situation. Their listening habits rather compare to musical "omnivores" (e.g., Neuhoff 2001; Elvers et al. 2015), who do not really exhibit any musical socialization in the sense of internalization (object constancy) of one or more music genres (Behne 1997, 2001; von Appen 2007; Korte 2007) but are characterized by a more adaptive-situational form of music preference (von Georgi 2013). Such a distinction between an adaptive-situational and an integrative-habitual, trans-situational form of music preference also corresponds to action-theoretically oriented approaches to interest development in psychology (e.g., Holodynsky and Oerter 2008).

Finally, it is worth noting that substance abuse, regardless of the preferred genre, is not only associated with increased use of music in everyday life for positive stimulation but also with general positive affectivity. Studies show that general positive affectivity and other extraversion-equivalent constructs are related to a positive attitude toward life, subjective well-being, and health (e.g., Costa and McCrae 1980; Emmons and Diener 1985; McCrae and Costa 1991; Watson and Clark 1992; Watson 2000; Vittersø 2001; Steel and Ones 2002; Hayes and Joseph 2003; Schutte et al. 2003; Williams et al. 2004; von Georgi 2006). These findings raise the question of whether increased substance abuse among adolescents necessarily entails a generally negative mental state. As the present chapter itself has shown, the data suggest that different clusters of psychological and somatic behaviors and disorders appear to be associated with different preconditions (e.g., emotional responsiveness vs. positive affectivity). An increased correlation between substance abuse and a particular music genre should thus—barring some exceptions, of course—not necessarily be interpreted negatively in terms of an indication of impaired mental health (Arnett 1991a, b).

Certainly, this is not to negate the health-damaging effects of substance abuse in any way. However, the present findings suggest that some adolescents are able to use both various substances and music as a means of positive activation or at least attempt to do so. With the help of positive stimulation through music, they seek to elicit emotional effects equivalent to those of substance abuse—in a manner comparable to addicts (Gebhardt et al. 2012).

29.4 Can Listening to Certain Genres of Music Make You Ill?

To date, the answer to this question may only be most likely not; although, conclusive evidence for this has yet to be provided. On the other hand, the existing studies on the postulated harmful effect of certain music genres frequently reveal methodological flaws, so that these studies, too, can hardly be regarded as evidence of any adverse effects, as has already been discussed. Besides, longitudinal studies and/or cohort sequence designs, which may shed light on age and generation effects that have been too readily disregarded, are almost entirely missing in music psychology research. Adding to the problems and criticism already mentioned, the following aspects should be taken into account when evaluating and interpreting research on the relationship between music preference and mental and/or physical problems in adolescents:

- *Number of reference samples used*

  Many of the effects observed to date can be attributed to methodological artifacts resulting from the use of just a single reference sample. Instead of juxtaposing multiple groups (music genres), many studies confine themselves to the comparison with one reference group only, which leads to an overestimation of existing differences both statistically and in terms of content.
- *Specific characteristics of the reference sample*

  As outlined above, the reference sample of pop music listeners classified as "normal" exhibits a number of specific characteristics that are not accounted for in the interpretation of the data and therefore further distort the conclusions drawn. Findings from research on popular music show very clearly that this particular group of listeners does not undergo any musical socialization in the sense of a specific development of music preferences. In fact, factors related to the situation (individual state of affect, peer group, processes of differentiation and identification, etc.) seem to play a far greater role for these recipients than specific music as an object of interest in itself. As such, one may question whether this group of listeners should be compared to individuals who, in contrast, have undergone a specific development of music preference (internalization, knowledge and expertise, historicization, etc.) and for whom their music preference represents much more than just a situational element (von Georgi 2013; von Georgi and Lothwesen 2014).
- *Differentiation level of health variables*

  As the second study presented here has shown already, it does not seem appropriate to adopt a generalized view in the sense of "a certain type of music makes people ill." It is rather very important in this context to have a close look at which construct dimensions of health and illness are being assessed. Substance abuse, for example, is primarily related to positive affect (extraversion, sensation seeking, impulsivity, etc.) in adolescents but not to negative affectivity (emotional lability, neuroticism, anxiety, etc.). The latter is to a greater extent associated with psychological and somatic distress. One must, therefore, assume that the findings of many studies are a result of an undifferentiated assessment of isolated health, behavioral, and personality variables.

- *Suggestion of linearity*

  The correlation coefficients employed in many studies suggest that there is a linear relationship between the consumption of hard music and the occurrence of certain abnormalities, implicitly leading to the following assumption: The more distinctive a music in terms of genre (in sense of stereotype), and the more dedicated its listener, the greater and more pronounced the resulting psychological and physical abnormalities will be. These patterns of thought, however, simply reflect the inherent property of linear correlation coefficients and do not necessarily correspond to reality, as has been demonstrated by von Georgi et al. (2011), who used a discriminant analytic approach to compare different listeners of hard music. In the present chapter, we chose to refrain from a detailed elaboration of the linearity problem, since it has already been discussed by von Georgi et al. (2011).

- *Mediating variables*

  Even though they are repeatedly found to play a significant part in the relationship between music preference and the examined parameters of health and illness, most studies to date have largely ignored the potential influence of mediating variables, such as the use of music in everyday life. In the last of the aforementioned studies, for example, it can be seen that the correlations between negative affectivity (NA) and somatic (SI) and psychological impairment (ME) within the Energetic & Rhythmic preference group weaken significantly when controlling for the variable "relaxing with music" (partial correlation: $r_{NA,SB} = .366$; $p = 0.033$ and $r_{NA,PE} = .122$; $p = 0.491$) (cf. Table 29.3). This lends support to the model of health-promoting effects of emotion modulation through music presented in Fig. 29.3 and further shows that particularly psychological stress can be compensated for by the use of music in everyday life. A similar finding along these lines is yielded by a study on mentally ill people, whose use of music in everyday life increased significantly in response to an intervention of music therapy (Silina et al. 2012). Likewise, a recent study indicates that feelings of stress and discomfort among active-duty police officers can be significantly reduced with the help of music that may be used for emotion modulation (Starcke et al. in preparation).

- *Age and cohort effects*

  Certainly, there may be more methodological and content-related problems and points of criticism (e.g., influence of culture, gender, etc.). Above all, however, it can be stated that the correlations and differences found are often a result of the use of specific reference samples, simplistic experimental designs and methods of analysis, along with the failure to account for mediator variables that create an apparent statistical relationship between a variety of different problem areas of adolescence and the respective youth-specific music genres. That the effects found meanwhile are not a matter of preference, but rather of generation, is indicated by the observable "trend reversal" within the scientific discourse on harmful music genres, which now increasingly focuses on urban music forms instead of heavy metal (Miranda and Claes 2004; van Havere et al. 2011).

In spite of the abovementioned problems, limitations and misinterpretations regarding a harmful effect of certain forms of music, it can be noted: If in the future a new generation of young people should decide to derive their "new youth music" from the stock of so-called occidental art music, all the youth-specific variables, from drug abuse to psychological and somatic symptoms and behavioral problems, will be associated with the reception of this very music. Yet it is unlikely that any of the figures of the last three decades would come to think of suggesting a causal relationship between this music and problematic adolescent behavior. Just as no one (any longer)—apart from a few exceptions—would attribute a (youth-)damaging effect to bebop or genuine rock 'n' roll. And so it remains to be concluded that the discussion about a supposedly illness-promoting effect of youth-specific music genres may be nothing other than a reflection of our own musical preferences and aversions, unconsciously being implicated in empirical practice.

References

Akiyama K, Sutoo D (2011) Effect of different frequencies of music on blood pressure regulation in spontaneously hypertensive rats. Neurosci Lett 487:58–60

Altenmüller E, Schlaug G (2012) Music, brain and health: exploring biological foundations of music's health effects. In: MacDonald R, Kreutz G, Mitchell L (eds) Music, health and well-being. Oxford University Press, Oxford, pp 12–24

Angelucci F, Ricci E, Padua L, Sabino A, Tonali PA (2007) Music exposure differentially alters the levels of brain-derived neurotrophic factor and nerve growth factor in the mouse hypothalamus. Neurosci Lett 429:152–155

Appen von R (2007) Der Wert der Musik. Zur Ästhetik des Populären. (= texte zur populären musik Bd. 4). Transcript, Bielefeld

Arnett J (1991a) Heavy metal music and reckless behavior among adolescents. J Youth Adolesc 20(6):573–592

Arnett J (1991b) Adolescents and heavy metal music: from the mouths of metalheads. Youth Soc 23(1):76–98

Arnett J (1995) Adolescents' uses of music for self-socialisation. J Youth Adolesc 24(5):519–533

Baacke D (1968) Beat. Die Sprachlose Opposition. Juventa, München

Baacke D (1993) Jugendkulturen und Musik. In: Bruhn H, Oerter R, Rösling H (Hrsg) Musikpsychologie. Rororo, Reinbeck, S 228–237

Baacke D (1998) Handbuch Jugend und Musik. Leske & Budrich, Opladen

Baker F, Bor W (2008) Can music preference indicate mental health status in young people? Australas Psychiatry 16:284–288

Bartlett D, Kaufman D, Smeltekop R (1993) The effects of music listening and perceived sensory experiences on the immune system as measured by interleukin 1 and cortisol. J Music Ther 30(4):194–209

Beck SL (1991) The therapeutic use of music for cancer-related pain. Oncol Nurs Forum 18:1327–1337

Behne K-E (1997) The development of "Musikerleben" in adolescence. How and why young people listen to music. In: Deliège I, Sloboda J (eds) Perception and cognition of music. Psychology Press, Hove, pp 143–159
Behne K-E (2001) Musik-Erleben: Abnutzung durch Überangebot? Eine Analyse empirischer Studien zum Musikhören Jugendlicher. Media Perspektiven 3:142–148
Bellstorf K (2009) Eine Studie zur Musikrezeption und Nutzung von Internetangeboten für musikinteressierte Jugendliche. Bachelorarbeit an der Hochschule für Angewandte Wissenschaften Hamburg (verfügbar unter). http://www.opus.hawhamburg.de/volltexte/2009/867/pdf/Bellstorf_Kathrin_090821.pdf
Biley F (2000) The effects on patient well-being of music listening as a nursing intervention: a review of the literature. J Clin Nurs 9:668–677
Bradt J, Dileo C, Grocke D, Magill L (2011) Music interventions for improving psychological and physical outcomes in cancer patients (Review). PLoS One 7(9):e44611
Chan MF, Wong ZY, Onishi H, Thayakam NV (2011) Effects of music on depression in older people: a randomised controlled trial. J Clin Nurs 21:776–783
Chen M-J, Miller BA, Grube JW, Waiters ED (2006) Music, substance use, and aggression. J Stud Alcohol 67(3):373–381
Connell J, Gibson C (2002) Sound tracks: popular music, identity and place. Routledge, New York
Corr PJ (ed) (2008) The reinforcement sensitivity theory of personality. Cambridge University Press, Cambridge
Costa PT, McCrae RR (1980) Influence of extraversion and neuroticism on subjective well-being: happy and unhappy people. J Pers Soc Psychol 38(4):668–678
DeNora T (1999) Music as a technology of self. Poetics 27:31–56
DeNora T (2000) Music in everyday life. Cambridge University Press, Cambridge
DeNora T (2001) Aesthetic agency and musical practice: new directions in the sociology of music and emotion. In: Juslin PN, Sloboda AA (eds) Music and emotion. Oxford University Press, Oxford, pp 161–180
Dillman Carpentier F, Knobloch S, Zillmann D (2003) Rock, rap, and rebellion: comparison of traits predicting selective exposure to defiant music. Personal Individ Differ 35:1643–1655
Dollase R (2005) Musikalische Sozialisation. In: Stoffer TH, Oerter R (Hrsg) Enzyklopädie der Psychologie: Spezielle Musikpsychologie. Hogrefe, Göttingen, S 151–204
Dunn PG, de Ruyter B, Bouwhuis DG (2012) Toward a better understanding of the relation between music preference, listening behavior, and personality. Psychol Music 40:411–428
Elvers P, Omigie D, Fuhmann W, Fischinger T (2015) Exploring the musical taste of expert listeners: musicology students reveal tendency toward omnivorous taste. Front Psychol 6:1252
Emmons RA, Diener E (1985) Personality correlates of subjective well-being. Personal Soc Psychol Bull 11:89–97
Escobar-Chaves SL, Tortolero SR, Markham CM, Low BJ, Eitel P, Thickstun P (2005) Impact of the media on adolescent sexual attitudes and behaviour. Pediatrics 116(1):303–326
Gebhardt S, von Georgi R (2010) Beeinflussung des Schmerzempfindens durch Musik bei depressiven Patienten. Jahrestagung der Deutschen Gesellschaft für Musikpsychologie. 8.-10. Oktober: Würzburg
Gebhardt S, von Georgi R (2019) Emotion modulation in obsessive-compulsive spectrum symptoms: the role of music in everyday life. Psychol Behav Sci Int J 14(1):181–184
Gebhardt S, Kunkel M, von Georgi R (2012) Emotionsregulation mittels Musik im Alltag von Suchtpatienten. Jahrestagung der Deutschen Gesellschaft für Musikpsychologie, 28.-30. September: Bremen
Gebhardt S, Kunkel M, von Georgi R (2015) Emotion modulation in everyday life and the subjective valence of music in mental disorders. In: Byant ML (ed) Handbook on emotion regulation: processes, cognitive effects and social consequences. Nova Science, New York, pp 143–156
Gebhardt S, Dammann I, Loescher K, Vedder H, von Georgi R (2018) The effects of music therapy on the interaction of the self and emotions—an interim analysis. Compl Ther Med 41:61–66
Good M (1996) Effects of relaxation and music on postoperative pain: a review. J Adv Nurs 24:905–914

Gray JA, McNaughton N (2000) The neuropsychology of anxiety: an enquiry into the function of the septo-hippocampal system. Oxford University Press, Oxford

Gullone E, Taffe J (2012) The emotion regulation questionnaire for children and adolescents (ERQ–CA): a psychometric evaluation. Psychol Assess 24(2):409–417

Hargreaves DJ, North AC (1999) The functions of music in everyday life: redefining the social in music psychology. Psychol Music 27:71–83

Hayes N, Joseph S (2003) Big 5 correlates of three measures of subjective well-being. Personal Individ Differ 34:723–727

Hays T, Minichiello V (2005) The meaning of music in the lives of older people: a qualitative study. Psychol Music 33(4):437–451

Holodynsky M, Oerter R (2008) Tätigkeitsregulation und die Entwicklung von Motivation, Emotion und Volition. In: Oerter R, Montada L (Hrsg) Entwicklungspsychologie (6. vollständig überarbeitete Auflage). Beltz PVU, Weinheim, S 535–571

John OP, Gross JJ (2004) Healthy and unhealthy emotion regulation: personality processes, individual differences, and life span development. J Pers 72(6):1301–1334

Juslin PN, Laukka P (2004) Expression, perception, and induction of musical emotions: a review and a questionnaire study of everyday listening. J New Music Res 33:217–238

Juslin PN, Sloboda AA (eds) (2001) Music and emotion. Oxford University Press, Oxford

King P (1988) Heavy metal music and drug abuse in adolescents. Postgrad Med 83:295–304

Klein JD, Brown JD, Childers KW, Oliveri J, Porter C, Dykers C (1993) Adolescents' risky behaviour and mass media uses. Pediatrics 92:24–31

Kleinen G (2008) Musikalische Sozialisation. In: Bruhn H, Kopiez R, Lehmann AC (Hrsg) Musikpsychologie. Das Neue Handbuch. Rowohlt, Reinbeck, S 37–66

Knobloch S, Zillmann D (2002) Moodmanagement via Digital Jukebox. J Commun 52(2):351–366

Korte H (2007) Was heisst: „Das bleibt"? Bausteine zu einer kulturwissenschaftlichen Kanontheorie. In: Helm D, Phleps T (Hrsg) No Time for Losers—Charts, Listen und andere Kanonisierungen in der populären Musik. Transcript, Bielefeld, S 11–23

Kreutz G, von Georgi R (2017) Musikhören, Singen, Tanzen und Musizieren: Beiträge zum Wohlbefinden. In: Lehmann AC, Kopiez R (Hrsg) Handbuch Musikpsychologie. Göttingen, Hogrefe, S 641–661

Krohne HW, Egloff B, Kohlmann C-W, Tausch A (1996) Untersuchungen mit einer deutschen Form der Positive und Negative Affect Schedule (PANAS). Diagnostica 42:139–156

Kurdek L (1987) Gender differences in the psychological symptomatology and coping strategies of young adolescents. J Early Adolesc 7:395–410

Lacourse E, Claes M, Villeneuve M (2001) Heavy metal music and adolescent suicidal risk. J Youth Adolesc 30(3):321–332

Laiho S (2004) The psychological function of music in adolescence. Nordic J Music Ther 13(1):49–65

Lazarus RS, Folkman S (1984) Stress appraisal and coping. Springer, New York

Leming JS (1987) Rock music and the socialisation of moral values in early adolescence. Youth Soc 18:363–383

Lester D, Whipple M (1996) Music preference, suicide preoccupation, and personality. Suicide Life Threat Behav 26:68–70

Litle P, Zuckerman M (1986) Sensation seeking and music preferences. Personal Individ Differ 7:575–577

Lohaus A, Klein-Heßling J (2008) Gesundheitsrisiken und Gesundheitsverhalten. In: Silbereisen RK, Hasselhorn M (Hrsg) Entwicklungspsychologie des Jugendalters. Enzyklopädie für Psychologie, Themenbereich C: Theorie und Forschung, Serie V: Entwicklungspsychologie. Hogrefe, Göttingen, S 663–695

Martin G, Clarke M, Pearce C (1993) Adolescent suicide: music preference as an indicator of vulnerability. J Am Acad Child Adolesc Psychiatry 32:530–535

Martin-Albo J, Valdivia-Salas S, Lombas A, Jimenez TI (2020) Spanish validation of the emotion regulation questionnaire for children and adolescents (ERQ-CA): introducing the ERQ-SpA. J Res Adolesc 30(1):55–60

McCrae RR, Costa PT (1991) Adding liebe und arbeit: the full five factor model of well-being. Personal Soc Psychol Bull 17:227–232
McCraty R, Atkinson M, Rein G, Watkins AD (1996) Music enhances the effect of positive emotional states on salivary IgA. Stress Med 12(3):167–175
McCraty R, Barrios-Choplin B, Atkinson M, Tomasino D (1998) The effects of different types of music on mood, tension, and mental clarity. Altern Ther Health Med 4(1):75–84
McDonald RAR, Mitchell LA, Dillon T, Serpell MG, Davies JB, Ashley EA (2003) An empirical investigation of the anxiolytic and pain reducing effects of music. Psychol Music 31(2):187–203
Miehling K (2006) Gewaltmusik—Musikgewalt. Königshausen & Neumann, Würzburg
Miranda D, Claes M (2004) Rap music genres and deviant behaviours in French-Canadian adolescents. J Youth Adolesc 33:113–122
Miranda D, Gaudreau P, Debrosse R, Morizot J, Kirmayer LJ (2012) Music listening and mental health: variations on internalizing psychopathology. In: MacDonald R, Kreutz G, Mitchell L (eds) Music, health, and wellbeing. Oxford University Press, New York, pp 513–529
Moore SA, Zoellner LA, Mollenholt N (2008) Are expressive suppression and cognitive reappraisal associated with stress-related symptoms? Behav Res Ther 46(9):993–1000
Mulder J, Ter Bogt T, Raaijmakers Q, Vollebergh W (2006, in press) Music tast groups and problem behavior. Journal of Youth and Adolescence. (published online first)
Mulder J, Ter Bogt T, Raaijmakers Q, Vollebergh W (2007) Music taste groups and problem behavior. J Youth Adolesc 36(3):313–324
Müller R, Glogner P, Rhein S, Heim J (Hrsg) (2002) Wozu Jugendliche Musik und Medien gebrauchen. Jugendliche Identität und musikalische und mediale Geschmacksbildung. Juventa, Weinheim, München
Müller R, Glogner P, Rhein S (2007) Die Theorie musikalischer Selbstorganisation. In: Auhagen W, Bullerjahn C, Höge H (Hrsg) Musikpsychologie. Jahrbuch der Deutschen Gesellschaft für Musikpsychologie (Band 19). Hogrefe, Göttingen, S 11–30
Neuhoff H (2001) Wandlungsprozesse elitärer und populärer Geschmackskultur? Die "Allesfresser-Hypothese" im Ländervergleich USA/Deutschland. Kölner Zeitschrift für Soziologie und Sozialpsychologie 53:751–772
Nilsson U (2008) The anxiety- and pain-reducing effects of music interventions: a systematic review. AORN J 87(4):780–807
Nilsson U (2009) Soothing music can increase oxytocin levels during bed rest after open-heart surgery: a randomised control trial. J Clin Nurs 18:2153–2161
North AC, Hargreaves DJ (1996) Situational influences on reported musical preferences. Psychomusicology 15:30–45
North AC, Hargreaves DJ (2007) Lifestyle correlates of musical preference: 1. Relationships, living arrangement, beliefs, and crime. Psychol Music 35(1):58–87
North AC, Hargreaves DJ, Hargreaves JJ (2004) Uses of music in everyday life. Music Percept 22(1):41–77
Núñez MJ, Mañá P, Liñares D, Riveiro MP, Balboa J, Suárez-Quintanilla J, Maracchi M, Méndez MR, López JM, Freire-Garabal M (2002) Music, immunity and cancer. Life Sci 71(9):1047–1057
Ochsner KN, Gross JJ (2005) The cognitive control of emotion. Trends Cogn Sci 9:242–249
Panksepp J, Bernatzky G (2002) Emotional sounds and the brain: the neuro-affective foundation of musical appreciation. Behav Process 6:133–155
Pape W (1998) Jugend, Jugendkulturen, Jugendszenen und Musik. In: Rösing H, Phlebs T (Hrsg) Beiträge zur Popularmusikforschung—NEUES zum Umgang mit Rock- und Popmusik (Band 23). CODA, Karben, S 233–252
Pape W (2001) Jugend, Jugendkulturen, Jugendszenen und Musik—die Fortsetzung. In: Phlebs T (Hrsg) Beiträge zur Popularmusikforschung—Populäre Musik im kulturwissenschaftlichen Diskurs II (Band 27/28). CODA, Karben, S 99–122
Pfaus JG, Myronuk LD, Jacobs WJ (1986) Soundtrack contents and depicted sexual violence. Arch Sex Behav 15(3):231–237

Phumdoung S, Good M (2003) Music reduces sensation and distress of labor pain. Pain Manag Nurs 4(2):54–61

Pickles V (2003) Music and the third age. Psychol Music 31(4):415–423

Preece DA, Becerra R, Robinson K, Gross JJ (2019) The emotion regulation questionnaire: psychometric properties in general community samples. J Pers Assess 4:1–9

Rawlings D, Hodge M, Sherr D, Depsey A (1995) Toughmindedness and preference for musical excerpts, categories and triads. Psychol Music 23(1):63–80

Rawlings D, Twomey F, Burns E, Morris S (1998) Personality, creativity and aesthetic preference: comparing psychoticism, sensation seeking, schizotypy and openness to experience. Empir Stud Arts 16:153–178

Rawlings D, Barrantes i Vidal N, Furnham A (2000) Personality and aesthetic preference in Spain and England: two studies relating sensation seeking and openness to experience to liking for paintings and music. Eur J Personal 14:553–576

Rentfrow PJ, Gosling SD (2003) The do re mi's of everyday life: the structure and personality correlates of music preferences. J Pers Soc Psychol 84(6):1236–1256

Robinson TO, Weaver JB, Zillmann D (1996) Exploring the relation between personality and the appreciation of rock music. Psychol Rep 78(1):259–269

Roth M, Hammelstein P (Hrsg) (2003) Sensation Seeking—Konzeption, Diagnostik und Anwendung. Hogrefe, Göttingen

Roth M, Hammelstein P, Brähler E (eds) (2007) Beyond a youthful behavior style—age and sex differences in sensation seeking based on need theory. Personal Individ Differ 43:1839–1850

Rustad RA, Small JE, Jobes DA, Safer MA, Peterson RJ (2003) The impact of rock videos and music with suicidal content on thoughts and attitudes about suicide. Suicide Life Threat Behav 33:120–131

Saarikallio S, Erkkilä J (2007) The role of music in adolescents' mood regulation. Psychol Music 35(1):92–112

Schäfer T, Sedelmeier P (2009) From the functions of music to music preference. Psychol Music 37(3):279–300

Schramm H (2005) Moodmanagement durch Musik. Die alltägliche Nutzung von Musik zur Regulierung von Stimmungen. Herbert von Halem, Köln

Schutte NS, Malouff JM, Segrera E, Wolf A, Rodgers L (2003) States reflecting the big five dimension. Personal Individ Differ 34:591–603

Schwartz KD, Fouts GT (2003) Music preferences, personality style, and developmental issues of adolescents. J Youth Adolesc 32(3):205–213

Silina A, von Georgi R, Gebhardt S, Weber B (2012) Indirekte Wirkung der Musiktherapie: Transfereffekte auf die Verwendung von Musik im Alltag bei Personen mit psychischen Erkrankungen. Jahrestagung der Deutschen Gesellschaft für Musikpsychologie. 28.-30. September: Bremen

Sloboda JA, O'Neill SA (2001) Emotions in everyday listening to music. In: Juslin PN, Sloboda JA (eds) Series in affective science. Music and emotion: theory and research. Oxford University Press, pp 415–429

Sloboda JA, O'Neill SA, Ivaldi A (2001) Functions of music in everyday life: an exploratory study using the experience sampling method. Music Sci 5:9–32

Stack S, Gundlach J, Reeves JL (1994) The heavy metal subculture and suicide. Suicide Life Threat Behav 24:15–23

Starcke K, Zimmermann S, von Georgi R (in preparation). Play it Sam! Abstinence from music listening causes psychological and physiological discomfort

Steel P, Ones DS (2002) Personality and happiness: a national-level analysis. J Pers Soc Psychol 83(3):767–781

Steinhausen H-C, Winkler Metzger C (2001) Risk, compensatory, vulnerability, and protective factors influencing mental health in adolescence. J Youth Adolesc 30(3):159–280

Teixeira A, Silva E, Tavares D, Freire T (2015) Portuguese validation of the emotion regulation questionnaire for children and adolescents (ERQ-CA): relations with self-esteem and life satisfaction. Child Indic Res 8(3):605–621

Took KJ, Weiss DS (1994) The relationship between heavy metal and rap music and adolescent turmoil: real or artifact. Adolescence 29:613–621

van Havere T, Vanderplasschen W, Lammertyn J, Broekaert E, Bellis M (2011) Drug use and nightlife: more than just dance music. Subst Abuse Treat Prev Policy 7(1):36

Vittersø J (2001) Personality traits and subjective well-being: emotional stability, not extraversion, is probably the important predictor. Personal Individ Differ 31:903–914

von Georgi R (2006) Theorie und Messung subjektiver Beschwerden. Der Andere Verlag, Tönning, Lübeck, Marburg

von Georgi R (2007) Das Inventar zur Messung der Aktivations- und Arousal-Modulation mittels Musik (IAAM). In: Schramm H (Hrsg) Medien und Kommunikationswissenschaft—Sonderband 1 „Musik und Medien". Baden-Baden, Nomos, S 138–156

von Georgi R (2011) Buchrezension: Gewaltmusik—Musikgewalt (Miehling, K. (2006, Königshausen & Neumann)). In: Auhagen W, Bullerjahn C, Höge H (Hrsg) Musikpsychologie. Jahrbuch der Deutschen Gesellschaft für Musikpsychologie (Band 22). Göttingen, Hogrefe, S 210–214

von Georgi R (2013) Anwendung von Musik im Alltag: Theorie und Validierungsstudien zum IAAM. Tectum-Verlag, Marburg

von Georgi R, Lothwesen KS (2014) Use of music for emotion modulation—testing the validity of the IAAM-scales within different groups of musical preference indicates different qualitative music preference types. In: 13th international conference on music perception and cognition and 5th conference for the Asian-Pacific Society for Cognitive Sciences of Music (ICMPC 13-APSCOM 5), 4–8 August, Seoul (South Korea)

von Georgi R, Grant P, von Georgi S, Gebhardt S (2006) Personality, emotion and the use of music in everyday life: measurement, theory and neurophysiological aspects of a missing link. Der Andere Verlag, Tönning

von Georgi R, König C, Gebhardt S (2007) Harte Musik, Persönlichkeit und normabweichendes Verhalten. Jahrestagung der Deutschen Gesellschaft für Musikpsychologie, 14.-16. September: Gießen und Tagung des Arbeitskreises Studium populärer Musik (ASPM). 2.-4. November: Barendorf

von Georgi R, Steinbrück J, Schütz M, Rein P (2008) Musik und Emotionsbeeinflussung: Eine Querschnittstudie zur Anwendung von Musik in unterschiedlichen Altersklassen. Jahrestagung der Deutschen Gesellschaft für Musikpsychologie. 12.-14. September: Hannover

von Georgi R, Cimbal K, von Georgi S (2009) Aktivations- und Arousal-Modulation mittels Musik im Alltag und deren Beziehungen zu musikalischen Präferenzen, Persönlichkeit und Gesundheit. In: Auhagen W, Bullerjahn C, Höge H (Hrsg) Musikpsychologie. Jahrbuch der Deutschen Gesellschaft für Musikpsychologie (Band 20). Göttingen, Hogrefe, S 141–183

von Georgi R, Kraus H, Cimbal K, Schütz M (2011) Persönlichkeit und Emotionsmodulation mittels Musik bei Heavy-Metal Fans. In: Auhagen W, Bullerjahn C, Höge H (Hrsg) Musikpsychologie. Jahrbuch der Deutschen Gesellschaft für Musikpsychologie (Band 21). Göttingen, Hogrefe, S 90–118

von Georgi R, Kunkel M, König C, Steinbrück J (2015) Kann Musik auch krank machen? Ein kritischer Beitrag zur krankheitsfördernden Wirkung von jugendspezifischen Musikgenres. In: Kreutz G, Bernatzky G (Hrsg) Musik und Medizin. Springer Verlag, Wien, S 247–271

Wanamaker CE, Reznikoff M (1989) Effects of aggressive and nonaggressive rock songs on projective and structured tests. J Psychol 123(6):561–570

Wass H, Miller MD, Redditt CA (1991) Adolescents and destructive themes in rock music: a follow-up. J Death Dying 23:199–206

Watson D (2000) Mood and temperament. The Guilford Press, New York

Watson D, Clark LA (1992) On traits and temperament: general and specific factors of emotional experience and their relation to the fife-factor model. J Pers 6:441–476

Weidinger CK, Demi AS (1991) Music listening preferences and preadmission dysfunctional psychosocial behaviors of adolescents hospitalized on an in-patient psychiatric unit. J Child Adolesc Psychiatr Nurs 4:3–8

Wells A, Hakanen EA (1991) The emotional use of popular music by adolescents. J Quart 68:445–454
Williams PG, O'Brien CD, Colder CR (2004) The effects of neuroticism and extraversion on self-assessed health and health-relevant cognition. Personal Individ Differ 37(1):83–94
Xu F, Cai R, Xu J, Zhang J, Sun X (2007) Early music exposure modifies GluR2 protein expression in rat auditory cortex and anterior cingulate cortex. Neurosci Lett 420:179–183
Zillmann D (1988a) Mood management through communication choices. Am Behav Sci 31(3):327–370
Zillmann D (1988b) Mood management: using entertainment to full advantage. In: Donohew L, Sypher HE, Higgins ET (eds) Communication, social cognition and affect. Lawrence Erlbaum, Hillsdale, pp 147–171
Zuckerman M (1994) Behavior expressions and biosocial bases of sensation seeking. Cambridge University Press, New York
Zuckerman M (1996) Item revisions in the sensation seeking scale form V (SSS-V). Personal Individ Differ 20:51

30 Hearing Damage Due to Music Consumption

Eckhard Hoffmann and Bernhard Richter

Does hearing loud music endanger one's ability to hear? While the answer in public discourse appears to be an unequivocal "yes" and a generation of hearing-impaired music listeners is often prophesied, the scientifically supported studies present a much more diverse picture. In the present chapter, the effect of music on hearing is discussed based on studies for music listeners and musicians. Moreover, mechanisms of damage are presented, as are factors relating to the protection of the ears. Taking into account the scientifically proven state of knowledge, a simple comparison of music with noise at the workplace is inadequate, even though the legislator does not differentiate concerning this point in the relevant regulations covering noise and vibration protection.

As a fascinating organ of the senses, the ear has always had an important monitoring function: way back in the misty past, signals that were received via the ear could warn of dangers as well as help in hunting prey. The sound-related events in these situations—both the noises created by wild animals creeping up, as well as the rustling of an animal of prey in the undergrowth—were generally rather quiet acoustic incidents. As a result, the ear developed its greatest sensitivity in the quiet range. As there were genuinely no loud noises in nature that were significant from an evolutionary viewpoint, the ear did not develop any protective mechanisms to cope with loud acoustic occurrences.

Exposure to sound has dramatically increased in the last 200 years due to the intrusion of noise on our environment created by machines and traffic. Moreover, in the last 150 years, a clear increase in loud musical events has been observed. Thus, opera and concerts developed from a courtly tradition in the sixteenth through

E. Hoffmann (✉) · B. Richter
Freiburg Institute for Musicians' Medicine, University of Music Freiburg, Medical Center and Faculty of Medicine – University of Freiburg, Freiburg Centre for Music Research and Teaching, Freiburg, Germany
e-mail: Eckhard.hoffmann@htw-aalen.de

G. Kreutz, G. Bernatzky (eds.), *Music and Medicine*, Neurocultural Health and Wellbeing, https://doi.org/10.1007/978-3-662-72175-9_30

eighteenth centuries, which took place in rather small rooms with comparatively few instruments and singers, to a bourgeois culture in the nineteenth century with a significant increase in the size of performance halls. Running parallel to this, the spectral composition of the orchestral sound, in particular on account of the continuous rise in orchestral tuning, changed due to the tendency towards ever greater orchestration and the introduction of new and louder orchestral instruments (Mahling 1997). Over the course of millennia, music could only be played and enjoyed live, without electronic amplification. A new era of music recording and consumption began with the development of recording devices, such as the phonograph (1877) invented by Thomas Alva Edison (1847–1931) and the electron tube, likewise initiated by Edison, which led to the first tube amplifiers at the beginning of the twentieth century. An early protagonist of this development was Enrico Caruso, who owed part of his great popularity—and considerable wealth—to his recordings. After the Second World War, the introduction of the vinyl record resulted in an ever-increasing dissemination of music recordings, and especially the 45 single brought new energy to the music market. Music amplifiers and loudspeaker systems, connected with such instruments as the electric guitar (e.g., the 1954 "Stratocaster" by Fender), opened up the opportunity to develop new musical styles, such as Rock 'n' Roll, which quickly established themselves, especially among the then-young generation, fundamentally changing the consumption of music. Bands like The Beatles achieved levels of popularity in the 1960s hitherto unknown for music ensembles. Thanks to further developments in amplifier and loudspeaker technology, it proved possible to stage ever-larger concerts. Besides these live events, vinyl records also created the technical basis for discotheques, in which the music of the day was played. Since the 1960s, a lively discussion has been conducted on the question of how to assess the risk of damage to hearing for musicians and their audience as posed by amplified music. Parallel to this debate, early studies were also published almost at the same time concerning the hazard to hearing among musicians caused by classical musical instruments (Flach and Aschoff 1966).

30.1 Music = Noise?

The question as to whether music can be regarded as noise cannot be clearly answered in the affirmative in every case. According to DIN 1320, noise is unwanted sound. It frequently arises as a waste product, e.g., as the sound of machinery, traffic, trains, or airplanes. The term "noise abatement" indicates that this noise should be avoided or controlled as far as possible. Thus, in industrialized settings, numerous sources of noise can be found that reduce the quality of the environment on account of the waste product of noise or that endanger people's hearing due to a high level of sound. In contrast, music is not a waste product for the musician, nor for the (willing) listener, nor is it undesirable noise. Music is made in order to render the sound audible and give pleasure to the listener. Despite this fundamental difference, no distinction is made in labor law between noise and music. Troublesome noise is sound conveying a message that is undesired. This may be the noise of traffic but also be the neighbor making music. In this, the degree of annoyance depends less on the level of sound, more on the message of the same, the control one has over the source of the sound, understanding of its necessity, the time of day, the cultural context, expectations in terms of quality of environment, and one's personal attitude towards the source of the sound. Thus, a buzzing mosquito in the bedroom is perceived as highly annoying, even though the sound level is not especially high, as it conveys the message that it will soon sting the person there. Troublesome noise can disturb one's sleep, among other things, impairing one's concentration and influencing the atmosphere. Two effects above all of sound on humans can be distinguished. Troublesome noise annoys the person, yet does no harm to the hearing organ, while it may cause general health disorders, such as raised blood pressure, for example (Babisch 2006). In the case of high sound levels, noise can even damage the hearing organ.

30.2 Noise-Induced Damage to the Ear

The problem that exposure to high sound levels can lead to hearing impairment has long been known. In this, a distinction is made essentially between two patterns of damage: chronic and acute noise-induced damage.

30.2.1 Chronic Noise Damage

As early as the nineteenth century, researchers were concerned with noise-induced hearing loss, differentiating here between noise created by acoustic trauma (e.g., rifle shot) and loss of hearing resulting from long-term work, e.g., in boilermakers' and locksmiths' workshops (Habermann 1890). As early as 1929, "deafness or hearing impairment bordering on deafness caused by noise" was taken up in the list of occupational diseases (currently BK Nr. 2301 on the List of Occupational Diseases in Germany). The working group of Beck and colleagues was already able to show more than 60 years ago that chronic exposure to noise leads to structural damage to the inner ear (Beck and Michler 1960). In the annual statistics of occupational diseases recognized as mandatorily eligible for compensation, hearing impairment continues to occupy a place near the top. After skin diseases and infectious diseases, noise-induced hearing loss was the third most common group, with around 15,000 suspected cases in 2022. Among the occupational diseases recognized as eligible for compensation, noise-induced hearing loss was the second most common in 2022, with 6637 cases (DGUV 2022).

30.2.2 Acute Noise-Induced Damage

For acute noise-induced damage, normally a very high sound level of ≥135 dB is required, such as trauma caused by a bang or an explosion. When regularly playing in an orchestra, such acute sound damage is not to be expected, as the maximum levels of individual instruments or of the whole orchestra do not reach the thresholds that characterize this kind of acoustic trauma. However, hearing impairment can arise as acute noise-induced damage with much lower sound pressure levels of <120 dB, if at the same time as the sound event, there also exists an unnatural posture of the head, causing abnormal strain on the cervical spine. In such cases, one speaks of an "acoustic accident." For musicians, acute sound-induced trauma may be observed in acoustic accidents if sudden sound events, such as an unexpected clash of cymbals, occur near to the ear while simultaneously the person affected turns their head. In the case of musicians, however, the more common cause of sound-induced damage is chronic exposure to noise. A sound pressure level above 80–85 dB(A) as a weekly exposure value can damage the hearing organ in the long term. The damage shows in so-called noise-induced hearing loss, which is characterized by hearing loss mainly in the high-frequency range with a maximum hearing loss at 4–6 kHz. The anticipated hearing loss can be calculated independently of the sound level and the exposure time in accordance with the ISO-Norm 1999 "Acoustics; determination of occupation-driven noise exposure and assessment of noise-induced hearing impairment." Rules, limit values, and consequences for safety at work are set down in the Noise and Vibration Health and Safety Regulation (LärmVibrationsArbSchV) (Table 30.1).

Table 30.1 Noise and vibration health and safety regulation (LärmVibrationsArbSchV) in the version of 19.07.2010)

Sound level at the workplace measures
Lower trigger value:
Daily exposure level to noise: LEX,8 h = 80 dB(A)
This is the exposure level to noise averaged over time, based on an 8-h shift
It covers all sound events occurring at the workplace
or
Reaching the peak sound pressure level:
LpC, peak = 135 dB(C)
This is the peak value of the momentary sound pressure level, e.g., in the event of a bang
Primarily, the sound emission should be prevented at the place of origin or be reduced as much as possible. Technical measures take priority over organizational measures
Duty to inform and instruct on the part of the employer
Provision of appropriate personal hearing protection on the part of the employer
Upper trigger value:
Daily exposure level to noise:
LEX,8 h = 85 dB(A)
or
Reaching the peak sound pressure level:
LpC, peak = 137 dB(C)
Identification of the workspace as a noise area
Mandatory wearing of hearing protection
Development and implementation of a program with technical and organizational measures for the reduction of exposure to noise

30.3 Musicians' Exposure to Sound Pressure Levels

With regard to the exposure, it could be shown that in professional classical symphony orchestras, the sound pressure levels already lie above the lower and upper trigger values for individual instruments: 80 dB(A) and 85 dB(A). In the group, they exceed the exposure threshold of 87 dB(A) (Behroozi and Luz 1997; Hohmann et al. 2003). The main sound exposure is created by the musician's own instrument, as this produces the sound close to the ear. For the assessment of the individual sound pressure exposures from the various groups of instruments, we were able to draw upon the systematic investigations carried out by Beat Hohmann for the Schweizerische Unfallversicherungsanstalt (SUVA, Lucerne), in which the individual practicing and teaching times of musicians are also taken into account. Measurement results are also available for musicians active in the rock/pop sector or in light music, which attest to an increased exposure through sound pressure levels of 105–110 dB (Rintelmann and Borus 1968). One exception to these sound pressure levels that are generally increased seems to exist among musicians who make music on historical instruments (e.g., the baroque construction method using gut strings, etc.) in line with the historically informed performance practice. Here, in measurements taken from one of the world's leading ensembles in the baroque music scene, the levels lay mostly below 85 dB (A) (Richter et al. 2011).

30.4 Noise and Vibration Health and Safety Regulation (LärmVibrationsArbSchV)

In the Noise and Vibration Health and Safety Regulation (LärmVibrationsArbSchV), which has been effective in Germany since 2008, it is laid down that in case of limit values being exceeded, a graduated plan with technical and organizational measures has to be drawn up before individual hearing protection must be worn. However, exposure cannot be significantly lowered by means of organizational measures either (e.g., better distribution of weekly working hours or optimization of the rehearsal plans), as musicians have to practice every day and must also frequently teach alongside their orchestral work. Technical measures with the costly rebuilding of an orchestra pit according to optimized sound protection conditions are likewise unable to sink the levels to below the limits (Drotleff and Leistner 2007). The law (LärmVibrationsArbSchV), conceived for the industrial waste product of noise and for the avoidance of noise-induced hearing loss at noise-intensive workplaces, applies to musicians and orchestras, too. However, the regulation does not cater for the special situation of music as a deliberately created product and often ensures a spectrum of tension within orchestras, in which musicians, conductors, orchestral managers, and those responsible for work safety adopt in part very different positions in this regard. This is especially the case for the regulations concerning the wearing of individual hearing protective gear. This was made clear in a study that was carried out on behalf of the Federal Museum of Labor and Social Affairs among 429 orchestral musicians from 9 professional orchestras in Germany (Richter et al.

2007; Zander et al. 2008). The goal of this survey was to investigate, within the framework of the introduction of the LärmVibrationsArbSchV, the current state of information and practice as relating to the subject of potential damage to and protection of hearing in German orchestras. More specifically, data were collected in the questionnaire concerning what musicians know about excessive sound exposure and potential damage to hearing, whether they know the various means of protecting hearing available on the market, and whether they have used such equipment in their daily work to date, whether the subjects of volume, excessive strain on hearing and protection of the same is important in the orchestra, and whether the musicians themselves are concerned for their hearing.

The various hearing protection models were known by around three-quarters of the orchestral musicians. Less than half of those questioned had personal experience in the usage of the various types, however. In reality, hearing protection—specifically for practicing, rehearsing, and performing—is only used by approximately one-sixth of those questioned.

Private music consumption is not covered by the LärmVibrationsArbSchV, as the work safety regulation is valid only for professional activities and does not extend into the private sphere. Here, however, when attending a concert, for example, the DIN 15905 Part 5, "Audio engineering in theaters and multipurpose halls, measures for the avoidance of endangerment to the public's hearing on account of high sound emissions from electro-acoustic sound technology" comes into effect. In it, a guide value of 99 dB is defined as the rating level LAr, which may not be exceeded at concert events at any location accessible to the public within a rating time Tr of 30 min. Limit values for private exposure to sound using MP3 players are under discussion. A level limitation to 100 dB(A) for MP3 players seems to be reasonable here from a prevention point of view, but a direct implementation of limit values from occupational health and safety does not.

Making and enjoying music are thereby governed not only by artistic aspects and personal preferences, but also affected by regulations that are, for the most part, aimed at the avoidance of noise and only insufficiently take into account the special nature of music as an artistic product.

30.5 Hearing Impairment Caused by Music?

With regards to popular music styles, the hazards were emphasized in early publications by Lebo et al. (1967) and Lipscomb (1969), for example, while others, such as Rintelmann and Borus (1968), considered concerns about damage to hearing unwarranted. In classical music, too, many studies describe the risk of suffering hearing impairment on account of the high levels of sound pressure, without providing evidence of the actual damage done to the musicians' hearing by means of audiometric measurements (Jansson and Karlsson 1983). Less clear, however, is the data regarding damage induced by and proven to be from music on the basis of audiometric investigations (cf. the following surveys: Marquard and Schäcke 1998; Behar et al. 2006). Here, a series of studies confirming a music-induced hearing loss among orchestral musicians contrasts with other studies that deny any such damage caused by noise. Interestingly, several authors found less damage than would have been expected according to ISO 1999 and 7029 (Obeling and Poulsen 1999; Kähäri et al. 2001).

30.6 Factors for the Protection of Ears

This raises the question of whether factors exist for the protection of ears among musicians (Richter et al. 2011). These factors have been little researched to date. It is possible that in this case an emotional attitude towards the pieces performed is significant: for musicians who can assign a positive affective link to the music they are playing, there seems to be damage to a lesser extent for the same exposure (Lindgren and Axelsson 1983; Swanson et al. 1987).

One possible anatomical–physiological correlation for the ability of musicians to protect their hearing more than nonmusicians could lie in the different expression of efferent nervous suppression mechanisms that have a moderating effect on the function of the outer hair cells in the inner ear (Richter et al. 1995; Guinan 2006). The inner ear is not only a recipient of sound, it also produces sounds itself during its active sound processing through the mobile outer hair sensory cells, which are transmitted into the auditory canal via the middle ear. The eardrum works here as a loudspeaker membrane. Otoacoustic emissions were first demonstrated by physicist David Kemp in 1977/78, and their measurement has meanwhile become an established part of audiological diagnostics.

Micheyl and colleagues, in their comparative measurement of transitorily evoked otoacoustic emissions (TEOAE) in musicians vs. nonmusicians, found that intensity perception decreased less over time in musicians than in nonmusicians, and in the case of contralateral stimulation, TEOAE was reduced more in musicians than in nonmusicians (Micheyl et al. 1995). Moreover, in their study of olivocochlear efferent suppression by measurement of TEOAE in 29 classical orchestral musicians vs. 28 control subjects, Brashears and colleagues showed a significantly more pronounced suppression of TEOAE to broadband noise in musicians than in nonmusicians (Brashears et al. 2003).

A further factor that may have an effect on protecting the ear is the fact that the strain on hearing through music is characterized by constant fluctuations and small breaks in exposure. Yet the concept of LEQ measurements determining an average overlooks the positive effect of recovery periods that presumably exist, often recurring during orchestral rehearsals and performances—depending on the work—thanks to the quiet passages (Richter et al. 2011).

30.7 Loss of Hearing Among Young Adults?

With the introduction of the Walkman in 1979 by the Sony Corporation, enjoyment of music became further personalized, as the listener's own music became available in portable form almost everywhere, and the music volume could be individually adjusted through the headphones. Visiting the discotheque also grew in popularity from the 1970s onward, and in the 1990s, according to a special study, 79% of young adults questioned visited a disco for around 4 h (Hoffmann 1997).

The potential consequences for young people's ability to hear were the subject of controversial discussion in numerous articles (Axelsson 1991; Hellbrück and Schick 1989; Hoffmann 1997; Ising et al. 1994; Krähenbühl et al. 1987; Rudloff et al. 1996; Turunen-Rise et al. 1991; Zenner et al. 1999). This led to the prognosis that one could expect that latest by the age of 50, every third person would need a hearing aid as a result of the noise encountered in leisure time (103. Deutscher Ärztetag, in 2000). Investigations with a large number of test subjects (>1500) found no significantly increased risk of damage to hearing among young adults who regularly visit the discotheque (Struwe et al. 1995; Hoffmann 2006). While every fourth young adult could be shown to have hearing loss, no correlation with the individual consumption of music through the Walkman or visits to concerts or the disco could be shown (Hoffmann 1997).

The first MP3 player was launched on the mass market in 1998, while the first Apple iPod was presented in 2001. MP3 players subsequently conquered the market with remarkable speed. Today, the memory of typical MP3 players contains music collections with thousands of songs, and every Smartphone can be used for storing and playing MP3 files, too. About 36% of elementary school pupils and 81% of students in classes 5–10 own an MP3 player. In the "Schnecke" screening project with a screening examination of more than 3000 school pupils, students with MP3 players showed no greater risk of hearing impairment. Taking into account the daily listening time and set volume, no increased risk of hearing loss could be shown, either (Hoffmann et al. 2008). However, publications also exist with contrary results (Hoover and Krishnamurti 2010), though in many publications, an assessment of the risk was undertaken only in accordance with work protection guidelines (Vogel et al. 2010; Danhauer et al. 2009).

In discussions, a constantly growing number of young people with hearing impairment due to the increasing noise in leisure time is postulated (WHO 2015; Pienkowski 2021). Rabinowitz and colleagues (Rabinowitz et al. 2006) analyzed hearing ability in attitudinal surveys in the United States over two decades (1985–2004) and found no significant increase in the prevalence of hearing loss over time but rather a slight decrease in prevalence rates for high-frequency hearing loss over the years. Likewise, the annual investigations undertaken by the Schweizerische Unfallversicherungsanstalt (SUVA) show a clear reduction in the prevalence of high-frequency hearing loss for youths in the period covering 1975–2011 (SUVA 2011). After half a century of rock and pop music with live concerts and discotheques, more than four decades after the launch of the Walkman, and around two decades after the triumphal march of the MP3 player, it should now be possible to better assess the long-term effects of loud music on the ability to hear. The presumably largest study on hearing ability covering all age groups comes from Nord-Trøndelag County in Norway. From 1995 to 1997, a standardized survey by means of a questionnaire was carried out on 51,975 test subjects (also concerning music consumption), as well as a hearing test.

It was not possible to demonstrate an effect of loud music on hearing ability both among Walkman users and those visiting discotheques and rock concerts (Tambs et al. 2003).

The authors clearly pointed out that, contrary to widespread belief, they found no music-related hearing loss at the time of the study in the late 1990s.

The study "How does Germany hear?" showed similar results (Hoffmann 2008). In this cross-sectional study to determine the hearing ability in the German population in age groups ranging from 10 to 85 years of age, the median of the hearing ability in the individual age groups corresponded broadly with expectations in accordance with ISO 7029, which describes the development of hearing ability regardless of gender and age. Although the audiometric data on which the formulas of ISO 7029 are based are already up to 50 years old, no systematic deterioration of the hearing threshold in the individual age groups was shown in the current study. It was not possible to observe a worrying increase in hearing impairment in any age group.

These results were also confirmed by a follow-up study by Engdahl and Aarhus, who had the opportunity to reexamine more than 12,000 of the people who had already taken part in the Norwegian study in 1998 after more than 20 years (Engdahl and Aarhus 2021). Age, gender, initial hearing threshold, education, noise exposure, ear infections, head injuries, and daily smoking were considered as possible influencing factors. Although personal music player (PMP) use increased from 8% of respondents in 1998 to 30% in 2018, neither use nor duration of use was associated with pure-tone average thresholds at 3, 4, and 6 kHz when compared with nonusers. In terms of loudness, listening at low levels was even associated with better thresholds (on average 2.5 dB), while listening at high levels was associated with slightly worse thresholds (on average 1.4 dB). The authors conclude that their large population study showed no association between normal PMP use and 20-year hearing progression; only among high-volume users was there a modest, measurable hearing deterioration.

The effect of loud music on hearing ability is, therefore, mostly overestimated in general discussion. The study results do not point to a dramatic deterioration in hearing ability on the part of the population due to discos, pop concerts, and the use of the Walkman, MP3 players, and smartphones. This does not exclude the possibility that in single cases hearing loss and tinnitus can result following a visit to a concert or disco. A specially developed prevention program can encourage heavy users of loud music to adopt healthy listening habits (Thulin et al. 2023).

30.8 Conclusion

Even though the sensory organ that is the ear is rarely still employed for the detection of prey, it forms a vital interface between man and his environment. It is an organ of communication, delivering control over the world around us and enabling the enjoyment of music. Protecting this sensitive organ of the senses by the consistent use of hearing protection during high-level sound generation that undoubtedly can be categorized as din, such as the usage of a circular saw, for example, should be self-evident. The goal is to preserve one's own ability to hear in order to be able to enjoy music over a long period and to retain one's ability to communicate.

References

103. Deutscher Ärztetag (2000) Entschließung zum Tagesordnungspunkt VI. Tätigkeitsbericht der Bundesärztekammer. Gesundheitliche Folgen von Freizeitlärm auf Seite A-1392. In: Deutsches Ärzteblatt (Dtsch Arztebl), Jg. 97, H. 20, S. A-1384 bis A-1392 bzw. C-1062 bis C-1069

Axelsson A (1991) Leisure noise exposure in adolescents and young adults. J Sound Vib Jg. 151, H. 3, S 447–453

Babisch W (2006) Transportation noise and cardiovascular risk: updated review and synthesis of epidemiological studies indicate that the evidence has increased. Noise Health 8:1–29

Beck C, Michler H (1960) Feinstrukturelle und histochemische Veränderungen an den Strukturen der Cochlea beim Meerschweinchen nach dosierter Reintonbestrahlung. Arch Ohren Nasen Kehlkopfheilkunde 174:496–567

Behar A, Wong W, Kunov H (2006) Risk of hearing loss in orchestra musicians: review of the literature. Med Probl Perform Art 21:164–168

Behroozi KB, Luz J (1997) Noise-related ailments of performing musicians: a review. Med Probl Perform Art 12:19–22

Brashears SM, Morlet TG, Berlin CI, Hood LJ (2003) Olivocochlear efferent suppression in classical musicians. J Am Acad Audiol 14:314–324

Danhauer JL, Johnson CE, Byrd A, DeGood L, Meuel C, Pecile A, Koch LL (2009) Survey of college students on iPod use and hearing health. J Am Acad Audiol Jg. 20, H. 1, 5–27, quiz 83–4

DGUV (Deutsche Gesetzliche Unfallversicherung) (2022) Anerkannte Berufskrankheiten. https://www.dguv.de/de/zahlen-fakten/bk-geschehen/anerkannte-bken/index.jsp

Drotleff H, Leistner M (2007) Room acoustic design of orchestra pits. Dokumentation der Tagung »Music—Safe and Sound« am 16./17.01.2007. www.baua.de/de/Themen-von-A-Z/Laerm-und-Akustik/Safe-and-Sound.html

Engdahl B, Aarhus L (2021, Trends Hear, 2021) Personal music players and hearing loss: the HUNT cohort study. 25:23312165211015881. https://doi.org/10.1177/23312165211015881

Flach M, Aschoff E (1966) Zur Frage berufsbedingter Schwerhörigkeit bei Musikern. Zeitschrift für Laryngologie 45:595–605

Guinan JJ (2006) Olivocochlear efferents: anatomy, physiology, function, and measurement efferent effects in humans. Ear Hear 27:589–607

Habermann J (1890) Über die Schwerhörigkeit der Kesselschmiede. Arch Ohrenheilk 30:1

Hellbrück J, Schick A (1989) Zehn Jahre Walkman—Grund zum Feiern oder Anlaß zur Sorge? Z Lärmbekämpfung 36:121–129

Hoffmann E (1997) Hörfähigkeit und Hörschäden junger Erwachsener. Unter Berücksichtigung der Lärmbelastung, Median/Heidelberg

Hoffmann E (2006) Auditory disorders among dance club visitors. Inter Noise Proc 1:1657–1664

Hoffmann E (2008) Wie hört Deutschland? In: Verband Deutscher Tonmeister (VDT) (Hrsg) 25. Tonmeistertagung 2008. VDT International Convention: November 2008. Verlag VDT, Bergisch-Gladbach, S 506–514

Hoffmann E, Silberzahn J, Limberger A, Beigel D (2008) Hör-, Seh- und Gleichgewichtsstörungen bei hessischen Schulkindern: Ein Screening bei über 3.000 Schülern im Alter zwischen 5 und 18 Jahren. Poster, 79. Jahresversammlung der Deutschen Gesellschaft für Hals-Nasen-Ohren-Heilkunde, Kopf- und Hals-Chirurgie e. V

Hohmann B, Dupasquier S, Billeter T (2003) Fortissimo mit Folgen. In: Stulz P, Landau A (Hrsg) Musik und Medizin. Chronos, Zürich, S 53–58

Hoover A, Krishnamurti S (2010) Survey of college students' MP3 listening: habits, safety issues, attitudes, and education. Am J Audiol 1:73–83. Online verfügbar unter. https://doi.org/10.1044/1059-0889(2010/08-0036)

Ising H, Hanel J, Pilgramm M, Babisch W, Lindthammer A (1994) Gehörschadensrisiko durch Musikhören mit Kopfhörern. HNO 42:764–768

Jansson E, Karlsson K (1983) Sound levels recorded within the symphony orchestra and risk criteria for hearing loss. Scand Audiol 12:215–221

Kähäri KR, Axelsson A, Hellstrom PA, Zachau G (2001) Hearing development in classical orchestral musicians. A follow-up study. Scand Audiol 30:141–149

Krähenbühl D, Arnold W, Fried R, Chüden H (1987) Hörschaden durch Walkman? Laryngol Rhinol Otol 66:286–289

Lebo CP, Oliphant KS, Garrett J (1967) Acoustic trauma from rock-and-roll music. Calif Med 5:378–380

Lindgren E, Axelsson A (1983) Temporary threshold shift after exposure to noise and music of equal energy. Ear Hear 4:197–201

Lipscomb DM (1969) Ear damage from exposure to rock and roll music. Arch Otolaryngol 5:545–555

Mahling CH (1997) Orchester. In: MGG. Sachteil, Bd 7. Bärenreiter u. Metzler, Kassel, Stuttgart, S 811–812

Marquard U, Schäcke G (1998) Gehörgefährdung durch Musizieren im Orchester. Zentralblatt für Arbeitsmedizin 48:188–204

Micheyl C, Carbonnel O, Collet L (1995) Medial olivocochlear system and loudness adaptation: differences between musicians and non-musicians. Brain Cogn 29:127–136

Obeling L, Poulsen T (1999) Hearing ability in Danish symphony orchestra musicians. Noise Health 1:43–49

Pienkowski M (2021) Loud music and leisure noise is a common cause of chronic hearing loss, tinnitus and hyperacusis. Int J Environ Res Public Health 2021(18):4236. https://doi.org/10.3390/ijerph18084236

Rabinowitz PM, Slade MD, Galusha D, Dixon-Ernst C, Cullen MR (2006) Trends in the prevalence of hearing loss among young adults entering an industrial workforce 1985 to 2004. Ear Hear 4:369–375. Online verfügbar unter. https://doi.org/10.1097/01.aud.0000224125.12338.9a

Richter B, Hauser R, Löhle E (1995) Der Einfluß kontralateraler Beschallung auf otoakustische Distorsionsprodukt-Emissionen des Menschen. Laryngo-Rhino-Otol 74:160–166

Richter B, Zander M, Spahn C (2007) Gehörschutz im Orchester. Schriftenreihe des Freiburger Instituts für Musikermedizin (Spahn C, Hrsg) »Freiburger Beiträge zur Musikermedizin«, Bd 4. Projektverlag, Freiburg/Bochum

Richter B, Zander M, Hohmann B, Spahn C (2011) Gehörschutz bei Musikern. HNO 59:538–546

Rintelmann WF, Borus JF (1968) Noise-induced hearing loss and rock and roll music. Arch Otolaryngol 4:377–385

Rudloff F, Specht HV, Penk S, Pethe J, Schuschke G (1996) Untersuchungen zu Ausmaß und möglichen Folgen jugendlichen Musikkonsums. Teil III—Ergebnisse von Schallpegelmessungen und audiologischen Untersuchungen. Zeitschrift für Lärmbekämpfung 43:9–14

Struwe F, Jansen G, Schwarze S, Schwenzer C, Nitzsche M (1995) Untersuchung von Hörgewohnheiten und möglichen Gehörrisiken durch Schalleinwirkungen in der Freizeit unter besonderer Berücksichtigung des Walkman-Hörens—Auszug. Herausgegeben von Bundesgesundheitsamt. Institut für Arbeitsmedizin der Heinrich-Heine-Universität Düsseldorf, Düsseldorf, S 94–97, 106

SUVA (2011) Hören Jugendliche wirklich schlechter als früher? Pressemitteilung vom 20.04.2011. Luzern

Swanson SJ, Dengerink HA, Kondrick P, Miller CL (1987) The influence of subjective factors on temporary threshold shifts after exposure to music and noise of equal energy. Ear Hear 8:288–291

Tambs K, Hoffman HJ, Borchgrevink HM, Holmen J, Samuelsen SO (2003) Hearing loss induced by noise, ear infections, and head injuries: results from the Nord-Trøndelag Hearing Loss Study. Int J Audiol 2:89–105

Thulin A, Kähäri K, Malmberg M (2023) The development and evaluation of an online hearing loss prevention program. Prev Med Rep 35:102298. https://doi.org/10.1016/j.pmedr.2023.102298

Turunen-Rise I, Flottorp G, Tvete O (1991) Personal cassette players (»Walkman«). Do they cause noise-induced hearing loss? Scand Audiol 4:239–244

Vogel I, Verschuure H, van der Ploeg CPB, Brug J, Raat H (2010) Estimating adolescent risk for hearing loss based on data from a large school-based survey. Am J Public Health 6:1095–1100. Online verfügbar unter. https://doi.org/10.2105/AJPH.2009.168690

World Health Organization (WHO) (2015) Hearing loss due to recreational exposure to loud sounds. A review. World Health Organization, Geneva

Zander M, Spahn C, Richter B (2008) Employment and acceptance of hearing protectors in classical symphony and opera orchestras. Noise Health 10:14–126

Zenner HP, Struwe V, Schuschke G, Spreng M, Stange G, Plath P, Babisch W et al (1999) Gehörschäden durch Freizeitlärm. HNO 4:236–248

The Soul Sung to Destruction: Music as an Instrument of Torture

31

M. J. Grant, Anna Papaeti, and Stephanie Leder

Somebody tell me frankly
what times are these
what kind of world
what country?
Ariel Dorfman, from the poem "Hope" (1988), cited here from Dorfman (2004).

When the author Ariel Dorfman wrote these lines, Chile was still under the rule of the dictatorship of Augusto Pinochet. In the poem, Dorfman describes the paradoxical situation in which the parents of the many people detained, tortured and killed in this period (1973–1990) found themselves. What kind of times are we living in, writes Dorfman in the first person, what kind of world is this, in which the news that my son is being held in a particular prison and tortured there—thus, is still alive at least—is a source of hope?

Dorfman's literary reflections on Chile's dictatorship of terror have become well-known through another of his works. The play *Death and the Maiden* (1990), famous not least through Roman Polanski's film version starring Sigourney Weaver and Ben Kingsley, takes its title from Franz Schubert's String Quartet No. 14, which is also known under this name. In Dorfman's play, the character Paulina Salas, a Chilean survivor of torture, encounters one of the men who had repeatedly raped her during her detention, after a period of many years. She had never seen this man's face: she recognises him, however, through his voice and habits. This man had raped her while the Schubert piece was playing on cassette in the background.

M. J. Grant (✉)
Reid School of Music, University of Edinburgh, Edinburgh, UK
e-mail: mj.grant@ed.ac.uk

A. Papaeti
Institute of Historical Research, National Hellenic Research Foundation, Athens, Greece
e-mail: apapaeti@eie.gr

S. Leder
Bamberg, Germany

G. Kreutz, G. Bernatzky (eds.), *Music and Medicine*, Neurocultural Health and Wellbeing, https://doi.org/10.1007/978-3-662-72175-9_31

That Dorfman chooses a musical motif here is not just poetic licence, for there is nothing fictional about the use of music in torture. Former prisoners from Chile's prisons in this period, and also representatives of the military, have reported that music was using during torture there (Comité de Defensa de los Derechos del Pueblo 1989; Bauer 2009; Chornik 2013, 2018); indeed, according to Katia Chornik's research, high-ranking officers—like the character in Dorfman's play—used classical music during torture, as opposed to low-ranking officers (Chornik 2013, pp. 57–58).[1] Chile is not alone here: the use of music in torture can be historically documented for many hundreds of years, and today as well occurs across the world (Grant and Papaeti 2013; Papaeti and Grant 2013; Grant 2014a, b). Only recently, however, has music torture become an object of scholarly research and only recently has it been explicitly recognised in law as a form of torture.

This chapter offers an overview of known forms, contexts and effects of the use of music as an instrument of torture. The first part of the chapter discusses definitions of torture and the impacts of torture, as well as describing the most well-known forms of music torture. In the second part, we discuss this further through three case studies of the use of music in torture: the Nazi concentration and death camps, detention centres for political prisoners in Greece under the military dictatorship (1967–1974), and the US "War Against Terror". The third part of the chapter summarises initial findings of research in this area and outlines possible consequences for practice as well as areas for future research.

The potential of music therapy for survivors of torture—which is indeed employed by various rehabilitation centres—is not discussed here (for more on this topic see Dixon 2002). Music can, in fact, be a source of strength for some people during torture and not only during rehabilitation (Papaeti 2020a, b). However, the widespread tendency to regard music in the first instance as something entirely positive, while simultaneously explaining away or trivialising negative impacts of music is in our opinion, one of the reasons why music torture was not taken seriously for so long.

31.1 Torture and Music Torture

31.1.1 Torture

The impacts of torture can be felt in almost every country in the world.[2] These impacts are not limited to the many states which have used torture systematically in the present day or within the last few generations: the consequences of torture can

[1] See also the online database *Cantos Cautivos*, which collects testimony from survivors and their representatives on aspects of music in detention under the Pinochet dictatorship, including many accounts of self-directed uses of music by prisoners as a strategy of survival. The database was developed by Katia Chornik in collaboration with the Museum of Memory and Human Rights in Santiago, Chile. https://www.cantoscautivos.org/en/index.php

[2] For further information see e.g. http://www.atlas-of-torture.org

also be felt in states which have to deal with traumatised refugees. The long-term effects of torture impact not only the victims of torture, who often live with the consequences for the rest of their lives, but also their close relations, so that the impacts of torture are felt over generations (Rothkegel 2011). States that do not themselves practice torture can nevertheless be implicated for many reasons, among them the following: when states deport people to countries in which they are at risk of torture; when they admit evidence gained under torture in court; when they export weapons and other relevant technology to countries with a known track record of using these in torture.

What, however, is actually meant by "torture"? In academic research, there are many different approaches to defining what is and is not covered by the term (Green et al. 2010). The *UN Convention Against Torture and other forms of Cruel, Inhuman or Degrading Treatment or Punishment* (1984, often referred to by the acronym CAT) gives the following, much-quoted legal definition:

> For the purposes of this Convention, the term "torture" means any act by which severe pain or suffering, whether physical or mental, is intentionally inflicted on a person for such purposes as obtaining from him or a third person information or a confession, punishing him for an act he or a third person has committed or is suspected of having committed, or intimidating or coercing him or a third person, or for any reason based on discrimination of any kind, when such pain or suffering is inflicted by or at the instigation of or with the consent or acquiescence of a public official or other person acting in an official capacity. It does not include pain or suffering arising only from, inherent in or incidental to lawful sanctions.

This definition emphasises the intentional infliction of severe pain, and this violence is *only* considered torture for the purposes of the Convention when it is carried out by or with the consent of someone acting on behalf of the state. It does not, however, cover practices that are legally sanctioned, although this part of the definition is controversial and has been interpreted in several different ways. The Convention does not offer definitions for the other types of treatment which, since the *Universal Declaration of Human Rights* (1948) and the human rights standards that build on this, have generally been named and prohibited along with torture: the "cruel, inhuman and degrading treatment or punishment" (CID punishment) referenced in the full title of the Convention (c.f. Nowak and McArthur 2006; Nowak 2006). Today, many forms of ill-treatment which may not be classed as torture in the narrower sense are, however, frequently classed as cruel, inhuman and degrading by human rights organisations: these include unacceptable living conditions in places of detention. Increasingly, academics and advocates have argued that practices which may not individually meet the test of torture can, when combined, amount to torture; in consequence, they argue that the distinction between torture and CID punishment is problematic (Başoğlu et al. 2007; Başoğlu 2017; Grant 2013b).

Despite these limitations, the existence of a legal definition of torture is highly significant: the development, adoption and monitoring of international, legally binding standards is a huge step in the fight against torture. And international law is very clear on one point: the prohibition of torture and CID punishment is absolute—there are no exceptions. Thus, the right not to be tortured is one of relatively few so-called non-derogable rights.

Although there may seem to be widespread international consensus in support of the prohibition of torture, this does not mean the fight against torture is over. More or less simultaneously with the establishment of regional and international human rights standards against torture, some states—including the superpowers and their close allies—began to develop various methods and practices that seemed to get round the prohibition of torture (see here especially McCoy 2006; on the ubiquity of torture, see also Conroy 2001). Moreover, attempts to justify torture as constituting the lesser of two evils continue apace. For this reason, it is imperative that the reasons why torture can never be allowed are made clear. Torture is not only a horrific attack on the body and mind of the victim: its primary aim is to destroy that person's subjectivity, their sense of self. Thus, torture is nothing less than a direct attack on that which is supposed to be inviolable: human dignity. As Heiner Bielefeldt has commented,

> The absolute status of the prohibition of torture is based not just on normative considerations, but on the actual experience of what happens when this law is not upheld. Again and again it has been shown that torture not only disregards the principle of human dignity (as is the case with all human rights violations), but that it constitutes the complete and systematic negation of this principle. Like slavery, and possibly only like slavery, in torture a human being is transformed completely into an object, is degraded to the status of a "thing" to be used as one likes. The aim of torture is to break the will of the victim, to reduce them to a helpless bundle of pain, fear and shame for the purposes of information retrieval, terrorisation, or demoralisation. The black hoods that can be seen in the torture pictures from Abu Ghraib demonstrate how torture literally makes its victims faceless and in this way seeks to destroy them as individual subjects. The consequences of such an experience for the victim are profound. As Jean Amery famously said, those who have been tortured are no longer at home in the world. Self-respect, self-confidence, and the basic ability to trust other people are so fundamentally broken through torture that in many cases they can never be repaired, and life-long trauma is the result. (Bielefeldt 2004, p. 6; our translation)

31.1.2 Music Torture

"Music torture" is used here as a collective term for different practices that constitute torture and in which music plays a central role. The dividing line between practices in which music itself constitutes the main aspect of the torture, and where music accompanies other practices, is fuzzy, particularly since how music is experienced in torture can vary significantly from individual to individual.

There are as yet very few legal foundations specifically dealing with music as torture. The UN Committee Against Torture has, however, classed the use of continuous loud music in detention as a contravention against the Convention against Torture in at least one case (UN Committee Against Torture 1997), especially when used with other practices of torture. The specific case concerned Israel and led to these practices being prohibited by the Israeli Supreme Court. The practices named also included stress positions, hooding and sleep deprivation, amongst others: there are significant similarities here to the practices used just a few years later by the USA in the so-called "War Against Terror" (see Sect. 31.2.3, below). In part, these practices derive from experiments with so-called sensory deprivation that were conducted in the first decades of the Cold War. These experiments aimed to isolate the test participants as far as possible from any social or sensory contact with the outside world. For example, the complete silence of an anechoic chamber or the use of a loud monotonous noise were used to undermine spatial orientation; simultaneously, sight was hindered through hooding, and touch through wrapping the participants in thick material (see Smith and Lewty 1959; Zubak et al. 1961). The supposed purpose of these experiments was to research psychiatric disorders; however, it has been established that in many cases this research was in part supported by the US secret services (McCoy 2006, pp. 20–59). Today, some experts also use the terms *sensory overload* (Center for Victims of Torture 2023) or *sensory bombardment* (Physicians For Human Rights 2008) to describe practices in which the senses are subjected to too many and too extreme stimuli, such as through exposure to continuous, loud music.

Apart from these developments, there are ample indications that music has long been used in practices that may amount to or come close to torture. Music has frequently been used in practices of so-called "re-education", for example in the Soviet Gulag (Klause 2013), in Franco's Spain (Calero-Carramolino 2023) and in Greek prison camps from the 1940s onward (Papaeti 2013a, 2019). In addition, public executions and other forms of public punishment have been accompanied by music for centuries (Grant 2013a); in the European Middle Ages, music and references to music played a role in practices of public ill-treatment (Herzfeld-Schild 2013). It is likely that, over time, different forms and functions of music torture have emerged in part through the influence of older practices, in part through new discoveries (Grant 2014a, b).

The reasons given for why music torture is used, and its actual impacts, can diverge. For example, it is often claimed—including by the Israeli state with regard to the case discussed above—that music is used simply to make communication among detainees difficult. Many sources suggest that music is intended to mask the screams of people being tortured: this should not be taken at face value; however, as further analysis sometimes reveals that very different kinds of logic are at work (Grant 2013b, 2019; see also Sect. 31.2.2, below). That music itself can be experienced as a form of torture, and not only as something which accompanies or seeks to conceal torture, is apparent primarily from testimony given by survivors. It is exactly this discrepancy between the superficial justifications and explanations often given and the experiences of those directly affected that makes it imperative to look at case studies in more detail. In this regard, we vehemently disagree with the musicologist Jonathan Pieslak's claim that the soldiers carrying out such practices, and not the prisoners themselves, are best placed to decide when and how the use of music constitutes torture (Pieslak 2009, pp. 90–99).[3]

[3] Pieslak's statement came in response to a 2007 joint resolution by the Society for Ethnomusicology, the American Musicological Society and the Society for American Music, which spoke out against the use of music in connection with torture by US security forces. Problematic is Pieslak's assumption that soldiers who took part in such practices would publicly admit to having committed such a serious human rights abuse as torture.

31.2 Three Case Studies

The following case studies are based largely on survivor testimony. They demonstrate how music is used during torture and ill-treatment, and what the impacts on individuals can be. Particularly in the second and third case studies, music is often used in connection with other types of sound. All the examples discussed here suggest, however, that music has its own specific impacts, not least as a method of humiliating and making fun of detainees.

31.2.1 The Concentration and Death Camps of the National Socialist Regime

Perhaps no other regime in history has used music so consciously and strategically as the National Socialist regime in Germany. This extends to the often systematic use of music in the concentration and extermination camps, including as an instrument of violence and of torture (see here especially Fackler 2000; Brauer 2009, 2016; Gilbert 2005; Naliwajek-Mazurek 2013). Forced singing ("singing on command") was already in use in the first work camps set up by the regime and can be regarded as a horrific counterpart to the ubiquitous use of songs and singing under National Socialism generally. A particular feature of the camp system, meanwhile, was the camp orchestras, in which those prisoners with the necessary skills were forced to play. The use of these camp orchestras in particular reveals connections to older military traditions: just as military bands had done in field camps since the eighteenth century, the concentration camp orchestras played to accompany the daily routine of the camps and at more specific events as well—according to many reports, this included executions. Survivors also recounted how they were forced to play to accompany the torture and humiliation of their fellow prisoners.

Singing on command, in particular at the *Appellplatz* or parade ground, was part of life in the camps from the very beginning. Studies on the early work camps (Fackler 2000) and Sachsenhausen (Brauer 2009), based on reminiscences from survivors, official records from court cases against camp commanders, and on the content of songs created in the camps, provide evidence of the different repertoires used in this forced singing. Brauer (2009) characterises singing on command in the first years of the concentration camp system as something that could on occasion be a source of strength for many prisoners, as long as they were able to identify with the songs sung—and most of the songs would have been familiar. However, this situation changed dramatically after the outbreak of the War due to the transformed demographics of the camp and the significant increase in the number of foreign prisoners (Brauer 2009, p. 94). In addition, in the later years of the war, more and more cases emerge of singing being used intentionally to humiliate and torture specific groups of prisoners: this included the use of singing in so-called stress positions (Brauer 2009, p. 98). Brauer quotes, for example, from the reminiscences of the famous Polish songwriter and camp survivor Aleksander Kulisiewicz, who described the practice known as the "singing horse" as follows:

> Here, the unlucky victims were strapped to a heavily laden cart, which they had to pull; when pulling it they were bent over almost double, with the head down low to the ground, and the whole time they had to sing as loud as they possibly could. The intention was to wreck muscles, lungs, rib cage, nervous system and vocal chords all at one and the same time. (quoted from Brauer 2009, p. 99, our translation from the German)

In the camps, singing fulfilled many functions that are characteristic of how music is used as an instrument of torture more generally. In addition to humiliating the prisoners, music served to mask the reality of the camps in two different ways. On the one hand, and especially in the early camps, music was supposedly used to communicate "German" values in an attempt to maintain the appearance that the camps merely served the purpose of re-education. On the other hand, survivors reported being made to sing very loudly in order to make the screams of other prisoners inaudible. In reality, singing was a form of psychological and physical violence, since prisoners were made to do it for hours regardless of how physically exhausted they were. Those who did not sing along properly were sometimes compelled to do so under pain of death. Guido Fackler quotes here from the testimony of Karl Röder, who, in his reminiscences of his time in Dachau and Flössenburg, described the constant obligation to sing as being a particularly severe form of treatment:

> The singing had to be done with a militaristic swagger—and most importantly of all, it had to be loud. They made absolutely sure that everyone shouted as loud as he could. After hours of singing we were often completely hoarse. They loved our bright, happy singing, they couldn't get enough of it. They knew we regarded it as punishment, that's why they always had us sing when we were doing punishment drill. We sang as soon as this started, and we sang when we were already completely exhausted; even the half-dead ones, lying on the ground, had to sing. Since it was life-threatening not to sing the way they wanted, we had to practice again and again. That was only possible in our free time. (quoted from Fackler 2001, pp. 143–144, our translation)

This necessity of singing even when no guards were present seems to have been particularly damaging for Röder: "I constantly gagged on hate and anger and had the feeling I was choking. I'd have preferred corporal punishment" (ibid.)

31.2.2 The Greek Junta, 1967–1974

The Greek military dictatorship of 1967–1974 is one of the earliest documented examples of a new, cutting-edge combination of torture methods that emerged in the Cold War period and used music and sound as an integral part of their ritual. According to testimonies from political prisoners, these methods included continuous standing, sleep, drink and food deprivation, stress positions and exposure to continuous loud music and/or sounds (Papaeti 2013b). Based on psychological research conducted in British, US and Canadian Universities, these rather banal methods constitute a holistic attack on the minds and bodies of prisoners. They must be understood in the context of both the international human rights treaties signed in the post-war period and also psychological warfare in the context of the Cold War. Codified in the CIA KUBARK Counterintelligence Interrogation Manual (1963), these methods form the basis of a new kind of interrogation practices used internationally not only in the 1960s and 1970s but also more recently in the so-called War on Terror (see Sect. 31.2.3).

On 21 April 1967, a military Junta came to power in Greece, bringing to a climactic end 30 years of conflict between right-wing and left-wing forces. Lasting 7 years, it fell in July 1974. To sustain the Junta in power, a brutal police state was developed. Its opponents were intimidated, detained, sent into internal exile and systematically tortured. The main bodies responsible were the Security Forces (*Asfalia*) and Greek Military Police (*Elliniki Stratiotiki Astynomia* or ESA).

The use of torture by the Junta has been a subject of great scrutiny and debate in Greece. Already during the dictatorship many testimonies circulated abroad, sparking international debate. Testimonies were also crucial to a complaint brought by Scandinavian countries and the Netherlands to the Council of Europe's Commission of Human Rights at the end of 1967 (Hammarberg 2007; European Commission of Human Rights 1969). As a result, Greece left the Council in 1969 in order to avoid suspension. With the restoration of democracy in the aftermath of the dictatorship, a series of trials took place to prosecute the crimes and abuses of the Junta. In this context, some Junta torturers were brought to court by private lawsuits initiated by survivors and not by the state.

Despite copious information available on the subject, until very recently music was absent from the debates on the dictatorship's use of torture. The fact that non-physical torture was not considered an offence under Greek law at the time is probably one of the reasons that the use of music was not clarified in the trials. The emphasis on bodily harm and physical violence continued in the ensuing decades. However, from the transcripts of the torturers' trials, an elliptic picture emerges of how music and sounds were used to break and humiliate prisoners. Music from radio and loudspeakers, noise, songs and forced singing recurs often enough in trial testimonies, though in passing, while witnesses were interrupted and asked to limit themselves to the list of alleged charges. The cases mentioned here took place between March and June 1973 at the headquarters of the Special Interrogation Unit of the Greek Military Police (hereafter EAT/ESA) in Athens (see Papaeti 2013b).

One of the first testimonies to mention music and sound is from A, an admiral and the retired Chief of the Navy.[4] A was arrested on 24 May 1973 and detained for 60 days in EAT/ESA. Before his interrogation began, he was kept in total isolation for 2 days. During that time, he started hallucinating and lost any sense of reality. In his testimony, he says "The loudspeaker started playing loudly. The shouts began.

[4] Pseudnoyms are used to protect the identity of the individuals concerned.

This situation transformed me in 2 days from a human being to a corpse" (in Rodakis 1976, p. 128)[5]; hallucinations are one of the main side effects experienced in this combination of torture techniques.

Sound is emphasized by B who was arrested in March 1973 and was detained for 40 days in EAT/ESA. She was put in a cell and given paper to write her statement. She recalled:

> Then the noises began. Part of the suffering was the noises. Noises caused by the guards' raids, noises caused by technical means: you thought that you were surrounded by radios and televisions with many, uncoordinated programmes. You'd go crazy. I have to repeat that what they wanted from me and my fellow-detainees was to exhaust us as human beings.

Similar was the testimony of C, an Air-Force Major, arrested on 2 June 1973:

> Needless to say that I did not sleep all these nights, because they did not let you sleep. Banging the doors, noise, cursing. Like [the song]… 'Charon is on the prowl' and other similar vulgarities.[6] The cursing, noises, radio at maximum volume, and the threats created a hellish atmosphere. (Rodakis 1976, p. 225)

The most detailed account of the use of music in the trials described the use of the song "Tarzan" (1972), a popular hit of the time. Singled out by D, a university student arrested in May 1973, it is encountered in all recent testimonies by political prisoners collected by Anna Papaeti that recall the use of music in torture. Most survivors found it hard to come to terms with the fact that the song was by left-wing composer Yannis Markopoulos and not a regime sympathizer. Released in 1972, "Tarzan" contained veiled anti-Junta lyrics that describe an urgent fantasy of insurgency and resistance but had successfully managed to pass the regime's censorship: "I'll go to the jungle with Tarzan/I'll have a ball/And if the wild beasts eat me/It will be written in history/that I was eaten by animals/and not by the century's disaster". D recounts:

> In the afternoon, somewhere outside, there were a lot of beatings, and I heard the torturers' shouts. They played a loudspeaker, so the voices would not be heard. The motif of the time was [the song] 'I will go to the jungle with Tarzan'. It was the song we heard all the time until we left. The military policemen were shouting 'Wait for your turn'. Waiting was worse than to be beaten. (Rodakis 1976, p. 448)

When D was interviewed in Athens in 2010,[7] he did not remember the "Tarzan" song from the loudspeakers but recalled the guards singing it while beating them at night. "In the evening", he said, "the soldiers would return to the prisons drunk and

---

[5] All translations are by Anna Papaeti.

[6] The popular song "Charon is on the prowl" was released in 1972. Originally a failure in terms of sales, it became a hit in 1973. After a highly publicized massacre in a nightclub by Nikos Koemtzis, the song was accused by journalist Dimitris Psathas of inciting young people to commit crime, making the song instantly famous. http://www.musicheaven.gr/html/modules.php?name=Splatt_Forums&file=viewtopic&topic=1494&start=80, accessed on 15 June 2012.

[7] All interviews were conducted by Anna Papaeti.

they would sing the Tarzan song in order to terrorize us. They would enter the cells for the so-called tea party or tea party with toast". Tea party here refers to a ritual during which several guards surrounded a detainee, shouting and cursing. While beating him, they would throw him against the bed or the chair. Its variant "tea party with toast" denoted more brutal beatings "This was not music", he said. "This was terror. It was part of the system".

Similar testimonies from three people held at EAT/ESA in May and June 1973 and interviewed in spring 2010 and 2012 state clearly that certain songs were repeated continuously day and night. All three interviewees mentioned "Tarzan" as one of the songs played to them. The most graphic case is that of Z. During the first trial, Z described one of the most standard ESA torture methods. After his arrest in June 1973, he was forced to stand upright—sometimes on one foot—for 9 days in a small, empty cell. He suffered beatings and interrogations, conducted at irregular intervals to subvert his sense of time. He was also deprived of drink. This ordeal resulted in excruciating pain and hallucinations. During this time, Z describes how he was forced to sing while holding his head back as far as possible for an extended amount of time. Suffering from drink deprivation, he would choke on his saliva: "The dry thick saliva would block my larynx and I thought that I was choking", he said (Rodakis 1976, p. 398).

When asked about music during an interview in 2010, Z did not mention this particular event. However, he gave a rather detailed account of the continuous use of loud music during torture. Just like D, he singled out "Tarzan" as well as the song "The guys, the guys". These were played continuously day and night. A third song, "Stephanos" (1972), describing the death of Stephanos the good man, mourned by his friends, was played right at the end of torture and had a strong ironic resonance. He said: "My ears still buzz 'the guys, the guys, the good buddies' from 100 radios. I don't know how many radios played this little song of the time by Kinousis.[8] 'The guys, the guys', and 'I will go to the jungle with Tarzan'". He said:

> They were constantly the same songs. They played them during torture so that the screams would not be heard, and at night when the guards came back drunk [...]. Imagine to be standing for days without water, to be hit by globs and then to hear this music, what kind of a situation was formed. You felt like going crazy. [...] In the end I had hallucinations. They hit me and their faces would transform. I thought that they were my friends and family. I'd tell them, Gianni why do you hit me? Such a situation was formed. And with all this, to hear this music 'the guys, the guys, the good buddies' and 'I will go to the jungle with Tarzan'. When the torture time was up, for it never occurred at fixed times, they would play, 'There goes Stefanos, the good man'.

At first, Z thought that these songs were played on the radio in order to mask the cries of those tortured. However, after a series of questions, he came to realize in the process of the interview that these songs were repeated in a loop without any interludes from a radio presenter. That the detention centres of EAT/ESA did not have any civilian buildings directly adjacent to them, but simply military and naval

[8] Giorgos Kinousis was a popular singer. His song "The guys, the guys" (1972) was a hit of the time.

hospitals, underlines the fact that there was no need to drown the sounds of torture. In the torture context, the songs' lyrics and their order are mocking and demeaning. Z did not consider the choice of songs a coincidence. Even four decades on from this experience, hearing this music would make him melancholic. Interesting in this interview is that Z did not recall being forced to sing although he had mentioned it in his trial testimony. He simply stated that probably, he was not asked to do so "because they knew my reaction to it". Lapses of memory and other discrepancies from trial testimonies are an important issue in such research. Survivors of torture, on many occasions, tend to suppress memories as a defence mechanism from traumatic events they have not been able to sufficiently symbolize or cope with. The description of forced singing by Z was painful, though no more traumatic than his descriptions of hallucinations and physical torture. However, his phrase "they never asked me, because they knew my reaction" implies more than the interviewee wishes to say. In EAT/ESA, there was no sense of logic that would have prevented his torturers from asking him to do anything. It is well documented that any refusal would simply result in more torture. This phrase says more about himself and how *he* values dignity rather than about his torturers. As a Cavalry Captain, Z probably viewed forced singing as more humiliating than any physical torture he was subjected to, a subject about which he was very forthcoming. In this sense, the memory lapse seems to be a defence mechanism, betraying his sensitivity on the issue of humiliation and loss of dignity. It also shows how the use of music in torture, understood by some as "benign" or mild, can in fact scar the person subjected to it more than physical torture.

31.2.3 The US "War Against Terror"

The use of music as part of the interrogation practices employed by US security services in the so-called "War Against Terror" is probably the most well-known example of music torture in the world today. According to various sources—including statements from current and former prisoners as well as members of the security services, and official military documents—the practices tersely termed "enhanced interrogation" were used in a whole series of institutions, including the Bagram military base in Afghanistan, the detention camps in the US naval base in Guantánamo, Cuba, as well as in various prisons and camps in Iraq (Human Rights Watch 2004, 2006; Feinstein 2012–14; see also Cusick 2006, 2008). The examples discussed below relate to only a few of these places of detention, but it has since been established that music was used systematically in torture in others as well. This is clear even from the *Army Field Manual for Human Intelligence Collector Operations, FM 2-22.3 (34-52)* which describes the standard procedures for various places of detention (Cusick 2008, p. 14). In addition, as mentioned previously, the techniques used are in many regards developed from practices that were already being tested and employed in the 1950s (McCoy 2006) and that have been used regularly since then—not only by US security forces.

Marwan Jabour, a Palestinian who grew up in Saudi Arabia, moved to Pakistan to study and was detained there on 9 May 2004. Human Rights Watch reported that

> during the first six months he was held at the secret prison they would sometimes play rock music at ear-blasting levels, which could last an hour, a day, a few days, or even a week. "It was loud, awful music," he said, "like the soundtrack from a horror movie." (Human Rights Watch 2007, p.16)

Another prisoner, held in the same prison, reported that the music once played continuously for 4 months (Human Rights Watch 2007, pp. 22–23). As well as music, Jabour also reported hearing a constant, low-level white noise that sounded as if it came from a generator.[9] Jabour himself was of the opinion that this strategy served primarily to prevent the prisoners from communicating with one another (Human Rights Watch 2007, p. 16). One of the consequences, however, was that prisoners were unable to sleep: sleep deprivation is a well-known technique of torture, with severe side-effects (Physicians for Human Rights 2007, p. 22). At other locations, the music was not played constantly but at irregular intervals; in these cases, prisoners lived with the fear of not knowing when it would start again. Moazzem Begg, who was detained both in Bagram and in Guantánamo, told Suzanne Cusick about the effects of this situation on him in Bagram:

> every single night, particularly toward the end of my time there [the music played and] it became almost impossible to sleep […] If even footsteps echoed in the building, you can imagine what full blast Marilyn Manson would sound like. Sometimes it would stop at 3 am or so, but your ability to sleep was already disturbed. You lose the ability to have a routine sleep … The other thing that they did was play the music at various times, … the random aspect of when it would start or end was frustrating, makes you tired, agitated, upset, on top of all the other situations of not knowing when you're going to be released, interrogated, or moved to those cells. Many people suffered from various kinds of anxiety attacks. People hyperventilated, losing control of their senses, hitting their bottle of water against the cell, against other people, trying to scrape their hands against the concertina wire, sometimes breaking down and crying. (Begg in conversation with Cusick, quoted from Cusick 2008, 7. Ellipses in square brackets are our addition)

Several reports from Guantánamo indicate that music was used in conjunction with stress positions and, in some cases, also together with strobe lighting. For example, an FBI agent described in an email that prisoners were chained to the floor in a foetal position for 18–20 h and were exposed to extremes of heat and cold and to very loud rap music; food and water were withheld. This treatment led one prisoner to literally pull out his hair: he "was almost unconscious on the floor, with a pile of hair next to him" (Borchelt 2005, p. 52). Tarek Dergoul, who was held in Guantánamo and released in March 2004, reported in detail his experience of these techniques:

---

[9] Similar noises have been reported in a number of other cases of torture using what are basically the same set of practices, including the case of the so-called "five techniques" used by British security forces in Northern Ireland (see Grant 2014a, b; Newbery 2015).

> One practice … was "short shackling" where we were forced to squat without a chair with our hands chained between our legs and chained to the floor. If we fell over, the chains would cut into our hands. We would be left in this position for hours before an interrogation, during the interrogations (which could last as long as 12 hours), and sometimes for hours while the interrogators left the room. The air conditioning was turned up so high that within minutes we would be freezing. There was strobe lighting and loud music played that was itself a form of torture. Sometimes dogs were brought in to frighten us… Sometimes detainees would be taken to the interrogation room day after day and kept short-shackled without interrogation ever happening, sometimes for weeks on end. (quoted from Human Rights Watch 2004, p. 17. Ellipses in original)

Dergoul later reported that, as a consequence of how he was treated in this detention, he suffers from somatic and psychological complaints: "I get migraines, I'm depressed and I suffer from memory loss. There's stuff that happened, embedded in my head, that I can't remember" (Dergoul as quoted in Borchelt 2005, p. 54). A further Guantánamo detainee, Benyam Mohammad, a British citizen who was born in Ethiopia, described his experiences in a so-called "dark prison" in 2004:

> It was pitch black, no lights on in the rooms for most of the time.… They hung me up. I was allowed a few hours of sleep on the second day, then hung up again, this time for two days. My legs had swollen. My wrists and hands had gone numb.… There was loud music, [Eminem's] "Slim Shady" and Dr. Dre for 20 days.… [Then] they changed the sounds to horrible ghost laughter and Halloween sounds. [At one point, I was] chained to the rails for a fortnight.… The CIA worked on people, including me, day and night.… Plenty lost their minds. I could hear people knocking their heads against the walls and the doors, screaming their heads off. (quoted from Human Rights Watch 2005, p. 2. Ellipses, bracketed insertions in original)

On another occasion, after he had been transported from Pakistan to Morocco and held in a further dark prison there, he reported:

> They cuffed me and put earphones on my head. They played hip-hop and rock music, very loud. I remember they played Meat Loaf and Aerosmith over and over. A couple of days later they did the same thing. Same music. (Grey and Cobain 2005; also quoted in Cusick 2006)

In the examples just discussed, there is a certain amount of consistency in the types of music played. However, other prisoners and also prison guards report the use of other types of music as well—for example, the use of songs from the children's TV programmes *Barney* and *Sesame Street*.[10] In some cases, the choice of music was left to the guards themselves; in others, however, the choice was linked to conscious strategies of humiliation and physical torture. This is particularly noticeable in the case of Mohammed al-Qatani, which Cusick reconstructed using information from interrogation records ("Interrogation Log, Detainee 063"; Cusick 2008).

Al-Qatani was detained in Guantánamo. According to Cusick, music formed part of a strategy which the logs referred to as "the bad Muslim theme", the aim of which

[10] On the latter, see especially the documentary *Songs of War* (Chytroschek 2010), which follows *Sesame Street* composer Christopher Cerf as he attempts to find out more about this.

was to prevent al-Qatani from practising his religion in the proper manner (Cusick 2008, p. 12). For example, one morning, al-Qatani asked if he could pray; he was told that he could pray if he drank some water first, which he had not done that morning as he was fasting for Ramadan. He began praying regardless, at which point "Sergeant R" said to him "'If you continue to chant, I'll turn on the music'. Detainee stopped chanting" (quoted from "Interrogation Log, Detainee 063" by Cusick 2008, p. 12).

This act of playing recorded music was particularly distressing for al-Qatani due to his Islamic beliefs. On 7 December 2002, the first day of Ramadan, Arabic music was played to him, and al-Qatani complained that listening to this would constitute a transgression against Islamic law. In response, the interrogation personnel ordered him to cite a passage from the Koran that forbade music (Cusick 2008, p. 12).[11] In the days that followed, more and more of his time was filled with music, on the one hand as a method of sleep deprivation, on the other to prevent him from answering questions during interrogation; in addition, the topic of the prohibition of music in Islam was raised again and again (Cusick 2008, p. 13). The result was that al-Qatani "broke down crying and asking God for forgiveness and … stated that he could do nothing about the music that was played in the [interrogation] booth" (quoted in Cusick 2008, pp. 13–14; ellipsis and insertion in original).

Al-Qatani was also sexually humiliated. Cusick describes how, to the sound of Christina Aguilera, he was forced to wear women's clothes or teased for being homosexual because he refused to look at images of scantily clad women (Cusick 2008, p. 12). Strategies of sexual degradation, including the threat of rape, have often been reported from Abu Ghraib (Borchelt 2005, p. 31).

31.3 Conclusions and Recommendations

In all of the examples discussed here, music appears in conjunction with other practices of torture and ill-treatment. This does not mean, however, that the music as such does not amount to a form of torture in these cases. Investigating music with no regard to the contexts in which it occurs is questionable at the best of times: this is particularly clear when dealing with music torture, which cannot be understood without considering the dynamic that exists between people in the case of torture. That music can result in serious physical and psychological damage is known from other contexts as well: disturbances from the neighbour's music have pushed some people to violence and even murder (Cloonan and Johnson 2008, pp. 164–167); noise pollution in everyday life has been the subject of many studies on the health impacts (Murphy and King 2022); last but not least, the field of musicians' medicine addresses the question of physical damage that can result from long-term musical practice. It should not surprise us, therefore, that in the context of torture and other

[11] There are many, often widely diverging opinions amongst scholars of Islam as regards the correct interpretation of teachings on music. Cusick goes into these issues in her article; for a further, general discussion, see also Nasr (1997).

forms of CID treatment, some musical practices constitute a significant danger, and increasingly, music psychologists and others are providing convincing explanations as to why this is the case (Windsor 2019).

General investigations into the health impacts of music and sound may give some indications as to potential impacts and diagnostic characteristics of music torture. This is important not least because there are still few studies that look at the short-term and long-term impacts of these practices. At present, however, some conclusions can be drawn which can also help us identify possible priorities both for future research and for clinical practice:

1. Even where the use of music in torture is conceived of or presented as being merely auxiliary to the main act of torture (for example, to acoustically mask the screams of victims), the victims themselves often experienced the music as a form of torture. The exact responses can be very individual, as can the extent to which people talk about this aspect of their treatment: some survivors do not mention music at all, or mention it only in passing, while others describe this as being the worst of all the torture practices to which they were subjected. Therefore, when survivors mention music and also other sounds or noise, this must always be taken seriously, including in therapy sessions or in meetings with legal advisers. Survivors of torture do sometimes report musical hallucinations, so that it may be advisable in some contexts to try and verify these statements, while respecting the truth of the experience for the survivor themself.
2. To the extent that it is ever possible to differentiate between physical and psychological violence in the case of torture, it must be borne in mind that various forms of music torture can be considered as forms of psychological *and* physical violence; Brauer (2009) uses the term "musical violence" to make this clear. Generally speaking, the distinction between physical and psychological violence is often highly artificial in the case of torture: the helplessness felt by the person affected is often a significant factor in the degree of psychological stress they experience; psychological aspects and methods of torture may actually increase the likelihood of the person affected developing a post-traumatic stress disorder (Başoğlu et al. 2007).
3. Known practices of music torture can be investigated for the likelihood of certain physiological impacts resulting from them. Damage to hearing from continuous exposure to loud noise, as well as damage to the vocal apparatus resulting from forced singing, are obvious examples. If such indicators are not present, however, this does not mean that music did not play a role during the torture. As we have seen, the use of music in connection with humiliation and degradation is of great importance. Findings on the various physiological impacts of music that until now have generally featured in studies focusing on therapeutic interventions with music could provide some foundations for further research here.
4. It is worth considering whether the use of centrally regulated music in prisons and other places of detention should not per se be prohibited. At the very least, those charged with monitoring prison conditions should be made aware that any indication that music has been used in places of detention should be probed in

some detail. Prisoners should not be denied the chance of voluntary participation in music and associated services and resources: any form of compulsion, however, whether through exposure to music or through singing on command, is highly questionable.[12]

There remain various desiderata for research into this topic. In particular, a larger range of case studies is needed, and also more work on systematising the forms, contexts and typical impacts of these types of torture. The results of such research could be of significance for all who are engaged in preventing torture and rehabilitating survivors. The tasks associated with such research require inter- and indeed multidisciplinary approaches on many different levels: these tasks require wide-ranging specialist knowledge and methodological expertise. There are, of course, many ethical issues raised by this research as well (Papaeti and Grant 2023). Preference should always be given to methods of data collection that exclude any risk at all of (re-)traumatising survivors. Therapists and doctors could play a significant role in such data collection to the extent that they are legally and ethically able to share information that arises in the course of diagnosis and therapy. In addition, more work on the existing historical sources could open up new perspectives and constitute an additional source for case studies that could be used for comparative work on music torture.

References

Başoğlu M (ed) (2017) Torture and its definition in international law: An interdisciplinary approach. Oxford University Press, Oxford/New York

Başoğlu M, Livanou M, Crnobarić C (2007) Torture vs. other cruel, inhuman and degrading treatment: is the distinction real or apparent? Arch Gen Psychiatry 64:277–285

Bauer S (2009) The meaning of music in a german sect in chile: colonia dignidad. Voices: a world forum for music therapy. http://voices.no/?q=colbauer200409. Last accessed 14 Aug 2014

Bielefeldt H (2004) Das Folterverbot im Rechtsstaat. Policy paper no. 4. Deutsches Institut für Menschenrechte, Berlin. https://www.institut-fuer-menschenrechte.de/fileadmin/_migrated/tx_commerce/policy_paper_4_das_folterverbot_im_rechtsstaat.pdf. Last accessed 28 June 2024

Borchelt G (2005) Break them down: systematic use of psychological torture by US forces. https://phr.org/wp-content/uploads/2005/05/break-them-down.pdf. Last accessed 28 June 2024

Brauer J (2009) Musik im Konzentrationslager Sachsenhausen. Metropol, Berlin

Brauer J (2016) How can music be torturous? Music in Nazi concentration and extermination camps. Music and Politics 10/1. https://doi.org/10.3998/mp.9460447.0010.103

Calero-Carramolino E (2023) Loss of place, loss of self: musical heterotopias in Franco's prisons (1938–1945). Ethnomusicology Forum 32(3):440–445. https://doi.org/10.1080/17411912.2023.2268086

Center for Victims of Torture (2023) Hidden harm. https://www.cvt.org/resources/hidden-harm/. Last accessed 28 June 2024

Chornik K (2013) Music and torture in Chilean detention centers: conversations with an ex-agent of Pinochet's secret police. The world of music (new series) 2(1), Special Issue: Music and Torture | Music and Punishment:51–65

[12] See also the resources on www.detentionconditions.org

Chornik K (2018) Memories of music in political detention in Chile under Pinochet. J Lat Am Cult Stud 27(27):157–173. https://doi.org/10.1080/13569325.2018.1450742
Chytroschek T (dir) (2010) Songs of war. Documentary film. A & O Buero
Cloonan M, Johnson B (2008) Dark side of the tune: popular music and violence. Ashgate, Aldershot
Comité de Defensa de los Derechos del Pueblo (1989). Las últimas técnicas de tortura aplicadas en Chile. In: Persona, Estado, Poder. Estudios sobre Salud Mental Chile 1973–1989. http://www.derechos.org/nizkor/chile/libros/poder/cap6.html. Last accessed 28 June 2024
Conroy J (2001) Unspeakable acts, ordinary people: the dynamics of torture. University of California Press, Berkeley
Cusick S (2006) Music as torture/Music as weapon. TRANS-transcultural music review 10. http://www.sibetrans.com/trans/a152/music-as-torture-music-as-weapon. 28 June 2024
Cusick S (2008) "You are in a place that is out of the world…": Music in the detention camps of the "global war on terror". J Soc Am Music 2:1–26
Dixon M (2002) Music and human rights. In: Sutton JP (ed) Music, music therapy and trauma: international perspectives. Jessica Kingsley Publishers, London/Philadelphia, pp 119–132
Dorfman A (2004) The tyranny of terror: is torture inevitable in our century and beyond? In: Levinson S (ed) Torture: a collection. Oxford University Press, Oxford, pp 3–18
European Commission of Human Rights (1969) Yearbook of the European convention on human rights: The Greek case. Martinus Nijhoff, The Hague
Fackler G (2000) "Des Lagers Stimme": Musik im KZ. Alltag und Häftlingskultur in den Konzentrationslagern 1933 bis 1936. Bremen, Edition Temmen
Fackler G (2001) Lied und Gesang im KZ. Lied und populäre Kultur/Song and Popular Culture 38:141–198
Feinstein D (chair) (2012–14) Senate select committee on intelligence: Committee Study of the Central Intelligence Agency's Detention and Interrogation Program. Findings and conclusions. Executive summary. Approved 2012, updated and released in a declassified version in 2014. US Senate, Washington. https://www.intelligence.senate.gov/sites/default/files/publications/CRPT-113srpt288.pdf. Last accessed 16 Nov 2020
Gilbert S (2005) Music in the holocaust: confronting life in the Nazi ghettos and camps. Clarendon Press, Oxford
Grant MJ (2013a) Music and punishment in the British Army in the eighteenth and nineteenth centuries. The world of music (new series) 2(1), Special Issue: Music and Torture | Music and Punishment:9–30
Grant MJ (2013b) The illogical logic of music torture. Tor J 23(2), Special Issue Music in Detention:4–13
Grant MJ (2014a) Pathways to music torture. Transpositions: Musiques et Sciences Sociales 4: music and armed conflict since 1945. http://transposition.revues.org/494. Last accessed 14 Aug 2014
Grant MJ (2014b) Rein, schön, fürchtbar: Musik als Folter. In: Paul G, Schock R (eds) Sound der Zeit: Geräusche, Töne, Stimmen—1889 bis heute. Wallstein, Göttingen, pp 546–553
Grant MJ (2019) Understanding perpetrators' use of music. In: Knittel S, Goldberg Z (eds) The Routledge international handbook of perpetrator studies. Routledge, London Abingdon/New York, pp 206–216
Grant MJ, Papaeti A (eds) (2013) The world of music (new series) 2(1), Special Issue: Music and Torture | Music and Punishment
Green D, Rasmussen A, Rosenfeld B (2010) Defining torture: a review of 40 years of health science research. J Trauma Stress 23(4):528–531
Grey S, Cobain I (2005) One of them made cuts in my penis. I was in agony. The Guardian, 2 August 2005. http://www.guardian.co.uk/uk/2005/aug/02/terrorism.humanrights1. Last accessed 16 Nov 2020
Hammarberg T (2007) The Greek case became a defining lesson for human rights policies in Europe. Website of the Council of Europe Commissioner for Human Rights. https://www.

coe.int/az/web/commissioner/-/the-greek-case-became-a-defining-lesson-for-human-rights-policies-in-europe. Last accessed 28 June 2024

Herzfeld-Schild ML (2013) 'He plays on the pillory'. The use of musical instruments for punishment in the middle ages and the early modern era. Torture Journal 23/2, Special Issue Music in Detention, pp 14–23

Human Rights Watch (2004) The road to Abu Ghraib. https://www.hrw.org/reports/2004/usa0604/usa0604.pdf. Last accessed 16 Nov 2020

Human Rights Watch (2005) U.S. operated secret, 'dark prison' in Kabul. https://www.hrw.org/news/2005/12/19/us-operated-secret-dark-prison-kabul. Last accessed 16 Nov 2020

Human Rights Watch (2006) „No blood, no foul": soldiers' accounts of detainee abuse in Iraq. In: Report 18 No. 3(G). http://www.hrw.org/reports/2006/07/22/no-blood-no-foul. Last accessed 14 Aug 2014

Human Rights Watch (2007) Ghost prisoner: two years in secret CIA detention. In: Report 19 No. 1(G). https://www.hrw.org/reports/2007/us0207/us0207webwcover.pdf. Last accessed 16 Nov 2020

Klause I (2013) Music in radio broadcasts in the gulag. In: Grant MJ, Stone-Davis FJ (eds) The soundtrack of conflict: the role of music in radio broadcasting in wartime and in conflict situations. Olms Verlag, Hildesheim, pp 13–23

McCoy A (2006) A question of torture: CIA interrogation, from the cold war to the war on terror. Metropolitan Books, New York

Murphy E, King EA (2022) Environmental noise pollution: noise mapping, public health, and policy, 2nd edn. Elsevier, Amsterdam

Naliwajek-Mazurek K (2013) Music and torture in Nazi sites of persecution and genocide in occupied Poland 1939–1945. The world of music (new series) 2(1), Special Issue: Music and Torture | Music and Punishment:31–50

Nasr SH (1997) Islam and music: the legal and the spiritual dimensions. In: Sullivan LE (ed) Enchanting powers: music in the world's religions. Harvard University Press, Cambridge, MA, pp 219–235

Newbery S (2015) Interrogation, intelligence and security: controversial British techniques. Manchester University Press, Manchester

Nowak M (2006) What practices constitute torture? US and UN standards. Hum Rights Q 28:809–841

Nowak M, McArthur E (2006) The distinction between torture and cruel, inhuman and degrading treatment or punishment. Tor J 16(3):147–151

Papaeti A (2013a) Music and 're-education' in Greek prison camps: from Makronisos (1947–1955) to Giaros (1967–1968). Torture Journal 23/2, Special Issue Music in Detention, pp 34–43

Papaeti A (2013b) Music, torture, testimony: reopening the case of the Greek Military Junta (1967–1974). The world of music (new series) 2(1), Special issue: music and torture | music and punishment:51–65

Papaeti A (2019) The undoing of music (podcast). Museo Nacional Centro de Arte Reina Sofía, Madrid. https://radio.museoreinasofia.es/en/papaeti

Papaeti A (2020a) Singing out terror: music communities in the detention centers of the military dictatorship in Greece (1967–74). In: Theodosiou A, Kallimopoulou E (eds) Music communities in Greece of the 21st century: ethnographic listening and perspectives. Pedio, Athens, pp 289–312

Papaeti A (2020b) On music, torture and detention: reflections on issues of research and discipline. Transposition. Musique et Sciences Sociales. Hors-série 2 | 2020: sound, music and violence. https://journals.openedition.org/transposition/5289

Papaeti A, Grant MJ (eds) (2013) Tor J 23(2), Special issue music in detention

Papaeti A, Grant MJ (2023) Musicological research with refugees: theoretical and ethical considerations. In: Gratzer W, Grosch N, Präger U, Scheiblhofer S (eds) The Routledge handbook of music and migration: theories and methodologies. Taylor and Francis, London, pp 223–252

Physicians for Human Rights (2007) Leave no marks: enhanced interrogation techniques and the risk of criminality. https://phr.org/wp-content/uploads/2007/08/leave-no-marks-1.pdf. Last accessed 20 Dec 2020

Physicians For Human Rights (2008) Broken laws, broken lives: medical evidence of torture by US personnel and its impact. https://s3.amazonaws.com/PHR_Reports/BrokenLaws_14.pdf. Last accessed 28 June 2024

Pieslak J (2009) Sound targets: American soldiers and music in the war in Iraq. Indiana University Press, Bloomington

Rodakis P (1976) The trials of the junta: the trials of torturers, vol I. Democratic Press, Athens

Rothkegel S (2011) The long-term impact of physical and psychological torture. Lecture at the workshop music torture: research perspectives, University of Göttingen, April 2011

Smith S, Lewty W (1959) Perceptual isolation using a silent room. Lancet 2(7098):342–345

UN Committee Against Torture (1997) Concluding observations of the Committee Against Torture: Israel. 05/09/1997, A/52/44, paras 253–260

Windsor L (2019) Music in detention and interrogation: the musical ecology of fear. In: Grimshaw-Aagaard M, Walther-Hansen M, Knakkergaard M (eds) The Oxford handbook of sound and imagination, vol 2. Oxford University Press, New York/Oxford, pp 281–300. https://doi.org/10.1093/oxfordhb/9780190460242.013.71

Zubek JP, Pushkar D, Sansom W, Gowing J (1961) Perceptual changes after prolonged sensory isolation (darkness and silence). Can J Psychol 15(2):83–100

Practical Music Practice in Times of Corona

32

Bernhard Richter, Manfred Nusseck, Carolin Neukamm, and Claudia Spahn

32.1 The Corona Pandemic at a Glance

32.1.1 Challenges for Medicine

At the end of 2019, the World Health Organization (WHO) was informed by Chinese authorities of the increased incidence of severe pneumonia of unknown cause in the city of Wuhan (WHO 2020a). A previously unknown coronavirus was identified as the cause of the illnesses. As this virus resembled a pathogen that had led to severe respiratory illnesses in 2002 (severe acute respiratory syndrome—SARS), the new virus was given the name SARS coronavirus-2 (SARS-CoV-2) (Coronaviridae Study Group of the International Committee on Taxonomy of Viruses 2020). As the disease was first described at the end of 2019, the disease caused by the virus was named CORONA VIRUS DISEASE-2019 (COVID-19) (WHO 2020b).

The virus was new to humans, and the population's immune system had not yet built up any protection worldwide. The spread of such a new pathogen against which there is no immunity is referred to as an *epidemic* as long as the event remains localized. However, SARS-CoV-2 spread rapidly worldwide, so that according to the WHO, the criteria for a *pandemic* were met from March 11, 2020 (WHO 2023). The number of cases increased worldwide in waves of infection, which showed an exponential increase.

The SARS-CoV-2 pandemic and the COVID-19 disease posed an unusual challenge for medicine, the doctors treating patients, and healthcare providers. Doctors

B. Richter (✉) · M. Nusseck · C. Neukamm · C. Spahn
Freiburg Institute for Musicians' Medicine, University of Music Freiburg, Medical Center and Faculty of Medicine – University of Freiburg, Freiburg Centre for Music Research and Teaching, Freiburg, Germany
e-mail: bernhard.richter@uniklinik-freiburg.de; manfred.nusseck@uniklinik-freiburg.de; carolin.neukamm@uniklinik-freiburg.de; claudia.spahn@uniklinik-freiburg.de

G. Kreutz, G. Bernatzky (eds.), *Music and Medicine*, Neurocultural Health and Wellbeing, https://doi.org/10.1007/978-3-662-72175-9_32

had no experience with the course of the disease, and the effectiveness of treatment measures was unclear. Doctors were confronted with seriously ill patients, who initially could not be treated adequately due to a lack of pathophysiological understanding and the absence of effective medication. The healthcare system was stretched to its limits by the sudden emergence of large numbers of cases requiring intensive medical care, including ventilation. In some countries, during the waves of illness—especially at the beginning of the pandemic—the capacity of intensive care beds was not sufficient to care for all patients seriously ill with COVID-19.

As the number of cases rose exponentially at the beginning of 2020 and the death rate quickly doubled, the Robert Koch Institute considered the situation to be so threatening to public health that the federal government—in close consultation with the federal states—decided on a first coronavirus lockdown in Germany, which came into force on March 22, 2020. Schools and daycare centers remained closed, church services, concerts, and gatherings were canceled. There was a ban on contact. From April 29, 2020, masks were compulsory in stores and on public transport. A social distancing requirement of 1.50 m also came into force on May 15, 2020.

32.1.2 Basic Information on the Transmission of Viruses in Respiratory Infections

The main transmission of viruses that cause respiratory infections generally occurs via smear infections, direct contact with droplets or aerosols that are produced when coughing and sneezing. These are absorbed by the other person via the mucous membranes of the nose, mouth, and deep respiratory tract when inhaled, and possibly via the conjunctiva of the eye. Figure 32.1 shows the transmission routes schematically.

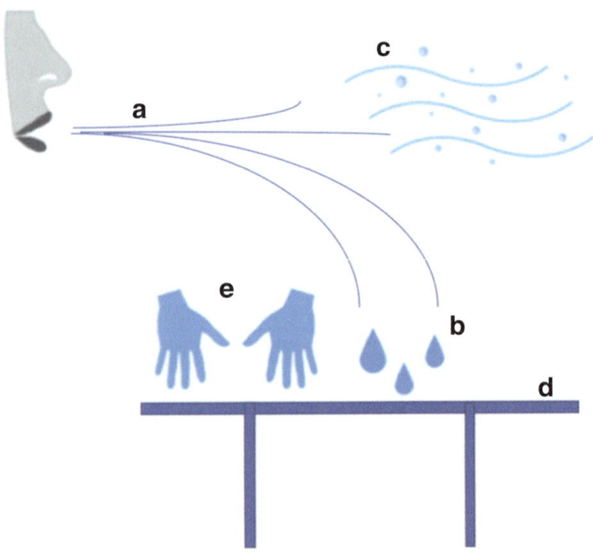

Fig. 32.1 Schematic representation of the possible transmission routes. Droplets (**b**) and aerosols (**c**) enter the environment with the exhaled air (**a**). The droplets can get onto surfaces (e.g., a table (**d**)). From there, they can be picked up by the hands (**e**). If the hands then come into contact with the mouth, nose, or eye, contact transmission (smear infection) can occur

An aerosol (artificial word from ancient Greek ἀήρ, English "Air" and Latin *solutio* "solution") is a heterogeneous mixture of very small solid or liquid suspended particles in a gas. Droplets in this context are *larger particles* (diameter of more than 5 µm). Some of them can be so large that they are visible when coughing or sneezing and can be felt on the skin. Some of the droplets fall to the ground at a distance of up to approx. 1 m due to gravity. Another part of the droplets evaporates—depending on their composition, size, and the condition of the surrounding air (saturation). The finest droplet nuclei remain, which spread very quickly around the source and in the (closed) room. If an infected person expels viruses when coughing, it can be assumed that the viruses are still detectable in the air after several minutes and possibly hours, even if the sick person has already moved away again. Other people can then inhale the airborne viruses (Vuorinen et al. 2020a, b).

Asymptomatic individuals usually emit aerosols <10 µm and produce very few droplets. The aerosols are more concentrated near the emitter. When aerosols are emitted from the mouth opening, it is to be expected that they first rise due to the lower specific density (approx. 37 °C and >95% relative humidity) and then mix with the room air. Sedimentation plays practically no role for aerosols below a particle size of approx. 4 µm. As a result, aerosols in closed rooms initially accumulate on the ceiling of the room. Over time, they spread throughout the room, similar to a gas. In terms of exposure, a distinction is, therefore, made between direct exposure in the near field (distance <1.5 m) and the increasing concentration of aerosols in the room air.

Viruses can also be transmitted from surfaces if they reach the hands by touching these contaminated surfaces, and the hands then touch the face without being cleaned—provided the viruses have retained their infectious properties by this time (contact transmission).

32.1.2.1 Spread of SARS-CoV-2

SARS-CoV-2 can be spread via droplet infection or aerosols (Meselson 2020; Santarpia et al. 2020). The aerosol transmission route is considered to be the most important (Morawska and Cao 2020; Morawska and Milton 2020). SARS-CoV-2 could remain viable in aerosols for up to several hours (van Doremalen et al. 2020). The lower the temperature and the lower the humidity, the longer the aerosols can remain in the enclosed space and also on surfaces. Further considerations on the importance of aerosols in the infection process of SARS-CoV-2 were published by the expert group "Aerosols" of the state government of Baden-Württemberg (Brockmann et al. 2021).

32.1.3 Medical Measures to Contain the Pandemic

As neither effective medication nor a vaccine to build up immunity in the population was available in the first year of the pandemic and as there also insufficient information and knowledge about the severity of the disease, the age structure of those infected, and the vulnerability of certain people with preexisting conditions in the first few months, the top priority in this phase of the pandemic was to avoid infection. In the subsequent phases of the pandemic, *vaccination* was added in December 2020 (in Germany from December 27, 2020) as an essential pillar for improving immunity in the population. Initially, vaccination was prioritized for older and previously ill people as well as for people in particularly exposed occupational fields, which was lifted on June 7, 2021. Since then, every adult has been able to be vaccinated. Subsequently, the Standing Committee on Vaccination (STIKO) also advocated that children and adolescents should be vaccinated (STIKO 2022).

As a further measure for the prompt detection and treatment of infections, for the interruption of infection chains, and for protection against overloading our healthcare system, *testing* was an essential component of a comprehensive pandemic response in accordance with the National Testing Strategy (Ministry of Health 2020). Since January 2021, there has been an entitlement to testing with regard to direct pathogen detection of the SARS-CoV-2 coronavirus (Coronavirus Testing Ordinance 2021). Tests based on the polymerase chain reaction (PCR) were available as the gold standard. The PCR test detects the virus with a high degree of accuracy—it has a high sensitivity. In addition, this test detects exactly the desired virus—the test has a high specificity. The results of PCR tests are not immediately available, as they have to be evaluated in specialized laboratories. In addition, the costs of the individual tests are not insignificant. Rapid antigen tests (AG test) for SARS-CoV-2 detect certain proteins of the SARS-CoV-2 coronavirus in the event of an infection. They offer the possibility of providing results within a very short time (approx. 15 min) and thus represent a possible preventive measure. They are significantly cheaper than PCR tests. However, the sensitivity of AG tests is the subject of controversial debate (Cerutti et al. 2020).

32.2 Making Music During the Corona Pandemic

32.2.1 Challenges for the Music World

The task facing society as a whole of overcoming the coronavirus pandemic through measures such as contact bans, social distancing, testing, and vaccination also posed major challenges for the music industry, which are described below.

The general restrictions imposed by the ban on contact and social distancing posed a completely new challenge for all areas of music-making. From a musician's medicine point of view, it was, therefore, necessary to collect evidence-based information for musicians as quickly as possible and to make this available to all those involved in the amateur and professional music sector, including the audience.

An initial risk assessment from the Freiburg Institute for Musicians' Medicine was carried out on April 25, 2020. Also in the first phase of the pandemic, working groups from the Charité (Mürbe et al. 2020; Willich et al. 2020), the German Society for Music Physiology and Musicians' Medicine ("Deutsche Gesellschaft für Musikphysiologie und Musikermedizin" DGfMM, Firle et al. 2020), the Institute of Fluid Mechanics and Aerodynamics at the Bundeswehr University Munich (Kähler and Hain 2020), and the Health and Prophylaxis Working Group of the German Orchestra Association ("Deutsche Orchestervereinigung" DOV) with commentary from the Association of German Company and Works Physicians (VDBW AG Bühnen und Orchester) (Böckelmann et al. 2020) presented risk assessments for musicians and singers.

The following statements are based on the risk assessment of our institute in the version of the tenth update from July 2022. They are based on the scientific findings of our own investigations, expert recommendations, and the information available in the literature.

From the authors' point of view, risk assessments with regard to specific issues relating to the practice of music should be based on the *additional* risk posed by the practice of music. The risk assessments of our working group thus followed the guiding principle that, on the one hand, the risks of coronavirus infection in the field of music were named in detail and, on the other hand, specific measures were recommended for the risks which, individually and in combination, appeared suitable for reducing the risk of infection. The explanations were intended to help define framework conditions under which music-making can take place in times of the pandemic with the greatest possible risk reduction.

32.2.2 Practicing Music in Times of Corona: Factors Influencing the Risk of Infection

In order to be able to take specific measures for the practical practice of music, it seems sensible to identify as many influencing factors as possible that can contribute to the concept of risk reduction.

32.2.2.1 Aerosol Formation When Singing and Playing a Wind Instrument

As increased infection rates were reported during choir rehearsals at the beginning of the pandemic (Hamner et al. 2020; Miller et al. 2021; Reichert et al. 2022; Axon et al. 2023), it is an important question for music practice whether singing or playing a wind instrument leads to increased aerosol formation. Studies by Mürbe et al. suggest that singing can lead to significantly higher aerosol emission rates compared to mouth breathing and speaking (Mürbe et al. 2020). A wide range of variation was found in this respect, with an average emission rate 30 times higher when singing compared to mouth breathing. Higher emission rates are also found when playing a wind instrument than when breathing or speaking (Firle et al. 2022).

In a study on aerosol emissions during singing by children, the working group of Mürbe et al. found higher aerosol emissions in children during singing than during speaking, in line with the results from adults (Mürbe et al. 2021). There is also great variability in aerosol emissions in children. A correlation between particle emissions and vocal loudness was confirmed, especially in the phonation type of "screaming." Compared to the previously published data on speaking/singing of adult professional singers, the values for children were in a similar range for speaking, but the values for singing were lower for children than for adult singers. Interestingly, individual children achieved higher emission values when "shouting" compared to the values achieved by adult singers when singing loudly. There were no significant differences between the two groups when shouting.

32.2.2.2 Indoor Air

The floor area and height of the room and the number of people in the room, as well as the activity and length of time people spend in an enclosed space appear to play an important role in the spread of viruses and the risk of infection they pose (Tellier 2006). The epidemiological findings from the course of the SARS-CoV-2 pandemic show that room and air conditions as well as the duration of exposure when people congregate have a decisive influence on the risk of infection (Leung et al. 2020; Chia et al. 2020; Liu et al. 2020; Miller et al. 2021). Infections primarily occur in people who spend long periods of time in enclosed spaces. In a study by Qian et al. in January and February 2020 on a total of 7324 cases of infected persons in China, the authors found that there was only one case of outdoor infection (Qian et al. 2021). It can be assumed that aerosols spread more quickly outdoors, the inactivation process of the pathogens is greatly accelerated (UV, ozone, hydroxyl radicals, nitrogen oxides), and the overall risk of infection is much lower as a result.

For music-making with several people, the open-air situation can, therefore, be considered when the weather is favorable. There is a long cultural tradition here, think of the ancient amphitheater. The term chorus (ancient Greek χορός choros) originally referred to the dance floor of an amphitheater, where people also sang. Brass band music in rural areas also traditionally takes place outdoors. Outdoor concerts are the predominant setting for pop and rock music.

When making music together in enclosed spaces, it makes sense to use very large rooms such as churches, concert halls, or town halls as rehearsal rooms. Generally speaking, this room constellation can be described as a "cathedral situation." Church rooms with a ceiling height of 10 m or more usually have such large indoor air volumes that they can be considered comparable to smaller rooms with a powerful ventilation system (air exchange rate 6/h) in terms of the risk of infection. In addition, many church rooms are equipped with modern ventilation systems. Where this is not the case, the air quality and the effectiveness of the ventilation can be checked directly on site using the CO_2 traffic light—as described below. The ventilation concept should be optimized on the basis of the values recorded on site.

32.2.2.3 Air Quality: CO_2 Content and Manual Ventilation Measures

The CO_2 content of the air provides an important starting point for assessing the risk of infection through aerosols. It can be used as an indicator for the accumulation of aerosols that may contain SARS-CoV-2 viruses (Kriegel and Hartmann 2020). The fact that gaseous carbon dioxide (CO_2) is an important measure of air quality was already established by Max Pettenkofer in the mid-nineteenth century. He recognized that CO_2 is not only a measure of air quality but that other substances in the air also behave proportionally to the CO_2 content (Pettenkofer 1858). According to Pettenkofer, the so-called *Pettenkofer number* of the CO_2 content was set at 1000 parts per million (ppm), compliance with which is required indoors, especially in a school context, even independently of singing and corona (Federal Environment Agency 2008).

In fall 2020, our own working group conducted a series of measurements with 141 musicians at the Freiburg University of Music (Nusseck et al. 2020). The CO_2 concentrations were determined during 47 teaching units and rehearsals. For this purpose, simple, relatively inexpensive CO_2 measuring devices were used, which also visually represent the air quality in the sense of a "traffic light." The duration after which a defined musical activity must be interrupted and ventilated was determined according to the time after which the air quality threshold defined by the European standard for indoor spaces (EN 13779) is reached (IDA 1: high indoor air quality) at a CO_2 concentration of 800 ppm. Wind players showed the highest CO_2 emissions, while singers showed low emission rates, comparable to those of the control group, which only spoke and listened. This meant that it was possible to define for each room at the University of Music how many people were allowed to stay in the room for how long, depending on their musical activity, until the limit value of 800 ppm for CO2 concentration was reached. In addition, measurements were taken to determine how many minutes each room had to be ventilated manually until the initial value of 400 ppm was reached again. Furthermore, it was measured how many minutes the respective room had to be ventilated with manual cross-ventilation until the initial value of 400 ppm was reached again (Nusseck et al. 2020).

A general rule as to when ventilation should take place has not proven to be sufficiently precise. Rather, based on the size of the room, the activity, and the number of musicians, the CO_2 curve indicates the time periods after which manual ventilation is required.

Bauer et al. also used CO_2 measurements as indicators of how to design a choir rehearsal with minimal risk of infection (Bauer et al. 2022). The measurements showed a linear relationship between the duration of singing, the size of the room, and the number of singers, so that this working group was also able to calculate when the threshold of 800 ppm was reached for a defined number of singers, taking into account the size of the room. Manual shock ventilation also led to the basic concentration of 400 ppm CO prevailing in the outside air being reached quickly[2].

32.2.2.4 Mechanical Ventilation

If singing and music-making take place in closed rooms with mechanical ventilation (ventilation and air conditioning systems, HVAC), the air exchange rate and the direction of the ventilation flow are important factors. With natural ventilation, aerosols are removed via the air exchange rate in the range of approx. 0.5–2/h even with closed windows; with air handling systems, e.g., in concert halls or halls, the air exchange rate is approx. 4–8/h; from an air exchange rate of 6/h, it can be assumed that aerosols are sufficiently removed. A reduced risk of infection from aerosols can be assumed in particular if the air conditioning system enables a high air exchange rate, and displacement ventilation takes place. The performance of an air conditioning system can be checked with CO_2 measurements.

32.2.2.5 Distance

Maintaining distance between people is important when making music to protect against droplet infection. Since maintaining this distance requires a great deal of attention, especially as physical proximity and social connection are an intuitive part of music-making situations, and since singing and instrumental music-making do not take place from a fixed body position but require a certain amount of movement in the room, the distance between people should be chosen according to evidence-based criteria in such a way that, on the one hand, the aspects of infection protection and, on the other hand, the communicative requirements of making music together are taken into account.

Droplets sink quickly to the ground due to their size and weight and normally reach a maximum distance of 1 m. This is the basis for the distance rule of 1.5 m in everyday situations (stores, offices, etc.).

In vocal physiology, it has long been known that during phonation (sound production during singing), there is no significant additional air movement in front of the singer's mouth, as sound waves propagate physically without flow. The flame of a burning candle does not move in front of a singer's mouth, even if he sings loudly.

This observation was again confirmed by measurements carried out by our working group with three singers in the Bamberg Symphony Orchestra (Richter et al. 2021). The artificial fog directed directly in front of the singers' mouths was not visibly deflected by singing at different pitches, volumes, and singing styles. During forced articulation with plosive sounds, slight turbulence could be observed at close range. The situation was similar when playing different wind instruments (Spahn et al. 2021). When measuring the air velocity with sensors at a distance of 2 m from the players of the wind instruments recorder, flute, clarinet, oboe, horn, trumpet, trombone, tuba, and saxophone, no air movement could be measured. Thus, in the measurements of our working group, the distance of 2 m to the front could be regarded as a safe distance for droplet infection even during forced vocal articulation and blowing. These observations are consistent with other research groups that have used different optical methods to visualize air dispersion when playing a wind instrument and when singing. Echternach et al. state that the aerosol clouds spread forward up to a distance of 1.4 m when singing and playing a wind instrument. Laterally, the dispersion distance was significantly smaller (Echternach et al. 2020). Becher et al. report a maximum propagation distance of 1.2 m based on studies using the Schlieren method and the Background Oriented Schlieren (BOS) method for wind players and singers (Becher et al. 2021).

Therefore, in our opinion, the distance—taking into account an additional safety distance—should be 2 m to the front and 1.5 m to the side when singing and blowing. By maintaining this distance for a single person, if there are several people in a closed room at the same time, the positive additional effect is that, according to this rule, only a few musicians can be present in small rooms. For larger formations, compliance with this rule requires a larger room size. This reduces not only the risk of transmission by droplets but also the risk of an increased accumulation of aerosols indoors. However, compliance with the distance recommendation could not replace regular ventilation and a reduction in the duration of sampling.

If, in exceptional cases, the distance between musicians cannot be maintained due to confined spaces, individual protective measures to protect against droplets, such as spit guards and partitions between singers and accompanists, may also be worth considering in individual cases.

32.2.2.6 Incoming Check: Vaccination Status and Testing

An incoming check may include the collection and intensive monitoring of several relevant characteristics such as vaccination and symptom status, testing, and other individual protective measures.

Since vaccination began in December 2020, vaccination can be seen as an essential pillar of coping with the coronavirus pandemic. Vaccination status must, therefore, be taken into account as a key input parameter.

A study by our working group examined vaccination rates and general attitudes towards vaccination in the cultural/music sector in June/July 2021 (Spahn et al. 2022a, b). A total of 4341 people from four different sectors took part in this study. The four areas included visitors to classical concerts and musicals, professional musicians, and those involved in amateur music. The results showed a significantly higher vaccination rate compared to the general population at the time of the study. The number of those who were still reluctant or refused to be vaccinated was only about half that of the general population. The results of this sample can serve as an indication that there appears to be a very high willingness to be vaccinated and a very low refusal to be vaccinated in the area of music culture.

Musicians of all musical genres should also check their own symptom status and take care to avoid contact with other musicians if they have unspecific symptoms such as fever plus respiratory symptoms or symptoms such as acute loss of smell and taste function. The same applies in the event of proven infection or contact with a person infected with coronavirus.

In addition, daily testing can be carried out before samples and performances. Both rapid antigen tests (AG test) and PCR tests are part of the national testing strategy (Federal Ministry of Health 2020). The tests differ in terms of specificity and sensitivity, time until the test result is available, and cost. Despite lower specificity and sensitivity, AG tests were frequently used in everyday life because the results were available quickly, and the costs were significantly lower. In order to increase safety and still keep costs within reasonable limits, so-called lollipop PCR tests can also be used in larger music formations, in which up to 30 samples per pool are evaluated together as a PCR test. Only if this pool is positive does each person in the pool have to be tested individually. Scientific studies can demonstrate the effectiveness and practicability of Lolli tests in a school context (Joachim et al. 2021). This pool testing strategy has also been transferred to the cultural sector.

32.2.2.7 Individual Protective Measures: Masks

Particularly for older people or those at risk due to preexisting conditions (see the risk list of the Robert Bosch Institute 2021), especially in the area of active music practice, particularly strict precautionary measures apply. For this group, wearing a mouth and nose protector can also be an important way of reducing risk in the music sector. It has been known for some time that masks are suitable for protecting against infection in the case of various respiratory diseases (van der Sande et al. 2008). The main issue with face masks is that it is used even though it may be spontaneously perceived as inappropriate or disruptive when singing or playing a string, plucked, or keyboard instrument, for example. From an infectiological point of view, a distinction is made when wearing face masks as to whether the aim is to protect a person from infection by droplets or aerosols from other people (self-protection) or whether the aim is to prevent the spread of infectious material from one person to others (external protection). When wearing an face mask, both possible effects are combined. The WHO has also been recommending the wearing of masks as a component of infection protection for the general population in a document (Interim Guidance) since June 5, 2020 (WHO 2020c). Studies have shown that wearing such masks can effectively reduce the spread of droplets and aerosols (Leung et al. 2020).

32.2.3 Opportunities for Risk Reduction in the Music Sector

If the influencing factors described above can be brought into an optimal relationship with regard to their risk and their protective effect, it is possible to achieve a meaningful risk reduction for the "music sector" system. In the view of our working group, the measures summarized in Fig. 32.2 play a decisive role, particularly in

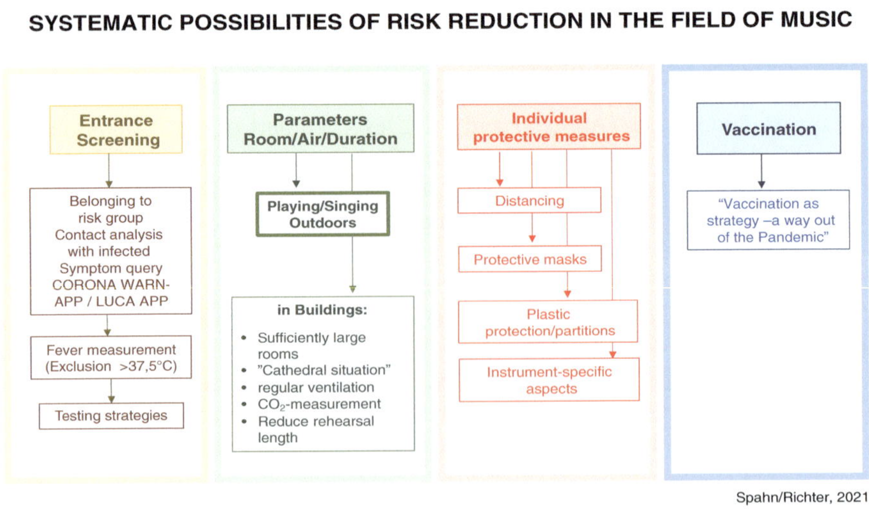

Fig. 32.2 Overview of systemic measures for risk reduction in the music sector

formations with a larger number of people (choir and community singing, orchestra, big band).

In the field of amateur music, especially in wind music and choirs, music associations and academies have taken up these ideas and developed hygiene concepts (see BdB Academy Staufen 2022). These include modular measures for both the active musicians and the audience and have been implemented very meticulously. The music associations were supported in developing the concepts as part of the German government's "Neustart Kultur" initiative. The hygiene concepts are available for download on the homepages of the associations (see BMCO 2022a, b).

32.2.4 Risk Management as a Central Approach

The course of the pandemic to date has seen a significant reduction in case mortality (Dennler et al. 2022). According to the S3 guideline on recommendations for the treatment of patients with COVID-19, the reasons for this are the significant increase in immunocompetence in the population, the increasing progress of vaccination, the infections experienced and the occurrence of the omicron variant, which is often less severe (Kluge et al. 2023). In addition, a reduction in mortality has been demonstrated for several drugs in randomized controlled trials.

Since the outbreak of the coronavirus pandemic, we also have experience of the epidemiologically important factors in the spread of SARS-CoV-2. In the meantime, the pandemic has developed into an endemic as a result of the build-up of basic immunity in the population through vaccinations and recoveries. The term endemic is used when the product of the basic reproduction rate (basic reproduction number R_0) and the susceptibility rate (susceptibility number S) is equal to one ($R_0 \times S = 1$). In the case of endemicity, the disease has not disappeared, but the number of cases in the population remains approximately the same and no longer increases exponentially (Lavine et al. 2021).

From the very beginning of the coronavirus pandemic, our risk management concept aimed to identify specific risks in the field of music and at the same time offer risk-reducing measures. In the case of newly emerging risks, the risk management process has been established in quality management—for example, in industry—for years. Separate ISO standards have been developed for this (ISO 31000:2018). Effective risk management usually requires a precise risk analysis with associated probabilities of occurrence and knowledge of how effective certain risk-reducing measures are. This has made it possible to develop flexible risk management concepts adapted to the respective musicians and music-making situations and to integrate the issues relating to the practice of music appropriately into the overall social framework. In order to enable individualized advice in the amateur sector, the Ministry of Science, Research and the Arts Baden-Württemberg has already set up an advice center for making music under corona conditions at the Freiburg Institute for Musicians' Medicine in July 2020. Using a contact form (https://fim.mh-freiburg.de/beratung-amateurmusik/), it is possible to answer questions from a musician's medicine perspective according to the latest scientific knowledge. The experience gained from the extensive consulting activities to date can also be transferred to the professional sector—concert halls, opera houses, and theaters as well as music schools. A differentiated analysis of the respective circumstances and the search for appropriate ways to reduce risk during the consultation has proven its worth.

In our opinion, if levels 1 & 2 are reached, the risk is reduced to such an extent that the practice of music is possible if the risk-reducing measures are strictly observed. If only level 3 can be achieved, it is not advisable to play music. The practice of music is prohibited at level 4 (Fig. 32.3).

Our risk management in practice envisaged that each institution would develop its own risk management system for its specific music-making setting based on the aforementioned stages. It is to be expected that the higher and more effective the number of risk-reducing measures and the more people are vaccinated, the greater the reduction in the risk of infection.

However, it must be clearly pointed out that a residual risk remains according to the ALARP principle (As Low As Reasonably Practicable).

In order to make the risk numerically assessable, our working group has contributed to the development of an assessment of the SARS-CoV-2 infection risk at indoor venues based on experimental and statistical data (Siebler et al. 2023). A simulation tool was programmed to assess the risk of infection, which incorporates

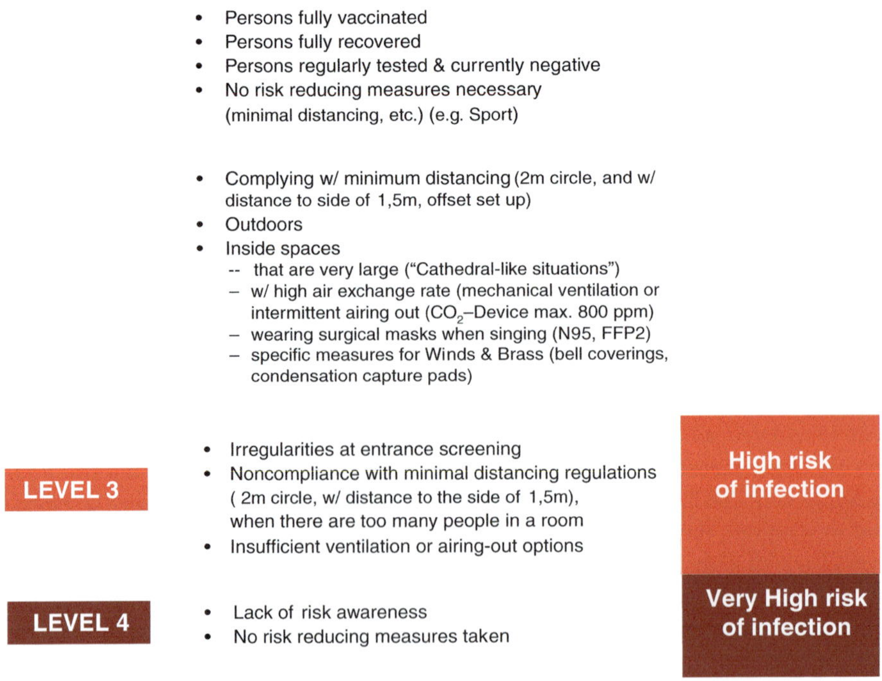

Fig. 32.3 Four levels with assessment of the reduction in the risk of infection depending on the risk-reducing measures (based on the risk matrix according to Nohl 2019)

epidemiological data such as incidences, vaccination rates, test sensitivities, and audience characteristics such as age structure and mask wearing, as well as experimentally determined indoor air and ventilation parameters of the venue. This tool enables cultural event organizers to gain an impression of the possible incidence of infection at the venue so that they can take appropriate measures.

32.3 Consequences of the Corona Pandemic in the Music Sector

32.3.1 General Psychosocial Consequences

The longer the coronavirus pandemic lasts and the measures it necessitates, the more negative psychosocial consequences can be observed.

Dealing with the pandemic has led to a stress syndrome that is triggered and intensified by factors such as unpredictability, helplessness, and being at the mercy of others (Heitzman 2020; Petzold et al. 2020). Several reviews consistently describe psychosocial consequences, including depression, anxiety, anger, stress, post-traumatic stress, social isolation, loneliness, and stigmatization (Brooks et al. 2020; Röhr et al. 2020; Bonati et al. 2022).

32.3.2 Music Studies and Music Students

The mental health of the students—the young musicians who will shape our musical culture in the future—is particularly crucial. Students, entire cohorts of whom have experienced studying under the conditions of the coronavirus pandemic, must be given special attention and care. It was, therefore, the primary goal of the Freiburg Institute for Musicians' Medicine to provide students and teachers at the Freiburg University of Music with effective hygiene concepts in order to be able to offer face-to-face teaching with lively artistic experiences even in times of the coronavirus pandemic.

In our working group, we investigated how music students perceived the different conditions during three semesters under coronavirus conditions (Spahn et al. 2022a, b). It was found that the music students were able to adapt well to the lockdown situation (summer semester 2020) and the new digital communication formats, but above all they greatly missed the social interaction and making music together, which was restricted at times. In this respect, they hardly differed from other peers (Bonati et al. 2022), but they were doubly affected by the loss of social contacts and the limited study content of ensemble music-making. The three semesters during the coronavirus pandemic phase from March 2020 to July 2021 were perceived differently. The winter semester 2020/2021 was experienced as the most challenging, as in this semester with online and face-to-face events, distances, and changes of location had to be combined with rapidly changing public corona regulations (Spahn et al. 2022a, b).

Our working group also looked at the effects of the coronavirus pandemic on study ability and practice behavior (Nusseck and Spahn 2021). With regard to their average practice time, music students stated that they practiced less during the lockdown than before the pandemic. However, the way they practiced revealed more self-regulated musical learning strategies. The results indicate that the music students developed certain self-regulated learning skills during the lockdown and that they were able to find suitable strategies to continue their musical development.

Since the coronavirus pandemic, there has been an increased demand from music students for offers to promote resilience in dealing with the demands of studying. For example, the Freiburg Institute for Musicians' Medicine offered a seminar entitled "Resilience for music students" at the Freiburg University of Music in the summer semester of 2022, which was in high demand and very well received (Spahn et al. 2023).

32.3.3 Freelance Musicians, Music Teachers, and Orchestral Musicians

The coronavirus pandemic has plunged the entire music culture into a state of instability. Professional musicians in all professional fields were faced with economic, psychological, and organizational challenges that required new strategies for dealing with them.

In orchestral musicians, it was shown that intrinsic self-motivation was linked to greater resilience to possible threats from the pandemic and that these musicians were better able to maintain routines even without concerts (López-Íñiguez et al. 2022).

Instrumental and vocal teachers were confronted with constantly changing regulations between online and face-to-face teaching. Pupils and parents were unsettled, and new formats and methods of teaching had to be found in the online setting. Many music teachers lost some of their students during the coronavirus pandemic.

Above all, however, the pandemic affected freelance musicians. While these musicians had a busy and successful portfolio career before the pandemic, they were no longer able to perform and earn a living due to the restrictions imposed during the pandemic (Cohen and Ginsborg 2021). In addition, many musicians were worried about the future. One year after their first survey (Cohen and Ginsborg 2021), the same working group found that the biggest challenges facing musicians were the possible loss of their career, financial constraints, emotional stress, motivation to practice, and confusion about career plans (Cohen and Ginsborg 2022). It was also found that musicians in the middle of their careers remained committed to their careers as musicians, older musicians aspired to a new field of musical activity without concert appearances, and musicians at the end of their careers—at the age of 65 and older—had inwardly "retired."

32.3.4 Singing and Making Music in Society

Society suffered during the coronavirus pandemic due to the loss and restriction of concert attendance and cultural events. The coronavirus pandemic hit amateur music particularly hard. All those who do not live from making music and are otherwise financially secure, but whose social contacts and enjoyment of life lie in making music together, were cut off from their important purpose in life.

Participation practices played a particularly important role for choirs during the pandemic. Above all, this included the desire for continuity in the choir, which arose from a sense of responsibility to somehow maintain choir activities (Daffern et al. 2021). However, the psychosocial importance of choral singing also became clear during the pandemic. It showed how important the choral experience is for personal well-being and a sense of community. The pandemic made the value of the musical experience tangible, and many people became more aware of what makes singing in a group a meaningful experience.

The fact that singing and making music are extremely positive and important for mental health must be reestablished as the risk of coronavirus decreases. Singing in particular has been labeled as dangerous due to the coronavirus pandemic, and this barrier must first be overcome.

Encouraging children and young people to sing and make music is a particularly important task and an ethical responsibility. The effects that the coronavirus pandemic can have on children and young people have already been studied since the first lockdown (Ravens-Sieberer et al. 2021). This makes a rapid return to "normality," in which children and young people also participate in cultural activities again, all the more important.

Singing together is an integral part of cultural school life and is an important factor in the socio-emotional development of children and young people. This also applies to music schools and children's and youth choirs.

Music is an extremely important psychological resource. This is particularly true for audiences interested in music. In a survey of over 1000 visitors to the Staatstheater Stuttgart as part of a pilot project by the Freiburg Institute for Musicians' Medicine, 95% of visitors stated that they had missed attending cultural events that could not take place during the coronavirus pandemic to a great or very great extent.

It is, therefore, extremely important for our society to promote music culture in all its facets in a responsible and socially responsible way after the coronavirus pandemic. Many people are finding it difficult to reconnect with life before corona, even though activities are once again permitted without restrictions.

32.4 Conclusion

Making music is a fundamental anthropological dimension and also represents an extremely important psychological resource. This applies not only to professional musicians—whether they are studying or working—but also to the many people for whom making music represents a central purpose in life and a social focus. Music also plays an important role for the public. The coronavirus pandemic has shown that interpersonal contact and live music is a staple for us humans that we cannot do without.

References

Axon CJ, Dingwall R, Evans S, Cassell JA (2023) The Skagit County choir COVID-19 outbreak—have we got it wrong? Public Health 214:85–90. https://doi.org/10.1016/j.puhe.2022.11.007

Bauer K, Hardege R, Neumann S, Schwarze R, Fuchs M, Heinrich Pieper L (2022) How safe is singing under pandemic conditions?—CO_2-measurements as simple method for risk estimation during choir rehearsals. J Voice:S0892-1997(22)00136-9. https://doi.org/10.1016/j.jvoice.2022.05.003

Bdb Academy Staufen (2022) Hygiene concepts in amateur music and professional ensembles. https://www.bdb-akademie.com/wp-content/uploads/2022-04-05_-BW-Schutzmassnahmen-Amateurmusik.pdf

Becher L, Gena AW, Alsaad H, Richter B, Spahn C, Voelker C (2021) The spread of breathing air from wind instruments and singers using Schlieren techniques. Indoor Air 31(6):1798–1814

BMCO (2022a) Protective measures. http://bundesmusikverband.de/schutzmassnahmen/

BMCO (2022b) Scientific foundations for a new start in amateur music. http://bundesmusikverband.de/grundlagen/

Böckelmann I, Böttcher S, Fendel M, Hartjen A, Neuber M, Höfting I, Richter A, Schlaich C, Wanke E (2020) DOV statement. Commentary on the proposal for measures submitted by the Health and Prophylaxis Working Group of the German Orchestra Association (DOV) dated 30.4.2020—Verband Deutscher Betriebs und Werksärzte VDBW Arbeitsgruppe Bühnen und Orchester. https://www.dov.org/projekte-kampagnen/musikergesundheit/corona-krise

Bonati M, Campi R, Segre G (2022) Psychological impact of the quarantine during the COVID-19 pandemic on the general European adult population: a systematic review of the evidence. Epidemiol Psychiatr Sci 31(e27):1–19. https://doi.org/10.1017/S2045796022000051

Brockmann S, Dittler A, Grün G, Haibel M, Iftner T, Kräusslich HG, Mizaikoff B, Niessner J, Richter B, Spahn C, Stergiaropoulos K, von Baum H (2021) Statement of the "Expert Group Aerosols": aerosols and SARS-CoV-2—origin, infectivity, spread and mitigation of airborne virus-containing particles in the respiratory air. Public Health 83(3):231–234. https://doi.org/10.1055/a-1363-0972

Brooks SK, Webster RK, Smith LE, Woodland L, Wessely S, Greenberg N, Rubin GJ (2020) The psychological impact of quarantine and how to reduce it: rapid review of the evidence. Lancet 395:912–920. https://doi.org/10.1016/S0140-6736(20)30460-8

Cerutti F, Burdino E, Milia MG, Allice T, Gregori G, Bruzzone B, Ghisetti V (2020) Urgent need of rapid tests for SARS CoV-2 antigen detection: evaluation of the SD-biosensor antigen test for SARS-CoV-2. J Clin Virol 132. https://doi.org/10.1016/j.jcv.2020.104654

Chia PY, Coleman KK, Tan YK, Ong SWX, Gum M, Lau SK et al (2020) Detection of air and surface contamination by severe acute respiratory syndrome coronavirus 2 (SARS-CoV-2) in hospital rooms of infected patients. Nat Commun 11:2800. https://doi.org/10.1038/s41467-020-16670-2

Chu DK, Akl EA, Duda S, Solo K, Yaacoub S, Schünemann HJ (2020) Physical distancing, face masks, and eye protection to prevent person-to-person transmission of SARS-CoV-2 and COVID-19: a systematic review and meta-analysis. Lancet 395(10242):1973–1987. https://doi.org/10.1016/S0140-6736(20)31142-9.Epub

Cohen S, Ginsborg J (2021) The experiences of mid-career and seasoned orchestral musicians in the UK during the first COVID-19 lockdown. Front Psychol 12:645967. https://doi.org/10.3389/fpsyg.2021.645967

Cohen S, Ginsborg J (2022) One year on: the impact of COVID-19 on the lives of freelance orchestral musicians in the United Kingdom. Front Psychol 13:885606. https://doi.org/10.3389/fpsyg.2022.885606

Communications of the ad hoc working group on indoor air guideline values of the Indoor Air Hygiene Commission of the Federal Environment Agency and the supreme state health authorities. Health assessment of carbon dioxide in indoor air Bundesgesundheitsbl. Gesundheitsforsch. Health Prot 2008 51:1358–1369. https://doi.org/10.1007/s00103-008-0707-2

Coronaviridae Study Group of the International Committee on Taxonomy of Viruses (2020) The species severe acute respiratory syndrome-related coronavirus: classifying 2019-nCoV and naming it SARS-CoV-2. Consensus statements. Nat Microbiol 5:536–544. https://doi.org/10.1038/s41564-020-0695-z

Coronavirus Test Ordinance—TestV (2021). https://www.bundesanzeiger.de/pub/publication/rjv0GJUnP0bov4hKuas/content/rjv0GJUnP0bov4hKuas/BAnz%20AT%2027.01.2021%20V2.pdf?inline

Daffern H, Balmer K, Brereton J (2021) Singing together, yet apart: the experience of UK Choir members and facilitators during the Covid-19 pandemic. Front Psychol 12:624474. https://doi.org/10.3389/fpsyg.2021.624474

Dennler U, Geisler F, Spinner CD (2022) Declining COVID-19 morbidity and case fatality in Germany: the pandemic end? Infection 2022:1–2. https://doi.org/10.1007/s15010-022-01873-0

Echternach M, Gantner S, Peters G, Westphalen C, Benthaus T, Jakubaß B, Kuranova L, Döllinger M, Kniesburges S (2020) Impulse dispersion of aerosols during singing and speaking: a potential COVID-19 transmission pathway. Am J Respir Crit Care Med 202(11):1584–1587. https://doi.org/10.1164/rccm.202009-3438LE

Federal Ministry of Health (2020) The national testing strategy—Corona tests in Germany. https://www.bundesgesundheitsministerium.de/coronavirus/nationale-teststrategie/faq-covid-19-tests.html

Firle C, Jabusch HC, Grell A, Fernholz I, Schmidt A, Steinmetz A (2020) Making music during the SARS-CoV-2 pandemic—recommendations of the German Society for Music Physiology and Musicians' Medicine (DGfMM) on infection protection when making music. https://dgfmm.org/fileadmin/DGfMM_Musizieren_waehrend_der_SARS_Cov2_Pandemie_14.05.2020.pdf

Firle C, Steinmetz A, Stier O, Stengel D, Ekkernkamp A (2022) Aerosol emission from playing wind instruments and related COVID-19 infection risk during music performance. Sci Rep 12:8598. https://doi.org/10.1038/s41598-022-12529-2

Hamner L, Dubbel P, Capron I, Ross A, Jordan A, Lee J, Lynn J, Ball A, Narwal S, Russell S, Patrick D, Leibrand H (2020) High SARS-CoV-2 attack rate following exposure at a choir practice—Skagit County, Washington, March 2020. MMWR Morb Mortal Wkly Rep 69:606–610. https://doi.org/10.15585/mmwr.mm6919e6

Heitzman J (2020) Impact of COVID-19 pandemic on mental health. Psychiatr Pol 54(2):187–198. https://doi.org/10.12740/PP/120373

ISO 31000:2018. Risk management—guidelines. https://www.iso.org/standard/65694.html

Joachim A, Dewald F, Suárez I, Zemlin M, Lang I, Stutz R, Marthaler A, Bosse H, Lübke N, Münch N, Bernard M, Jeltsch K, Tönshoff B, Weidner N, Kräusslich H, Birzele L, Hübner J, Blacksmith P, Meyer-Bühn M, HoremhebHoremheb-Rubio G, Cornely O, Haverkamp H, Wiesmüller G, Fätkenheuer G, Hero B, Kaiser R, Dötsch J, Rybniker J (2021) Pooled RT-qPCR testing for SARS-CoV-2 surveillance in schools—a cluster randomized trial. icalMedicine 39:101082. https://doi.org/10.1016/j.eclinm.2021.101082

Kähler CJ, Hain R (2020) Making music during the pandemic—what does science advise?—on infection risks when singing in choirs and making music with wind instruments. Institute of Fluid Mechanics and Aerodynamics. https://www.unibw.de/home/news-rund-um-corona/musizieren-waehrend-der-pandemie-was-raet-die-wissenschaft

Kluge S, Janssens U, Welte T, Weber-Carstens S, Schälte G, Spinner CD, Malin JJ, Gastmeier P, Langer F, Bracht H, Westhoff M, Pfeifer M, Rabe KF, Hoffmann F, Böttiger BW, Weinmann-Menke J, Kersten A, Berlit P, Krawczyk M, Nehls W, Haase R, Müller OJ, Specker C, Nothacker M, Skoetz N, Marx G, Karagiannidis C (2023) S3 guideline—recommendations for the treatment of patients with COVID-19. AWMF register no. 113/001

Kriegel M, Hartmann A (2020) Indoor risk assessment of virus-laden aerosols. https://doi.org/10.14279/depositonce-10343.2

Lavine JS, Bjornstad ON, Antia R (2021) Immunological characteristics govern the transition of COVID-19 to endemicity. Science 371(6530):741–745. https://doi.org/10.1126/science.abe6522

Leung NH, Chu DK, Shiu EY, Chan K-H, McDevitt JJ, Hau BJ et al (2020) Respiratory virus shedding in exhaled breath and efficacy of face masks. Nat Med:1–5. https://doi.org/10.1038/s41591-020-0843-2

Liu Y, Ning Z, Chen Y, Guo M, Liu Y, Gali NK et al (2020) Aerodynamic analysis of SARS-CoV-2 in two Wuhan hospitals. Nature:1–6. https://doi.org/10.1038/s41586-020-2271-3

López-Íñiguez G, McPherson GE, Zarza Alzugaray FJ (2022) Effects of threat and motivation on classical musicians' professional performance practice during the COVID-19 pandemic. Front Psychol 13:834666. https://doi.org/10.3389/fpsyg.2022.834666

Meselson M (2020) Droplets and aerosols in the transmission of SARS-CoV-2. N Engl J Med. https://doi.org/10.1056/NEJMc2009324

Miller SL, Nazaroff WW, Jimenez JL, Boerstra A, Buonanno G, Dancer SJ, Kurnitski J, Marr LC, Morawska L, Noakes C (2021) Transmission of SARS-CoV-2 by inhalation of respiratory aerosol in the Skagit Valley Chorale superspreading event. Indoor Air 31(2):314–323. https://doi.org/10.1111/ina.12751

Morawska L, Cao J (2020) Airborne transmission of SARS-CoV-2: the world should face the reality. Environ Int 139:105730. https://doi.org/10.1016/j.envint.2020.105730

Morawska L, Milton DK (2020) It is time to address airborne transmission of COVID-19. Clin Infect Dis:ciaa939. https://doi.org/10.1093/cid/ciaa939

Mürbe D, Bischoff P, Fleischer M, Gastmeier P (2020) Assessment of the risk of infection with SARS-CoV-2 viruses during singing. Charité Berlin, https://audiologie-phoniatrie.charite.de/fileadmin/user_upload/microsites/m_cc16/audiologie/Allgemein/Singen_und_SARS-CoV-2_Prof._Mürbe_et_al._04052020.pdf

Mürbe D, Kriegel M, Lange J, Rotheudt H, Fleischer M (2021) Aerosol emission in professional singing of classical music. Scientific Reports 11(1):14861. https://doi.org/10.1038/s41598-021-93281-x

Nohl J (2019) Risikomatrix. https://www.dguv.de/medien/ifa/de/pra/container/pdf/risikomatrix-nohl.pdf

Nusseck M, Spahn C (2021) Musical practice in music students during COVID-19 lockdown. Front Psychol 12:643177. https://doi.org/10.3389/fpsyg.2021.643177

Nusseck M, Richter B, Holtmeier L, Skala D, Spahn C (2020) CO2 measurements in instrumental and vocal closed room settings as a risk reducing measure for a coronavirus infection. https://www.medrxiv.org/content/10.1101/2020.10.26.20218354v1

Pettenkofer (1858) Besprechung Allgemeiner auf die Ventilation bezüglicher Fragen über den Luftwechsel in Wohngebäuden. J.G. Cotta bookshop, Munich

Petzold MP, Plag J, Ströhle A (2020) Dealing with mental stress in healthcare professionals in the context of the Covid-19 pandemic. Nervenarzt. https://doi.org/10.1007/s00115-020-00905-0

Qian H, Miao T, Liu L, Zheng X, Luo D, & Li Y (2021) Indoor transmission of SARS-CoV-2. Indoor air, 31(3), 639–645. https://doi.org/10.1111/ina.12766

Ravens-Sieberer U, Kaman A, Otto C, Adedeji A, Napp AK, Becker M, Blanck-Stellmacher U, Löffler C, Schlack R, Hölling H, Devine J, Erhart M, Hurrelmann K (2021) Mental health and psychological distress of children and adolescents in the first wave of the COVID-19 pandemic—results of the COPSY study. Fed Health J. https://doi.org/10.1007/s00103-021-03291-3

Reichert F, Stier O, Hartmann A, Ruscher C, Brinkmann A, Grossegesse M, Neumann M, Werber D, Hausner M, Kunze M, Weiß B, Michel J, Nitsche A, An der Heiden M, Kriegel M, Corman VM, Jones TC, Drosten C, Brommann T, Buchholz U (2022) Analysis of two choir outbreaks acting in concert to characterize long-range transmission risks through SARS-CoV-2. Berlin, Germany, 2020. PLoS One 17(11):e0277699. https://doi.org/10.1371/journal.pone.0277699

Richter B, Hipp A, Schubert B, Axt M, Stratmann M, Schmölder C, Spahn C (2021) From classic to rap: airborne transmission of different singing styles, in times of Covid-19. medRxiv preprint. https://doi.org/10.1101/2021.03.25.21253694

Robert Koch Institute (2021) Risk list. https://www.rki.de/DE/Content/InfAZ/N/Neuartiges_Coronavirus/Steckbrief.html#doc13776792bodyText3

Röhr S, Müller F, Jung F, Apfelbacher C, Seidler A, Steffi G, Riedel-Heller SG (2020) Psychosocial consequences of quarantine measures in severe coronavirus outbreaks: a rapid review. Psychiatr Prax 47:179–189. https://doi.org/10.1055/a-1159-5562

Santarpia JL, Rivera DN, Herrera V, Morwitzer MJ, Creager H, Santarpia GW et al. (2020) Transmission potential of SARS-CoV-2 in viral shedding observed at the University of Nebraska Medical Center. medRxiv

Siebler L, Rathje T, Calandri M, Stergiaropoulos K, Donker T, Richter B, Spahn C, Nusseck M (2023) A coupled experimental and statistical approach for an assessment of SARS-CoV-2 infection risk at indoor event locations. Under review

Spahn C, Hipp A, Schubert B, Axt M, Stratmann M, Schmölder C, Richter B (2021) Air flow and air velocity measurements while playing wind instruments, with respect to/in times of Covid-19. Int J Environ Res Public Health 18(10):5413

Spahn C, Hipp AM, Richter B, Nusseck M (2022a) Coronavirus vaccination rates in cultural areas in Germany. Epidemiol Infect 150:e34. https://doi.org/10.1017/S0950268822000085

Spahn C, Immerz A, Hipp AM, Nusseck M (2022b) Social contact, practice, organization and technical knowledge: experiences of music students in the course of the COVID-19 pandemic. Front Psychol 13:885890. https://doi.org/10.3389/fpsyg.2022.885890

Spahn C, Schmirl J, Immerz A, Nusseck M (2023) Resilience in music students—conception, evaluation and effect of a teaching program to promote resilience. In: Nusseck M, Spahn C (eds) Gesundheit von Musikstudierenden—Beiträge aus dem Musikhochschulen-Netzwerk (DFG) "Gesundheit und Prävention", vol 10. Projektverlag

STIKO (2022). https://www.rki.de/DE/Content/Infekt/EpidBull/Archiv/2022/Ausgaben/21_22.pdf?__blob=publicationFile

Tellier R (2006) Review of aerosol transmission of influenza A virus. Emerg Infect Dis 12(11):1657–1662

van der Sande M, Teunis P, Sabel R (2008) Professional and home-made face masks reduce exposure to respiratory infections among the general population. PLoS One 3:e2618. https://doi.org/10.1371/journal.pone.0002618

van Doremalen N, Bushmaker T, Morris DH, Holbrook MG, Gamble A, Williamson BN, Tamin A, Harcourt JL, Thornburg NJ, Gerber SI, Lloyd-Smith JO, de Wit E, Munster VJ (2020) Aerosol and surface stability of SARS-CoV-2 as compared with SARS-CoV-1. N Engl J Med 382:1564–1567. https://doi.org/10.1056/NEJMc2004973

Vuorinen V et al (2020a) Researchers modelling the spread of the coronavirus emphasise the importance of avoiding busy indoor spaces. https://www.aalto.fi/en/news/researchers-modelling-the-spread-of-the-coronavirus-emphasise-the-importanceof-avoiding-busy

Vuorinen V et al (2020b) Modelling aerosol transport and virus exposure with numerical simulations in relation to SARS-CoV-2 transmission by inhalation indoors. Safety Science 130:104866. https://doi.org/10.1016/j.ssci.2020.104866

WHO (2020a) Pneumonia of unknown cause—China. Disease Outbreak News(DONs). https://www.who.int/emergencies/disease-outbreak-news/item/2020-DON229

WHO (2020b) Situation report—22nd Novel Coronavirus (2019-nCoV). February 11, 2020. Accessed 29 Mar 2023

WHO (2020c) Advice on the use of masks in the context of COVID-19: interim guidance, 5 June 2020. World Health Organization. https://apps.who.int/iris/handle/10665/332293. License: CC BY-NC-SA 3.0 IGO

WHO (2023). https://www.who.int/europe/emergencies/situations/covid-19

Willich SN, Berghöfer A, Wiese-Posselt MK, Gastmeier P (2020) Statement on the performance of orchestras during the COVID-19 pandemic. https://epidemiologie.charite.de/fileadmin/user_upload/microsites/m_cc01/epidemiologie/downloads/Stellungnahme_SpielbetriebOrchester_17-8-2020.pdf

Index

G. Kreutz, G. Bernatzky (eds.), *Music and Medicine*, Neurocultural Health and Wellbeing, https://doi.org/10.1007/978-3-662-72175-9

MIX
Papier aus verantwortungsvollen Quellen
Paper from responsible sources
FSC® C105338

If you have any concerns about our products,
you can contact us on
ProductSafety@springernature.com

In case Publisher is established outside the EU,
the EU authorized representative is:
Springer Nature Customer Service Center GmbH
Europaplatz 3, 69115 Heidelberg, Germany

Printed by Libri Plureos GmbH
in Hamburg, Germany